COSMETIC OCULOPLASTIC SURGERY

COSMETIC OCULOPLASTIC SURGERY

Third Edition

Eyelid, Forehead, and Facial Techniques

ALLEN M. PUTTERMAN, MD

Professor of Ophthalmology and Director of Oculoplastic Surgery
University of Illinois at Chicago College of Medicine

Clinical Professor of Maxillofacial Surgery
Northwestern University

Chief of Ophthalmology
Michael Reese Hospital Medical Center

Consultant in Oculoplastic Surgery
Mercy Hospital, West Side Veterans Administration Hospital, and
Illinois Masonic Hospital
Chicago, Illinois

LINDA A. WARREN

Medical Illustrator
Department of Ophthalmology and Visual Sciences
University of Illinois at Chicago College of Medicine
Chicago, Illinois

W.B. SAUNDERS COMPANY
A Division of Harcourt Brace & Company
Philadelphia London Toronto Montreal Sydney Tokyo

W.B. SAUNDERS COMPANY
A Division of Harcourt Brace & Company

The Curtis Center
Independence Square West
Philadelphia, Pennsylvania 19106

Library of Congress Cataloging-in-Publication Data

Cosmetic oculoplastic surgery: eyelid, forehead, and facial techniques / [edited by] Allen M. Putterman; [illustrated by] Linda A. Warren.—3rd ed.

p.   cm.

Includes bibliographical references and index.

ISBN 0–7216–7076–8

I. Putterman, Allen M.   [DNLM: 1. Blepharoplasty.   2. Eyebrows—surgery.   3. Face—surgery.   4. Forehead—surgery.   5. Reconstructive Surgical Procedures—methods.   WW 205 C834 1999]

RD119.5. E94C67 1999   617.7′1—dc21

DNLM/DLC   98-12905

COSMETIC OCULOPLASTIC SURGERY: EYELID, FOREHEAD,
AND FACIAL TECHNIQUES   ISBN 0–7216–7076–8

Printed in the United States of America.

Last digit is the print number: 9   8   7   6   5   4   3   2   1

In memory of my father, Mayer Putterman,
for his inspiration, support, and encouragement.

Contributors

JAMES ALEX, M.D.
Associate Professor of Surgery, Yale University School of Medicine. Surgeon, Yale–New Haven Hospital, New Haven, Connecticut.
Rejuvenation of the Aging Brow and Forehead

RICHARD L. ANDERSON, M.D.
Professor of Ophthalmology, University of Utah School of Medicine, Salt Lake City, Utah.
Upper Blepharoplasty Combined with Levator Aponeurosis Repair

HENRY I. BAYLIS, M.D.
Founding Chief, Division of Ophthalmic Plastic Surgery, University of California, Los Angeles, UCLA School of Medicine, Los Angeles, California.
Simplified Face and Neck Lift; Complications of Upper Blepharoplasty; Complications of Lower Blepharoplasty

C. BRADLEY BOWMAN, M.D.
Assistant Clinical Professor of Ophthalmology, University of Texas Southwestern Medical Center at Dallas Southwestern Medical School, Dallas, Texas.
Internal Brow Lift: Browplasty and Browpexy

WILLIAM P. CHEN, M.D.
Associate Clinical Professor of Ophthalmology, University of California, Los Angeles, UCLA School of Medicine; Jules Stein Eye Institute, Los Angeles; and University of California, Irvine College of Medicine, Irvine. Senior Attending Surgeon, Ophthalmic Plastic Surgery Service, Harbor-UCLA Medical Center, Torrance, California.
Upper Blepharoplasty in the Asian Patient

JOSEPH A. EVIATAR, M.D.
Assistant Clinical Professor of Ophthalmology, New York University School of Medicine. Adjunct Surgeon, New York Eye and Ear Infirmary, New York, New York.
Patient Selection for Cosmetic Oculoplastic Surgery

STEVEN FAGIEN, M.D., FACS
Assistant Clinical Professor, University of Florida College of Medicine, Gainesville. Director, The Boca Raton Center for Ophthalmic Plastic and Reconstructive Surgery, Boca Raton, Florida.
Facial Soft-Tissue Augmentation with Autologous Injectable Collagen; Treatment of Hyperkinetic Facial Lines with Botulinum Toxin

DAVID R. FETT, M.D.
Assistant Clinical Professor, University of California, Los Angeles, UCLA School of Medicine, and the Jules Stein Eye Institute, Los Angeles, California.
Cosmetic Oculoplastic Surgery Marketing

TONY S. FU, M.D.
Clinical Assistant Professor of Dermatology, University of Illinois at Chicago College of Medicine. Lecturer, Department of Dermatology, Northwestern University Medical School, Chicago, Illinois.
Dermatopathology in the Cosmetic Oculoplasty Surgery Patient

ROBERT A. GOLDBERG, M.D.
Associate Professor of Ophthalmology, University of California, Los Angeles, UCLA School of Medicine. Chief, Orbital and Ophthalmic Plastic Surgery Division, Jules Stein Eye Institute, Los Angeles, California.
Complications of Upper Blepharoplasty; Complications of Lower Blepharoplasty; Fat Repositioning

MICHAEL J. GROTH, M.D.
Assistant Clinical Professor, Department of Ophthalmology, Division of Ophthalmic Plastic and Reconstructive Surgery, University of California, Los Angeles, UCLA School of Medicine, and the Jules Stein Eye Institute. Clinical Instructor, Wadsworth Veterans Affairs Hospital, Los Angeles, California.
Complications of Lower Blepharoplasty

DAVID HENDRICK, M.D.
Clinical Instructor, Veterans Administration Medical Center, Denver, Colorado. Private Practitioner, Vail, Colorado.
Rejuvenation of the Aging Brow and Forehead

JONATHAN A. HOENIG, M.D.
Clinical Assistant Professor of Ophthalmology, Department of Orbit and Ophthalmic Plastic Surgery, Drew-King Medical Center. Clinical Instructor, Jules Stein Eye Institute, University of California, Los Angeles, UCLA School of Medicine, Los Angeles, California.
Simplified Face and Neck Lift; Chemical Peel: Eyelid, Periorbital, and Facial Skin Rejuvenation in Conjunction with or Independent of Cosmetic Blepharoplasty

ALBERT HORNBLASS, M.D.
Clinical Professor of Ophthalmology, State University of New York, Brooklyn, New York. Director of Ophthalmic Plastic Orbital and Reconstructive Surgery, Manhattan Eye, Ear, and Throat Hospital, New York, and Hackensack University Medical Center, Hackensack, New Jersey.
Patient Selection for Cosmetic Oculoplastic Surgery

ROBERT HUTCHERSON, M.D.
Assistant Clinical Professor, University of California, Los
Angeles, UCLA School of Medicine, Los Angeles. Private
Practitioner, Beverly Hills, California.
Endoscopy-Assisted Small-Incision Forehead and Brow Lift

LAWRENCE B. KATZEN, M.D.
Clinical Assistant Professor, Bascom Palmer Eye Institute,
University of Miami School of Medicine, Miami, Florida.
Medical Director, Katzen Eye Care Center, West Palm Beach
and Boynton Beach, Florida.
*The History of Cosmetic Oculoplastic Surgery; Anesthesia,
Analgesia, and Amnesia*

GREGORY S. KELLER, M.D.
Assistant Clinical Professor, University of California, Los
Angeles, UCLA School of Medicine, Los Angeles. Private
Practitioner, Santa Barbara, California.
Endoscopy-Assisted Small-Incision Forehead and Brow Lift

CHARLES R. LEONE, JR., M.M.Sc., M.D.
Clinical Professor of Ophthalmology, University of Texas
Medical School at San Antonio, San Antonio, Texas.
Treatment of a Prolapsed Lacrimal Gland

MARK R. LEVINE, M.D.
Clinical Professor of Ophthalmology, Case Western Reserve
University School of Medicine. Chief of Ophthalmology,
Mount Sinai Medical Center. Head, Oculoplastic and Orbital
Surgery Service, University Hospitals of Cleveland,
Cleveland, Ohio.
Blepharopigmentation

CLINTON D. McCORD, JR., M.D.
Attending Physician, Southeastern Oculoplastic Clinic and
Paces Plastic Surgery Clinic, Atlanta, Georgia.
Internal Brow Lift: Browplasty and Browpexy

WILLIAM M. McLEISH, M.D.
Assistant Professor of Ophthalmology, Mayo Medical School,
Rochester, Minnesota. Attending Physician, Mayo Clinic,
Scottsdale, Arizona.
*Upper Blepharoplasty Combined with Levator Aponeurosis
Repair*

ARTHUR L. MILLMAN, M.D.
Assistant Professor, The New York Eye and Ear Infirmary,
New York Medical College. Surgeon Director, Manhattan
Center for Facial Plastic Surgery. Attending Surgeon and
Consultant, Oculoplastic Surgery, Lenox Hill Hospital,
Mount Sinai Medical Center, and Beth Israel Medical Center,
New York, New York.
*Eyelid and Facial Laser Skin Resurfacing; Carbon Dioxide
Laser Blepharoplasty*

DAVID M. MORROW, M.D
Jules Stein Eye Institute, Division of Ophthalmic Plastic
Surgery, University of California, Los Angeles. Director,
Foundation for the Advancement of Specialty Surgery, and
Director, The Morrow Institute, a Multispecialty Aesthetic
Medicine and Surgery Group, Los Angeles, California.
*Simplified Face and Neck Lift; Chemical Peel: Eyelid,
Periorbital, and Facial Skin Rejuvenation in Conjunction
with or Independent of Cosmetic Blepharoplasty*

MARIANNE NELSON O'DONOGHUE, M.D.
Associate Professor of Dermatology, Rush Medical College of
Rush University, Rush–Presbyterian–St. Luke's Medical
Center, Chicago, Illinois. Attending Physician, West
Suburban Hospital, Oak Park, Illinois.
Ocular and Facial Cosmetics

J. JUSTIN OLDER, M.D., FACS
Clinical Professor and Director, Oculoplastic Service
Department of Ophthalmology, University of South Florida
College of Medicine, Tampa, Florida.
Treatment of Upper Eyelid Retraction: External Approach

ALLEN M. PUTTERMAN, M.D.
Professor of Ophthalmology and Director of Oculoplastic
Surgery, University of Illinois at Chicago College of
Medicine. Clinical Professor of Maxillofacial Surgery,
Northwestern University. Chief of Ophthalmology, Michael
Reese Hospital Medical Center. Consultant in Oculoplastic
Surgery, Mercy Hospital, West Side Veterans Administration
Hospital, and Illinois Masonic Hospital, Chicago, Illinois.
*Evaluation of the Cosmetic Oculoplastic Surgery Patient;
Treatment of Upper Eyelid Dermatochalasis and Orbital Fat:
Skin Flap Approach; Treatment of Upper Eyelid
Dermatochalasis with Reconstruction of Upper Eyelid Crease:
Skin-Muscle Flap Approach; Internal Brow Lift: Browplasty
and Browpexy (Putterman Modification of Internal Brow
Lift); Müller's Muscle–Conjunctival Resection–Ptosis Procedure
Combined with Upper Blepharoplasty; Treatment of Upper
Eyelid Retraction: Internal Approach; Treatment of Lower
Eyelid Dermatochalasis, Herniated Orbital Fat, Abnormal-
Appearing Skin, and Hypertrophic Orbicularis Muscle: Skin
Flap Approach; Treatment of Lower Eyelid Dermatochalasis,
Herniated Orbital Fat, and Hypertrophic Orbicularis Muscle:
Skin-Muscle Flap Approach; Transconjunctival Approach to
Resection of Lower Eyelid Herniated Orbital Fat; Tarsal Strip
Procedure Combined with Lower Blepharoplasty; Lateral
Canthal Plication; Treatment of Eyelid Varicose Veins with
Blepharoplasty; Cheek and Midface Lift Combined with Full-
Thickness Temporal Lower Eyelid Resection; Treatment of
Lower Eyelid Retraction with Recession of Lower Lid
Retractors and Hard-Palate Grafting; Lateral Tarsorrhaphy
in the Treatment of Thyroid Ophthalmopathy; Endoscopy-
Assisted Small-Incision Forehead and Brow Lift (Putterman
Upper Blepharoplasty Approach to Endoscopic Forehead and
Brow Lift); Blepharoplasty with Neodymium:YAG Laser,
Cautery, or Colorado Needle; Patient Satisfaction in Cosmetic
Oculoplastic Surgery; Excision of Corrugator Muscles: Upper
Blepharoplasty Approach*

NORMAN SHORR, M.D.
Clinical Professor of Ophthalmology, University of California,
Los Angeles, UCLA School of Medicine. Director,
Fellowship in Orbital and Ophthalmic Plastic and
Reconstructive Surgery, and Director, Aesthetic
Reconstructive Surgery Service, Jules Stein Eye Institute, Los
Angeles, California.
*Chemical Peel: Eyelid, Periorbital, and Facial Skin
Rejuvenation in Conjunction with or Independent of Cosmetic
Blepharoplasty*

BERNARD H. SHULMAN, M.D.
Former Clinical Professor of Psychiatry, Northwestern
University Medical School. Director of Psychiatry, Diamond
Headache Clinic, Columbus Hospital, Chicago, Illinois.
Psychiatric Issues in Cosmetic Eyelid and Facial Surgery

ROBERT B. SHULMAN, M.D.
Instructor, Department of Psychiatry, Rush Medical College of Rush University, Chicago, Illinois. Attending Psychiatrist, Rush North Shore Medical Center, Skokie, Illinois.
Psychiatric Issues in Cosmetic Eyelid and Facial Surgery

BERND SILVER, M.D.
Assistant Clinical Professor, Washington University School of Medicine. Attending Physician, Jewish Hospital of St. Louis; Barnes Hospital, and Missouri Baptist Hospital, St. Louis, Missouri.
Photographing the Blepharoplasty Patient

MYRON TANENBAUM, M.D.
Associate Clinical Professor of Ophthalmology, Bascom Palmer Eye Institute, University of Miami, School of Medicine, Miami, Florida.
Internal Brow Lift: Browplasty and Browpexy

M. EUGENE TARDY, M.D.
Professor of Clinical Otolaryngology–Head & Neck Surgery, and Director, Division of Facial Plastic Surgery, University of

Illinois College of Medicine. Attending Physican, Saint Joseph Hospital, Chicago, Illinois.
Rejuvenation of the Aging Brow and Forehead

MARTHA C. WILSON, M.D.
Clinical Instructor, University of Texas Medical School at San Antonio. Attending Physician, Baptist Memorial Hospital System, St. Luke's Lutheran Hospital, Southwest Texas Methodist Hospital, and Health Care Santa Rosa Corporation, San Antonio, Texas.
Complications of Upper Blepharoplasty

MATTHEW W. WILSON, M.D.
Assistant Professor, Department of Ophthalmology, University of Colorado School of Medicine, Denver, Colorado.
Eyelid and Facial Anatomy

JOHN L. WOBIG, M.D., M.B.A.
Lester T. Jones Chair of Oculoplastics, Chief, Oculoplastics, Casey Eye Institute, Oregon Health Sciences University School of Medicine, Portland, Oregon.
Eyelid and Facial Anatomy

Preface

With the first edition of *Cosmetic Oculoplastic Surgery* in 1982, it was my intent to provide a complete and detailed reference to cosmetic eyelid and cosmetic eyebrow surgery. That text had 21 chapters and included everything I could possibly think of in this field. In 1993, the second edition of *Cosmetic Oculoplastic Surgery* was published to update the textbook. That edition was expanded to 27 chapters. Since publication of the second edition, the field of cosmetic oculoplastic surgery has rapidly expanded, necessitating another update. The third edition includes additional new material, to continue the philosophy of providing a complete and detailed reference to this field. This new text has 43 chapters, double the size of the first edition.

One of the first changes was to rename the book. The title, *Cosmetic Oculoplastic Surgery: Eyelid, Forehead, and Facial Techniques,* reflects that the field of oculoplastic surgery has expanded beyond the confines of the eyelids to that of the entire face.

All of the chapters continue to include a detailed and complete description of the surgical techniques. The contributors provide thorough documentation of the results, explanation of complications of each procedure, preoperative and postoperative photographs, and selected references. Discussions of other aspects of plastic surgery, including history, psychiatry, cosmetology, anesthesia, patient satisfaction, and dermatopathology, are included.

In addition to updating all of the chapters, I have added chapters dealing with the treatment of upper and lower eyelid retraction, lateral canthal plication, treatment of eyelid varicose veins, cheek and midface lift, lateral tarsorrhaphy, endoscopy-assisted small-incision forehead and brow lift, face lifting, eyelid and facial laser skin resurfacing, facial soft-tissue augmentation, treatment of hyperkinetic facial lines with botulinum toxin, and carbon dioxide blepharoplasty. I have also added a new chapter on cosmetic surgery marketing because this has become an important consideration in developing a practice in cosmetic surgery.

As the manuscript was nearing completion, new developments occurred and were added at the end of the text to keep it up to date and comprehensive. These new techniques include repositioning of orbital fat and excision of the corrugator muscles through an upper blepharoplasty approach. I excluded discussion of another technique that I have only recently begun to use: the injection of fat into the face to decrease furrows and hollowing of the lower eyelid, especially in the nasojugal area. This technique has not yet been tested adequately, and further studies are required to determine its efficacy and safety.

As in the previous editions, a strength of this text lies in its numerous illustrations. The illustrations in most multiauthored medical books vary greatly from chapter to chapter in style, tone, and meaning. This makes some contributions more interesting and easier to follow and attracts the reader to some parts of the book more than to others, according to the impressiveness of the drawings rather than the importance of the techniques described. To avoid this flaw, I have again had one talented medical illustrator prepare all the artwork for this textbook. Linda Warren took the sketches and ideas provided by the different contributors and transformed them into complete, meaningful, complementary illustrations. Ms. Warren spent numerous hours working on these drawings, and I did my best to supervise the production of each one. The effort resulted in beautifully detailed illustrations that are consistent in clarity and quality. More than 100 new illustrations were added to update this text, bringing the total number of illustrations to over 350. They will, I believe, hold your interest and add to your ease and skill in performing surgery.

Additionally, many of the photographs have been replaced and updated.

My medical editor, Kathleen Louden, ELS, reviewed all of the written material in the text, and I believe her editing has made the book both easier to read and more understandable.

It is my hope that you enjoy this book and that you gain an improved understanding and success in performing cosmetic oculofacial plastic surgery.

Contents

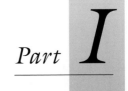

PREOPERATIVE CONSIDERATIONS

Lawrence B. Katzen

Chapter 1

The History of Cosmetic Oculoplastic Surgery

I am always amazed that so many of the medical procedures we think of as innovative actually have roots far back in time. In this chapter, Larry Katzen traces the origin of cosmetic oculoplastic surgery. He found that the first resection of excessive upper eyelid skin was performed 2000 years ago. Resection of herniated orbital fat, the formation of the upper eyelid crease, and the importance of photography in cosmetic surgery also have a long history.

Before the technicalities of cosmetic surgery are presented, Dr. Katzen's chapter provides an interesting background. It adds to our appreciation of what has gone into the development and advances of modern cosmetic eyelid and facial surgery and demonstrates that our current techniques are merely modifications of those developed long ago.

This chapter has been updated to include the many new advances in cosmetic eyelid and facial surgery over the last 15 years. This includes the origins of laser surgery and skin resurfacing, subperiosteal brow and midface lifts, and botulinum toxin and autologous collagen injections.

ALLEN M. PUTTERMAN

ANCIENT MEDICINE

Gather a fold of lid skin between a couple of fingers, or raise it up with a hook, and lay the fold between two small wooden bars or rods as long as the lid and as broad as a lancet. Bind their ends very tight together. The skin between these small pieces of wood, deprived of nutrient, dies in about ten days, the enclosed skin falls off, leaving no scar.

The Tadhkirat of Ali ibn Isa of Baghdad

Cosmetic eyelid surgery today has the benefit of 2000 years of development and refinement of surgical techniques and instruments. Ali ibn Isa (A.D. 940–1010) described the procedure just quoted more than 1000 years ago (Fig. 1–1), at a time when his medical treatment for "oedema of the lids" was "letting blood from the head, and treating the eye with a preparation of celandine, sandalwood, and endives. . . ."[1]

Aulus Cornelius Celsus, a Roman encyclopedist and philosopher in the first century, was probably the first to comment on the excision of skin of the upper eyelids when he described the treatment of "relaxed eyelid" in his *De re Medica* (A.D. 25–35).[2] *De re Medica* was not published until 1478, following its rediscovery by Pope Nicholas V.

Even before Celsus, the Hindus were known to have referred to cosmetic and reconstructive surgery about the face. The accepted form of corporal punishment in India 2000 years ago was amputation of the nose. The surgeons of this time became so skilled in reattaching this appendage that officials began to throw the amputated nose into the fire to ensure their goal of disfigurement. It is interesting that the skilled surgeons who were able to reattach the nose successfully were actually members of the lowly tile makers' caste.[3]

MODERN COSMETIC EYELID SURGERY

Blepharoplasty (Greek *blepharon*, meaning eyelid, and *plastos*, meaning formed) was originally used by von

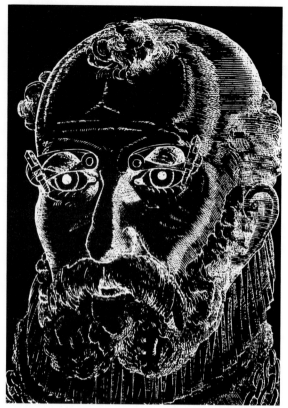

figure 1–1

Early technique of excision of excess skin of the upper eyelid.

Graefe[4] in 1818 to describe a case of eyelid reconstruction that he had performed in 1809. This meaning prevailed for the next 150 years.

In the 1913 *American Encyclopedia of Ophthalmology,*[5] blepharoplasty is defined as the re-formation, replacement, readjustment, or transplantation of any of the eyelid tissues. In contemporary usage, blepharoplasty refers to the excision of excessive eyelid skin, with or without the excision of orbital fat, for either functional or cosmetic indications. The cosmetic indications have been recognized by physicians only since the turn of the twentieth century but are now the most common reasons for such surgery on the eyelids. This change followed the development of improved operative techniques, better surgical results, and control of sepsis as well as changing social mores.

It is difficult to determine whether the "relaxed eyelid" described by Celsus was a true ptosis or an excess skin fold. In any event, by the late 1700s, reports began to appear in Germany[6] specifically identifying the excess fold of the upper eyelid. Beer's 1817 text is credited with providing the medical literature with the first illustration of this eyelid deformity.[7] Many different authors from the first half of the nineteenth century began advocating excision of this excess skin, including Mackenzie,[8] Alibert,[9] Graf,[10] and Dupuytren.[11]

The first accurate description of "herniated orbital fat," written in 1844 by Sichel,[12] did not create a wave of surgical excisions because surgery at that time was performed only for functional reasons. The case of *Fett-hernien* reported in 1899 by Schmidt-Rimpler,[13] which described herniated orbital fat, was clouded by the later report by Elschnig,[14] who called the same patient's condition a lipoma.

Near the turn of the nineteenth century, Ernest Fuchs[15] attempted to decipher the confusing terminology that had developed in the literature. "Ptosis adiposa," the misnomer used by Sichel, and "ptosis atonica," used by Hotz,[16] had been introduced earlier in the nineteenth century. Sichel[12] had claimed that the excess upper lid fold was filled with fat, which caused it to hang down over the lid margin. Hotz believed that the skin was normally attached to the top of the tarsus, and that the loss of this attachment created an excessive upper lid skin fold with a pseudoptosis. It was Fuchs who recognized the importance of the weakening of the fascial bands connecting the skin and orbicularis with the tendons of the levator in the development of the excess skin fold. In his 1892 text, Fuchs[15] wrote:

> So also the ptosis adiposa of Sichel, which consists in the fact that the covering fold of the upper lid is of unusual size, so as to hang down over the free border of the lid in the region of the palpebral fissure, does not belong under the head of ptosis proper. It was formerly assumed that this enlargement was caused by an excessive accumulation of fat in the covering fold, for which reason the name of ptosis adiposa was given to it. Its true cause, however, depends upon the fact that the bands of fascia connecting the skin with the tendon of the levator . . . and with the upper margin of the orbit are not rigid enough; consequently the skin is not properly drawn up when the lid is raised, but hangs down in the form of a flabby pouch (Hotz). Except for the disfigurement it causes ptosis adiposa entails no disagreeable symptoms. It can be removed by simple ablation of the excess of skin, but it is better, although also more tedious, to attach the skin to the upper border of the tarsus by Hotz's operation, and thus prevent its drooping.

And so Fuchs was the first to recognize the cosmetic value of re-formation and elevation of the eyelid crease. Fuchs[17] is also credited with originating the often misused term *blepharochalasis* in 1896. Sometimes used to describe the changes associated with herniated orbital fat, this term should be reserved for those cases of thickened and indurated eyelids, most often found in younger women, and associated with recurrent episodes of idiopathic edema.[18, 19] The term *dermatochalasis* was introduced 56 years later by Fox[20] to describe the apparent excess eyelid skin associated with aging.

In the early 1900s, the historical focus on cosmetic eyelid surgery shifted to the United States, where Conrad Miller,[21] in 1907, produced *Cosmetic Surgery: The Correction of Featural Imperfections,* the first published book on cosmetic surgery. This edition, which covered many aspects of plastic surgery, contained the first photograph in medical history to illustrate the lower eyelid incision for removing a crescent of excess skin. It is interesting to note Miller's surgical technique. In his discussion of the lower eyelid incision, Miller stated that "just sufficient skin is left along the margin of the lid to permit the stitches being passed in closing. The line of union is brought in this way under the shadow of the lashes, and is entirely invisible." On excision of the fold above the eye, Miller wrote that "the fold above the eye after infiltration is picked and trimmed away. The line of closure here is at the upper extremity of the lid so that the slight line of the union is hidden in the fold between the lid and the brow when the eye is open, and only shows slightly when the eye is closed." Miller's enlarged text,[22] which followed in 1924, provided diagrams of incision sites for upper and lower eyelid blepharoplasty that are remarkably similar to those commonly used today (Fig. 1–2).

Frederick Kolle,[23] in a 1911 text on plastic and cosmetic surgery, wrote about wrinkled eyelids in a chapter on blepharoplasty. He probably was the first to recognize and note the safety and value of marking the skin preoperatively to determine the amount of excess skin to excise.

Adabert Bettman[24–26] added to the contributions by Miller and Kolle in his publications in the 1920s, in which he described precautions, specifically related to surgery about the eyelids, to be taken in minimizing postoperative scarring. He emphasized gentle treatment of the tissues, exact apposition of wound edges, elimination of tension on all wound edges, and timely suture removal. These, of course, are concepts that are still important today.

The first work in English devoted solely to oculoplastic surgery was written by Edmund Spaeth.[27] *Newer Methods of Ophthalmic Plastic Surgery*, published in 1925, deals entirely with eyelid reconstruction and does not mention cosmetic surgery.

By the late 1920s, still no mention had been made in the United States of the excision of herniated orbital fat for cosmetic reasons. Although advances and progress in medicine (including antibiotics, finer suture materials, improved technology, and better control of sepsis) allowed for the beginnings of the public desire for and acceptance of cosmetic surgery, it was still frowned on by the majority of physicians.

In the same decade in Europe, Julian Bourguet[28] was also developing new techniques in cosmetic eyelid surgery. In 1924, he was probably the first to describe transconjunctival resection of the pockets of herniated orbital fat. In the following year, he published probably the first before-and-after photographs of patients who had undergone cosmetic lower eyelid surgery (Fig. 1–3).[29] In 1929, Bourguet[30] described the two separate fat compartments of the upper lid and advocated their removal. Many surgeons followed his lead, including Claoué[31] and Passot.[32] Passot[32, 33] is also credited as being the first to name the supraciliary brow incision for the correction of brow ptosis. It is interesting that Passot expressed his objections to the secrecy of techniques practiced by some of his contemporaries: "By keeping their methods secret, they allow a certain suspicion to exist about their procedures."[34, 35]

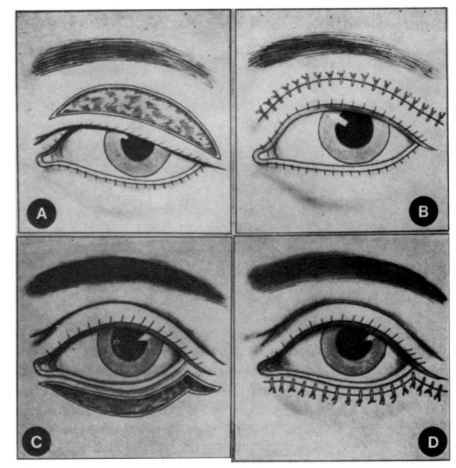

figure 1–2

A, An upper eyelid incision. *B*, An upper eyelid closure. *C*, A triangular resection modification to lower eyelid incision to prevent ectropion. *D*, A lower eyelid closure. (From Miller CC: Cosmetic Surgery: The Correction of Featural Imperfections. Philadelphia, FA Davis, 1924. With permission.)

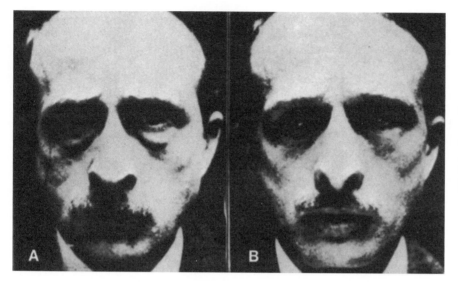

figure 1–3
Earliest photographs illustrating preoperative *(A)* and postoperative *(B)* appearances of lower eyelid blepharoplasty. (From Bourguet J: Chirurgie esthétique de la face: Les nez concaves, les rides et les "poches" sous les yeux. Arch Franco-Belges Chir 1925; 28:293. With permission.)

At the same time, one of the first female surgeons to appear in the history of cosmetic surgery was perfecting her techniques in Paris.[36, 37] A. Suzanne Noel's 1926 book on cosmetic eyelid surgery[38] was the earliest to include numerous preoperative and postoperative photographs.[36] Noel also initiated the emphasis, for the benefit of other surgeons, on the advantages and the importance of looking at these photographs and showing them to one's patients. She was also the first to be photographed performing a blepharoplasty. Thanks to the contributions of Noel and others and to the development of photography as an art and science, photographic documentation is now an integral part of the practice of the cosmetic oculoplastic surgeon. In addition, Noel must certainly be credited for recognizing the importance of the psychological implications of cosmetic surgery for both the patient and the patient's family. She distinguished between the attitudes of American and European men: "American men are anxious to encourage their wives to have such an operation. . . . [S]uch is not the case with the European male; as a result, French women have the operation performed and do not talk about it."

In the first two decades of the 1900s, a surgical technique widely used in Europe was commonly known as the "temporal lift." In current literature, this technique is known as the "mini-lift." Its benefits remain controversial. Bourguet,[39] in 1921, was the first to condemn this type of surgery. In 1926, Hunt[40] described a coronal skin resection to achieve a forehead lift. Joseph,[41] in 1931, described hairline and forehead crease incisions to raise the brows. The coronal brow lift lost favor because the results were thought to be too transient.

A number of authors then recognized the importance of interrupting the frontalis muscle action to achieve lasting results with the forehead lift.[35, 42–45] The importance of attenuating the action of the procerus and corrugator muscles was recognized by Salvadore Castanares in 1964.[46]

Since the 1930s, additional individual contributions have been made to cosmetic eyelid surgery. An offering in 1951 by Castanares[47] of a detailed description of the

fat compartments of the upper and lower orbit and their relationship to the eyelids cannot be overlooked. It was also Castanares[48–50] who recognized the importance of the orbicularis muscle (including its hypertrophy and excision, when indicated) as part of the overall evaluation and technique in cosmetic blepharoplasty.[48–50]

In 1954, Sayoc[51] reported on the use of the Hotz trichiasis procedure for the cosmetic alteration of the Asian upper eyelid crease-fold complex. Pang's 1961 report on the Far Eastern method of the surgical formation of the upper lid fold[52] was the first to advocate the technique of supratarsal fixation, although this term was introduced 13 years later by Jack Sheen.[53] Khou Boo-Chai's 1963 report[54] was the initial description of eyelid crease elevation with upper eyelid blepharoplasty, but he advocated dermal fixation to the tarsal plate and referred only to the Asian eyelid.

Significant contributions to cosmetic eyelid surgery in the 1970s focused on the levator aponeurosis and crease-fold complex.[55] In 1974, Sheen[53] recognized the low eyelid crease as the cause of apparent failure in many white patients undergoing upper lid blepharoplasty. He advocated orbicularis fixation to the levator aponeurosis 16 mm above the lid margin; 3 years later, iatrogenic postoperative ptosis prompted him to lower it to 12 mm.[56] At that time, observing postoperative lid retraction, he inadvertently discovered a way to strengthen the levator aponeurosis by tucking it. The next year, Dryden and Leibsohn[57] reported on intentional levator advancement for simultaneous blepharoplasty and repair of ptosis.

Putterman and Urist[58] recognized the role of the crease-fold complex in upper eyelid asymmetry associated with ptosis, trauma, and other eyelid abnormalities. Sheen[59] advocated tarsal fixation in the lower eyelid to achieve a "youthful" appearance.

In the last 25 years, there have been significant additional contributions to the development of cosmetic oculoplastic surgery. With the increased frequency of operations, there has been a growing awareness of potential complications. The importance of the preoperative evaluation has been emphasized as essential to minimizing complications; this also has resulted in the development of adjunctive surgical procedures.

Preoperative evaluation of the blepharoplasty patient should detect the presence of a prolapsed lacrimal gland. In 1978, Smith and Petrelli[60] described the surgical repair of a prolapsed lacrimal gland. Specific adjunctive dacryoadenopexy in upper eyelid blepharoplasty was described in 1983 by Smith and Lisman.[61] This technique is used frequently in geriatric blepharoplasty.

In 1975, Putterman[62] recommended that the eyes not be patched after cosmetic blepharoplasty so that a potential sight-threatening retrobulbar hemorrhage could be more easily identified. Putterman and Urist[63] also demonstrated that baggy eyelids can occur as a true hernia resulting from detachment of the septum from capsulopalpebral fascia and levator aponeurosis.

In the 1970s, reports first appeared in the plastic surgery literature describing and confirming the existence of the dry eye syndrome after blepharoplasty.[64–66] In 1976, Tenzel[67] recommended that each patient be given a Schirmer tear test to evaluate basic tear secretion before cosmetic blepharoplasty. He recommended that function take precedence over cosmesis in patients with decreased tear function. The decade of the 1980s witnessed the development and widespread use of temporary and permanent punctal occlusion as an adjunct to blepharoplasty and as a treatment of dry eye symptoms after blepharoplasty.

The recognition in 1972 of lower eyelid laxity as a cause of postblepharoplasty ectropion has significantly reduced the incidence of this complication.[68] Tenzel[67] recommended combined horizontal shortening and lower eyelid blepharoplasty when lower eyelid laxity is recognized preoperatively. In 1979, Webster and colleagues[69] described a temporary lateral canthal suspension suture in cases of minimal to moderate horizontal eyelid laxity. In 1982, Putterman[70] edited the first textbook dedicated to cosmetic oculoplastic surgery. In it, he described and illustrated the use of Byron Smith's modification of the Kuhnt-Szymanowski procedure for tightening the lower eyelid at the time of cosmetic blepharoplasty. This involved a full-thickness resection at the eyelid margin. Katzen and Tenzel[71] were the first to recommend that horizontal shortening be performed at the lateral canthus at the time of cosmetic lower eyelid blepharoplasty, thus eliminating the need for eyelid margin sutures. The lateral canthus remains the favored location for treating horizontal laxity.

Historical developments in the 1980s have sometimes seemed less significant. Blepharopigmentation was introduced more by industry and in the lay press than in the scientific literature. The technique, introduced to ophthalmologists by Giora G. Angres,[72] was initially developed for aphakic and presbyopic patients and by handicapped persons who were unable to accurately apply their own eyeliner. It has since been used as an adjunct to cosmetic blepharoplasty[73] as well as eyebrow enhancement[74] for cosmesis and in patients with alopecia. The consumer demand for the cosmetic procedure was predicted to be great by the equipment manufacturers but never really developed. In 1980, Orkan Stasior[75, 76] first described posterior eyebrow fixation, a technique for brow elevation through a blepharoplasty incision.

In 1982, trichloroacetic acid (TCA) exfoliation was first described in the ophthalmic literature by Allan Lorincz[77] as a "superficial chemical cautery for circumscribed eyelid skin lesions." Ten years earlier, Wolport and colleagues[78] had described a chemical peel with trichloroacetic acid for fine wrinkles of aging skin. This technique has been gaining popularity as a "light chemical peel" to reduce the fine wrinkle lines in the periorbital area. The efficacy and duration of chemical peels with this acid remain uncertain.

RECENT ADVANCES IN COSMETIC EYELID AND FACIAL SURGERY

In 1985, Bosniak and Sachs[79] described lipolytic diathermy as a technique for fat pad "sculpting" in cosmetic blepharoplasty. Putterman[80] described scalpel–YAG laser blepharoplasty in 1990. Rapid-absorbing gut sutures were introduced for skin closure around the same time. These techniques have not gained widespread acceptance.

Baker and associates[81] first described carbon dioxide (CO_2) laser blepharoplasty in 1984. This technique involved skin and fat excision using continuous-energy laser output, which was the only power mode available at the time. The work of Baylis and colleagues[82] and their multiple courses, exhibits, and presentations were responsible for popularizing and reintroducing the oculoplastic community to the benefits of transconjunctival blepharoplasty. David[83] was the first, in 1988, to describe the use of the CO_2 laser for transconjunctival lower eyelid fat excision.

Botulinum Toxin A

Botulinum toxin A was initially developed as an alternative to the surgical treatment of strabismus. In the early 1970s, many ophthalmologists participated in the Food and Drug Administration (FDA)–approved study of the efficacy of botulinum toxin A in the treatment of benign essential blepharospasm and hemifacial spasm. Noting the beneficial side effects on periocular wrinkles and glabellar frown lines, oculoplastic surgeons began using botulinum toxin A for cosmetic purposes in the early 1990s. It was not until 1994 that initial reports describing cosmetic use of botulinum by Keen and associates[84] and Buyuron and Huddleston[85] appeared in the literature. That same year, Keen and Blitzer[86] performed a double-blind study confirming the efficacy of botulinum toxin A for the treatment of hyperkinetic facial lines.

Laser Resurfacing

Many of the oculoplastic surgical advances in the last 10 years have been technology-dependent. Refinements in our understanding and delivery of laser energy, combined with development of new lasers and endoscopic equipment, have had a dramatically favorable impact on the art of cosmetic oculoplastic surgery. Interdisciplinary exchange of knowledge, equipment, and techniques has contributed to improved patient results and satisfaction. This is well illustrated by the introduction and refinement of laser resurfacing procedures.

The use of the CO_2 laser for surface vaporization began in 1987 as a treatment modality for localized cutaneous tumors and more diffuse dermal disease. The incidental finding of cosmetic benefit led to the initial report of cosmetic facial resurfacing in 1989.[87] The initial use of a computer-assisted scanning device to achieve uniform and smooth depth vaporization was reported in 1987 by Brauner and Schifman.[88] The technique was not initially successful because of inadequate energy levels and a gaussian laser beam distribution.

At about the same time, dermatologists began understanding the importance of laser tissue interaction and the theoretical thermal relaxation time of skin.[89] Hobbs and colleagues[90] described the use of superpulsed laser and high-irradiation, short-duration pulses (1 ms) to minimize thermal damage. In 1989, David and Lask[91] demonstrated histologic evidence of the cosmetic benefit that was being observed clinically. They showed reduction in atypical keratocytes and solar elastosis with a histologically normal epithelium 4 weeks after laser resurfacing.

In the early 1990s, the medical laser industry responded by producing a variety of superpulsed, ultrapulsed, and scanning lasers with and without computer-generated pattern delivery systems. In 1994, Weinstein[92] was the first to describe laser resurfacing of periocular wrinkles in the literature. At the 1994 American Academy of Ophthalmology annual meeting, many oculoplastic surgeons were skeptical as they viewed Sterling Baker's videos, live surgery, and postoperative patients. Since that time, cosmetic laser resurfacing is now widely accepted by the medical community and the public. It is a significant advance in improving the appearance of periocular rhytids ("crow's feet").

Hibst and Kaufman[93–95] have been working with and recommending the erbium:YAG laser for cosmetic resurfacing. The erbium laser's shorter pulsed time, higher pulsed power, and increased laser light absorption in tissue water may make it more efficacious for surface ablation. More clinical experience is necessary to make that determination.

The Facelift

Laser resurfacing has been a great advance in tightening the facial dermal envelope. Other dramatic and significant developments have occurred in lifting the soft tissues to their original youthful bony positions. The subperiosteal rhytidectomy was first described for facial rejuvenation by Tessier[96] in 1979. Psillakis and associates[97] pointed out the high incidence of frontal nerve injury along with loss of scalp sensation associated with this technique. He also noted the difficulty involved in elevating the midface. Adams and Miller[98] should be

credited with introducing the sensory nerve–sparing biplanar forehead lift. Ramirez[99] deserves great credit for his influence in introducing the endoscope to aesthetic facial procedures. He was the first to describe the endoscopically assisted biplanar forehead lift.[100]

May and colleagues[101] in 1990 described sculpting and resection of the retro-orbicularis oculi fat. In 1995, Aiche and Ramirez[102] described the excision of the suborbicularis oculi fat. Knize[103] and Guyuron and colleagues[104] described resection and/or interruption of the corrugator supercilii and procerus muscles through eyelid incisions. Owsley[105] initially described a cheek lift by elevating the malar fat pad to reduce prominent nasolabial folds. This was performed through a preauricular incision. May and associates[106] described malar augmentation and a cheek lift through a subciliary incision. That same year, McCord and colleagues[107] described a subperiosteal malar cheek lift combined with lower eyelid blepharoplasty. There were similarities to the "Madame Butterfly" procedure described 10 years earlier by Shorr and Fallor[108] as a corrective procedure for complications of blepharoplasty.

THE FUTURE OF COSMETIC EYELID AND FACIAL SURGERY

We look forward to new techniques and refinements in existing techniques to further reduce the already low complication rate associated with cosmetic oculoplastic surgery. Ancillary medications and new adhesive dressings that can reduce perioperative edema and accelerate healing may be developed. Enhanced laser delivery systems and new wavelengths such as the erbium laser may further improve surgical results. Future historical developments may focus on prevention through the use of antiaging medications to reverse solar damage and increase skin elasticity. There is also a potential for autologous collagen and botulinum toxin A to become more useful. The day may come when scientific evidence will support the use of nutritional therapy and topical skin care products.

References

1. Wood C (trans): The Tadhkirat of Ali ibn Isa of Baghdad, pp 98, 115, 118–119. Chicago, Northwestern University, 1936.
2. Arrington G: A History of Ophthalmology. New York, MD Publications, 1959.
3. Tieck GJ, Hunt HL: Plastic and cosmetic surgery of the head, neck, and face. Am J Ophthalmol 1921; 35:173–176.
4. von Graefe CF: De Rhinoplastice, p 13. Berlin, Reime, 1818.
5. Wood CA (ed): The American Encyclopedia of Ophthalmology. Chicago, Cleveland Press, 1913.
6. Beer GJ: Lehre der Augenkrankheiten. Vienna, CF Wappler, 1792.
7. Dupuis C, Rees TD: Historical notes on blepharoplasty. Plast Reconstr Surg 1971; 47:246–251.
8. Mackenzie W: A Practical Treatise of the Diseases of the Eye, pp 170–171. London, Longman, 1830.
9. Alibert JL: Monographie des Dermatoses ou Précis Théorique et Practique des Maladies de la Peau, p 795. Paris, Daynac, 1832.
10. Graf D: Oertliche erbliche Erschlaffung der Haut. Wochenschr Gesamte Heilkd 1836; 4:225–227.

11. Dupuytren G (ed): De l'oedeme chronique des tumeurs enkystées des paupières. In Leçons Orales de Clinique Chirurgicale, 2nd ed, vol 3, pp 377–378. Paris, Germer-Bailliere, 1839.

12. Sichel A: Ptosis adiposa. Ann Ocul 1844; 12:187.

13. Schmidt-Rimpler H: Fett-hernien der oberen Augenlider. Cent Blatt Prak Augenheilkd 1899; 23:297.

14. Elschnig A: Fett-hernien, Sog, Tränensacke, der Unterlider. Klin Monatsbl Augenheilkd 1930; 84:763.

15. Fuchs E: Textbook of Ophthalmology, pp 501–502, 720–722. New York, D Appleton, 1892.

16. Hotz FC: Ueber das Wesen und die Operation der sogenannten Ptosis Atonica. Arch Augenheilkd 1880; 9:95.

17. Fuchs E: Ueber blepharochalasis (Erschlaffung der Lidhaut). Wien Klin Wochenschr 1896; 9:109.

18. Benedict WL: Blepharochalasis: Report of three cases. JAMA 1926; 87:1735.

19. Panneton P: Le blepharochalazis: A propos de 51 cas dans la même famille. Arch Ophtalmol 1936; 53:724.

20. Fox SA: Ophthalmic Plastic Surgery. New York, Grune & Stratton, 1952.

21. Miller CC: Cosmetic Surgery: The Correction of Featural Imperfections, 2nd ed, pp 40–42. Chicago, Oak Printing, 1908.

22. Miller CC: Cosmetic Surgery: The Correction of Featural Imperfections, pp 30–32. Philadelphia, FA Davis, 1924.

23. Kolle FS: Plastic and Cosmetic Surgery. New York, D Appleton, 1911.

24. Bettman AG: Plastic and cosmetic surgery of the face. Northwest Med 1920; 19:205.

25. Bettman AG: Plastic surgery about the eye. Ann Surg 1928; 88:994–1006.

26. Bettman AG: The Minimum Scar. Portland, Ore, Medical Sentinel, 1926.

27. Spaeth EB: Newer Methods of Ophthalmic Plastic Surgery. Philadelphia, P Blackiston's Son and Co, 1925.

28. Bourguet J: Les hernies graisseuses de l'orbite: Notre traitement chirurgical. Bull Acad Med 1924; 92:1270.

29. Bourguet J: Chirurgie esthétique de la face: Les nez concaves, les rides et les "poches" sous les yeux. Arch Franco-Belges Chir 1925; 28:293.

30. Bourguet J: La chirurgie esthétique de l'oeil et des paupières. Monde Med 1929; 39:725–731.

31. Claoué C: Documents de Chirurgie Plastique et Esthétique: Compte Rendu des Séances de la Société Scientifique Française de Chirurgie Plastique et Esthétique, pp 344–353. Paris, Maloine, 1931.

32. Passot R: La Chirurgie Esthétique Pure: Technique et Résultats, pp 176–180. Paris, Gaston Doin et Cie, 1931.

33. Stephenson K: The history of face, neck and eyelid surgery. In Masters F, Lewis J (eds): Symposium on Aesthetic Surgery of the Face, Eyelid, and Breast, pp 13–21. St. Louis, CV Mosby, 1972.

34. Passot R: La chirurgie esthétique des rides du visage. Presse Med 1919; 27:258.

35. Rees TD (ed): History. In Aesthetic Plastic Surgery. Philadelphia, WB Saunders, 1980.

36. Rogers BO: A brief history of cosmetic surgery. Surg Clin North Am 1971; 51:265–288.

37. Rogers BO: A history of cosmetic surgery. Bull NY Acad Med 1971; 47:265–299.

38. Noel A: La Chirurgie Esthétique: Son Role Social. Paris, Masson et Cie, 1926.

39. Bourguet J: La Chirurgie esthétique de la face, pp 1657–1670. Le Concours Médical, 1921.

40. Hunt HL: Plastic Surgery of the Head, Face and Neck, p 198. Philadelphia, Lea & Febiger, 1926.

41. Joseph J: Nasenplastik und sonstige Gesichtsplastik: Nebst einen Anhang über Mammaplastik, pp 507–509. Leipzig, Curt Katizch, 1931.

42. Bames HO: Frown disfigurement and ptosis. Plast Reconstr Surg 1957; 19:337.

43. Eitner E: Weitermitteilungen über kosmetische Faltenoperationen in Gesicht. Wein Med Wochenschr 1935; 85:244.

44. Gonzalez-Ulloa M: A trend of new operations to improve the results of rhytidectomy. Int Micr J Aesth Plast Surg 1974A.

45. Regnault P: Complete face and forehead lifting with double traction on "crow's feet." Plast Reconstr Surg 1972; 49:123–129.

46. Castanares S: Forehead wrinkles, glabellar frown and ptosis of the eyebrows. Plast Reconstr Surg 1964; 34:406.

47. Castanares S: Blepharoplasty for herniated intraorbital fat. Plast Reconstr Surg 1951; 8:46.

48. Castanares S: Baggy eyelids: Physiological considerations and surgical techniques. In Broadbent TR (ed): Transactions of International Congress of Plastic Surgery, p 499. Amsterdam, Excerpta Medica, 1963.

49. Castanares S: A comparison of blepharoplasty techniques. In Masters F, Lewis JR (eds): Symposium on Aesthetic Surgery of the Face, Eyelid, and Breast. St. Louis, CV Mosby, 1972.

50. Castanares S: Correction of the baggy eyclids deformity produced by herniation of orbital fat. In Smith B, Converse M (eds): Proceedings of the Second International Symposium on Plastic and Reconstructive Surgery of the Eye and Adnexa. St. Louis, CV Mosby, 1967.

51. Sayoc BT: Plastic reconstruction of the superior palpebral fold. Am J Ophthalmol 1954; 38:556–559.

52. Pang RG: Surgical formation of upper lid fold. Arch Ophthalmol 1961; 65:783–784.

53. Sheen JH: Supratarsal fixation in upper blepharoplasty. Plast Reconstr Surg 1974; 54:424–431.

54. Boo-Chai K: Plastic construction of the superior palpebral fold. Plast Reconstr Surg 1963; 31:74–78.

55. Beard C, Obear M, Tenzel R, et al: Symposium: Cosmetic blepharoplasty. Trans Am Acad Ophthalmol Otolaryngol 1969; 73:1141–1149.

56. Sheen JH: A change in the technique of supratarsal fixation in upper blepharoplasty. Plast Reconstr Surg 1977; 59:831–834.

57. Dryden R, Leibsohn J: The levator aponeurosis in blepharoplasty. Ophthalmology 1978; 85:718–725.

58. Putterman AM, Urist MJ: Reconstruction of the upper eyelid crease and fold. Arch Ophthalmol 1976; 94:1941–1954.

59. Sheen JH: Tarsal fixation in lower blepharoplasty. Plast Reconstr Surg 1978; 62:24–31.

60. Smith B, Petrelli R: Surgical repair of prolapsed lacrimal glands. Arch Ophthalmol 1978; 96:113–114.

61. Smith B, Lisman R: Dacryoadenopexy as a recognized factor in upper lid blepharoplasty. Plast Reconstr Surg 1983; 771:629.

62. Putterman AM: Temporary blindness after cosmetic blepharoplasty. Am J Ophthalmol 1975; 80:1081–1083.

63. Putterman AM, Urist M: Baggy eyelids: A true hernia. Ann Ophthalmol 1973; 5:1029–1032.

64. Graham WP, Messner KH, Miller SH: Keratoconjunctivitis sicca symptoms appearing after blepharoplasty. Plast Reconstr Surg 1976; 57:57–61.

65. Rees TD: Dry eye complications after blepharoplasty. Plast Reconstr Surg 1975; 56:375–380.

66. Scholtz RC, Swartz S: "Dry eye" following blepharoplasty. Plast Reconstr Surg 1974; 54:644–647.

67. Tenzel RR: Cosmetic blepharoplasty. In Soll DB (ed): Management of Complications in Ophthalmic Plastic Surgery, pp 119–131. Birmingham, Ala, Aesculapius, 1976.

68. Edgerton M: Causes and prevention of lower lid ectropion following blepharoplasty. Plast Reconstr Surg 1972; 49:367–373.

69. Webster RC, Davidson TM, Reardon EJ, Smith RC: Suspending sutures in blepharoplasty. Arch Otolaryngol 1979; 105:601–604.

70. Putterman AM: Cosmetic Oculoplastic Surgery, pp 187–208. New York, Grune & Stratton, 1982.

71. Katzen LB, Tenzel RR: Canthal laxity and eyelid malpositions. Adv Ophthalmol Plast Reconstr Surg 1983; 2:229–243.

72. Angres GG: Angres permalid-liner method: A new surgical procedure. Ann Ophthalmol 1984; 16:145–148.

73. Angres GG: The Angres permalid-liner method to enhance the result of cosmetic blepharoplasty. Ann Ophthalmol 1985; 17:176–177.

74. Angres GG: Blepharopigmentation and eyebrow enhancement techniques for maximum cosmetic results. Ann Ophthalmol 1985; 17:605–611.

75. Stasior OG: Posterior eyebrow fixation. Presented at the 1980 Scientific Symposium of the American Society of Ophthalmic Plastic and Reconstructive Surgery, Chicago.

76. Stasior OG, Lemke BN: The posterior eyebrow fixation. Adv Ophthalmic Plast Reconstr Surg 1983; 2:193–197.

77. Lorincz A: Chemexfoliation. In Putterman AM (ed): Cosmetic Oculoplastic Surgery, p 246. New York, Grune & Stratton, 1982.
78. Wolport FG, Dalton WE, Hoopes JT: Chemical peel with trichloroacetic acid. Br J Plast Surg 1972; 25:333–334.
79. Bosniak SL, Sachs ME: Lipolytic diathermy. Orbit 1985; 44:157.
80. Putterman AM: Scalpel neodymium:YAG laser and oculoplastic surgery. Am J Ophthalmol 1990; 109:581–584.
81. Baker S, Muenzler W, Small R, Leonard J: Carbon dioxide laser blepharoplasty. Ophthalmology 1984; 91:238–244.
82. Baylis HI, Long JA, Groth MF: Transconjunctival lower eyelid blepharoplasty, techniques and complications. Ophthalmology 1989; 96:1027–1032.
83. David LM: The laser approach to blepharoplasty. J Dermatol Surg Oncol 1988; 14(7):741–746.
84. Keen M, Kopelman JE, Aviv JE, et al: Botulinum toxin A: A novel method to remove periorbital wrinkles. Facial Plast Surg 1994; 10(2):141–146.
85. Buyuron B, Huddleston SW: Aesthetic indications for botulinum injection. Plast Reconstr Surg 1994; 93:913–918.
86. Keen M, Blitzer A, Aviv J, et al: Botulinum toxin A for hyperkinetic facial lines: Results of a double-blind, placebo-controlled study. Plast Reconstr Surg 1994; 94(1):94–99.
87. Spadoni D, Cain CL: Facial resurfacing using the carbon dioxide laser. Am Operating Room Nurses J 1989; 50:1007, 1009–1013.
88. Brauner G, Schifman A: Laser surgery in children. J Dermatol Surg Oncol 1987; 13:178–186.
89. Anderson RR, Parrish JA: Selective photothermolysis: Precise microsurgery by selective absorption of pulsed radiation. Science 1983; 220:524–527.
90. Hobbs ER, Balin PT, Wheeland RG, et al: Superpulsed lasers: Minimizing thermal damage with short duration, high irradiance pulsed. J Dermatol Surg Oncol 1987; 13:955–964.
91. David LM, Lask GP, Glassberg E, et al: Laser abrasion for cosmetic and medical treatment of facial actinic damage. Cutis 1989; 43(6):583–587.
92. Weinstein C: Ultrapulse carbon dioxide laser removal of periocular wrinkles in association with laser blepharoplasty. J Clin Laser Med Surg 1994; 12(4):205.
93. Hibst R, Kaufman R: Effects of laser parameters on pulsed erbium:YAG laser skin ablation. Laser Med Sci 1991; 6:391–397.
94. Kaufman R, Hibst R: Pulsed 2.94 μm erbium:YAG laser skin ablation: Experimental results and first clinical application. Clin Exp Dermatol 1990; 15:389–393.
95. Kaufman R, Hibst R: Pulsed erbium:YAG laser ablation in cutaneous surgery. Lasers Surg Med 1996; 19:324–330.
96. Tessier P: Face lifting and frontal rhytidectomy. In Ely FJ (ed): Transactions of the Seventh International Congress of Plastic and Reconstructive Surgery, Rio de Janeiro, September 1979.
97. Psillakis JM, Rumley TO, Camargos A: Subperiosteal approach as an improved concept for correction of the aging face. Plast Reconstr Surg 1988; 82:383–394.
98. Adams JR, Miller PA: The biplane forehead lift: A technique for preservation of sensory innervation to the scalp and vascular supply to the forehead skin. Plast Surg Forum 1993; 16:109.
99. Ramirez O: Endoscopically assisted biplanar forehead lift. Plast Reconstr Surg 1995; 96:323–333.
100. Ramirez O: Endoscopic techniques in facial rejuvenation: An overview, part I. Aesthetic Plast Surg 1993; 91:463–476.
101. May JW, Feason J, Zingarelli P: Retro-orbicularis oculus fat (ROOF) resection in aesthetic blepharoplasty: A 6-year study in 63 patients. Plast Reconstr Surg 1990; 86:682–689.
102. Aiche AE, Ramirez OH: The suborbicularis oculi fat pads: An anatomic and clinical study. Plast Reconstr Surg 1995; 95:37–42.
103. Knize DM: Transpalpebral approach to the corrugator supercilii and procerus muscles. Plast Reconstr Surg 1995; 95:52–60.
104. Guyuron B, Michelow BJ, Thomas T: Corrugator supercilii muscle resection through blepharoplasty incision. Plast Reconstr Surg 1995; 95:691–696.
105. Owsley J: Lifting the malar fat pad for correction of prominent nasolabial folds. Plast Reconstr Surg 1993; 91:463–476.
106. May JW, Zenn MR, Zingarelli P, et al: Subciliary malar augmentation and cheek advancement: A 6-year study in 22 patients undergoing blepharoplasty. Plast Reconstr Surg 1995; 96:1553–1559.
107. Hester TR Jr, Codner MA, McCord CD Jr: Subperiosteal malar cheek lift with lower lid blepharoplasty. In McCord CD Jr (ed): Eyelid surgery: Principles and Techniques, pp 210–215. New York, Lippincott-Raven, 1995.
108. Shorr N, Fallor M: "Madame Butterfly" procedure: Combined cheek and lateral canthal suspension procedure for post blepharoplasty "round eye" and lower eyelid retraction. Ophthalmic Plast Reconstr Surg 1985; 1:229–235.

Allen M. Putterman

Chapter 2

Evaluation of the Cosmetic Oculoplastic Surgery Patient

The preoperative evaluation of the candidate for cosmetic oculoplastic surgery is extremely important and cannot be overemphasized. In addition to helping determine the specific procedures required by the patient, evaluation aids in selecting candidates for surgery. Moreover, the initial visit provides a setting in which to prepare patients for surgery and to inform them about its possible complications, thereby ensuring a smoother postoperative course.

In this chapter are the steps I follow in evaluating patients who desire cosmetic oculoplastic surgery: (1) examination of abnormalities of the forehead, eyebrows, eyelids, cheeks, face, and skin condition; (2) ocular assessment; (3) tear secretion measurements; and (4) photographs. Most important, the preoperative examination provides an opportunity for the surgeon to determine what the patient hopes to gain from this operation and to tell the patient what can be realistically accomplished.

This chapter has been updated by the addition of measurements for upper and lower eyelid retraction in patients with thyroid disease. A decrease in the palpebral fissure width on down gaze in the evaluation of blepharoptosis is emphasized. Evaluation of "cheek bags" (festoons) and depressions, facial sagging, and skin wrinkling is also newly added.

ALLEN M. PUTTERMAN

Evaluation of the patient who may be interested in cosmetic surgery is very important. The surgeon can decide which patients should or should not have surgery and can choose the appropriate procedures. A thorough evaluation also can help avoid postoperative complications and unhappiness.

One of the most important aspects of evaluation is to establish what patients find objectionable in their appearance and what they expect surgery to accomplish. I usually determine this by handing patients a mirror and asking them to hold it at eye level as they point out their objectionable features (Fig. 2–1). Frequently, patients emphasize their most minor blemishes and dismiss the major defects noted by the surgeon. The surgeon should therefore make sure that the patient has realistic expectations.

HISTORY

In taking a medical history, the surgeon questions the patient about illnesses, medications, allergies, and edema. Emphasis is on ruling out thyroid disease, heart failure, bleeding tendencies, and unusual edema. For example, patients with thyroid disease may look as if they need cosmetic surgery, but the treatment needed is frequently medical, not surgical. Also, patients with thyroid disease must be followed up for at least 6 months until their eyelid retraction measurements and amounts of eyelid edema and herniated fat are stable before surgery can be considered. Patients should also be questioned about intake of aspirin or anti-inflammatory medications, such as ibuprofen, vitamin E, and anticoagulants. These drugs must be discontinued for several

11

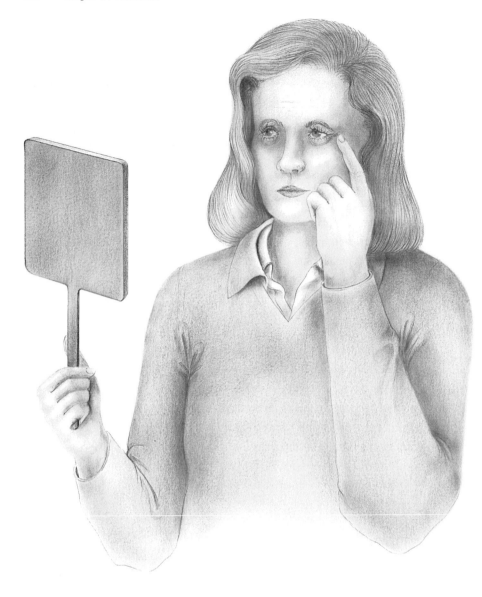

figure 2–1
Cosmetic oculoplastic surgery patients view themselves in a mirror and point out to the surgeon what changes they would like in their appearance. This may differ greatly from what the surgeon sees as the patients' problems.

weeks preoperatively to avoid the possibility of complications of bleeding during and after surgery.

The surgeon should also try to find out why the patient wants surgery now. In this way, the surgeon can differentiate patients who have realistic, mature reasons for requesting surgery from those who do not.

The examination includes an evaluation of the forehead, eyebrows, upper and lower eyelids, cheeks, face, and skin condition. I encourage all surgeons to step back and view the patient's entire face first before they focus on specific structures. The purpose of this examination is to determine which cosmetic problems are correctable so that they can be compared with the patient's expectations.

FOREHEAD AND EYEBROW EXAMINATION

In examining the forehead and eyebrows, the cosmetic surgeon is looking mainly for brow ptosis (drooping), which causes excessive upper eyelid folds. The surgeon also looks for asymmetric brow ptosis or ptosis of parts of the brow (e.g., nasal or temporal). In patients with apparent dermatochalasis (excess skin) of the upper eyelid that is actually due to a brow ptosis, excising upper eyelid skin without elevating the eyebrow only minimally improves appearance. Additionally, forehead wrinkles and frown lines caused by overactive corrugator and procerus muscles are examined.

Measuring the distance from the central upper eyelid margin to the central inferior brow edge with the patient gazing in primary position can help identify patients with brow ptosis. If this measurement is much less than 10 mm, especially in women, surgical elevation of the brow may be desirable.

Another useful measurement is the distance from the central inferior part of the eyebrow to the inferior corneal limbus as the patient gazes in primary position. The measurement is commonly about 22 mm. If this measurement is much less than that amount, especially in women, elevation of the brow is also suggested. Also, this measurement is frequently more reliable than that of the brow to upper eyelid, which varies with upper eyelid ptosis or retraction.

The amount of brow ptosis can be determined in several ways. The first is to line the zero mark of a millimeter ruler with the central superior brow edge (Fig. 2–2). The brow is then elevated to a cosmetically acceptable level with the examiner's finger, and the amount of excursion of the brow is noted on the ruler where the superior central brow edge meets the ruler. This measurement is repeated over the temporal and nasal aspects of the brow about 10 mm from the brow ends, and similar measurements are made over the opposite brow.

The same measurement can be made by first placing the brow in a cosmetically acceptable position with the examiner's finger, lining the 20-mm mark of the ruler with the superior central brow edge, and then releasing the brow and noting how many millimeters the brow drops as it assumes its ptotic position.

Still another method of measuring brow ptosis or asymmetry is to use the ocular asymmetry measuring device (Karl Ilg & Co., St. Charles, Ill.),[1] an instrument that Chalfin and I devised. It consists of a headband, a ruler, and a T-shaped crosspiece. When the band is placed around the patient's forehead, it fixes the ruler vertically over the midforehead. The crosspiece line intersects the medial canthus and levels the crosspiece. The crosspiece is then aligned with the central superior brow, and the location where the indicator is positioned on the ruler is noted (Fig. 2–3). The brow is elevated with the examiner's finger to a cosmetically acceptable level. The crosspiece is then elevated to the new superior central brow position, and the excursion of the indicator on the ruler is noted. The measurements are repeated temporally and nasally and on the opposite brow.

The ocular asymmetry measuring device is especially useful in unilateral brow ptosis. In these cases, the crosspiece is raised to the highest position on the arch of the lower eyebrow, and the position of the indicator on the millimeter ruler is noted. The crosspiece is then raised to the corresponding point on the opposite eyebrow, and the position of the indicator is again noted. The excursion of the indicator is a direct measurement of asymmetry, as the indicator is fixed to the crosspiece and they move as one unit. Measuring the amount of brow ptosis aids in determining the amount of skin that must be removed to elevate the brow surgically (see Chapters 27 and 28).

EXAMINATION OF THE UPPER EYELID

The upper eyelid is evaluated for excessive skin, herniated orbital fat, abnormal eyelid creases, ptosis, retraction, and prolapse of the lacrimal gland.

Eyelid Skin-Fat Examination

The amount of excessive skin and whether the skin is more redundant over part of the upper eyelid are determined. The surgeon finds herniated orbital fat by noting fullness in the upper eyelid, especially nasally and, at times, centrally. Lifting the lid fold by elevating the brow and simultaneously pushing on the eye through the lower eyelid can increase the fat herniation in the suspected areas and verify that the fullness is due to fat, not edema. Fat generally flows forward during this maneuver, whereas edema of the eyelids remains unchanged. Preoperative determination of excessive skin

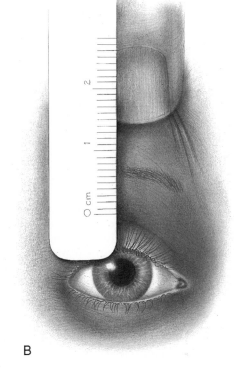

figure 2–2

Measurement of the amount of eyebrow ptosis. A, The zero (0) mark of a millimeter ruler is aligned adjacent to the top of the central ptotic brow. *B,* The surgeon lifts the ptotic brow to the desired postoperative position, and the amount of excursion of the central superior brow is noted by the level of the brow adjacent to the ruler. In this case, the brow has been elevated 7.5 mm.

A   B

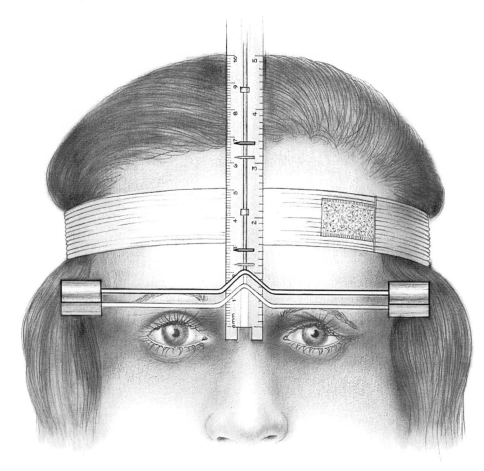

figure 2–3

Ocular asymmetry measuring device for determining the amount of brow ptosis. In asymmetric brow ptosis, the measuring rod is set at the central superior aspect of the more ptotic brow, and the point of indicator on the ruler is noted. The measuring rod is then elevated to a similar position on the more normal brow, and the millimeters of excursion of the indicator determine the amount of brow ptosis.

and herniated orbital fat establishes candidates who would benefit by the excision of these tissues.

Eyelid Crease Examination

The examiner can find the upper eyelid crease by lifting the eyebrow and asking the patient to look downward first, then slightly upward, and then downward again. The distance from the central upper eyelid margin to the central crease as the patient looks down and as the eyelid fold is elevated with the examiner's finger determines the margin crease distance (MCD) measurement (Fig. 2–4). Normally, this is 9–11 mm. If the distance is much less, reconstruction of the eyelid crease and excision of the skin fat should be considered (see Chapter 10). If the MCD is much greater than normal, a disinsertion of the levator aponeurosis should be suspected. As the levator aponeurosis recesses into the orbit, it frequently elevates the eyelid crease upward.

The surgeon must discuss reconstruction of an upper eyelid crease with the patient preoperatively. Although most patients find a high upper eyelid crease to be cosmetically appealing, some, especially Asians, may strongly dislike its appearance. It is therefore advantageous to be able to demonstrate to patients preoperatively how they will look with crease reconstruction and to predetermine the desired level at which to reconstruct the upper eyelid crease.

To predetermine the position at which to reconstruct an upper eyelid crease, the surgeon will need a curved instrument for compression of the upper eyelid skin. I formerly used an unwound, slightly curved paper clip and pressed it at various positions of the upper eyelid. Many of my patients reacted negatively to the use of a paper clip to determine the eyelid crease, saying how crude an instrument it was. This negative reaction led to my development of a more sophisticated instrument, the upper eyelid creaser (Karl Ilg & Co.).[2]

This creaser consists of a 4-cm, curved, thin metal wire attached to a handle (Fig. 2–5). The wire has a curvature similar to the normal upper eyelid crease, but it is flexible and can be bent by the examiner if the curve needs to be flattened or extended. The examiner holds the handle and presses the wire into the upper eyelid at various positions until the surgeon and patient agree on a desirable level at which the reconstruction is to be performed (Fig. 2–6). A measurement is made between the upper eyelid margin and the chosen position and is used intraoperatively to determine the position for reconstructing the crease.

Evaluation of Blepharoptosis

Ptosis of the upper eyelid is determined by measuring the palpebral fissure width and margin reflex distance–1

Evaluation of the Cosmetic Oculoplastic Surgery Patient

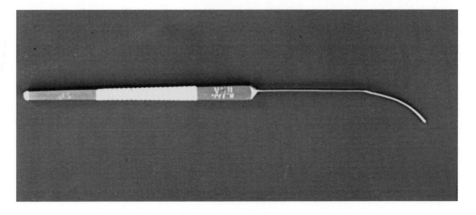

figure 2–4

The margin crease distance (MCD) is a measurement of the distance from the lid crease to the lid margin over the central upper eyelid on down gaze.

MCD

(MRD_1). Palpebral fissure width is the distance from the central lower eyelid to the central upper eyelid margins and is measured with the patient's eyes in the primary position of gaze (Fig. 2–7). Normally, this width is about 10 mm. If it is significantly less, a ptosis should be suspected and treated.

The MRD_1 is a quantitative measurement of ptosis and is determined as follows. With the eyes of the examiner and patient at the same level, an eye muscle light held between the examiner's eyes is directed at the patient. The MRD_1 is the number of millimeters from the light reflex on the patient's cornea to the central upper eyelid margin with the patient's eyes in the primary position of gaze; this is recorded in positive numbers (Fig. 2–8).[3] If the ptotic eyelid covers the corneal reflex, the eyelid is raised until the reflex is seen. The number of millimeters that the eyelid must be raised is recorded as the MRD_1 in negative numbers. The MRD_1 is a more accurate measurement of the amount of ptosis than the palpebral fissure width because the latter can be altered by abnormalities of the lower eyelid, including lower eyelid retraction. The normal MRD_1 is 4–4.5

figure 2–5

The upper eyelid creaser consists of a handle and a thin, slightly curved metal extension.

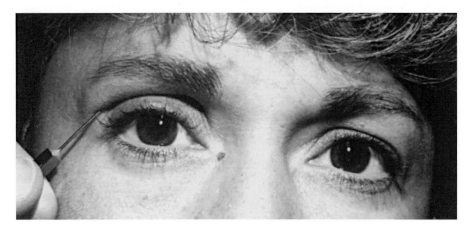

figure 2–6

A patient with upper eyelid dermatochalasis (excess skin) and poorly defined upper eyelid creases. The upper eyelid creaser is used to compress the upper eyelid skin to determine the desired position at which to reconstruct an upper eyelid crease.

mm. A smaller measurement usually means ptosis of the upper eyelid.

The palpebral fissure width on down gaze is another important measurement of blepharoptosis. The examiner uses his or her finger to fixate the patient's brow on the side being examined while raising the brow and upper eyelid on the opposite side. The patient is instructed to look to the extreme downward position of gaze while the distance between the upper and lower eyelids is measured. Normally, this distance is 2 mm or more. If the distance is 1.5 mm or less, patients frequently have difficulty reading because of the upper eyelid ptosis unless they raise their eyebrows, which is usually difficult to sustain. Olson and I[4] showed that approximately one third of patients with acquired ptosis of the upper eyelids have a zero palpebral fissure width on down gaze and are essentially blind unless they raise their eyebrows and thus their eyelids.

Evaluation of Upper Eyelid Retraction

Upper eyelid retraction occurs in some patients with thyroid ophthalmopathy. The retraction is determined by measurement of the palpebral fissure width in the primary position of gaze or by the MRD_1 (see previous paragraph). The measurements are helpful in the treatment of upper eyelid retraction (see Chapters 15 and 16).

Evaluation of Prolapsed Lacrimal Gland

Fullness of the upper eyelid in the temporal region should alert the surgeon to a possible prolapsed lacrimal gland because there is no orbital fat in the temporal upper eyelid. Pulling the upper eyelid fold upward by elevating the brow with the surgeon's finger helps to identify this abnormality. If prolapse exists, it is treated by repositioning the lacrimal gland into the lacrimal fossa at the time of the blepharoplasty (see Chapter 17).

EXAMINATION OF THE LOWER EYELID

The lower eyelid is evaluated for excessive skin, herniated orbital fat, retraction, and laxity.

Lower Eyelid Skin-Fat Examination

The excessive skin in the lower eyelid is considered as the patient looks upward. This position places the skin

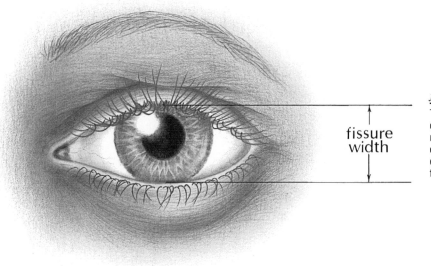

figure 2–7

The palpebral fissure width is measured over the central eyelid with the patient gazing in the primary position. This is a measurement from the central lower to the central upper eyelid, and the difference between the normal and ptotic lids determines the amount of eyelid ptosis.

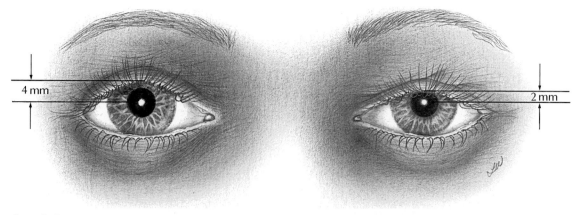

figure 2–8

The margin reflex distance–1 (MRD₁) is useful for determining the amount of ptosis. This is the distance from the light reflex on the patient's cornea to the central upper eyelid as the patient gazes in the primary position. The difference in MRD₁ between the normal and the ptotic lid determines the amount of ptosis.

on the stretch needed to look upward, and any extra skin with the eyelid in this position usually can be sacrificed without fear of producing a cicatricial ectropion postoperatively. If the amount of excessive skin is determined with the patient looking straight ahead or downward and if the excessive skin in these positions is excised, the patient might have an ectropion on up gaze.

Herniated orbital fat in the lower eyelid is judged by determining fullness in the medial, central, and temporal areas of the eyelids when the patient looks upward. To differentiate fat from edema, the examiner applies pressure to the eye through the upper eyelid. Increased fullness in the lower eyelid correlates with fat herniation; no change in fullness is seen if edema is present. Also, the examiner must consider hypertrophy of the orbicularis muscle, which can be emphasized by having the patient smile.

Evaluation of Lower Eyelid Retraction

Lower eyelid retraction occurs in some patients with thyroid ophthalmopathy. The amount of retraction is measured by the distance from the inferior limbus to the lower eyelid temporally, centrally, and nasally. Normally, the lower eyelid is at the level of the inferior limbus. This measurement is helpful in determining the size of the grafts used to treat lower eyelid retraction (see Chapter 25).

Another measurement is the margin reflex distance–2 (MRD₂) (Fig. 2–9).[5] The MRD₂ is the distance from a corneal light reflex to the lower eyelid as the examiner and patient's eyes line up at the same level and the examiner shines a muscle light at the patient's eyes. This distance normally is about 5.5 mm but increases with lower eyelid retraction. The MRD₂ also is helpful in determining the size of the grafts used to treat lower eyelid retraction (see Chapter 25).

Evaluation of Lower Eyelid Laxity

Laxity of the lower eyelid is evaluated when the surgeon pulls the lower eyelid downward and observes how quickly it snaps back to the eye (Fig. 2–10). Pinching full-thickness eyelid tissues together also helps in the evaluation of a redundant eyelid. In cases of marked horizontal lower eyelid laxity, redundant eyelid, or a

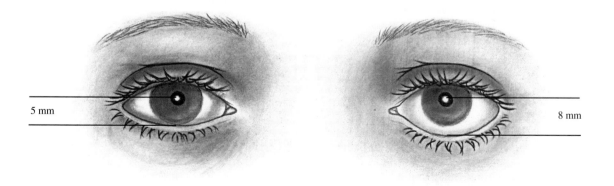

figure 2–9

The margin reflex distance–2 (MRD₂) is useful for measuring the amount of lower eyelid retracton. This is the distance from a corneal light reflex to the lower eyelid as the examiner and the patient's eye line up with each other and the examiner shines a muscle light at the patient's eyes.

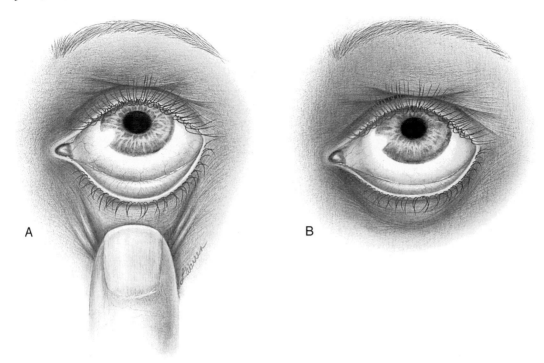

figure 2–10

A, The amount of horizontal laxity of the lower eyelid is determined by pulling the lower eyelid downward. *B,* Lack of elevation of the lower lid from the everted position on releasing the surgeon's finger indicates that the lower lid is horizontally lax
and that an ectropion is likely to complicate lower eyelid cosmetic surgery.

slowness in the eyelid to snap back after eversion, the
surgeon should consider a lower eyelid horizontal short-
ening/full-thickness temporal eyelid resection or tarsal
strip procedure in order to avoid a postoperative ectropion after resection of skin and fat (see Chapters 21
and 24).

The examiner measures laxity of the lateral canthal
tendon by pulling the lateral canthus nasally (Fig. 2–11).
Normally, the lateral canthus moves only minimally with
this maneuver; however, if the lateral canthus can easily
be pulled to or beyond the lateral limbus of the eye,
attenuation of the lateral canthal tendon must be suspected. Similarly, medial canthal tendon attenuation is
diagnosed by the ease in pulling the medial canthus
temporally. In either case, the surgeon should consider
a lateral or medial canthal tendon tuck procedure, combined with a cosmetic blepharoplasty, in order to avoid
a postoperative lower lid ectropion (see Chapter 21).

EXAMINATION OF THE CHEEK AND FACE

The cheek and face should be examined. Cheek bags
and cheek depressions occur with thyroid ophthalmopathy and aging; nasolabial fold depressions also occur.
These problems can be improved with a cheek or midface lift through a lower blepharoplasty approach (see
Chapter 24). Sagging of the face and neck also occurs
with aging and is treated with a facelift and liposuction
(see Chapter 29).

SKIN EVALUATION

The condition of the skin should be evaluated. Wrinkled
skin of the eyelids, lip area, and face are frequently due
to aging and sun exposure. Chemical peels and laser
resurfacing are methods that can be used to improve
skin texture (see Chapters 30 and 31).

DETERMINATION OF VISUAL ACUITY

Visual acuity is determined with the patient wearing
glasses or contact lenses. If the acuity is less than 20/
20, a refraction is performed to determine the best
vision. If visual acuity cannot be improved to 20/20, a
thorough eye examination should be performed to find
the cause.

If patients have poor vision postoperatively, they may
believe the operation to be the cause. If the postoperative visual acuity is the same as that recorded preoperatively, however, the operation undoubtedly is not at
fault.

OCULAR MOTILITY TESTING

The examiner can test oular motility by having the
patient follow a muscle light to the cardinal positions of
gaze. A *cover-uncover test* rules out tropia (deviation)
and phoria (movement). Phorias can become tropias,
and diplopia (double vision) can occur spontaneously as

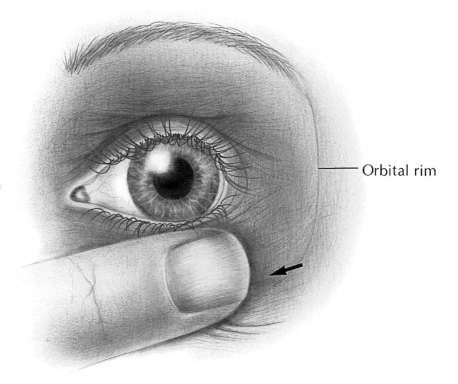

Orbital rim

figure 2–11

Lateral canthal tendon laxity is measured by the ease with which the lateral canthus can be pulled nasally when the lower lid is drawn in this direction. This signifies the need for a lateral canthal tuck.

a result of injury to the inferior or superior oblique tendons during a blepharoplasty.

EVALUATION OF BASIC TEAR SECRETION

A basic tear secretion test is performed to rule out hyposecretion of the basic tear secretors. Several drops of proparacaine topical anesthetic are applied to each eye and the lower cul-de-sac. The lower cul-de-sac and lower lid palpebral conjunctiva are blotted with a tissue paper. A Schirmer strip (SMP Division, Cooper Laboratories, San German, Puerto Rico) is bent at its notch, 5 mm from one end, and the strip is placed over the temporal palpebral conjunctiva of the lower eyelid (Fig. 2–12). The patient is instructed to look upward, and the lights are dimmed.

After 5 minutes, the strip is removed and a measurement is made from the notch to the end of wetting. (Theoretically, it is possible to do this test for 1 minute, rather than 5 minutes, and to multiply the amount of wetting in 1 minute by 3 to obtain an appraisal of the 5-minute level.) Normally, this measurement should be between 10 and 15 mm of wetting in 5 minutes. If it is significantly less, hyposecretion of the basic tear secretors should be suspected. The basic tear secretors consist of the conjunctival goblet cells, the meibomian oil glands, and the accessory lacrimal glands of Krause and Wolfring, and they are believed to keep the eyes moist during normal conditions.

If basic tear secretion is insufficient, symptoms of ocular irritation may develop or increase following a cosmetic blepharoplasty. In these cases, tightening the eyelid skin by excessive skin resection might lead to *lagophthalmos* (difficulty in completely closing the eyelids). Whereas a patient with normal tear-secreting eyes might tolerate this condition, a patient with dry eyes may not. This may be the ultimate condition that causes the asymptomatic patient to become symptomatic. If the basic tear secretion test result is low, it is important to ensure that the patient is not taking a diuretic or antihistamine because these drugs can cause a falsely low reading. If so, these drugs should be discontinued and the test repeated.

In a patient with low basic tear secretion, a cosmetic blepharoplasty might be contraindicated; if such a procedure is done, only a very conservative skin excision should be performed. In any case, patients must be fully aware that they have this problem and that after the blepharoplasty they may have to use artificial tears or a lubricating ophthalmic ointment for the rest of their lives. Some surgeons believe that the cause of the ocular irritation in this situation is excision of too much upper eyelid skin. In my experience, however, the more common cause is lower eyelid retraction secondary to excessive resection of lower eyelid skin.

Repair of blepharoptosis with the possibility of secondary lagophthalmos may also be contraindicated in patients with dry eyes.

EVALUATION OF VISUAL FIELDS

Peripheral visual fields are evaluated if a loss of peripheral vision is suspected. The purpose is to document any loss of peripheral vision from upper eyelid dermatochalasis or brow ptosis that causes the upper eyelid skin fold to overhang the upper eyelid margin. This skin fold acts as

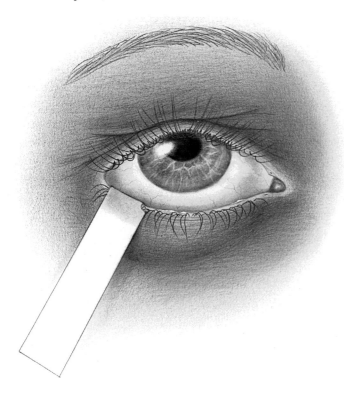

figure 2–12

A basic tear secretion test identifies patients with potentially dry eyes. Schirmer strips are placed over the temporal lower eyelids as the patient looks upward, and the amount of wetting on the strip is measured.

an "awning" that usually leads to a loss of vision in the superior or superotemporal periphery. Visual fields are also helpful in establishing the amount of peripheral vision loss in patients with blepharoptosis. Documentation of these problems can be helpful to patients in obtaining insurance benefits for surgery. Many insurance companies will pay for surgical excision of excessive upper eyelid skin or brow or upper eyelid elevation that results in a legitimate improvement in vision. Many companies, however, want proof in the form of peripheral visual field examination results and preoperative and postoperative photographs.

Many different perimeters can determine peripheral visual field loss. Many insurance companies require the use of automated equipment, such as the Goldman and Humphrey perimeters, with tests performed both with the upper eyelid taped upward and untaped (Fig. 2–13). Currently, I use the A-Mark perimeter, an arc that is moved to various positions as a light is shifted from the extreme peripheral visual field toward central areas and the patient notes when he or she first sees the light. In my experience, this method provides a satisfactory documentation of visual field loss.

ASSESSMENT BY PHOTOGRAPHY

Photographs are taken of every candidate for cosmetic oculoplastic surgery. Preoperative photographs have several advantages:

1. They provide a visual record for preoperative assessment of the patient's cosmetic problems,
2. New aspects of the patient's problems that were not appreciated at the initial examination become apparent on photographs,

3. They give the surgeon an opportunity to demonstrate to the patient the improvement in appearance postoperatively. It is amazing how easily patients forget how they appeared preoperatively when they are examined several months after surgery. Seeing their preoperative photographs gives them a renewed appreciation of their operation, which is beneficial to both the patient and surgeon.

Usually, I take photographs of both eyes in primary and in up and down positions of gaze preoperatively and 2–4 months after surgery at the last patient visit. I also take a left and right modified side view by focusing slightly in front of the side of the patient's face. Photography in cosmetic eyelid surgery is detailed further in Chapter 5.

EVALUATION OF THE CORNEA

Candidates are routinely tested for Bell's phenomenon and corneal staining. Corneal sensation is tested in selected patients whose corneas stain.

The examiner tests for Bell's phenomenon by having the patient tightly close the eyelids. The examiner then pries the eyelids open slightly and notes the position of the cornea and iris. Normally, the eye will elevate. If not, the patient may have a potential for ocular irritation after tightening the eyelids, and the surgery should be conservative or not performed at all. Certainly, patients should be warned of this possibility preoperatively because they may have to use artificial tears or ocular ointment for the rest of their lives.

Corneal sensation is tested while the patient gazes slightly upward. The examiner pulls up a wisp of cotton

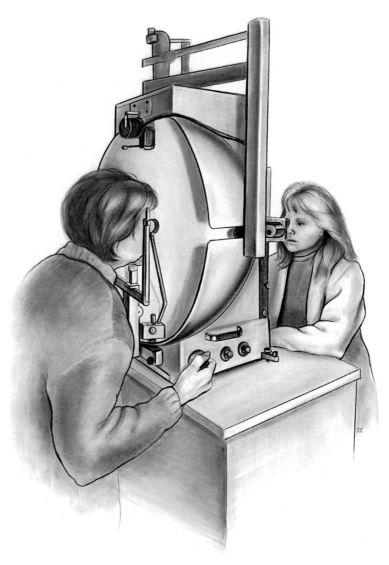

figure 2–13

Peripheral visual fields are performed in patients with upper eyelid ptosis and upper eyelid skin folds that hang over the upper eyelid margin. Loss of superotemporal vision is common in patients with marked upper eyelid dermatochalasis, and diffuse loss of superior vision is common in ptosis.

from a cotton applicator and touches the peripheral cornea with it. No response or a minimal response is abnormal, and surgery is contraindicated because of the possibility of postoperative corneal problems.

Fluorescein applied to the inferior cul-de-sac allows the examiner to study the cornea for staining under the cobalt blue light of the slit lamp. Marked keratopathy can be expected to increase after cosmetic eyelid surgery. Affected patients should not have surgery unless the keratopathy is minimal; even if it is minimal, the skin and fat should be resected very conservatively and the patient should be warned preoperatively of the possibility of postoperative ocular irritation and long-term need for ocular lubricants. The same is true for patients with blepharoptosis.

CONSULTATION

After the examination is complete, it is important to explain the findings to the patient. While the patient holds a mirror directly in front of his or her face, I point out the abnormalities. I demonstrate ptotic brows and a wrinkled forehead, low upper eyelid creases, excessive skin, herniated fat, skin discoloration and wrinkles, upper eyelid ptosis, orbicularis muscle hypertrophy, cheek bags and depressions, nasolabial folds, and facial sagging. Then I demonstrate sites for surgical incisions and postoperative scars. I correlate the patient's complaints with what I have found and discuss what can and cannot be accomplished surgically.

After bringing the patient into a consultation room, I discuss operating procedures, surgical fees, and potential complications. I explain to the patient who has a ptotic eyebrow that unless the brow is elevated, I can only minimally eliminate the excessive upper eyelid skin folds. Additionally, I emphasize that there will be a brow scar after a direct brow lift, which can be covered with cosmetics. I explain complications of upper eyelid surgery, such as cysts, ptosis, and asymmetry, and make an effort to put these complications into perspective. I tell the patient that upper eyelid cysts are common in the incision line postoperatively but that, to date, no patient of mine has had upper eyelid ptosis.

For surgery of the lower eyelid, I explain the possibility of ectropion postoperatively. I emphasize the potential for hair loss and sensory or motor dysfunction with forehead elevation, skin dimples with internal brow and cheek lifts, and redness and skin pigmentation with chemical peels and laser resurfacing. If the patient has a tendency for dry eyes, I discuss this problem and the possible need for artificial tears and ocular ointments after surgery.

If there is a need to resect herniated orbital fat, I inform patients that I prefer them to stay for 3 hours postoperatively in the surgical facility. With this type of surgery, it is possible to produce a hemorrhage, which can migrate to the retrobulbar position and cause blindness. The chance of this occurring, however, is rare, and I have not had a case of permanent blindness resulting from cosmetic surgery. If patients stay in the recovery area for several hours, they can be watched carefully for this complication; if a hemorrhage does occur, it can be detected quickly and treated.

For any surgery whose costs are not covered by insurance, I request that all surgical fees be paid in full 2 weeks preoperatively. This eliminates payment problems later. Insurance companies will not pay for the operation if it is purely cosmetic. Also, if patients are dissatisfied, they cannot withhold or reduce the surgeon's fees. The 2-week interval is enough time for checks to clear through bank processing and discourages patients from changing the date of surgery. This prepayment does not apply to blepharoptosis or eyelid retraction surgical procedures that are medically necessary and paid for by insurance companies.

A second consultation and examination are performed at the surgical center immediately before the operation. This meeting allows the surgeon to view the patient and reappraise the surgical approach. It also lets the surgeon review with the patient what the operation should accomplish, the hospital's procedures, and potential complications. The patient may also use this time to ask questions, which can lessen fears of surgery and decrease any chance of misunderstanding.

References

1. Putterman AM, Chalfin J: Ocular asymmetry measuring device. Ophthalmology 1979; 86:1203–1208.
2. Putterman AM: Eyelid creaser. Arch Ophthalmol 1990; 108:1518.
3. Putterman AM, Urist MJ: Müller muscle–conjunctival resection. Arch Ophthalmol 1975; 94:619–623.
4. Olson JJ, Putterman AM: Loss of vertical palpebral fissure height on downgaze in acquired blepharoptosis. Arch Ophthalmol 1995; 113:1293–1297.
5. Putterman AM: Basic oculoplastic surgery. In Peyman GA, Sanders DR, Goldberg MF (eds): Principles and Practice of Ophthalmology, pp 2248–2250. Philadelphia, WB Saunders, 1980.

Albert Hornblass
Joseph A. Eviatar

Chapter 3

Patient Selection for Cosmetic Oculoplastic Surgery

In this chapter, Albert Hornblass and Joseph Eviatar categorize the various problems in cosmetic oculoplastic surgery and help us select the appropriate surgical procedures to correct each of them. Photographs demonstrate the various aesthetic problems that require cosmetic oculoplastic surgery. This chapter should be beneficial to the reader in choosing specific techniques outlined in the following chapters to treat a particular patient's cosmetic deformity.

The chapter discusses eyebrow ptosis, eyelid dermatochalasis, blepharochalasis, eyelid edema, herniated orbital fat, prolapsed lacrimal gland, Asian eyelids, eyelash ptosis, blepharoptosis, pseudoptosis, festoons ("cheek bags"), hypertrophic orbicularis muscle, eyelid laxity and ectropion, scleral show, proptosis in thyroid disease, eyelid erythema, and "crow's feet" (rhytids). Thyroid disease and its treatment are now detailed in this book. I asked the authors to include a discussion in this chapter because it is important to differentiate patients with thyroid ophthalmopathy from those with the more traditional cosmetic oculoplastic surgical problems.

Differentiating functional from cosmetic blepharoplasty is also explained. The blepharoplasty procedure can improve vision by eliminating the "awning" effect of skin draping over the eyelid margin; it also can significantly reduce brow aches and headaches that result from the constant elevation of the brows as the patient attempts to reduce the excessive upper eyelid folds to see better.

The authors have added new material on selection of patients for face lifting.

ALLEN M. PUTTERMAN

Patients desiring cosmetic surgery present to the oculoplastic surgeon with a myriad of conditions and complaints. The surgeon must evaluate each patient's condition from cosmetic, functional, and psychological perspectives to determine whether surgical intervention would be appropriate. If surgery might be beneficial, the surgeon must choose the appropriate surgical procedure. This chapter outlines the types of defects and deformities seen in these patients and attempts to guide the oculoplastic surgeon toward a satisfying solution.

EYEBROW PTOSIS

Brow ptosis is a result of inferior migration of the eyebrow below its natural position at the level of the supraorbital bony rim. It often causes a tired appearance and an excessive upper eyelid fold. This condition usually results from age-related changes of the skin and connective tissues but may result from facial nerve paralysis or unilateral tumors. Brow ptosis is usually greater laterally.

Examination of the patient for brow ptosis is vital,

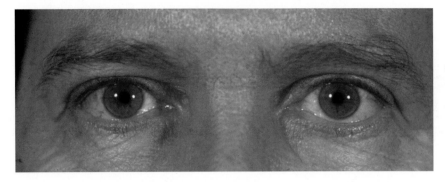

 figure 3–1

A 48-year-old man with upper eyelid dermatochalasis (excess skin) and ptosis of the eyebrows. An internal browpexy at the time of blepharoplasty would fixate his brows and prevent further downward migration.

especially when one is considering blepharoplasty, which can worsen preexisting brow ptosis and may lead to a more tired or an angry appearance. Manual elevation of the brow will determine the extent of ptosis and reveal the amount of excess skin present. (It is critical to remember that the normal female brow has a high arched contour, whereas the male brow is flatter and lower on the rim.)

Five different presentations of brow ptosis are seen, and each invites a unique surgical approach.

The patient presenting for blepharoplasty who has very mild ptosis, which often appears exaggerated after surgery, is an ideal candidate for *internal brow fixation* at the time of blepharoplasty (Fig. 3–1). In this type of ptosis, there is little redundant brow skin, and internal fixation of the brows through an eyelid crease incision prevents further downward migration without inducing visible forehead scarring (see Chapter 12).

The patient who has some redundant forehead skin or asymmetric brow ptosis usually benefits from a *direct brow lift* via a suprabrow incision (Fig. 3–2) (see Chapter 27). This technique is particularly well suited to men with a receding hairline in whom a coronal brow lift is not viable and who have prominent brow hair that may hide the faint scars. The direct approach would also benefit women with excess forehead skin and with a dark, full brow who are willing to hide these scars with makeup and who decline a more extensive surgical procedure.

The male patient with deep furrows in his forehead and excess brow skin may also be a candidate for a *midforehead brow lift* (Fig. 3–3) (see Chapter 27). By concealing the scars in the furrows, the surgeon can excise redundant skin and bypass the dilemma of hiding the surgical scars of coronal brow-lifting surgery in the patient with male-pattern baldness.

For the patient with brow ptosis and excessive fore-

head skin with a low hairline, the *coronal brow lift* permits an excellent surgical result without scars (Fig. 3–4) (see Chapter 27).[1] Alternatively, an *endoscopy-assisted brow lift* can be performed in many of these patients and allows the surgeon to elevate the brows and reduce forehead creases, with minimal scarring (see Chapter 28).

Finally, because brow ptosis is often greatest laterally, the *temporal brow lift* can be effective in patients in whom the hairline allows for such a procedure and a lateral lift is sufficient (see Chapter 27).

The surgeon must remember to treat brow ptosis surgically before attempting blepharoplasty procedures.

EYELID DERMATOCHALASIS

Redundant skin can occur in the upper or lower eyelids but is usually much more prevalent in the upper eyelids, where it may be a functional as well as a cosmetic concern. Hooding of the upper eyelids, a result of diminished skin elasticity and tone, can lead to a reduction in the visual field and to ptosis.

Patients with isolated dermatochalasis (excess skin) of the upper eyelids without herniated orbital fat need only a resection of skin from the upper eyelids (Fig. 3–5) (see Chapter 9). These patients usually do not present with a functional problem. The amount of skin to be removed can be determined with the pinch technique. The surgeon pinches the excess eyelid skin with a toothed forceps until the eyelashes begin to evert. This excess skin is then outlined on the skin with a marker. By gently pressing on the globe and observing for protrusion of the fat pockets, the surgeon can ensure that no fat needs to be removed. The redundant orbicularis muscle should be excised if found.

The upper eyelid crease does not need to be surgically

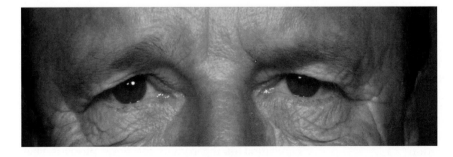

figure 3–2

A 55-year-old man with dermatochalasis and brow ptosis that is more marked laterally. Because of his receding hairline and irregular brow ptosis, he is a good candidate for a direct brow lift through a suprabrow incision.

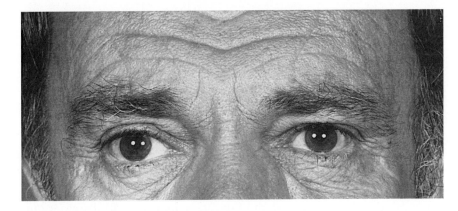

figure 3–3

A 57-year-old man with dermatochalasis, greater on his left eyelid, and with bilateral brow ptosis. His deep forehead furrows would allow for a midforehead brow lift to correct the brow ptosis.

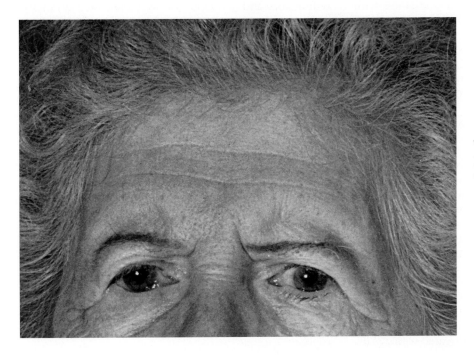

figure 3–4

A 65-year-old woman with marked brow ptosis and dermatochalasis. Depressions above the eyebrows indicate the location of the superior orbital rims. Because of her low hairline and excess forehead skin, she would benefit from a coronal brow lift as well as a blepharoplasty.

figure 3–5

A 38-year-old man with dermatochalasis of the upper lids requiring isolated removal of skin. Herniated fat can be appreciated in the lower lids without skin redundancy. A transconjunctival approach to remove the lower eyelid fat produced good cosmetic results.

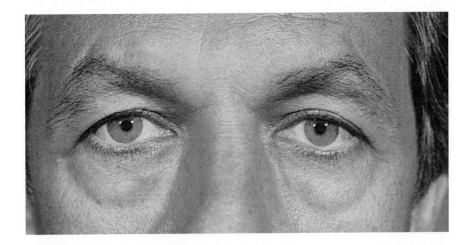

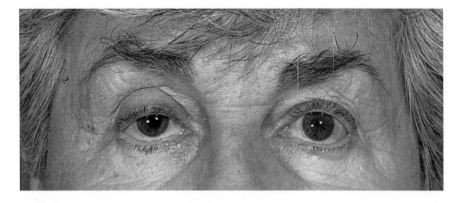

figure 3–6

A 65-year-old woman with dermatochalasis, right-sided ptosis, and a high right lid crease. For a good result, the ptosis and asymmetric lid crease should be corrected at the time of blepharoplasty.

reconstructed if the crease is close to normal (~10 mm above the eyelid margin), and the orbicularis muscle does not need to be excised in these patients. Patients with a low (0–8 mm) or asymmetric eyelid crease should undergo excision of the orbicularis muscle along with skin and fat (as needed) and a eyelid crease reconstruction (Fig. 3–6) (see Chapter 10). Less upper eyelid skin needs to be excised in patients with eyelid crease reconstruction, and the possibility of postoperative complications of lagophthalmos and exposure keratopathy is less likely. This may be helpful in blepharoplasty patients with keratitis sicca.[2]

A thorough preoperative evaluation to rule out dry eyes and an examination to ensure an adequate Bell's phenomenon enable the surgeon to determine how much skin can be safely removed from a given eyelid. For example, the patient with a rheumatic disease or the older patient with a dry eye must undergo more conservative removal of skin, and the cosmetic result is less satisfying.

The presence of excess skin of the lower eyelid without accompanying fat herniation is rare, but the surgeon can treat this by undermining skin from orbicularis muscle and removing excess skin laterally as needed (Fig. 3–7) (see Chapter 18).[3] Alternatively, laser skin resurfacing can sometimes be performed in these patients without the need for skin removal. Usually, patients with herniated fat and excess skin are best treated with a skin-muscle flap approach (see Chapter 19).

BLEPHAROCHALASIS

Blepharochalasis (relaxation of eyelid skin) is less common than dermatochalasis and is usually seen in patients with recurrent attacks of angioneurotic edema (Fig. 3–8). Rarely, it can be congenital. In patients with blepharochalasis, a stretching of the orbital septum and preseptal muscles because of recurrent edema causes skin redundancy and herniation of orbital fat. Blepharoplasty surgery with removal of orbital fat and excess skin can benefit these patients. At times, patients also need ptosis surgery and horizontal eyelid shortening.[4]

EYELID EDEMA

Eyelid edema may be caused by localized allergy or systemic conditions and cannot be treated surgically until the underlying cause is treated (Fig. 3–9). Systemic allergy, hypertension, sodium retention, low-grade infections, thyroid disease, toxins, renal disease, long-standing blepharospasm, anemia, lymphedema, and parasites are all possible causes. The laxity and distensibility of the subcutaneous connective tissue in the eyelids make them a ready site for the edematous accumulation of fluid. Attention must first be directed to any underlying medical condition. Patients with recurrent edema secondary to chronic systemic disease are poor candidates for cosmetic blepharoplasty. Once the systemic conditions have been treated and the eyelid edema resolves, patients often benefit from upper and/or lower blepharoplasty.

HERNIATED ORBITAL FAT

In addition to excess upper and lower eyelid skin, patients also have baggy eyelids, often a result of herniated

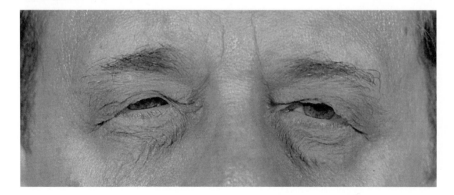

figure 3–7

A 64-year-old man with dermatochalasis far in excess of the herniated orbital fat. The patient desired only removal of the excess skin.

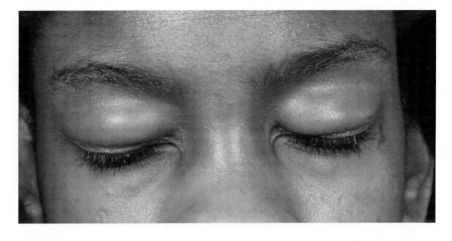

figure 3–8

A 27-year-old man with a history of multiple episodes of angioneurotic edema of the eyelids with skin redundancy and prolapsed fat. After the edema resolves, a blepharoplasty with removal of skin and fat may improve his appearance.

orbital fat (Fig. 3–10).[5] Atrophy and dehiscence of the orbital septum allow the orbital fat pads to prolapse forward, creating unsightly bulges. In the upper eyelid, the nasal fat pads are most commonly noticeable preoperatively and the central fat pads are less noticeable. Temporal brow fat may also herniate laterally and during surgery may appear in the area of the lacrimal gland. Preoperative photographs consulted in the operating room are needed to guide the surgeon in removal of fat because removing too much fat will result in deep superior sulcus deformities. Displaying the fat as it is removed from each eyelid allows the surgeon to remove equal amounts of fat and to achieve a symmetric result.

It is important to determine the need for removing skin. Patients without redundant skin may benefit from a transconjunctival approach to surgery (see Figs. 3–5 and 3–10) (see Chapter 20). This technique not only eliminates the possibility of noticeable scars but also reduces the chance of postoperative lower eyelid retraction. In patients who require removal of lower eyelid skin, a traditional skin-muscle flap approach (see Chapter

19) or a transconjunctival approach combined with laser skin resurfacing can be used.

PROLAPSED LACRIMAL GLAND

When evaluating eyelid bulging, the surgeon must remember that a temporal upper eyelid bulge is probably due to a prolapsed lacrimal gland (Fig. 3–11),[6] since there is no temporal orbital fat pad in the upper eyelid. At times, the gland may lie behind yellow herniated temporal fat. Fixation of the gland back into the temporal fossa is the proper surgical treatment (see Chapter 17). Removal of the gland may result in a severe dry eye. As in all blepharoplasty patients, an examination to rule out dry eyes is important both before and after surgery.[7]

ASIAN EYELIDS

In contrast to the Caucasian eye, the Asian eye has more fullness of the upper eyelid and a narrower palpebral

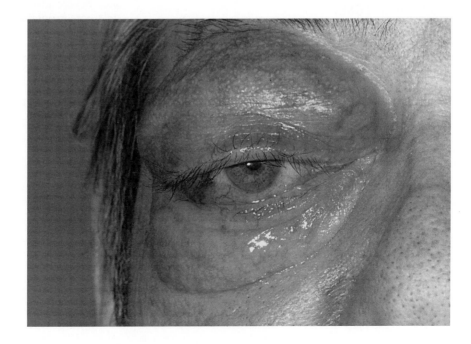

figure 3–9

A 48-year-old man with progressive Graves' orbitopathy resulting in marked swelling of both the upper and lower eyelids. Cosmetic surgery should not be performed on such a patient until the disease process has stabilized.

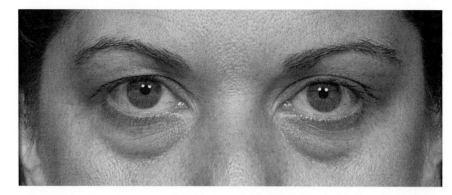

figure 3–10

A young woman with dermatochalasis, greater on the right upper eyelid, and with prominent inferior herniated fat pads. Minimally redundant lower eyelid skin allows for a transconjunctival approach for removal of the fat pads.

fissure (Fig. 3–12). There is no sharply outlined eyelid crease, and often there is an epicanthal fold. Patients may desire a more "Caucasian" appearance or may simply present for blepharoplasty or removal of an epicanthal fold. The surgical options must be thoroughly reviewed with each patient, and realistic expectations must be stressed. Suturing or incisional techniques may be used to create an eyelid crease 5–10 mm above the lash line, and the location of the crease should be determined preoperatively according to the patient's desires (see Chapter 11).[8]

EYELASH PTOSIS

In certain patients, the upper eyelid deformities include eyelash ptosis where there is downward pointing of the eyelashes (Fig. 3–13). During blepharoplasty or correction of blepharoptosis, placement of several sutures from orbicularis to levator aponeurosis during the formation of the eyelid crease rotates the lashes into a more natural position and provides a more satisfactory cosmetic result (see Chapter 10).

BLEPHAROPTOSIS

Blepharoptosis may be a concomitant condition in the patient who desires a blepharoplasty.[9] Ptosis may present as either a cosmetic or functional complaint (Fig. 3–14). When the complaint is functional, visual field testing reveals a constriction of the superior field in one or both eyes. Such testing is best performed at the end of the day, when the patient is fatigued.

To evaluate the presence and extent of ptosis, the surgeon measures the palpebral aperture in the primary, upward, and downward positions of gaze. The margin reflex distance (MRD) and the degree of levator function are also noted. The surgeon must determine whether the ptosis is congenital, neurogenic, traumatic, mechanical, or myogenic. If myasthenia is suspected, edrophonium chloride (Tensilon) testing should be performed. Bilaterality and the position of the brows must be noted to determine whether a ptosis procedure is required for both eyelids. Most cases of acquired ptosis are myogenic and involutional.

Patients with dermatochalasis, mild to moderate ptosis, and good levator function generally do well with a blepharoplasty in combination with either a Fasanella-Servat procedure (tarsoconjunctivomüllerectomy)[10] or a Putterman müllerectomy[11] (see Chapter 14). The latter can be used if preoperative instillation of 2.5 per cent phenylephrine (Neo-Synephrine) drops restored normal eyelid height.[12] A high eyelid crease and a thin eyelid suggest levator dehiscence; surgery on the levator aponeurosis often produces the best cosmetic result and allows restoration of a proper eyelid crease (see Chapter 13). Severe ptosis requires a maximal levator resection or a tarsofrontalis suspension in cases of poor levator function.[13]

PSEUDOPTOSIS

Pseudoptosis, in which ptosis appears to be present, occurs with enophthalmos, phthisis, microphthalmos,

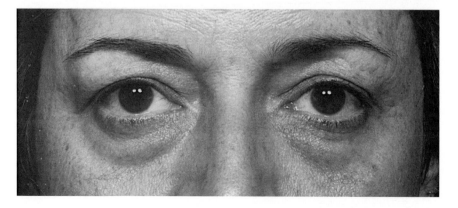

figure 3–11

In this woman, a prolapsed lacrimal gland in the right upper eyelid creates an unsightly bulge. The prolapsed gland was resuspended at the time of blepharoplasty of all four lids, with a good cosmetic result.

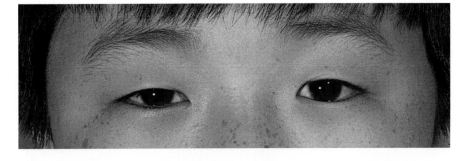

figure 3–12

An 18-year-old Asian man. Note the normal fullness of the upper lids, absence of a definite lid crease, and narrow palpebral fissure width. Discussing the height of the proposed lid crease with patients before surgery enhances patient satisfaction.

and hypotropia. It is a common problem in the anophthalmic socket (Fig. 3–15). It may also be the result of exophthalmos or eyelid retraction in the other eye. If the underlying problem (i.e., orbital correction of hypotropia or volume augmentation in the anophthalmic socket) cannot be addressed directly because of the risks of anesthesia or because the patient refuses the correction, eyelid surgery may improve cosmesis.

In patients with anophthalmia, the surgeon must be careful not to shorten the cul-de-sac. We have used the McCord tarsectomy[14] with good success. In this procedure, 1 mm of tarsus is excised for every 1 mm of eyelid ptosis.

FESTOONS ("CHEEK BAGS")

Malar bags should be noted in any patient presenting for blepharoplasty (Fig. 3–16).[15] These festoons result from attenuation, degeneration, and involution of the orbicularis muscle and overlying skin. Fat may also prolapse into these bags. Patients must be warned that a standard blepharoplasty cannot eliminate malar bags. Patients may benefit, however, from undermining of cheek skin and removal of excess orbicularis muscle at the time of blepharoplasty or from removal of both skin and muscle.[16] Patients also should be warned that surgical incisions may have to be made over the festoons, resulting in visible scars.

Patients with large "bags on bags" should be advised that they present a difficult surgical problem and that correction of the defect cannot be ensured. Laser skin resurfacing may help to diminish this appearance, although it does not usually eliminate festoons.

HYPERTROPHIC ORBICULARIS MUSCLE

A horizontal bulging of the lower eyelid immediately below the palpebral margin is often the result of a hypertrophic orbicularis muscle. This frequently occurs in patients who have an exaggerated smile or squint[17]; unlike with festoons, however, no pockets of edema or fat are found in this condition. The *squinch test*, which involves watching the contractions of the orbicularis as the eye is "squinched" during exaggerated smiling, is useful in distinguishing festoons with prolapsed fat from areas of hypertrophic orbicularis muscle (Fig. 3–17).[15] Treatment is directed to excising the prominent orbicularis muscle and redundant skin (see Chapters 18 and 19).

EYELID LAXITY AND ECTROPION

In the blepharoplasty patient, the aging changes that lead to redundant skin and bulges of fat may also result in lower eyelid laxity. This may manifest as epiphora, frank ectropion, or poor eyelid apposition to the globe and is common in patients older than 50 years of age (Fig. 3–18). Patients who present with seventh nerve palsy without aging changes require an isolated correction of eyelid laxity without blepharoplasty. Failure to identify this condition before blepharoplasty may result in exacerbation of the ectropion.

The *snap test* is useful for uncovering this problem. The patient tilts his or her head downward, and the surgeon pulls the lower eyelid away from the globe. A normal eyelid promptly retracts back toward the globe, whereas the lax eyelid retracts slowly or incompletely.

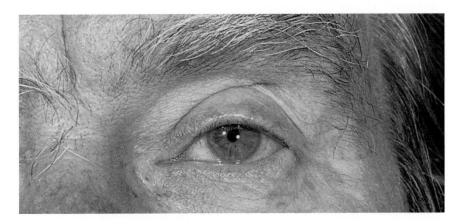

figure 3–13

A 50-year-old man with mild dermatochalasis and eyelid ptosis who also exhibits eyelash ptosis. Correction of eyelash ptosis at the time of surgery provided a good cosmetic result.

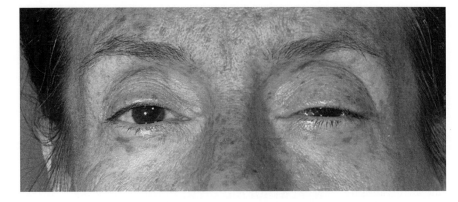

figure 3–14

A 48-year-old woman with marked involutional ptosis, greater on her left than on her right, when her eyebrows are relaxed. Note the high lid creases and the lack of significant dermatochalasis. Preoperative visual field examination revealed marked constriction of the superior fields.

figure 3–15

A woman with an enucleated left eye who presented with an enophthalmic socket and complaint of a drooping lid. This pseudoptosis was successfully treated with a conjunctivotarsomüllerectomy. The patient declined surgery to augment the orbital volume.

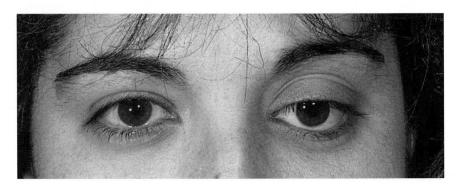

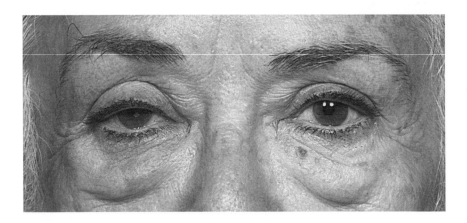

figure 3–16

A 68-year-old woman with festoons ("cheek bags") in addition to dermatochalasis and ptosis. Without undermining and excision of the skin and muscle on the cheek, prominent festoons will remain postoperatively.

figure 3–17

A man demonstrating the squinch test. Note the hypertrophied orbicularis muscle and lack of edematous festoons. Removing the hypertrophied orbicularis helped to diminish the lower lid fullness.

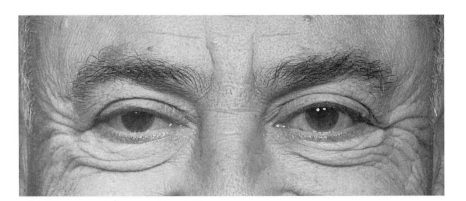

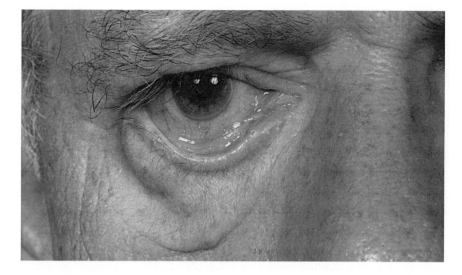

figure 3–18

A 70-year-old man with dermatochalasis and marked involutional ectropion of the right lower lid. Punctal eversion accounted for the patient's tearing. Removal of the excess skin without addressing the lid malposition would further aggravate the ectropion.

Patients with cicatricial ectropion do not appear to have lax eyelids during this test. Cicatricial ectropion must be repaired with skin grafts, in contrast to involutional ectropion, which requires tightening procedures.

Eyelid laxity should be treated at the time of blepharoplasty. Lateral tarsal strips, full-thickness horizontal eyelid shortening, and plication of the medial or lateral canthal tendons can correct this deformity (see Chapters 21 and 24).[18]

SCLERAL SHOW

Scleral show due to eyelid retraction may be unilateral or bilateral and may affect the upper and/or lower eyelids. It may result from thyroid disease (Fig. 3–19),[19] exophthalmos, trauma, or prior surgery. Patients may present with inferior punctate keratopathy. Evaluation involves identifying the underlying disease and measuring the amount of scleral show. The condition can be corrected with a tarsal strip procedure or with a V-to-Y-plasty or Z-plasty skin-muscle resection of the lower eyelid[20] with or without insertion of a scleral[21] or retro-auricular cartilage or hard-palate[22] graft (see Chapters 21 and 25).

PROPTOSIS AND THYROID DISEASE

Proptosis (bulging eye) is caused by thyroid disease, tumor, orbital inflammatory disease, and carotid cavernous fistula, among other conditions. Long-standing proptosis is most commonly due to thyroid disease (Fig. 3–20). After the cause of the process has been diagnosed and treated, cosmetic surgery can be considered.

The thyroid patient with optic nerve compression and proptosis can be treated with an orbital decompression for visual and aesthetic reasons; often a posterior decompression is required via a Caldwell-Luc operation. A combined decompression of the medial wall and floor of the orbit is currently the procedure of choice.[23] Patients with marked proptosis and extraocular muscle imbalance may benefit from a cosmetic decompression and, possibly, treatment of the muscle imbalance during a second procedure. Decompression for cosmetic indications only is somewhat controversial, and as in all decompression procedures, the risks of blindness and imbalance of extraocular motility should be carefully weighed.[24] Some patients may benefit from orbital fat decompression. When proptosis is not extreme, eyelid surgery may provide adequate cosmesis without the risks of orbital surgery.[25, 26] Procedures include canthoplasties, vertical muscle resections and recessions, scleral hard-

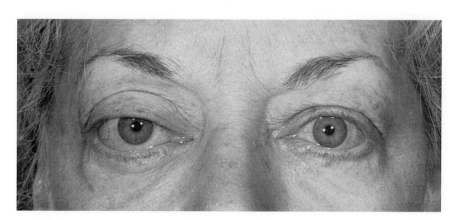

figure 3–19

A woman with Graves' orbitopathy demonstrating lower lid retraction as well as ptosis and proptosis of the right eye. Because both right eyelids (upper and lower) were malpositioned, the palpebral fissure width was 10 mm in both eyes.

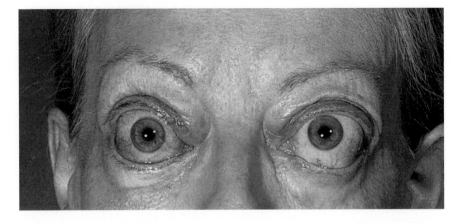

figure 3–20

A 42-year-old woman with marked proptosis, extraocular muscle imbalance, and eyelid retraction secondary to Graves' orbitopathy. This patient required bilateral orbital decompressions because of optic nerve compression.

palate and cartilage grafts, lateral tarsorrhaphies, removal of orbital fat, and blepharoplasty (see Chapters 15, 16, 25, and 26). Surgery should aim to eradicate the bulges in the eyelids, remove the scleral show, and suspend the herniated lacrimal glands. These types of eyelid procedures are also often useful to treat the thyroid patient with exposure keratopathy.

EYELID ERYTHEMA

Redness in the skin and eyelids may occur as a result of (1) overfilling of the arterial and capillary circulation due to fever, (2) local irritation, or (3) inflammation of the skin, eye, orbit, or lacrimal sac. Allergies and reflex vasodilation may also manifest as eyelid erythema. Vasomotor blepharitis, a condition seen in persons of fair complexion with delicate skin, manifests as eyelid hyperemia resulting from congestion of superficial eyelid blood vessels.

Medical therapy should be directed to the source of the problem[27] and might include vasoconstrictors and topical steroids. Surgery should be discouraged, but argon laser therapy may be used selectively to treat small vessels on the eyelids. Cosmetic makeup may be helpful in covering the erythema.

CROW'S FEET AND EYELID WRINKLES

Fine wrinkles in the skin under the lower eyelid and in the lateral canthal region cannot be corrected by blepharoplasty surgery, and this problem must be explained to patients preoperatively (Fig. 3–21). Deep crow's feet may be corrected with an orbicularis muscle flap.[28] In this surgical technique, a temporal coronal flap is used to spread out the excessive orbicularis muscle in the lateral canthal region. This muscle, some believe, accounts for the excessive wrinkling. The orbicularis muscle is then fixed to the periosteum in the splay position.

Fine rhytids and abnormal hyperpigmentation of the lower eyelids may be treated by chemexfoliation using phenol[29] or trichloroacetic acid, but patients must be warned of possible complications, especially with the use of phenol (see Chapter 30). The treatment of choice for crow's feet is often laser skin resurfacing (see Chapter 31).

PATIENT SELECTION FOR FACE LIFTING

Oculoplastic surgeons recently have become aware of the need to address the face as well as the periorbital area.

Facial aging becomes manifested by gravitational migration of the facial tissue that includes the skin, subcutaneous fat, and the superficial fascia that invests and interconnects the mimetic muscles. Patients with increasing prominence of the midface, nasolabial folds, drooping jowls at the midmandibular border, and increased laxity at the neck and chin tissue are good candidates for a facelift or at least a mini–cheek lift. The

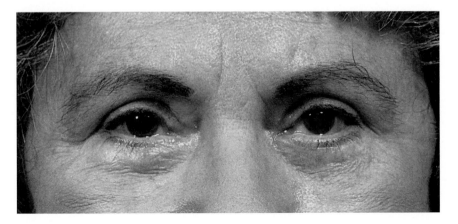

figure 3–21

A woman who underwent blepharoplasty and is left with residual fine rhytids ("crow's feet") of the lower eyelids. Chemexfoliation or laser skin resurfacing may decrease the prominence of these markings. Further removal of eyelid skin is not warranted.

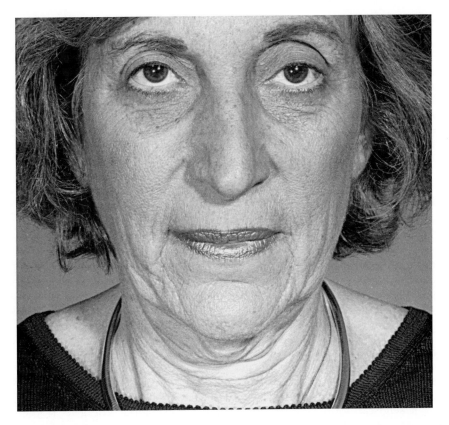

figure 3–22

A woman with redundant cervical subcutaneous fat in the submental and submandibular locations. Liposuction can achieve removal of this redundant fat.

removal of redundant cervical subcutaneous fat in the submental and submandibular locations can be achieved with liposuction (Fig. 3–22) (see Chapter 29).

Patients with a prominent nasolabial fold may require superolateral advancement of the malar fat pad and mid-face skin along a vector perpendicular to the nasolabial crease (see Chapter 24). Facial shape changes from a tapered, angular appearance in youth to one that is more square in elderly persons, with little distinction between malar highlights and midfacial fat (Fig. 3–23).

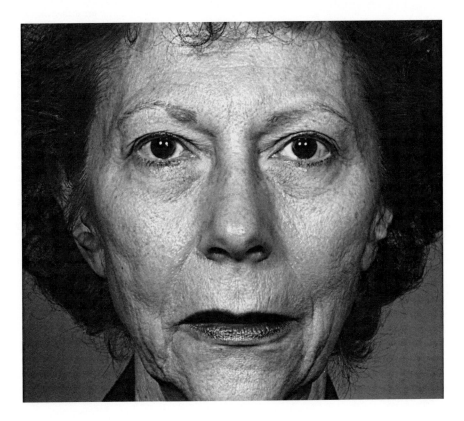

figure 3–23

An older woman's face shows little distinction between malar highlights and midfacial fat.

MALAR DEPRESSIONS

In some individuals, there is a flattening of the malar eminence resulting from previous trauma. These patients may have had a trimalar fracture. Orbital bone surgery or a cheek implant may be helpful in correcting this defect; however, malar depression may occur as a result of migration of fat. Surgery should be directed at redistributing orbital fat or performing a mini–cheek lift (see Chapter 24).

CONTRAINDICATIONS TO TREATMENT

The surgeon must always remember that cosmetic surgery is an elective procedure that may give the patient great comfort but that may also cause disappointment and even harm. Realistic expectations are vital if the patient is to be satisfied with the surgical result.[30] In addition, patients with unstable medical conditions should defer cosmetic surgery.

Patients with thyroid disease who plan to undergo strictly cosmetic surgery should await stabilization of the orbitopathy before surgery. Patients who form keloids should also be cautious about cosmetic surgery; in these patients, preoperative superficial radiation may be used to lessen scar formation. Finally, orbital fat excision should not be performed on a patient with monocular vision because there is a risk, albeit small, for orbital hemorrhage and blindness. Of the reported cases of visual loss after blepharoplasty, we are unaware of any that occurred in patients who underwent skin and muscle excision only.

References

1. Tabbal N: Special techniques in cosmetic surgery. In Smith BC (ed): Ophthalmic Plastic and Reconstructive Surgery, p 724. St. Louis, CV Mosby, 1987.
2. Putterman AM: Upper eyelid blepharoplasty. In Hornblass A (ed): Oculoplastic, Orbital and Reconstructive Surgery, vol 1, p 474. Baltimore, Williams & Wilkins, 1988.
3. Webster RC: Blepharoplasty. In Smith BC (ed): Ophthalmic Plastic and Reconstructive Surgery, p 708. St. Louis, CV Mosby, 1987.
4. Anderson RL, Donnis DG: The tarsal strip procedure. Arch Ophthalmol 1979; 7:2192–2196.
5. Tenzel RR: Cosmetic blepharoplasty. In Soll DB (ed): Management and Complications in Ophthalmic Plastic Surgery, pp 119–131. Birmingham, Ala, Aesculapius, 1976.
6. Smith B, Petrelli R: Surgical repair of prolapsed lacrimal glands. Arch Ophthalmol 1978; 96:113–114.
7. Hornblass A, Ingis JM: Lacrimal function tests. Arch Ophthalmol 1979; 97:1654–1655.
8. Liu D: Oriental eyelids: Anatomic differences and surgical consideration. In Hornblass A (ed): Oculoplastic, Orbital and Reconstructive Surgery, vol 1, p 513. Baltimore, Williams & Wilkins, 1988.
9. Hornblass A: Ptosis and pseudoptosis and blepharoplasty. In Rees TD (ed): Modern Trends in Blepharoplasty, pp 811–830. Philadelphia, WB Saunders, 1981.
10. Fasanella RM, Servat J: Levator resection for minimal ptosis: Another simplified operation. Arch Ophthalmol 1961; 65:493–496.
11. Putterman AM, Urist MJ: Müller muscle–conjunctiva resection. Arch Ophthalmol 1975; 93:619–623.
12. Glatt HJ, Fett DR, Putterman AM: Comparison of 2.5% and 10% phenylephrine in the elevation of upper eyelids with ptosis. Ophthalmic Surg 1990; 21:173.
13. Epstein GA, Putterman AM: Super maximal levator resection for severe unilateral congenital blepharoptosis. Ophthalmic Surg 1984; 15:971–982.
14. McCord CD Jr: An external minimal ptosis procedure: External tarsoaponeurectomy. Trans Am Acad Ophthalmol Otolaryngol 1975; 79:683–686.
15. Furnas DW: Festoons of orbicularis muscle as a cause of baggy eyelids. Plast Reconstr Surg 1978; 61:540–546.
16. Hornblass A, Gross ND: Ptosis and pseudoptosis in the blepharoplasty patient. In Hornblass A (ed): Oculoplastic, Orbital and Reconstructive Surgery, vol 1, p 572. Baltimore, Williams & Wilkins, 1988.
17. Furnas DW: The orbicularis oculi muscle: Management in blepharoplasty. Clin Plast Surg 1981; 8:687–706.
18. Soll DB (ed): Management of Complications in Ophthalmic Plastic Surgery, pp 295–344. Birmingham, Ala, Aesculapius, 1976.
19. Rees TD, Tabbal N: Lower blepharoplasty. Clin Plast Surg 1981; 8:643–661.
20. Iliff CE, Iliff JW, Iliff NT: Oculoplastic Surgery, pp 11–15. Philadelphia, WB Saunders, 1979.
21. Dryden RM, Soll DB: The use of scleral transplantation in cicatricial entropion and eyelid retraction. Trans Am Acad Ophthalmol Otolaryngol 1977; 83:669–678.
22. Tenzel RR: Complications of blepharoplasty: Orbital hematoma, ectropion, and scleral show. Clin Plast Surg 1981; 7:797–802.
23. Ogura TH, Lucente FE: Surgical results of orbital decompression for malignant exophthalmos. Laryngoscope 1974; 84:637–644.
24. DeSanto LW: The total rehabilitation of Graves' ophthalmopathy. Laryngoscope 1980; 90:1652–1678.
25. Henderson JW: Relief of eyelid retraction: A surgical procedure. Arch Ophthalmol 1965; 74:205–216.
26. Putterman AM: Surgical treatment of thyroid-related upper eyelid retraction: Graded Müller's muscle excision and levator recession. Ophthalmology 1981; 88:507–512.
27. Duke-Elder S, MacFaul PA: The: ocular adnexa. Diseases of the eyelid. In Duke-Elder S (ed): System of Ophthalmology, vol 13, pp 8–19. St. Louis, CV Mosby, 1974.
28. Aston SJ: Orbicularis oculi muscle flaps: A technique to reduce crow's-feet and lateral canthal skin folds. Plast Reconstr Surg 1980; 65:206–216.
29. Tabbal N: Chemabrasion of the periorbital area. In Hornblass A (ed): Oculoplastic, Orbital and Reconstructive Surgery, vol 1, p 540. Baltimore, Williams & Wilkins, 1988.
30. Courtiss AH: Selection of alternatives in aesthetic blepharoplasty. In Rees TD (ed): Modern Trends in Blepharoplasty, pp 739–754. Philadelphia, WB Saunders, 1981.

Bernard H. Shulman
Robert B. Shulman

Chapter 4

Psychiatric Issues in Cosmetic Eyelid and Facial Surgery

The psychiatric issues in cosmetic oculoplastic surgery are probably the most important and difficult problems with which the surgeon must contend. The differentiation of the ideal candidate for surgery from the emotionally disturbed patient with expectations beyond the surgeon's capabilities is frequently confusing. Dealing with the unsatisfied patient is another source of problems, and it is easy for both patient and surgeon to be led astray.

Bernard Shulman is a noted psychiatrist who has expertise with cosmetic surgical patients. In this chapter, he and his son, Robert Shulman, help us understand the motivation of patients seeking cosmetic oculoplastic surgery so that we can be wiser in our choice of surgical candidates. The authors also aid us in understanding patients who are unhappy postoperatively so that we can be more helpful in soothing them and less likely to be carried away with our own guilt. The authors also emphasize the need for friendship with our patients.

I have found that one of the best ways to avoid postoperative dissatisfaction is by spending a great deal of preoperative time discussing the procedure and possible complications with the patient. Honesty and reassurance about postoperative problems also can lessen the frustrations of both the patient and the physician.

ALLEN M. PUTTERMAN

Among the various cosmetic surgical procedures in common use, blepharoplasty and facial cosmetic surgery appear, to many prospective patients, to be relatively simple. These procedures are often performed in the office rather than in the hospital. Because these operations do not change the basic structure of the face, it is easy for patients to anticipate how they will look after surgery, and most of the time they are happy with the result.

Various authors have identified different psychiatric issues in cosmetic surgery.[1-4] The psychiatric issues are not many, and they need not be outside the surgeon's expertise. Mainly, the surgeon will want to know how to take these issues into account when planning surgery.

MOTIVATION

When a person has an eyelid deformity or growth, the motive for seeking eyelid surgery seems legitimate and self-evident. Ostensibly, the goals are to have the disfigurement repaired and to retain a properly functioning eyelid. The most common motive for blepharoplasty, however, is to have wrinkles or extra tissue removed in order to look younger and more attractive. The usual female candidate wants signs of aging removed or her eyes to appear larger. The male candidate may certainly want the same and is likely to be in a profession in which his facial appearance is an important consideration (e.g., acting). Women in the same occupations may have the same motivation.

35

The stated motive is not always the only motive or even the true motive. Polysurgical addicts have other hidden goals when they request surgery. The timing of surgery may carry a special motive. One woman decided to have blepharoplasty so that she would have a good reason for not attending a party honoring a hated rival. She made her impending surgery public knowledge and boasted that her surgeon was so busy that he could not take her at any other time. She hoped by this means to avoid the party without seeming envious and defeated.

Besides the peculiar preoccupation of the polysurgical addict or the inappropriate motives found in other psychologically disturbed patients, illegitimate motives are usually associated with inappropriate expectations. A good example of a well-motivated patient would be the person who had a blepharoplasty a decade earlier and was pleased with the results. Such a patient, now older, found the first operation satisfying enough to want it repeated.

The intensity and sincerity of the motive can be assessed by the surgeon. Candidates who have been thinking about the surgery for some time are generally more satisfying patients for the surgeon than candidates who are acting on impulse. Impulsive people are more likely to change their minds and are more likely to regret their impulsive behavior. Lubkin described an example of a newly widowed woman who came to a distant city for surgery and then canceled it.[5]

Still another factor to consider is whether the desire for surgery comes from the candidate or from some other person pushing the candidate. A passive older woman pushed by her husband may later regret the operation and become depressed.[2, 4] Another example of an illegitimate motive is the case of a physician who asked the surgeon for a cosmetic procedure for his teenage daughter. Two weeks after the surgery, the young woman was confined to a psychiatric unit, grossly psychotic. Her father had not confided in the surgeon about his daughter's mental illness because, he stated afterward, he thought the operation would help her.

EXPECTATIONS

Blepharoplasty can be expected to improve appearance by removing wrinkles and excess tissue. Whether or not the resulting appearance will be exactly what the patient wants is sometimes chancy. The face in the mirror does not always fit the face in the patient's imagination, and it is wise for the surgeon to be on guard against inappropriate expectations. Shulman[3] pointed out that the surgery "will not make the habitually shy person outgoing, will not remove other problems that lead to painful lack of confidence and feelings of inferiority and will not guarantee success in love and marriage."

Unrealistic expectations can also be found routinely in people with certain types of psychiatric disorders. These expectations range from the grossly unrealistic ("I thought the voices would stop bothering me if I changed my looks") to more plausible expectations ("I've been feeling so depressed lately, I thought the operation would give me a lift").

Although complications are rare in cosmetic eyelid and facial surgery, their occurrence does run counter to the patient's expectations and can lead to regret about an operation. Even with a good result in terms of facial appearance, a complication such as a dry eye may be irritating enough to make the patient angry with the surgeon. Such complications are always regrettable, and each prospective patient should be warned beforehand that they can occur.

PSYCHIATRIC CHARACTERISTICS OF THE CANDIDATE

Contraindications

Certain psychiatric disorders are contraindications to elective surgery. These are:

- Mental disorders, specifically the psychotic states
- Affective states
- Somatoform disorders
- States of severe anxiety

Mental Disorders

The psychotic states include the acute schizophrenic patient, who is not rational enough to cooperate with the surgeon, and the delusional or paranoid patient, who suspects and misinterprets the surgeon's behavior.

Affective States

The affective states are characterized by the manic patient, who may be overoptimistic or grandiose, may make unreasonable and impulsive demands, may be emotionally labile, and may fail to comply with instructions. In the depressed patient, the mood may improve for a few days after surgery; however, the patient most often will then experience a return of the depressed state.

Somatoform Disorders

The somatoform disorders include (1) hypochondriasis, (2) body dysmorphic disorder, and (3) factitious disorder.

Hypochondriasis is the unrealistic preoccupation with having a disease. The fear or belief that one has a disease persists despite medical reassurance, and the patient may have a great deal of underlying hostility. Hypochondriacs usually have a history of doctor shopping and may present with extensive lists of symptoms and medications.

Body dysmorphic disorder is a form of monosymptomatic hypochondriasis and is characterized by the exaggerated belief that the body is deformed. If a true defect is present, its significance is grossly and unrealistically exaggerated. As many as 2 per cent of plastic surgery consultations have been reported from patients with this disorder.[6]

Factitious disorders are characterized by the conscious, deliberate, and surreptitious feigning of symptoms to simulate illness or disease. These individuals have a psychological need to assume the sick role and an absence of an external incentive, such as economic gain or better care. This motivation is contrasted with *malingering*, which is the intentional production of symptoms, but with clearly identifiable and external incentives, such as avoiding work, obtaining financial compensation, and obtaining drugs. Factitious disorders are usually seen in relatively young, unmarried females, often with a history of medical or nursing training.

A special variant is *Munchausen syndrome*, characterized by pathological lying and a pattern of wandering from city to city, hospital to hospital, with the patient feigning illness. These patients are most often male and may have multiple abdominal scars or evidence of self-mutilation. True Munchausen syndrome is probably rare. The surgeon should beware of any patients with somatoform disorders, as these patients can easily be dissatisfied and may give even normal postoperative sequelae pathologic meaning.

Severe Anxiety

Anxiety can exist on its own, as in generalized anxiety disorder or panic disorder, or can be a major component of other psychiatric illness, such as obsessive-compulsive disorder, substance abuse, depression, or any of the previously discussed illnesses. When a highly anxious patient is encountered preoperatively, a thorough examination should be done to rule out other psychiatric illness. Patients addicted to drugs or alcohol pose a special problem because chronic intoxication or withdrawal symptoms may complicate postoperative care, as can inappropriate demands for excessive pain medication.

Other States

Other psychological states are less acute but still influence the motivation, the expectations, and the preoperative and postoperative behavior of the patient. These states are not always mental disorders but may be personality traits, that is, troublesome behaviors that complicate what should be a straightforward transaction between patient and surgeon and a relatively simple postoperative course. Although mentally ill patients can be recognized by their display of gross psychopathology, patients with these personality types do not show gross disturbance. Still, they can be recognized by certain behavioral clues.

Behavioral Clues to Psychopathology

Vagueness

When questioning a patient, the surgeon has the right to expect clear answers. An unclear history with unsatisfying answers is usually distressing to every physician and should alert the cosmetic surgeon. The patient with schizophrenia not only may be vague in answering but also may avoid eye contact with the surgeon. The stated reasons for coming are unclear ("I just felt like it," or "I thought I would look better") without any elaboration or explanation.

Vagueness can also be seen in responses by the patient with a histrionic personality, who gives considerable history but no clear picture of what is going on. The more "information" given, the more confusing the picture may become.

Secretiveness

A paranoid person generally gives information about certain matters but is uncommonly close-mouthed about others. Such a person seems suspicious and distrustful or unusually brittle or fragile. After talking to this type of patient for awhile, the surgeon will begin to feel that certain kinds of information are being deliberately concealed and that the inquiry is constantly being deflected away from certain sensitive areas.

Excessively Fastidious Appearance

Shulman[3] describes the patient who "enters the office, face somber, immaculately dressed, exquisitely manicured and without one hair out of place." Such patients seem excessively concerned with keeping themselves intact. Posture and gait give evidence of the attempt to maintain some kind of perfect image. This behavior implies considerable insecurity and is often found in the brittle, paranoid person.

Overactivity and Expansiveness

Overtalkativeness, exuberance, and overoptimism are common signs of a manic or hypomanic state. Patients in such a state seldom let the surgeon get a word in edgewise. They tell the surgeon what they want and also describe their plans in other matters. They may sound very plausible and organized, until the surgeon notices that they are beginning to skip from subject to subject and do not stick to any one issue for very long. Nevertheless, these people are affable, and the surgeon may be charmed into agreeing to perform surgery before realizing what type of people they are.

Obsessive and Detailed Questioning

Some people with intense anxiety constantly ask for information and may ask the same question repeatedly. The understanding surgeon will answer the question several times before becoming irritated. Depressed patients also sometimes show this kind of anxious behavior, and they also ask for repeated assurance that everything will turn out well, although their questions betray that they are pessimistic about the outcome. Obsessive-compulsive patients want to know all the details of the procedure, whereas hypochondriacs describe what they want in great detail and ask many questions about the pathologic meaning of minor events.

Excessive Emotional Expression

Unusual intensity or lability of emotional expressions should be a warning to the surgeon that the patient may be an irrational person. States of marked emotional arousal indicate that the person is in a frame of mind in which logic and reason may have little influence. Many of the major psychiatric disturbances, the anxiety states, affective disorders, and schizophreniform conditions are accompanied by emotional overintensity and wide fluctuations of mood. Such patients may become too frightened to permit surgery or may show troublesome mental states postoperatively.

Not all of these patients are mentally ill. Some have histrionic or borderline character traits that include excessive emotional display. Some are merely tense and betray the tension in increased emotional expression. The presence of increased emotional display is a warning that some disturbance exists, calling for further inquiry.

ASSESSMENT METHODS
Assessing Motivation

A direct question (e.g., "Why do you want this surgery?") does not always elicit the true motive. The surgeon can bring out more useful information by persuading patients to talk about themselves; judicious questions can prompt self-revelation. The surgeon may begin the inquiry by saying, "I like to know a little about my patients. Tell me about yourself," and then asking about the life situation, marriage, job, satisfaction with life, and so on. A patient with an orderly life situation is more likely to have a reasonable motive, such as simply wanting to look younger. The existence of a troubled life situation leads one to wonder whether the planned operation is suitably timed or whether it is intended to solve some problem in the patient's life.

The question "How long have you wanted to have this surgery?" permits the surgeon to investigate whether or not the patient is acting on a whim. Patients who are seeking surgery impulsively have a poorer prognosis in the sense that they are less likely to be satisfied with the result or are more likely to have remorse after the procedure.

Assessing Expectations

Expectations are closely tied to motives. In coming for cosmetic facial surgery, the patient is seeking a result and hopes to achieve it. A patient whose expectations are unreasonable will be unhappy with the outcome. The surgeon can ask direct questions about expectations, such as, "What do you hope to gain through this operation?" or "Can you put into words what you expect will be the result?"

Of course, the surgeon should warn the patient about a possibly unsatisfactory outcome and may ask, "What if you look in the mirror and what you see isn't quite what you expected? How will you feel then?"

PROGNOSIS

The patient with a good prognosis for surgery has an easily correctable problem and is also a rational person with a reasonable motive and expectations. In the assessment of the patient, certain factors in the history and examination suggest a poorer prognosis.

History of Hospitalization for Psychiatric Illness

Previous psychiatric hospitalizations suggest mental or emotional instability and point to a possible need for psychiatric consultation.

History of Repeated Surgery

If the patient has been satisfied with previous surgery, such a history need not be a contraindication. However, a patient who has not been satisfied with a previous outcome should give the surgeon pause. Some surgeons may be tempted to prove that they can succeed where others have failed, but it would be better for them to temper their vanity and to be wary of such patients.

Unreasonable expectations, suspect motives, and impulsive decisions are the other psychological factors that affect prognosis unfavorably. In general, the patient with a good prognosis is an older, emotionally stable person who has an obviously appropriate reason for the procedure.

AVOIDING PATIENT DISSATISFACTION

Even with careful patient selection and reasonably good potential outcome of surgery, some patients will be dissatisfied postoperatively. The most effective way to avoid such dissatisfaction is to establish a good patient-doctor relationship. By being cordial and friendly, displaying interest, and being attentive and approachable, the surgeon can invoke friendly feelings in the patient. The patient who feels friendly toward the surgeon is more apt to accept a slightly unsatisfactory result than the patient who is merely impressed with the expertise of the surgeon or is intimidated by the surgeon's commanding presence. If the patient then becomes dissatisfied, the surgeon can trade on his or her stock of friendship while seeing the patient through the period of dissatisfaction. This is easier if the surgeon has already become a person the patient is willing to trust.

References

1. Milani MR, Kornfeld DS: Psychiatry and other medical specialties. In Kaplan HI, Freedman AM, Sadock BJ (eds): Comprehensive Textbook of Psychiatry, sec 3, pp 2056–2069. Baltimore, Williams & Wilkins, 1980.
2. Olley P: Psychiatric aspects of cosmetic surgery. In Howells JG (ed): Psychiatric Aspects of Surgery, p 491. New York, Brunner/Mazel, 1976.
3. Shulman BH: Psychiatric assessment of the candidate for cosmetic surgery. Otolaryngol Clin North Am 1980; 13:383–389.
4. Thompson JA, Knorr NJ, Edgerton MT: Cosmetic surgery: The psychiatric perspective. Psychosomatics 1978; 19:7.
5. Lubkin V: Psychologic aspects of ophthalmic plastic surgery. In Silver B (ed): Ophthalmic Plastic Surgery, 3rd ed, pp 43–45. Rochester, Minn, American Academy of Ophthalmology and Otolaryngology, 1977.
6. Talbott JA, Hales RE, Yudofsky SC (eds): Textbook of Psychiatry, p 549. Washington DC, American Psychiatric Press, 1988.

Bernd Silver

Chapter 5

Photographing the Blepharoplasty Patient

In this chapter, Bernd Silver details all the aspects of photographing the cosmetic oculoplastic surgery patient. He informs us of cameras, lenses, films, lighting, and views needed to provide the best preoperative and postoperative photographs. He emphasizes the importance of consistency, alignment, and background in the production of excellent photographs. He also discusses the advantages and disadvantages of slides (transparencies) versus prints and mentions the new use of digital photography.

Photographing the patient who is seeking cosmetic blepharoplasty is important. Photography provides documentation of postoperative changes showing functional improvement, which at times needs to be proved in order for the patient to be compensated by the insurance company. It also provides a quick way to demonstrate the improvement in the appearance of our patients, who frequently forget their preoperative status and become overly concerned about and fixated on slight surgical blemishes.

I generally take five preoperative and postoperative photographs or slides—in primary, up, and down positions of gaze and right and left oblique views. The primary position of gaze demonstrates patients in the position they generally see themselves. The up-gaze view enhances lower eyelid herniated orbital fat, and the down-gaze view emphasizes upper eyelid dermatochalasis (excess skin). The oblique views demonstrate upper eyelid temporal excess skin, lower eyelid herniated orbital fat, and ptotic temporal brows.

I routinely take preoperative instant (Polaroid) pictures as well. I use these at surgery to view the patient's preoperative appearance so that I can judge more precisely the amount of tissue to remove. I also take a preoperative Polaroid photograph following the phenylephrine test in patients with upper eyelid ptosis in whom I choose to perform a Müller's muscle–conjunctival resection procedure. I also use a Polaroid photograph during surgery to help determine the amount of resection to perform. A preoperative Polaroid shot is also useful postoperatively to show patients what they looked like before surgery, especially when they have minor complaints about their appearance. Because most patients have forgotten their preoperative status, they usually better appreciate the improvement in their appearance when they see the Polaroid photograph.

After the final postoperative visit, I send preoperative and postoperative slides with a letter to the referring doctor and to the patient. This practice emphasizes the patient's improvement, which I believe leads to a more satisfied patient and a more satisfied referring physician.

I also use an instant slide printer (Vivitar) to transform slides to photographs. I use this method to produce preoperative and postoperative photographs to send to insurance companies for patients who have a functional problem. These photographs are aimed at persuading the insurance companies of the medical necessity of surgery and hence the need to compensate the patient.

ALLEN M. PUTTERMAN

Photographic documentation of the patient's preoperative appearance is imperative for the surgeon who performs cosmetic eyelid surgery. Photographs document the patient's problems for the surgeon's record, provide information for insurance purposes, and are helpful for resolving medicolegal disputes. With photographs, the surgeon can document the status of the patient at various stages during the surgical process for the patient, the insurance company, or an attorney. It is often amazing how little patients remember about their preoperative appearance, especially months after the procedure, when the bill arrives.

Preoperative photographs can help the surgeon explain the nature of the problem to the patient, demonstrate the proposed operation, and then document progress postoperatively. Studying the patient's appearance before surgery also provides clues that may resolve any lingering doubts about the condition, and if the postoperative result is less than ideal, further study of the photographs (sometimes in consultation with other surgeons) may be very useful.

CONSISTENCY

Consistent techniques in medical photography are absolutely necessary. Photographs taken under different conditions at different times may not be comparable. For comparative photographs, the lens, films, processing techniques, lighting, magnification, and viewing angle should be the same; altering any of these parameters can make follow-up pictures of limited value. This chapter reviews all of these items, the various kinds of photographs that are useful for the blepharoplasty surgeon, and, finally, the views that provide the most consistent and useful photographs.

SLIDES VERSUS PRINTS

Photographic documentation can be performed by the use of transparencies or prints. Slides are particularly useful for demonstrating techniques when the surgeon is involved in medical education. Slides also provide the largest, most vivid views. Slides need to be viewed through a mechanical device, such as a slide projector

or viewbox, but they can easily be made into prints if needed.

Photographic prints lend themselves best to recordkeeping and to general distribution. They can be seen with ordinary room illumination, are easily and inexpensively duplicated, and can be sketched on. The smaller sizes (i.e., 4 × 6 or 5 × 7 inches) are ideal for records. Copies can be submitted to insurance companies, patients, and anyone else concerned. When needed, prints can be made into transparencies and used for projection purposes, but the results are not as good.

For some oculoplastic surgeons, the simplest solution to the choice between slides and prints is to use a separate camera body for each.

A few photographers prefer a larger format than 35 mm. The usual choice of film size is 2¼ × 2¼ inches. The resulting images are photographically somewhat superior. The use of the larger-format cameras, however, makes the photographic process more cumbersome and expensive. For giving lectures, it is often difficult to obtain projectors that can show the larger format.

DIGITAL PHOTOGRAPHY

Digital photography has recently begun to be used in cosmetic surgery. This new technology allows the patient to see before-and-after pictures on a computer screen without the use of film. Within seconds after the photograph is taken with a digital camera, the image can be projected onto the screen. The image can then be manipulated to show the patient what the eyelids will look like after surgery.

Very high resolution can be obtained, especially with more expensive equipment that allows a close-up option. The Kodak DCS 460 is one type of digital camera, which can be attached to a Nikon, Canon, Minolta, or Olympus camera for use with close-up and other specialized lenses. A surgeon who does not want to purchase an expensive digital camera but wants to manipulate a photograph or slide on the computer can have a service bureau scan the image to digitize it.

SINGLE-LENS REFLEX CAMERA

The 35-mm single-lens reflex camera is ideal for the blepharoplasty surgeon. It is convenient in size and weight and is available in many price ranges. This type of camera permits the viewer to focus and compose the image through the same lens with which the picture will be taken; thus, the problem of parallax is eliminated. Surgeons who do their own photography can make adjustments in the angle of view and magnification. Today's better single-lens reflex 35-mm cameras permit such niceties as automatic exposure for flash and for ambient lighting. The best cameras can determine the correct amount of light and, at the right moment, can cut off the light for proper exposure. A specified lens aperture is set, and the camera performs the correct exposure compensation without assistance from the photographer.

Automatic focusing and automatic film speed indexing are common. By lining up a central spot on the camera screen with a landmark on the subject, the photographer can apply gentle pressure on the exposure button to enable instant correct focusing. Even the need to set the film speed has been eliminated by the placement of a bar code on the film cassette that the camera can read.

Many single-lens reflex cameras permit removal of the existing viewfinder screen and replacement with screens having grid lines (designed for architectural studies) (Fig. 5–1). These are helpful as guides to placing the subject in the picture for consistency.

The "autofocus" camera permits automatic focusing in the close-up range. Autofocusing works best at modest magnification (1:4 to 1:2), the most useful range for the blepharoplasty photograph. At higher magnification (i.e., 1:1 to 1:2) and at short distances, focusing depth is very shallow and autofocusing becomes less helpful. The focusing device may focus back and forth but may fail to lock in on a correct point of focus. For such instances, the autofocus device can be bypassed, and manual focusing used.

LENSES

Selecting the appropriate lens for close-up photography is more important than selecting the camera. The stan- dard lens is designed so that the distance between subject and lens is greater than the distance between lens and film. One can use the ordinary 50-mm lens that comes with the camera together with close-up, low-diopter lens attached to the front of the camera's lens to obtain an adequate magnification.

Macrolenses, or close-up lenses, are designed for optimum performance for the near focusing range (Fig. 5–2). These specialized lenses are designed so that the distance between subject and lens is about the same as the distance between lens and film ("balanced lenses").

There are various *zoom lenses*, which have limited macrolens capability. These lenses often go into the macro range at the wide-angle setting only, contrary to what is desirable for blepharoplasty photography. Zoom lenses are made of multiple lens elements and thus are heavier and more complex, with lower image quality.

For photographing the face, selection of focal length must be considered. Each focal length has its advantages and its disadvantages (see Fig. 5–2). Macrolenses come in the following focal lengths:

The *50–60-mm lens* is usually the smallest, lightest, and easiest to work with. Focusing is precise, with sharp end points. Photographers selecting this lens must work at close proximity to the subject, producing a mild degree of "wide-angle" distortion—the nose appears to be relatively long, and the ears appear to be set too far back. Also, the light source may be uncomfortably close to the patient, and in the operating room, it may be difficult for the photographer to avoid contamination.

The *90–100-mm lens* permits greater distance between lens and subject, thereby reducing distortion, and the photographer has a greater working distance (particularly useful in the operating room). Although these lenses tend to be heavier, larger, and longer than the 50–60-mm lenses, their focal length is ideal. With this focal length, autofocusing is most helpful.

The *200-mm lens* is probably the least useful. The lens

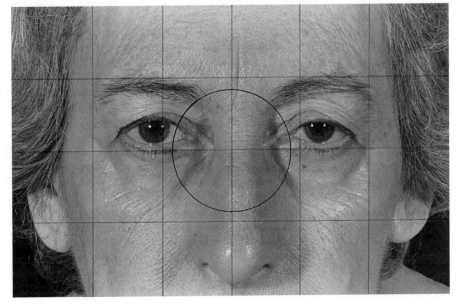

figure 5–1

Architecture-type viewfinder screen is superimposed on the photograph to demonstrate its usefulness in subject placement in the photograph.

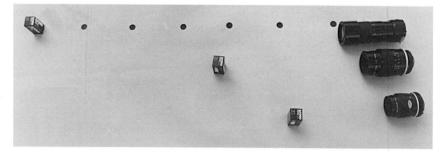

figure 5–2

Macrolenses of different focal lengths are arranged to demonstrate the relative working distances between the front of the lens and the subject (indicated by film boxes).

is much heavier and more difficult than the others to hold in the hands. Focusing can be vague, and the photographer is forced to use the smallest apertures to gain depth of focus.

In addition to excellent lenses dedicated for use on specific cameras, several generic lenses produce very fine images in the focal lengths just described. Such a lens may come with mounts made for a specific camera, or adapters may need to be added to the lens to permit its use on several different cameras. Often the price difference between dedicated and generic lenses is large.

Several lenses are made specifically for medical photography. They usually use a focal length of about *100 mm* and contain a variety of built-in light sources. They are macrolenses of excellent quality and are easy to use. Unfortunately, built-in light sources remain close to the axis of the lenses, producing flat illumination and less desirable modeling. The chief advantage of these lenses is found in the operating room because they are self-contained and can be used by a relatively untrained assistant.

FILM

Whether to use color or black-and-white film depends on the availability of sources for developing and printing the photographs. Although black-and-white film is much easier than color film to develop and print, the widespread use of color film has reduced the availability of laboratories that specialize in black-and-white work. A darkroom enthusiast can manipulate black-and-white photographs by varying the development of the film and printing, a possibility not available in color work. Color film development is universal, particularly with the availability of "mini-labs," which can be found in many camera stores. The quality of the resultant photographs varies, and it is worth the extra effort to find a good laboratory so that the color and quality of the results are consistent. Color photos are realistic and permit easier evaluation of skin color and texture changes.

Film selection also involves choosing film speed. Generally, the faster the speed of film (ISO 400 or faster), the less light required, but at a sacrifice in quality, with the resulting picture being more grainy, less detailed, and often with inferior colors. Such films permit adequate pictures using operating room illumination. To avoid blurring, the photographer must be skillful, and the patient must be cooperative and avoid movement. Slower film speeds (ISO 50–100) produce a finer image,

better color quality, and more detail. Artificial illumination and (usually) an electronic flash are necessary.

Many good films are available from Kodak, Fuji, and other major manufacturers.

Polaroid films are an interesting alternative. These films produce almost instant results but at a sacrifice in quality. Polaroid film allows the surgeon to discuss the problem almost immediately following the photographic session. The use of cameras for this purpose is very limited. The units designed for Polaroid photography use simple lenses and framing devices, which are not as good as those used for single-lens macrophotography (Fig. 5–3).

LIGHTING

Lighting is probably one of the most important considerations in medical photography. The choices are limited to continuous and electronic flash lighting.

Continuous lighting usually means ambient or tungsten floodlamps and is limited to use with the faster films, often with large lens apertures and very shallow depth of focus. The intensity of the light and heat associated with floodlamps can be very uncomfortable for the subject. The patient may be unable to avoid squinting or may move too rapidly to provide a sharp image. In addition, as a floodlamp ages, the color of its light becomes warmer, producing images that over time may be difficult to compare.

Electronic flash lighting is extremely fast (1/50,000 of a second), cool, and color-balanced for daylight illumination. The color is consistent (although it may vary with the manufacturer) and will not change significantly with aging of the flash tube. Because flash units can be light in weight, small, and portable, they are easily used in both the operating room and office. Small light sources tend to be harsher, with resultant shadows. Larger, studio-type electronic flash units, with modeling lights, are an alternative for the office, where compactness and mobility are less important.

The smaller, compact flash units, often sold as portable electronic flash devices for amateur use, offer the advantages of being lightweight, compact, portable, and hand-held. They can be used in the office and in the operating room. In the operating room, the smaller, on-camera light source is ideal. An autofocus camera fitted with an on-camera light source and through-the-lens metering markedly simplifies picture taking. The use of electronic flash in the operating room was once danger-

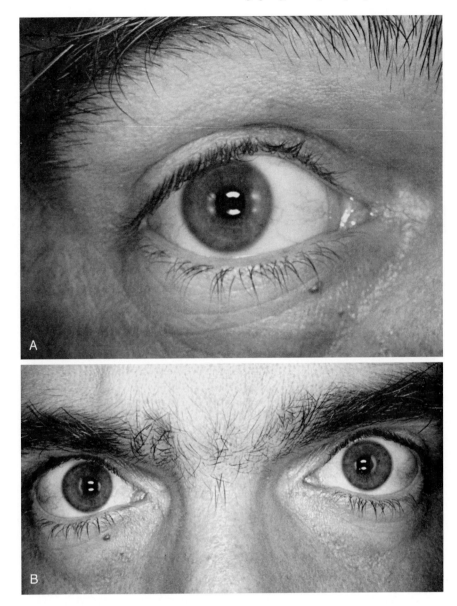

figure 5–3

Photographs made with a Polaroid CU5 unit reveal uneven lighting *(A)* and an exaggerated enlargement of the nose caused by wide-angle distortion *(B)*.

ous because of the explosive surgical gases, but such gases are rarely employed today. The photographer using flash illumination during surgery must follow operating room protocol, including avoidance of contamination and interference with surgery, and maintaining quiet.

Larger, more powerful studio flash units, positioned on light stands and placed farther from the subject, can produce particularly fine results, often approaching studio portraits. It is often possible to place these lights several feet from the subject, providing much better modeling and texture. Small modeling lights are a part of many of these units and can guide the positioning and placement of the light to reveal details and textures not possible with smaller flash units. The quality of these light sources can be modified by adding diffusing devices or by bouncing the light off or through photographic umbrellas. Such modifications provide pleasing, softer results. The easiest way to determine accurate exposure is with a flash meter. If a predetermined, fixed photo-

graphic location has been selected, exposure can be determined and the results tested. The photographer then simply keeps all parameters unchanged for each photography session.

For the on-camera portable light sources, it is important to understand a useful concept of exposure based on the *inverse square law.* For small details, greater magnification is needed, so the lens must be extended. With this added lens extension, more light is needed on the subject. If the light source is attached near the front of the lens, the light is closer to the subject. The increase in amount of light falling on the subject is the same order of magnitude as required by the additional lens extension. The closer the front of the lens is to the subject, the closer the light source is to the subject and proportionately more light illuminates the subject. This compensates for the additional light demanded by the greater extension of the lens.

Blepharoplasty photographs can be produced by a single flash unit on or near the camera or by two separate

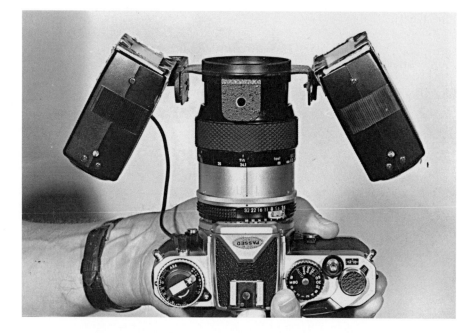

figure 5–4

A Jones bracket attached near the front element of the lens provides correct illumination of all degrees of extension.

units. No matter where a single flash unit is placed, a shadow will be cast somewhere on the face. If the flash unit is at the side, shadows will be produced by the nose and eye socket. If the flash is positioned above the camera, the upper face will tend to be overly highlighted, with the amount of light diminishing rapidly further down on the face, and eyebrows and sockets may be cast in shadows. The use of a longer lens (90–100 mm) can reduce this effect to some extent. A reflector can be positioned near the shadow side of the face to reduce shadows; however, the illumination will still be uneven and such devices are clumsy.

A more pleasing result can be obtained with the use of two flash units, one on either side of the camera; the units can be attached to it or mounted on separate light stands. Flash units can be attached to a camera by various coupling devices, such as "hot shoes" (slave units that fire a second unit when triggered by another flash exposure) or by cables designed to permit the camera's meter to control the amount of light output. Dedicated cables, which can fire both flash units while still controlling exposure through the camera lens, are available for many cameras. Using cables is probably the most foolproof method available because the camera controls the flash units no matter which type of extension or lens is used.

Probably one of the more difficult problems in oculoplastic surgery is finding a means of securing the small, portable flash units to the camera. A bracket available from Jones Photo Equipment Company (North Hollywood, Calif.) is attached to the front of the lens by a filter retaining ring (Fig. 5–4). The flash units are attached to this bracket, either from the sides or top. This device works well and is compact, but the entire weight of the flash unit is poorly supported by a lightweight retainer ring.

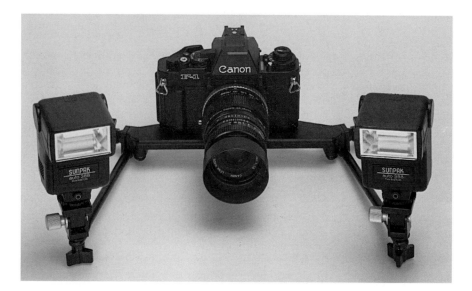

figure 5–5

Lepp bracket attached to camera and flash units.

A more satisfactory, recently available bracket is the Lepp II Dual Flash Macro Bracket, marketed by the Stroboframe Division of the Saunders Group (Rochester, N.Y.) (Fig. 5–5). This unit is securely attached to the base of the camera body by special plates, and the bracket arms are universally adjustable. The resulting unit, although bulky, is stable and can be readily collapsed and reexpanded as needed.

ALIGNMENT

Magnification and alignment should be determined according to the surgeon's preferences. For blepharoplasty photographs, there is often a temptation to concentrate on the eyelids only, to the exclusion of adjacent landmarks, such as ears, nose, and upper lips. Including these landmarks allows for easier viewer orientation. Such photographs can be supplemented with pictures at higher magnification. Orientation of the face to the camera must be consistent. If the face is photographed from varying viewpoints—from a higher or a lower angle—the abnormalities being studied may look different to the viewer. The "Frankfort" plane, aligning the bridge of the nose, outer canthi, and tragus of the ears, is recommended because of its repeatability.

BACKGROUND

Some consideration should be given to the photographic location. The background should be nondistracting. Head rests, slit lamps, or other office equipment is distracting. The patient should be encouraged to remove all jewelry as well as facial and eyelid makeup.

PHOTOGRAPHIC VIEWS

A final consideration in blepharoplasty photography is the photographic view. Blepharoplasty patients should be photographed looking directly at the viewer with

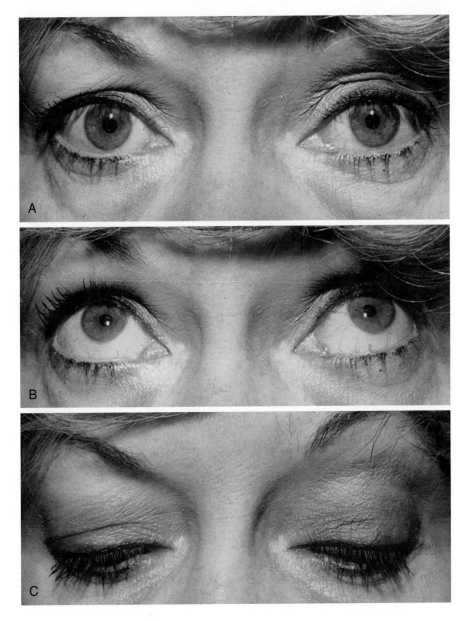

figure 5–6

Routine preoperative photographs of both eyes. *A*, Looking straight ahead. *B*, Looking up. *C*, Looking down.

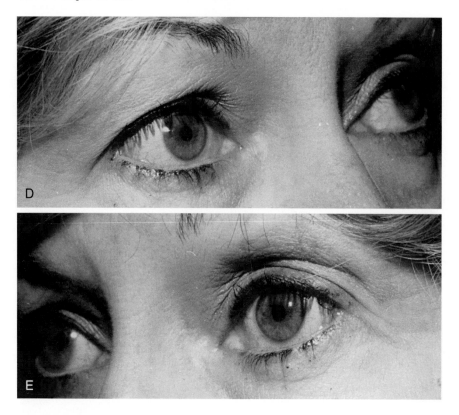

D, Right oblique view. *E,* Left oblique view. (Courtesy of Allen M. Putterman, M.D.)

the eyes open and then closed. Patients can also be photographed looking up and down, and in oblique axes, particularly when such positions reveal fatty protu-berances, scleral show, and bony irregularities; this view is also helpful if extraocular motility problems are pres-ent (Fig. 5–6).

Tony S. Fu

Chapter 6

Dermatopathology in the Cosmetic Oculoplastic Surgery Patient

Dermatochalasis (excess skin) is an important problem that is correctable with cosmetic oculoplastic surgery. In this chapter, Tony Fu, a dermatopathologist, outlines the changes that occur in the skin leading to redundancy, inelasticity, and wrinkling.

Dr. Fu demonstrates that dermatochalasis is the result of changes in the collagen fibers, elastic fibers, and ground substances in the dermis as well as in the epidermis. His most striking remark is that these changes are almost exclusively due to sun exposure rather than aging.

ALLEN M. PUTTERMAN

Dermatochalasis is a lack of elasticity of the skin that is manifest in looseness, wrinkling, and redundancy. Dermatochalasis frequently occurs in the eyelids. Because it represents unattractive and aging skin, it is a much feared condition in our vanity-conscious world. Yet this condition is unknowingly intensified by long-term exposure of skin to sunlight.[1, 2]

Dermatochalasis is also seen in general dermatologic conditions such as cutis laxa[3] and leprechaunism.[4] Usually, the eyelid skin does not droop in these conditions, which are often congenital. The change in skin elasticity occurs early in life, and aging and sun damage to the tissue are not primary causes. (These general forms of dermatochalasis are not within the scope of this chapter, however, and interested readers can consult the cited references.)

NORMAL SKIN

Microscopically, the eyelid skin can be divided into three distinct layers. From the surface inward, these are the epidermis, the dermis, and the subcutaneous fat tissue (Fig. 6–1A).[5–7] The epidermis is embryologically derived from ectoderm. It is mainly composed of keratinocytes, which act as a shield to protect the tissues from the external environment, and melanocytes, which guard these tissues from solar irradiation.

Tissues of ectodermal origin give rise to adnexal and nerve tissues in the dermis. The adnexal tissue includes pilosebaceous structures and apocrine and eccrine glands, which descend from the epidermis during fetal life. Most of the dermis is embryologically derived from mesoderm. The dermis layer contains blood vessels, lymphatics, muscles, collagen fibers, elastic fibers, and ground substances (e.g., mucopolysaccharides), which give strength and elasticity to the skin (Fig. 6–1B). It is this fibrous compartment that is studied for the events that occur in a loose and drooping skin.

In nonwhites, the innermost subcutaneous fat layer is mainly composed of fat cells derived from mesoderm. This layer does not possess many fibrous elements and works as a soft cushion to absorb shock. Energy is stored in the fat, which protects the body from heat loss in cold temperatures. Because of its softness, when the fat tissue protrudes into loose skin, the surface of the skin looks baggy. (There is almost no fat layer, however, in eyelid skin.)

AGING AND SUNLIGHT

All systems of the body, including the eyes, are involved in the aging process.[8] Aging alone will not cause many histologically evident alterations in the human skin without exposure to sunlight.[9, 10] Without the effects of

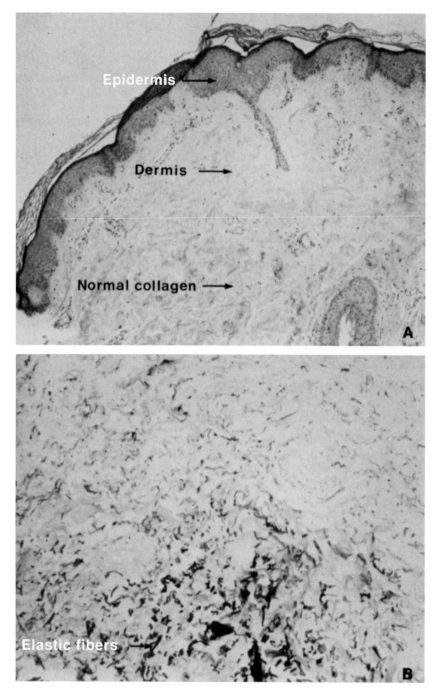

figure 6–1

A, Normal skin. No elastotic changes are seen. (Hematoxylin and eosin, × 40.) *B*, Elastic fibers appear between collagen fibers. (Elastic stain, × 100.)

sunlight, the aging process is also barely detectable on gross examination.

Pathologic Features

The main components involved in changes of the skin with age and exposure to sunlight are collagen fibers, elastic fibers, and ground substances in the dermis as well as the epidermis.

Collagen Fibers

Histochemically, with age alone without sun damage, only very mild thickening and coarsening can be seen in the collagen fibers.[10] With aging, new collagen formation and the turnover of older collagen are decreased,[11] but the total amount of collagen is increased.[12] Biochemically, the solubility of aging collagen is reduced in neutral salt, weak acids, and cold alkali as a result of cross-linking. Also, collagen-bound water is decreased. Yet, the nitrogen in collagen is increased.[11]

In sun-exposed tissue, the total amount of collagen is reduced.[12] Under an electron microscope, fibroblasts contain regular crystals in the mitochondria, dense particles in the matrix, and vesicular formation in the endoplasmic reticulum. In addition, collagen fibrils thicken into bundles, with reduced interfibrillar ground substance.[11]

Elastic Fibers

Histochemically, only a moderate increase in elastic fibers is noted in aging skin without sun exposure.[10] The most striking histologic feature, actinic elastosis, can be seen only in sun-damaged skin (Fig. 6–2).[13, 14] (Previously, actinic elastosis was called senile elastosis or basophilic degeneration.[15]) In early actinic elastosis, elastic fibers are only mildly increased and thickened. Gradually, the fibers become hyperplastic; then they form amorphous masses. Histochemically, they show an affinity for hematoxylin and create a bluish stain. The elastosis is located in the upper half of the dermis, with a clear zone below the epidermis.[16]

In one reported case, a loss of elastic tissue (focal elastolysis), instead of elastic hyperplasia, was observed.[17] Elastic hyperplasia occurs as early as the first decade of life and increases with age.[1] The degree of actinic elastosis depends also on the amount of melanin pigment in the epidermis. The relationship is in inverse proportion, which may explain the difficulty in judging the age of darkly pigmented people.[13]

Ultrastructurally, the elastic fibers in actinic elastosis show accumulations of dense grains and holes, which widen the diameter of the fibers. Also, the collagen fibrils are reduced.[18] Biochemically, lysine is decreased in aged skin, which probably causes an increase in the cross-linking process.[19] Sugars, lipids, glutamic acid, and aspartic acid can also be detected in aged skin, and patchy calcification can be found in the elastic tissue.[11]

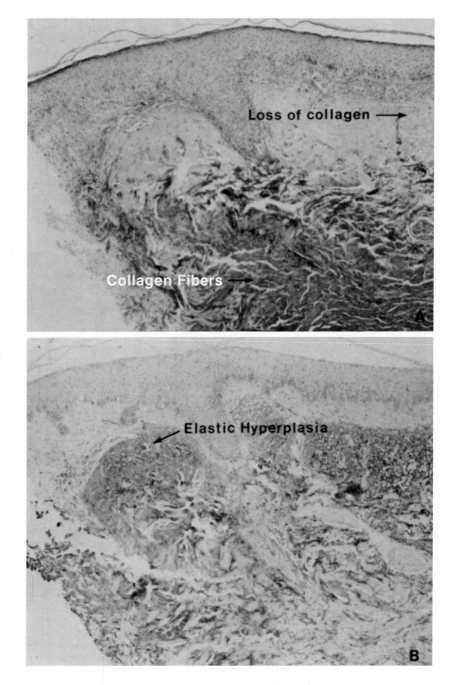

figure 6–2

A, Actinic elastosis. (Hematoxylin and eosin, × 40.) *B*, Same lesion showing elastic clumping and hyperplasia. (Elastic stain, × 40.)

Increased dermal elastin can be measured with greater age.[11] Similarly, enormously larger amounts of elastin have been noted in sun-damaged skin. Elastin occupies 13 per cent of the dry weight of skin, in contrast to 2 per cent of unexposed tissues.[12]

Ground Substances

The ground substances contain mucopolysaccharides, glycoproteins, water, and salts. Four types of acid mucopolysaccharides have been identified in the dermis[20]:

- Hyaluronic acid
- Dermatan sulfate
- Chondroitin-6-sulfate
- Heparin

As seen with special histologic stains, only mild decreases in neutral and acid mucopolysaccharides are present. This histologic change can be reflected in the reduced amount of hexosamine in the aged dermis. But biochemical research has shown more clearly that acid mucopolysaccharides, especially hyaluronic acid, decrease with age.[20-22] On the other hand, acid mucopolysaccharides, in particular hyaluronic acid, are increased in sun-damaged skin.[20-23] Similarly, nonfibrous proteins are reduced in aged dermis and are increased in actinically damaged skin.[24]

Most pathologic events in the three layers of the skin can probably be explained by the following mechanism.[10] Ultraviolet light below 3100 Å can labilize the lysosomes in the fibroblasts. In turn, collagenase in the lysosomes is released and digests and depletes the collagen. There is no elastase in the lysosome. Therefore, the elastic tissue is increased to replace the digested collagen. The total mechanism is more complicated than given here, but only further studies can completely elucidate all the subtleties involved in the process.

Epidermis

The epidermis is atrophic. There are atypical changes, loss of polarity of keratinocytes, and increased activity of melanocytes.[25] Studies show some effects of tretinoin on photodamaged skin.[25]

References

1. Kligman AM: Early destructive effect of sunlight on human skin. JAMA 1969; 210:2377–2380.
2. Kligman AM: Solar elastosis in relation to pigmentation. In Fitzpatrick TB, Pathak MA, Harber LC, et al (eds): Sunlight and Man, pp 157–163. Tokyo, University of Tokyo Press, 1974.
3. Goltz RW, Hult AM, Goldfarb M, et al: Cutis laxa: A manifestation of generalized elastosis. Arch Dermatol 1965; 92:373–387.
4. Patterson JH, Walkins WL: Leprechaunism in a male infant. J Pediatr 1962; 60:730–739.
5. Ackerman AB: Histological Diagnosis of Inflammatory Skin Diseases, pp 13–80. Philadelphia, Lea & Febiger, 1978.
6. Fitzpatrick TB, Eisen AZ, Wolff K, et al: Dermatology in General Medicine, 2nd ed, pp 164–195. New York, McGraw-Hill, 1979.
7. Montagna W, Parakkal PF: The Structure and Function of the Skin, 2nd ed. New York, Academic Press, 1980.
8. Rook A, Wilkinson DS, Ebling FJG: Textbook of Dermatology, 3rd ed, p 225. London, Blackwell Scientific, 1980.
9. Knox JM, Cockerell EG, Freeman RG: Etiological factors and premature aging. JAMA 1962; 179:630-636.
10. Smith JG Jr, Finlayson GR: Dermal connective tissue alterations with age and chronic sun damage. J Soc Cosmet Chem 1965; 16:527–535.
11. Solomon LM, Virtue C: The biology of cutaneous aging. Int J Dermatol 1975; 14:172–181.
12. Smith JG Jr, Davidson EA, Clark RD: Dermal elastin in actinic elastosis and pseudoxanthoma elasticum. Nature 1962; 195:716.
13. Pinkus H, Mehregan AH: A Guide to Dermatohistopathology, 3rd ed, p 302. New York, Appleton-Century-Crofts, 1981.
14. Loewi G, Glynn LE, Dorling J: Studies on the nature of collagen degeneration. J Pathol Bacteriol 1960; 80:1–8.
15. Lund HZ, Sommerville RL: Basophilic degeneration of the cutis. Am J Clin Pathol 1957; 27:183–194.
16. Gillman T, Penn J, Brooks D, et al: Abnormal elastic fibers. Arch Pathol 1955; 59:733–749.
17. Tsuji T: Loss of dermal elastic tissue in solar elastosis. Arch Dermatol 1980; 116:474–475.
18. Danielsen L: Morphological changes in pseudoxanthoma elasticum and senile skin. Acta Derm Venereol 1979; 83(Suppl):9–79.
19. Miller EJ, Martin GR, Piez KA: The utilization of lysine in the biosynthesis of elastin cross links. Biochem Biophys Res Commun 1964; 17:248.
20. Loewi G: The acid mucopolysaccharides of human skin. Biochim Biophys Acta 1962; 52:435.
21. Loewi G, Meyer K: The acid mucopolysaccharides of embryonic skin. Biochim Biophys Acta 1958; 27:453.
22. Prodi G: Effect of age on acid mucopolysaccharides in rat dermis. J Gerontol 1964; 19:128.
23. Sams WM Jr, Smith JG Jr: The histochemistry of chronically sun-damaged skin. J Invest Dermatol 1961; 37:447.
24. Smith JG Jr, Davidson EA, Sams WM Jr, et al: Alterations in human dermal connective tissue with age and chronic sun damage. J Invest Dermatol 1962; 39:347–350.
25. Bhawan J, Gonzalez-Serva A, Nehal K, et al: Effects of tretinoin on photodamaged skin: A histologic study. Arch Dermatol 1991; 127:666–672.

John L. Wobig
Matthew W. Wilson

Chapter 7

Eyelid and Facial Anatomy

Understanding basic anatomy is paramount to performing surgery on any region of the body. The eyelids are complex structures, and their parts, especially, must be known bycosmetic oculoplastic surgeons.

Because blepharoplasty commonly consists the removal of skin and fat, many doctors think that only a limited knowledge of eyelid anatomy is needed. As John Wobig and Matthew Wilson point out, however, there is always the possibility in cosmetic surgery of injuring vital structures of the eyelid and orbit. The authors indicate that removal of the orbicularis muscle can lead to injury of the levator aponeurosis; lack of knowledge of the upper eyelid fat compartments can result in excision of the lacrimal gland; and numbness of the eyelids is a likely complication when suborbicularis facial nerves are interrupted. Injury to almost all eyelid and orbital structures is certainly possible with excision of orbital fat.

In addition, the superior oblique muscle separates the medial and central lower orbital fat compartments. This is especially important to remember in the performance of transconjunctival (internal) blepharoplasties, in which the inferior oblique muscle must be identified to prevent injury. It is less evident, but no less important, in the external approach to lower blepharoplasty. Also, brow fat that exists beneath the orbicularis muscle can result in a fullness beneath the central and temporal brow. Excision of this fat can improve the cosmetic appearance in certain patients. The anatomy of the brow fat is illustrated in Chapter 12, and the higher attachment of the orbital septum to the levator aponeurosis in Caucasian compared with Asian eyelids is demonstrated in Chapter 11.

The anatomy of the corrugator, procerus, and frontalis muscles is important in improving the appearance of the brows and foreheads and is described in Chapters 27 and 28.

A discussion of facial anatomy has been added in this chapter because the third edition of this textbook covers midface and full facelifts in addition to endoscopic and full forehead lifts (see Chapters 24 and 27–29). There is also a chapter on treatment of hyperkinetic facial lines by injection of botulinum toxin into various facial muscles (see Chapter 33).

Before embarking on these procedures, the surgeon must be familiar with the anatomy of the face. Vulnerable structures, such as the fifth and seventh nerve branches and facial blood vessels, are emphasized to help the surgeon avoid injuring them during facial surgery. Also, the elaboration of various facial muscles should help the surgeon understand how to decrease hyperactivity of these structures during injection of botulinum toxin.

ALLEN M. PUTTERMAN

EYELID ANATOMY

For the purpose of cosmetic surgery, the eyelids can be divided into the following structural planes (Fig. 7–1): (1) skin and subcutaneous fascia, (2) orbicularis muscle and submuscular fascia, (3) septum orbitale, (4) preaponeurotic fat, (5) eyelid retractors, and (6) tarsus and conjunctiva.

Skin

The skin of the eyelid is stratified into three layers (Fig. 7–2):

1. The *epidermis*, or outer layer, which is devoid of lymphatics, blood vessels, and connective tissue,[1] depends on the corium for its nourishment.
2. The *corium*, or middle layer, is dense connective tissue that supports the appendages, vessels, and nerves.
3. The *intercushioning layer* is the subcutaneous tissue. The skin of the upper and lower eyelids is unique because it is the thinnest in the body and contains minimal fat.

Incisions for blepharoplasty are placed in the eyelid crease to conceal postoperative scars. Transverse palpebral creases exist in both the upper and lower lids. The upper palpebral crease roughly marks the superior edge

of the tarsus, the division between the pretarsal and preseptal orbicularis muscle in the area where fibers of the aponeurosis pass into the overlying pretarsal muscle and skin. The crease in the lower eyelid indicates the inferior edge of the tarsus. The thin, well-nourished skin allows for minimal scarring. Hypertrophic scars are rare but do occur. Hypertrophic scarring frequently responds to injections of betamethasone acetate (Celestone Soluspan) given intradermally and limited to 0.25–0.5 ml.

Orbicularis Muscle and Submuscular Fascia

The orbicularis muscle is divided arbitrarily into orbital and palpebral portions. The palpebral orbicularis muscle is subdivided into pretarsal and preseptal parts on the basis of underlying anatomic structures (Fig. 7–3). There are voluntary and involuntary actions to the palpebral part of orbicularis muscle and involuntary action to the orbital part. The orbital orbicularis is rarely encountered in blepharoplasty but is encountered in brow ptosis surgery.

The orbicularis muscle arises from the second branchial arch.[2] The migration of the muscle is like a horseshoe, with the open ends inserting into the medial orbital wall. The pretarsal muscle is firmly attached to the underlying tarsus. The only separation of the pretarsal muscle is in the upper eyelid, where the levator

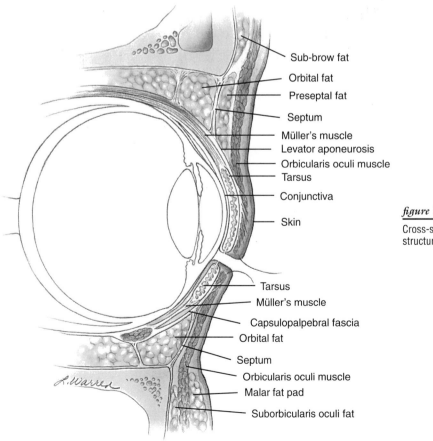

Sub-brow fat
Orbital fat
Preseptal fat
Septum
Müller's muscle
Levator aponeurosis
Orbicularis oculi muscle
Tarsus
Conjunctiva
Skin

Tarsus
Müller's muscle
Capsulopalpebral fascia
Orbital fat
Septum
Orbicularis oculi muscle
Malar fat pad
Suborbicularis oculi fat

figure 7–1

Cross-section of upper and lower eyelids depicting structures in various layers.

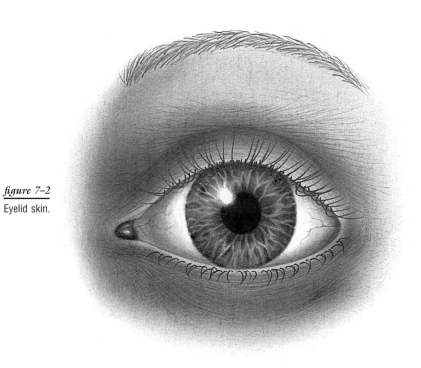

figure 7–2
Eyelid skin.

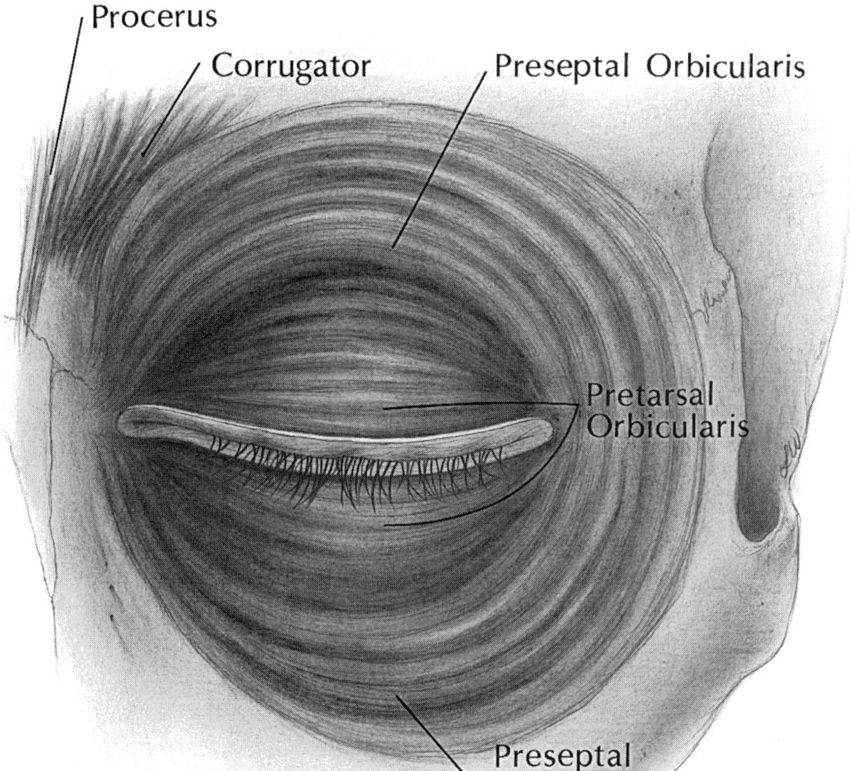

Procerus

Corrugator   Preseptal Orbicularis

Pretarsal
Orbicularis

figure 7–3
Eyelid muscle.

Preseptal
Orbicularis

aponeurosis attaches to the pretarsal muscle at the upper edge of the tarsus. The pretarsal muscles are attached laterally by a lateral canthal tendon to the lateral orbital tubercle. The medial insertion of the pretarsal muscle is by the medial canthal tendon to the medial orbital wall. The pretarsal muscle has deep heads that insert in the lacrimal bone behind the posterior lacrimal crest. Removal of the pretarsal muscle with blepharoplasty risks a chance of injury to the levator aponeurosis. The preseptal muscle, which overlies the septum, inserts medially on the medial orbital wall. Superficial fibers of the preseptal muscle join with the medial canthal tendon. Posterior fibers of the muscle insert in the lacrimal diaphragm. Laterally, the preseptal muscle is continuous and does not interdigitate. Therefore, no true raphe exists.

The submuscular fascia is immediately posterior to the orbicularis muscle. The network of branches of the facial nerve and maxillary division of the fifth cranial nerve are within the submuscular fascia. Cutting nerve branches in this region causes numbness after blepharoplasty. Fibers pass through the orbicularis muscles to the subcutaneous portion of the skin, which holds the skin and muscle together. Separation of the skin from the underlying muscle in blepharoplasty requires careful dissection.

Muscle resection in blepharoplasty must not be overzealous. The orbicularis muscle is necessary to move the marginal tear film toward the lacus lacrimalis. In addition, the deep heads of the preseptal muscle, with their insertion into the lacrimal diaphragm, pull the lateral wall of the tear sac laterally. Good postoperative apposition of the lids in the closed position is maintained by conservative removal of the orbicularis muscle with skin.

Septum Orbitale

The septum orbitale divides the eyelid into anterior and posterior portions (Fig. 7–4). The septum is a mesodermal layer of the embryonic eyelid.[3] The septum extends from the bony margin toward the tarsus. In the upper eyelid the septum attaches to the levator aponeurosis, generally 2–5 mm above the superior edge of the tarsus. However, the septal levator attachment can vary from 10 mm above to almost at the level of the superior tarsal border. The septum does not extend over the anterior surface of the tarsus. In the lower eyelid, the septum is attached to the inferior edge of the tarsus. There is a dense band at the bony margin, called the arcus marginale, where the periosteum and the periorbita fuse. The septum attaches medially to the spine at the lower end of the anterior lacrimal crest, called the lacrimal tubercle. The septum extends from the lower eyelid to the upper eyelid medially by passing under the attachments to the medial orbicularis muscle at the posterior lacrimal crest. The septum is difficult to trace laterally because it blends with the lateral canthal tendon and lateral horn of the levator. The septum forms an arch under the supraor-

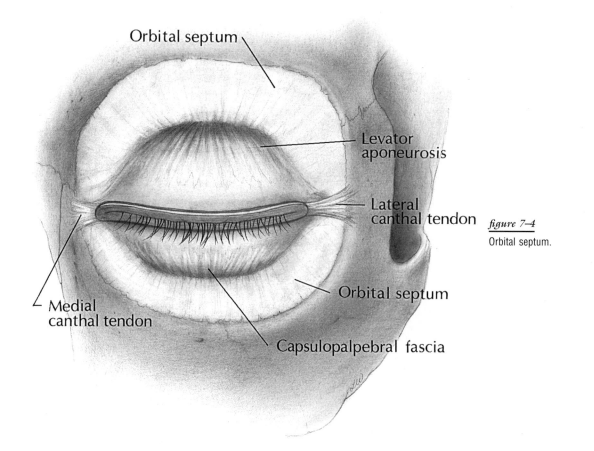

figure 7–4
Orbital septum.

bital notch and around the supratrochlear and infra-trochlear nerves and vessels.

The anatomic significance of the septum orbitale is that it keeps the orbital fat in its posterior location. If the septum is sutured in error to the tarsus during surgery, the eyelid will not close adequately. In addition, if the septum is sutured tightly, any posterior bleeding will be trapped in the orbit.

Preaponeurotic Fat

The preaponeurotic fat is an excellent surgical landmark (Fig. 7–5).[4] It acts as a cushion to the eyelid and divides the septum from the levator aponeurosis, allowing a certain amount of freedom to the movement of the levator. The upper eyelid has two fat pads: nasal and middle. The nasal fat pad is smaller. The lower eyelid is believed to have three fat compartments: a small medial fat pad, a large central fat pad, and a temporal fat pad. The temporal fat pad varies in size and may have more than one compartment.[5] The fat is separated by a small capsule and fibrous compartment. The significance of this structural plane in blepharoplasty is in the large blood vessels that transverse the fat and can cause extensive bleeding if the fat is not removed with extreme care. In addition, cautery is transmitted along the fat to the central surgical space and must be done with prudence.[6]

The nasal and middle fat pad are divided by the inferior oblique muscle. Identification of the inferior oblique muscle is important during transconjunctival blepharoplasty.

Eyelid Retractors

The retractors of the eyelids are located deep to the preaponeurotic fat and are essential for opening the eyelids (Fig. 7–6). The origin of the upper eyelid retractors is at the apex of the orbit from the undersurface of the lesser wing of the sphenoid bone. The levator palpebrae superioris overlies the superior rectus muscle. As the levator emerges from a horizontal to a vertical direction, it divides into an anterior aponeurosis layer and a posterior superior tarsal layer. The aponeurosis spreads medially and laterally to form the horns of the levator. The horns attach to the respective medial and lateral retinacula. The lower end of the aponeurosis inserts into the lower third of the anterior surface of the tarsus. In addition, the aponeurosis is attached to the pretarsal muscle and skin by fibrotic bands.

The superior transverse ligament, or Whitnall's ligament, extends from the lacrimal gland fossa laterally to the trochlea medially. It is thought to act as a fulcrum and to allow for the change in direction of the levator.

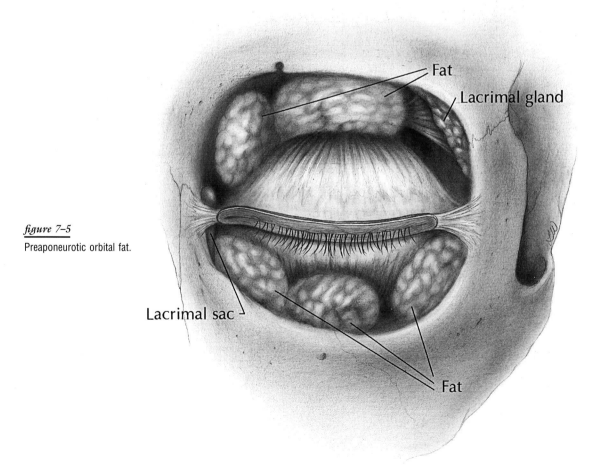

figure 7–5
Preaponeurotic orbital fat.

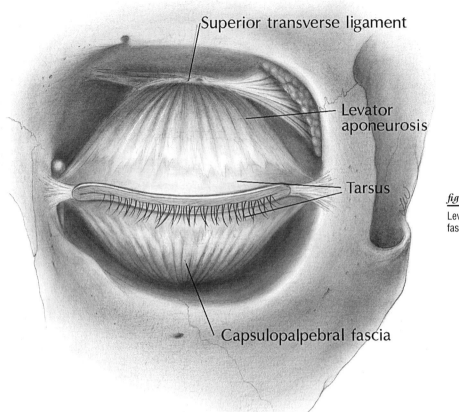

Superior transverse ligament

Levator aponeurosis

Tarsus

Capsulopalpebral fascia

figure 7–6
Levator aponeurosis and capsulopalpebral fascia.

It also has a suspensory role in the orbit and possibly acts as a check ligament of the levator muscle.

The inferior division of the levator (Müller's muscle) is a superior tarsal muscle. This smooth muscle is innervated by the cervical sympathetic system. Inferiorly the muscle attaches to the superior margin of the tarsus.

The lower eyelid retractors are like those in the upper eyelid, except that the inferior rectus muscle and the lower eyelid retractor are not separated. The inferior rectus muscle has a capsulopalpebral head (see Fig. 7–6), which is the peripheral extension of the inferior rectus muscle.

The three layers that form anterior to the inferior transverse ligament, or Lockwood ligament, are:

- The *superficial layer*, which is the aponeurosis and inserts into the inferior edge of the tarsus
- The *intermediate layer*, which is the inferior tarsal muscle (Müller's muscle) and attaches to the inferior border of the tarsus (Fig. 7–7)
- The *deepest layer*, which forms the anterior part of Tenon's capsule and attaches to the conjunctival fornix

The retractors are important to know in blepharoplasty because the surgeon should check for pathologic conditions in these layers. Vigorous removal of the orbicularis muscles can damage the underlying aponeurosis. Also, dehiscence of the aponeurosis can be repaired more easily if it is identified at the time of blepharoplasty.

Damage to the inferior rectus muscle can occur as a result of the peripheral extension of this muscle. Although not a retractor, the inferior oblique muscle must be identified in lower eyelid blepharoplasty, especially if the procedure is done transconjunctivally.

Tarsus and Conjunctiva

The most posterior layers of the eyelids are the tarsus and conjunctiva (Fig. 7–8). The tarsi are dense connective tissues that give form to the eyelids. The upper tarsus is approximately 29 mm long and extends from the lateral commissure to the punctum medially. The upper tarsus is 10 mm wide in the central eyelid and narrows medially and laterally. The lower tarsus is as long as the upper tarsus but is only 4–5 mm wide at the center of the eyelid. Each tarsus has numerous meibomian glands with orifices on the ciliary border.

The conjunctiva is firmly adherent to the overlying tarsus. The palpebral conjunctiva can be divided into marginal, tarsal, and orbital portions. The marginal conjunctiva joins with the skin at the eyelid margin. The tarsal conjunctiva is firmly adherent to the tarsus, and the orbital conjunctiva lies adjacent to the superior and inferior tarsal muscles. There is no reason for blepharoplasty to involve these structures unless there is combined horizontal shortening of the eyelid or an internal approach is used to remove herniated orbital fat (see Chapters 20 and 21).

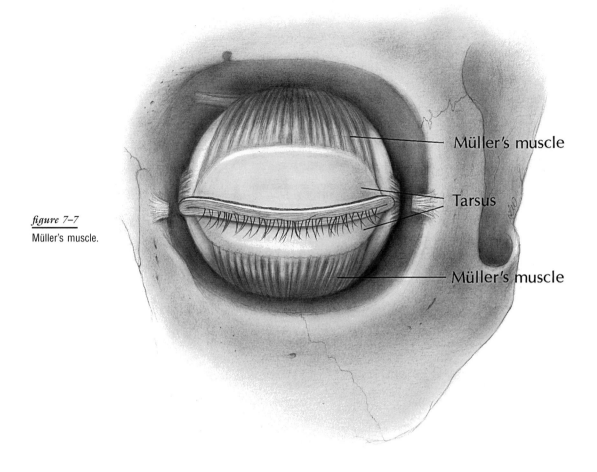

figure 7–7
Müller's muscle.

Müller's muscle

Tarsus

Müller's muscle

FACIAL ANATOMY

Recent advances in oculoplastic surgery require an understanding of facial anatomy and its relation to the eyelids. Ophthalmic plastic surgeons now perform forehead and brow lifts, midface lifts, full facelifts, and botulinum injections into facial muscles.

Bones

The bony architecture determines facial contour. Transition from forehead to temple and temple to cheek depends, in part, on the hard tissue foundations and bony prominences (Fig. 7–9). The skull is a composite of the cranium and midface. The frontal bone, parietal bones, and occipital bone form the roof of the cranium, whereas the greater wing of the sphenoid and the temporal bone form the lateral wall. The midface is defined as the area between the maxillary teeth and a line joining the two zygomaticofrontal sutures, the posterior limit of which is the sphenoethmoid junction and the pterygoid plates. The maxillary, palatine, zygomatic, ethmoid, and nasal bones form the midface, as do the turbinates and the zygomatic process of the temporal bones.

The mandible comprises the lower face. It articulates with the skull at the condyles, forming a synovial joint. A complexity of muscular attachments helps to stabilize the joint.

Skin and Subcutaneous Tissues

The skin and subcutaneous fat of the face have mechanical properties. Elastic and collagen fibers with surrounding ground substance make the skin a pliable medium with which to work. A keratinized stratified squamous epithelium overlies the dermis. The superficial papillary dermis contains thin randomly arranged collagen fibers. The deeper reticular dermis has coarser collagen bundles that run parallel to the surface of the skin. Subcutaneous fat lies beneath the dermis. The thickness is variable from individual to individual and from one area of the face to another. The cheeks, temples, and neck have the thickest subcutaneous fat pads. Connective tissue septa divide the subcutaneous fat into lobules.

In addition, a plane of submuscular nonseptate fat exists. A supraperiosteal submuscular fat pad is present over the zygoma, the suborbicularis oculi fat (SOOF) (Fig. 7–10). This is continuous superiorly with the retro-orbicularis fat (ROOF) situated in the upper eyelid and the eyebrow fat pad described by Lemke and Stasior.[7]

The skin and subcutaneous fat of the face can be divided in facial aesthetic units having similar color, texture, thickness, and mobility. The anatomy of the skin is important to consider in laser resurfacing and chemical peels (see Chapters 30 and 31). Incisions at the boundaries of these units result in minimal scarring. Relaxed skin tension lines are the lines of skin tension present when the skin is in a relaxed state. The relaxed

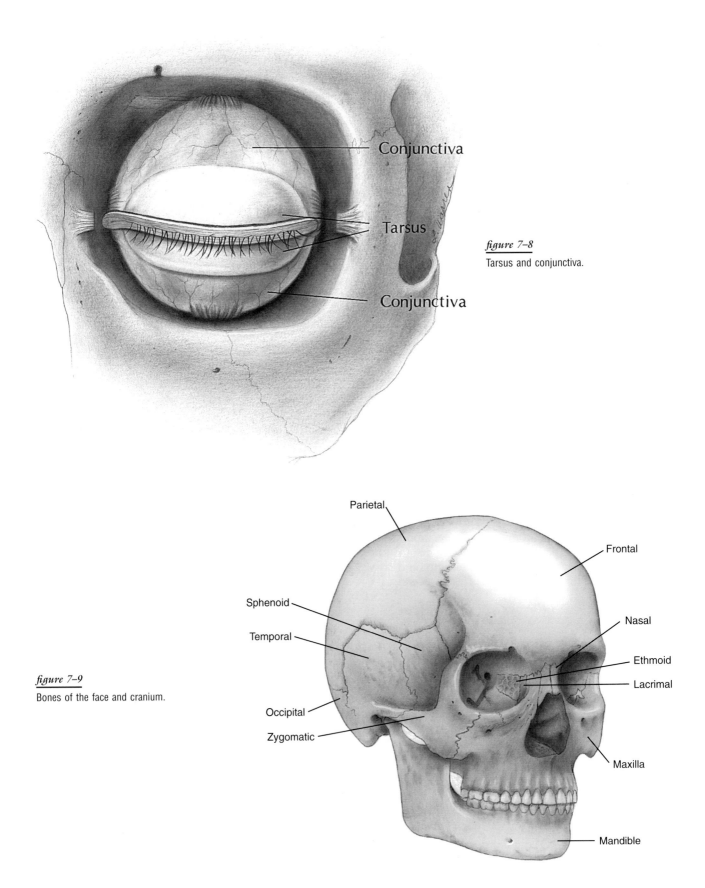

figure 7-8
Tarsus and conjunctiva.

figure 7-9

Bones of the face and cranium.

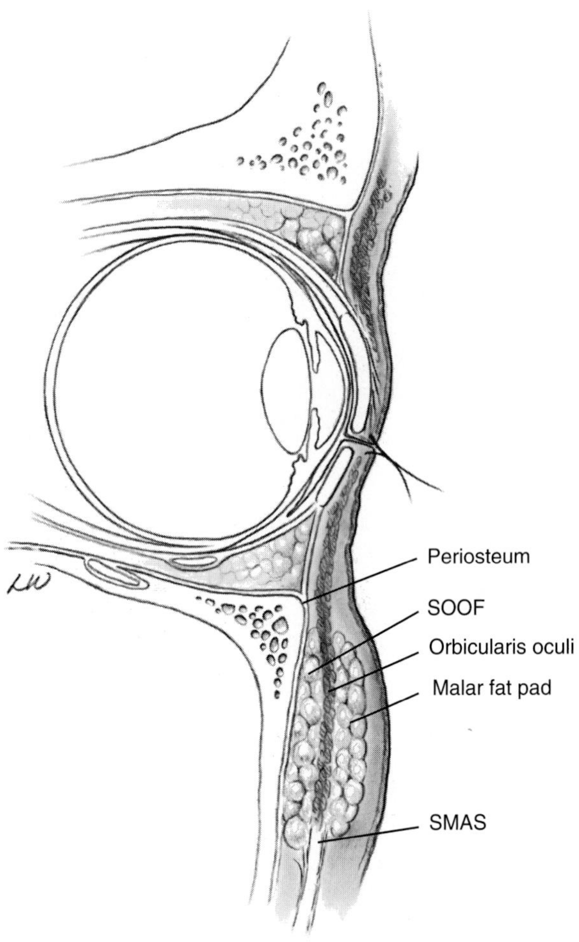

figure 7–10

Suborbicularis oculi fat (SOOF). SMAS, superficial musculoaponeurotic system.

Periosteum

SOOF

Orbicularis oculi

Malar fat pad

SMAS

skin tension lines follow the wrinkles of the face except in the glabellar area. Incisions along these tension lines produce minimal scarring.[8]

Superficial Musculoaponeurotic System

The muscles of facial expression are interconnected by a continuous fibromuscular layer known as the superficial musculoaponeurotic system (SMAS). The SMAS acts as a distributor of facial muscle contractions to the skin. Facial expressions result from the contraction of the facial muscles transmitted to the skin by the SMAS. Fibrous septa connect the dermis to the SMAS dividing the subcutaneous fat into lobules. The SMAS incorporates the orbicularis oculi muscle. Bony attachments help to stabilize it.

Specific criteria define the SMAS (Fig. 7–11)[9]:

1. It must divide the subcutaneous fat into two layers.
2. Fibrous septa extend from the dermis to the fat.
3. Fat is present deep to the SMAS, lying between deep facial muscles, and is not divided by fibrous septa.
4. The major neurovascular bundles lie deep to the SMAS.
5. The SMAS acts as a distributor of forces from associated contracting muscles.

The SMAS acts as stabilizer and coordinator of muscle

movement. Over time, the effects of gravity and age cause relaxation and laxity of facial soft tissues. Facial surgeons routinely perform a SMAS dissection during facial rejuvenation procedures to correct SMAS ptosis (see Chapter 29). The SMAS thus has important implications for cosmetic surgery and rhytidectomies.

Major vessels and nerves are deep to the SMAS, and their smaller branches perforate it (Fig. 7–12). The subdermal plexus lies superficial to the SMAS. There are important regional variations in the anatomy of the SMAS and associated neurovascular structures:

In the *lower face*, the facial nerve branches are deep to the SMAS, as are the sensory nerves. The facial muscles receive their innervation on their deep surfaces. Dissections superficial to the SMAS protect these structures.

In the *temporal area*, the temporal branch of the facial nerve crosses the superficial aspect of the zygomatic arch and continues within the SMAS to its entrance into the frontalis muscle (Fig. 7–13).[8, 9]

In the *upper face*, the supraorbital and the supratrochlear neurovascular bundles exit their respective foramina, penetrate the SMAS, and course superiorly beneath the skin's surface. Dissections beneath the SMAS temporally and the upper face protect key neurovascular structures.

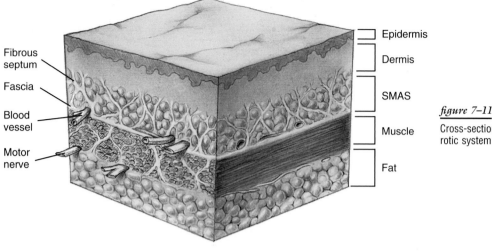

figure 7–11

Cross-section of the superficial musculoaponeurotic system (SMAS).

Labels: Fibrous septum, Fascia, Blood vessel, Motor nerve, Epidermis, Dermis, SMAS, Muscle, Fat

Muscles

Facial musculature can be divided into two groups: (1) the muscles of facial expression and (2) the muscles of mastication (chewing).

Facial Expression

The muscles of facial expression arise from the second branchial arch, the hyoid arch; these are thin, flat muscles innervated by the facial nerve. There is considerable variation in their anatomy.

The frontalis and corrugator muscles animate the forehead (Fig. 7–14). The frontalis muscle raises the eyebrows and causes transverse wrinkles of the forehead. The corrugator muscles bring the eyebrows toward each other. The frontalis is encased by the tendinous galea. The galea is continuous laterally with the superficial temporal fascia. A subcutaneous layer of dense connective tissue binds the skin to the galea. The nerves and blood vessels are present in this layer and are, therefore, superficial to the galea. The galea is separated from the periosteum by a loose areolar tissue, allowing movement of the scalp over the skull. Dissections performed in the subgaleal plane produce minimal bleeding.

The nasal muscles are the procerus, nasalis, and depressor septi. The procerus muscle pulls the forehead skin inferiorly, causing transverse creases between the brows. The nasalis muscle is composed of two parts: (1) the compressor naris and (2) the dilator naris, which open and close the nares, respectively. Excision of the corrugator and procerus muscles, or botulinum toxin

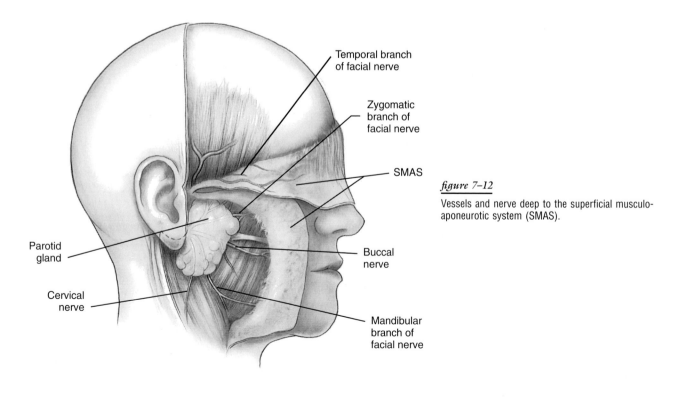

figure 7–12

Vessels and nerve deep to the superficial musculoaponeurotic system (SMAS).

Labels: Temporal branch of facial nerve, Zygomatic branch of facial nerve, SMAS, Buccal nerve, Mandibular branch of facial nerve, Cervical nerve, Parotid gland

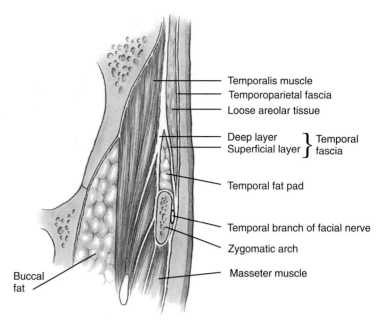

figure 7–13

Temporal branch of the facial nerve overlying the zygoma.

injection into them, can decrease the frowns of aging (see Chapters 27, 28, and 33).

Mastication

The buccinator muscle is the cheek muscle responsible for keeping food between the teeth during mastication. The mouth is encircled by the orbicularis oris muscle, which functions as a sphincter. Multiple lip elevators and depressors surround the mouth, providing a wide range of motion.

The muscles of mastication include (1) the masseter and (2) the temporalis (Fig. 7–15). The masseter muscle arises from the zygomatic arch and inserts into the mandible. The temporalis muscle arises from the temporalis fossa and inserts onto the medial side of the ramus of the mandible and the entire coronoid process. Both

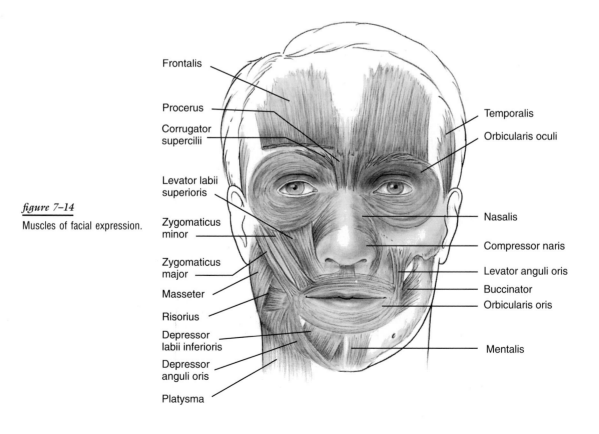

figure 7–14

Muscles of facial expression.

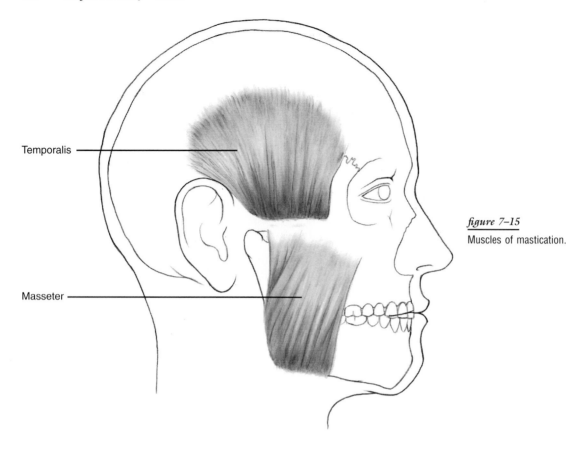

figure 7–15
Muscles of mastication.

Temporalis

Masseter

the masseter and temporalis receive their motor innervation from the third division of the fifth cranial nerve and thus can be used for facial reanimation in long-standing cases of facial paralysis. The medial and lateral pterygoids complete the muscles of mastication. They are of less significance surgically.

The temporalis muscle is covered by a dense, tough fascia, the deep temporalis fascia. The deep temporalis fascia is continuous with periosteum of the skull and is firmly attached to the temporal, parietal, and frontal bones. The deep temporalis fascia is relatively immobile. Superior to the zygomatic arch, the deep temporalis fascia splits into superficial and deep layers, which insert onto the superficial and deep aspects of the superior surface of the zygomatic arch. Between these two layers is the superficial temporal fat pad, a superior extension of the buccal fat pad.

The superficial temporalis fascia is superficial to the deep temporalis fascia. This fascial layer is continuous with the galea aponeurosis superiorly and the SMAS inferiorly. The temporal branch of the facial nerve is tightly adherent to the deep surface of this fascial layer. Dissection in the temporal region must be deep to the superficial temporalis fascia to avoid injury to the temporal branch of the facial nerve, which is present 1–2 cm posterior to the orbital rim. This avascular plane is continuous with the subgaleal space superiorly.

Nerves

The pathways of the facial nerve from the stylomastoid foramen to the undersurface of the muscles it innervates are quite variable. The main branch of the facial nerve exits the stylomastoid foramen and enters the parotid gland, where it divides into its major facial branches. The facial nerve is located 6–8 mm inferior to the tympanomastoid suture as it emerges from the stylomastoid foramen. The main trunk of the facial nerve can be found between the cartilaginous pointer of the external auditory canal and the posterior belly of the digastric, where it attaches to the mastoid tip.

The facial nerve has five major branches (Fig. 7–16):

- Temporal
- Zygomatic
- Buccal
- Mandibular
- Cervical

The temporal and mandibular branches are at greatest risk for injury. The temporal nerve leaves the superior border of the parotid gland and travels within the SMAS over the zygomatic arch and temporal area to insert on the undersurface of the temporalis. To avoid injury to the temporal nerve, the surgeon should carry out dissection deep to the SMAS.

The mandibular nerve most commonly passes above the inferior border of the mandible. Here, the nerve lies deep to the platysma muscle. En route it may pass either superficial or deep to the facial artery but is almost always superficial to the posterior and anterior facial veins. As the nerve approaches the mouth, it becomes more superficial and innervates the mouth depressors posteriorly.[10] Injury to the mandibular nerve paralyzes the depressors of the corner of the mouth, creating

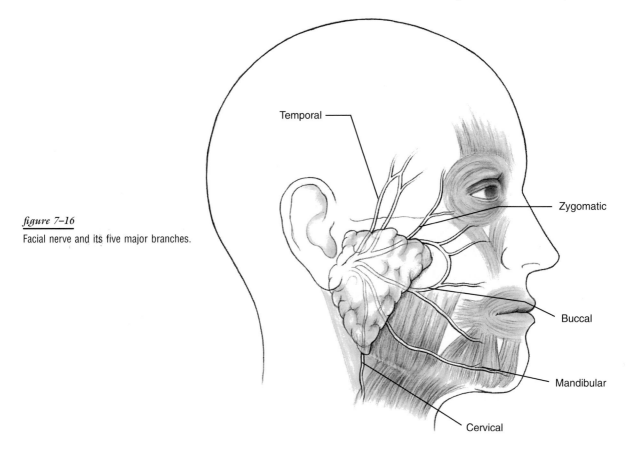

figure 7–16

Facial nerve and its five major branches.

a marked facial deformity. During facelift procedures, dissections performed just beneath the SMAS/platysma muscle complex protect the mandibular nerve at the angle of the mandible. Increasing adhesions between skin and muscle around the mouth, plus a more superficial course, places the terminal branches of the mandibular nerve at risk for injury during blunt dissection.[1] Perioral rhytids (wrinkles) are best treated by chemical peels, dermabrasion, or carbon dioxide laser resurfacing (see Chapters 30 and 31).

The face receives its sensory innervation from three branches of the fifth cranial nerve (Fig. 7–17):

The first division, or *ophthalmic nerve*, innervates the scalp, forehead, and nasal dorsum as well as the tentorium cerebella. The surgeon must take care to avoid injury to the supraorbital and supratrochlear nerves as they emerge from their respective foramina during brow-lifting or facelift procedures.

The second division, the *maxillary nerve*, innervates the lower eyelid, cheek, side of the nose, nasal vestibule, and the skin and mucosa of the upper lip. The infraorbital branch of this nerve innervates the maxillary sinus mucosa and upper teeth. Subperiosteal midface cheek lifts may injure the infraorbital nerve with subsequent paresthesia in the maxillary region. The pterygopalatine branch provides sensation to the mucoperiosteum of the nasal cavity, septum, palate, sphenoid, ethmoid sinuses, and nasopharynx.

The third division, or *mandibular branch*, innervates

the lower teeth, gingiva, and mandible. The mandibular branch also provides sensation to the temporal area and part of the external auditory canal, including the tympanic membrane. The mandibular branch also provides motor innervation to the temporalis, masseter, and medial and lateral pterygoid muscles. Other muscles receiving motor supply from the mandibular branch include the tensor tympani, tensor veli palatini, mylohyoid, and anterior belly of the digastric muscle.

Vasculature

The face receives its blood supply via the internal and external carotid arteries, which have multiple anastomoses.

The *internal carotid artery* gives off the ophthalmic artery, which supplies a mask-like area, including the eyelids, nasal dorsum, and forehead. The ophthalmic artery has numerous branches, including the supraorbital, supratrochlear, infratrochlear, anterior ethmoid, posterior ethmoid, medial and lateral palpebral, and marginal arteries (Fig. 7–18). The supraorbital and supratrochlear arteries may be injured during brow-lifting procedures. While releasing the corrugator muscles, the surgeon should pay attention to these arteries as they exit their foramina and pierce the frontalis muscle.

The *external carotid artery* gives off the facial, internal maxillary, and superficial temporal arteries (Fig. 7–19). The facial artery supplies superior and inferior labial

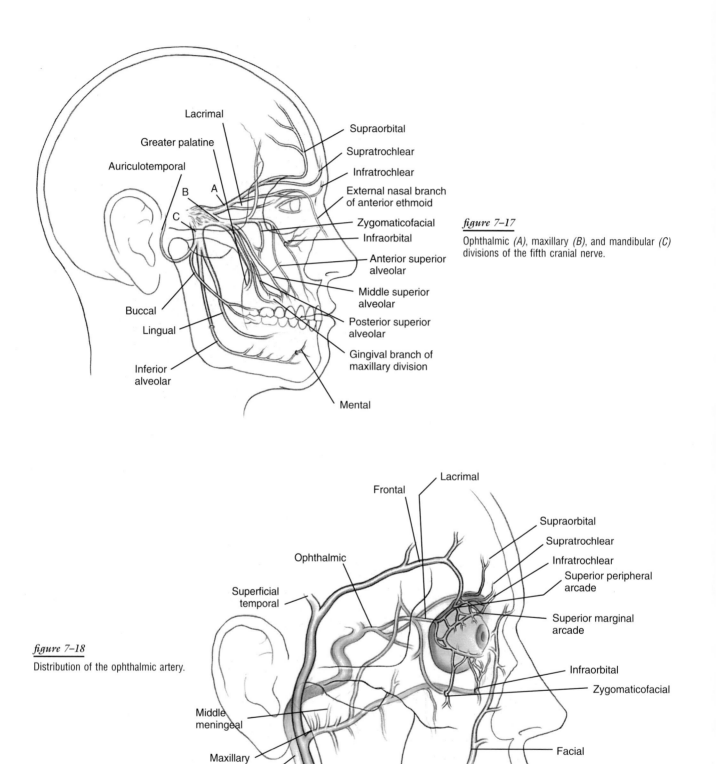

figure 7–17

Ophthalmic *(A)*, maxillary *(B)*, and mandibular *(C)* divisions of the fifth cranial nerve.

figure 7–18

Distribution of the ophthalmic artery.

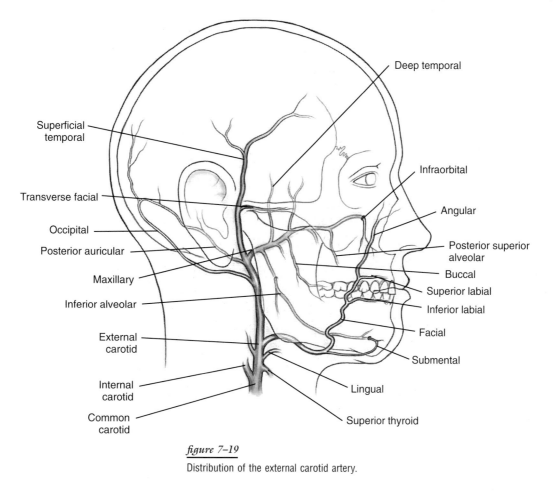

figure 7–19
Distribution of the external carotid artery.

arteries to the lips, and it also supplies the lateral aspect and dorsum of the nose. In addition, the sphenopalatine artery supplies lateral nasal mucosa. There is a rich anastomosis, with anterior and posterior ethmoid arteries. Inadvertent intra-arterial injections in this area may result in embolization and blindness.

The *internal maxillary artery* gives rise to the infraorbital artery in pterygopalatine fossa. The infraorbital artery passes through the infraorbital fissure into the orbit. It continues anteriorly in the infraorbital groove and infraorbital canal to emerge below the inferior orbital margin, where it supplies the lower eyelid. The infraorbital artery may be damaged during subperiosteal midface cheek lifts as it exits its foramen.

The *superficial temporal artery* is the terminal branch of the external carotid artery arising within the parotid gland. The superficial temporal artery travels in the SMAS across the zygomatic arch. Dissections deep to the SMAS protect the superficial temporal artery from injury. Before crossing the zygomatic arch, the superficial temporal artery gives off the traverse facial artery, which supplies the lateral canthal area. The transverse facial artery anastomoses with the medial and lateral palpebral arteries. At the superior border of the zygomatic, the superficial temporal artery gives off a second branch, the middle temporal artery. This artery supplies the superficial temporal fat pad, the deep temporalis fascia, and the temporalis muscle. The superficial tempo-

ral artery continues superiorly, giving off terminal branches that supply the parietal area and forehead, including the frontalis muscle. There are anastomotic connections with the ipsilateral supraorbital and supratrochlear arteries.

The scalp is extremely well vascularized because of the ample amount of collateral blood flow. Overzealous electrocautery, however, may result in scalp necrosis during coronal flap elevation. Unipolar cautery results in more extensive tissue damage than bipolar cautery. Bipolar cautery should be used for hemostasis of the scalp edges. Prior surgery or radiation increases the risk of scalp necrosis.[11]

The vascular supply to the face forms a series of subepidermal plexuses. These include the fascial plexus, the subcutaneous plexus, and the subdermal plexus. The dermis has a superficial and a deep vascular plexus. The *superficial plexus*, also known as the subepidermal or subpapillary plexus, runs in the papillary dermis and sends vascular loops into each dermal papilla. The *deep vascular plexus* surrounds the dermal appendages within the reticular dermis. The septocutaneous vessels travel within the fascia investing muscles, and the musculocutaneous plexus passes directly through the muscles. These plexuses are supplied by direct and indirect cutaneous vessels. The venous drainage flows from the subdermal plexus through the venae communicantes to the deep venous plexus.[8]

Lymphatics

The face contains 300 lymph nodes and has a vast lymphatic anastomotic plexus. The midface drains to the submental and submandibular lymph nodes onto the internal jugular chain. The lateral face drains to the parotid as well as the preauricular and retroauricular lymph nodes. The parietal area drains to both the parotid and retroauricular lymph nodes.

References

1. Pillsbury DM, Shelley WB, Kligman AM: A Manual of Cutaneous Medicine, p 4. Philadelphia, WB Saunders, 1961.
2. Jones TL, Wobig JL: Surgery of the Eyelids and Lacrimal System, pp 21–22. Birmingham, Ala, Aesculapius, 1976.
3. Jones LT, Reeh MT, Wirtschafter J: Ophthalmic Anatomy, pp 45–46. Rochester, Minn, American Academy of Ophthalmology, 1970.
4. Beard C: Ptosis. St Louis, CV Mosby, 1976, p 18.
5. Putterman AM: The mysterious second temporal fat pad. Ophthalmic Plast Reconstr Surg 1985; 1:73–74.
6. Zide BM, Jelks GW: Surgical Anatomy of Orbit, p 12. New York, Raven Press, 1985.
7. Lemke BN, Stasior GO: The anatomy of eye brow ptosis. Arch Ophthalmol 1982; 100:981–986.
8. Larabee WF, Makielski KH: Surgical Anatomy of the Face, pp 23–110. New York, Raven Press, 1993.
9. Kikkawa DO, Lemke BN, Dortzbach RK: Relations of the superficial musculoaponeurotic system to the orbit and characterization of the orbitomalar ligament. Ophthalmic Plast Reconstr Surg 1996; 12:77–88.
10. Leibman EP, Webster RC, Gaul JR, Griffin T: The marginal mandibular nerve in rhytidectomy and liposuction surgery. Arch Otolaryngol Head Neck Surg 1988; 114:179–181.
11. Alvi A, Carrau RL: The bicoronal flap approach in craniofacial trauma. J Cranio-Maxillofac Trauma 1966; 2:40–55.

Lawrence B. Katzen

Chapter 8

Anesthesia, Analgesia, and Amnesia

The cosmetic oculoplastic surgeon's reputation rests not only on the final results of the surgery but also on the degree of the patient's discomfort and anxiety. It is therefore very important that the apprehension created by the operating room setting and the discomfort of the local anesthetic injection and orbital fat excision be decreased as much as possible.

Larry Katzen has written an informative chapter on the subject of anesthesia, analgesia, and amnesia. He initially discusses premedication, which can be administered by the surgeon who chooses to operate without an anesthesiologist. Among the preoperative medications are narcotics, tranquilizers, and sedatives, including barbiturates and hypnotics. His preference is midazolam given intravenously in incremental doses 1 hour preoperatively. He then gives intravenous propofol before local infiltration of anesthetic and uses this continuously for long procedures. He supplements this agent with alfentanil before anticipated painful procedures and intravenous sedation with midazolam as needed. Additionally, he comments on EMLA cream to numb the skin.

Dr. Katzen and I agree that our preference, whenever possible and affordable, is to have an anesthesiologist give intravenous anesthesia while monitoring the patient's vital signs and providing comfort to the patient. Sedatives such as thiopental and methohexital (Brevital) can be given before injections of local anesthetic and excision of orbital fat to reduce discomfort. Because these drugs inhibit breathing, however, most anesthesiologists are reluctant to give very high doses during cosmetic oculoplastic surgery, in which access to the airway is not easy, especially if the patient's entire face is prepared and draped. Most anesthesiologists prefer tranquilizers, such as diazepam and midazolam, that can produce patient comfort with relative safeness.

Dr. Katzen also introduces conscious sedation using nitrous oxide–oxygen, which can produce deep sedation without general anesthesia. In addition, he details the various drugs used for intraoperative anesthesia, including tetracaine, lidocaine (Xylocaine), and bupivacaine (Marcaine). He demonstrates how epinephrine, hyaluronidase (Wydase), and sodium bicarbonate can enhance the effect of these injections and decrease the discomfort. He finds that mixing fresh solutions of lidocaine with epinephrine can produce an injectable solution that is less uncomfortable to the patient than the commercially available mixture, which is acidic. He also discusses the saline-balanced salt solution that Tenzel and colleagues dilute with an anesthetic agent to reduce the discomfort during infiltration. I believe this is preferable to the sodium bicarbonate method of reducing discomfort because unusual types of eyelid pigmentation developed in several of my patients following injection of sodium bicarbonate.

ALLEN M. PUTTERMAN

Contemporary cosmetic eyelid surgery can and should be performed without pain to the patient. Sensory anesthesia can be induced and maintained either with or without altering the patient's state of consciousness. The type of anesthesia used is ultimately the responsibility of the surgeon, and it is not chosen until the patient has been fully evaluated medically, psychologically, and socioeconomically.

Most cosmetic eyelid procedures can be performed with the use of local anesthesia alone. In most cases, nothing short of general anesthesia can substitute for an adequate local block; however, in an effort to minimize the anxiety and discomfort the patient must endure and to alter the patient's memory perception of the experience, it is often useful to have an anesthesiologist supplement local anesthesia with intravenous analgesia and sedation.

Careful titration of small intravenous doses enables the anesthesiologist to control the patient's level of awareness. With the concept of "aesthetic anesthesia"[1] kept in mind, it is apparent that the interaction involving anesthesiologist, patient, and medication is the key to caring for the patient's psyche as he or she passes through the surgical experience. The personal contact provided when the anesthesiologist holds the patient's hand during the operation has tremendous calming effects and eases the isolation of the operating room (Fig. 8–1). Postoperatively, patients often voluntarily express their appreciation for this tactile sedative as well as for their altered state of consciousness. Detailed communication between the surgeon and anesthesiologist helps to ensure optimal results. With the use of intravenous hypnotics before the administration of local anesthesia, there need not be any sensation or recall of the pain usually associated with infiltration anesthesia. The appropriately timed intravenous injection of narcotic or opioid analgesics inhibits the perception of painful stimuli. Strategic use of amnesic agents can help minimize recall of any perioperative pain.

The development of more potent, faster-acting hypnotic and narcotic agents as well as the universal shift to outpatient surgery have contributed to a marked decrease in the use of tranquilizers and intramuscular injections.

PREOPERATIVE EVALUATION

It is essential that the anesthesiologist personally evaluate the patient preoperatively. This initial interaction reassures the patient and instills confidence that he or she will indeed be cared for competently and with sensitivity. The anesthesiologist will also be a familiar face for the patient in the unaccustomed surroundings of the operating room.

A medical history should be obtained and should include information on any previous adverse reactions the patient or family members have had to anesthetic agents, the patient's previous favorable and unfavorable experiences with medications, a list of current medications, and details of any mental illness or seizure disorder. A relevant physical examination should be performed. The information obtained from this initial interaction enables the anesthetist to individualize a regimen for the patient's benefit; just as the surgeon chooses from an operative repertoire, the anesthesiologist selects or avoids certain drugs. The level of the patient's anxiety also may be assessed and appropriate measures planned.

PREMEDICATION

Close communication between surgeon and anesthetist (anesthesiologist or nurse-anesthetist) allows the patient

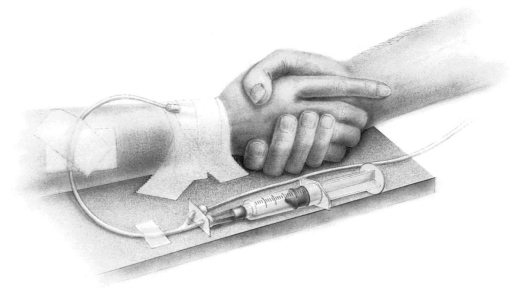

figure 8–1

The human contact of the anesthetist's holding the patient's hand during surgery has a tremendous calming effect and helps ease the isolation of the operating room.

to arrive in the operating room in the state of awareness desired by the surgeon. Some surgeons prefer a patient to be fully alert for marking of the skin incision lines before an upper eyelid blepharoplasty, but to be initially sedated for excision of herniated lower lid fat. The patient's response to initial medication may assist the anesthetist in choosing drugs and dosages for intraoperative administration. Drugs used for premedication for nongeneral anesthesia include narcotics, tranquilizers, and sedatives, including barbiturates and hypnotics. In general, I prefer to give midazolam (0.5–2 mg) intravenously in incremental doses of 0.5–1 mg 30–60 minutes preoperatively. Of course, drugs and dosages are adjusted for the individual patient.

When the surgeon is working without an anesthetist, oral premedication can be very effective. Diazepam (Valium), 10 mg given orally 45 minutes before surgery, relieves anxiety in most cases. Triazolam (Halcion), 0.25–0.5 mg by mouth, results in relaxation, sleep, and amnesia.

Narcotics

Meperidine, fentanyl, and alfentanil are the narcotics most commonly used today. Morphine is rarely used. Although not the narcotic of choice, meperidine is preferred over morphine because of the lower incidence of nausea and vomiting and a lesser depressive effect on respiration after its use. Fentanyl provides excellent analgesia but has the potential to cause severe respiratory depression; sometimes a patient under local anesthesia who is administered this drug may need to be reminded to breathe.

For analgesia, I prefer alfentanil. It has an immediate onset of action and a terminal elimination half-life equal to 20 per cent of fentanyl. It is potent enough to allow cataract surgery without the use of eye block or topical anesthesia.

Intramuscular administration of narcotics is discouraged because small incremental intravenous doses provide much better control.

Sedatives

Sedatives help to relieve anxiety and create a hypnotic state. Their hypnotic effect is enhanced by narcotics. Pentobarbital and secobarbital are commonly used for premedication in patients receiving general anesthesia; the usual adult dose is 75–100 mg. I prefer to avoid the use of long-acting sedatives in patients whose cooperation is needed or whose eyelid level must be assessed during surgery, because of the effects of the drugs and their tendency to produce a secondary transient intraoperative ptosis.

Tranquilizers

The tranquilizers constitute a group of drugs that consist of the phenothiazines. Although these drugs are

usually given to enhance the effects of narcotics and barbiturates and to reduce the amount of postoperative nausea and vomiting, their prophylactic value in preventing postoperative nausea and vomiting after the administration of noninhalation anesthesia is questionable. Because of this fact, they are rarely used with noninhalation anesthesia.

INTRAOPERATIVE ANESTHESIA

Local Anesthesia

Local anesthetic agents block the propagation of the sensory stimulus and motor impulse by preventing depolarization of the cell membrane, thereby impairing conduction.[2] When administered, a local anesthetic, like any drug, should be considered to be a controlled physiologic insult to the body. An intimate knowledge of proper concentrations, routes of administration, and maximum safe dosage as well as potential side effects, adverse reactions, and their management is mandatory for safe use. Anesthetics may be administered topically, infiltrated locally, or injected as a nerve block.

Most local anesthetic agents are chemically similar and are categorized as esters or amines, based on a chemical linkage present between two of the three parts (the intermediate chain and the aromatic residue). The third part is the amide group, which accounts for the enhanced tissue penetration in more alkaline solutions.

Topical Anesthetics

The two most widely used topical conjunctival anesthetics in ophthalmology today are tetracaine and proparacaine. These agents are useful preoperatively in evaluating basic tear secretion as well as intraoperatively for insertion and removal of protective corneal-scleral shells. A mixture of lidocaine and prilocaine for dermal application can be used for analgesia before infiltration anesthesia or injection of botulinum toxin (Botox).

Tetracaine. Tetracaine, available commercially in solutions of 0.5–2 per cent, may be instilled directly onto the cornea and conjunctiva. The onset of anesthesia occurs within 26 seconds, and the duration ranges from 9 to 24 minutes.[3] On instillation, most patients complain of a burning sensation that lasts until the anesthetic effect is established. The drug's side effect of transient punctate keratopathy is well known, and because this effect is dose-related, the 0.5 per cent solution is preferred.

Proparacaine. Proparacaine is commercially available in solutions of 0.5 per cent. Additives are 0.2 per cent chlorobutanol and 1:10,000 benzalkonium chloride, both of which help maintain sterility. Proparacaine produces anesthetic effects similar to those of tetracaine but has the advantage of producing less discomfort and, generally, less keratopathy. This feature has resulted in its current popularity, especially for use in the office. It is not currently available in peel packages for intraoperative use.

EMLA Cream. EMLA cream is a combination of 2.5 per cent lidocaine and 2.5 per cent prilocaine. It is an emulsion in which the oil phase exists as a eutectic mixture. This allows the anesthetics to exist as liquids facilitating dermal absorption. Contact with the conjunctiva and cornea should be avoided. The manufacturer recommends application with an occlusive dressing for 1–2 hours before treatment. I have found that application to the eyelids for 30 minutes without an occlusive dressing has an adequate analgesic effect.

Allergy. Allergic reactions to topical anesthetic agents are uncommon, and cross-sensitivity is not necessarily present. Allergic sensitivity to tetracaine or proparacaine usually follows repeated applications, as with glaucoma drops, and may manifest as signs and symptoms ranging from itching and swelling of the eyelids to conjunctival hyperemia and epithelial keratopathy. Use of EMLA cream often causes blanching, erythema, or edema.

Infiltration Anesthesia

Because of the ease and the relative safety associated with infiltration anesthesia, some surgeons perform many cosmetic eyelid procedures in the office without the aid of an anesthetist. These surgeons should have a working knowledge of the onset and duration of action as well as the maximum dosage for each anesthetic agent to be used for infiltration anesthesia (Table 8–1). Toxic reactions to anesthetic agents include convulsion, respiratory arrest, and cardiovascular collapse, making it mandatory for the surgeon to have the knowledge and materials to treat these complications: intravenous infusion setups and intravenous medications, the capacity to perform artificial ventilation, and a working knowledge of cardiopulmonary resuscitation. (The American Heart Association and the American Medical Association have published an excellent manual on cardiopulmonary resuscitation.[4]) Surgeons certainly should maintain current certification in these techniques, although judicious use of infiltration anesthesia should prevent the need to use these lifesaving measures.

Lidocaine. Lidocaine (Xylocaine) is probably the agent most commonly used for infiltration anesthesia because

it diffuses well through tissue and produces little irritation. It is available in solutions of 0.5–2 per cent, with and without epinephrine. When injected, the maximum dose is 500 mg, and the concentration may vary, depending on the desired area of anesthesia and the required volume of infiltration. I have found that patients who do not receive epinephrine often require a second injection after 60–90 minutes. It is my clinical impression that 2 per cent solutions with epinephrine provide more prolonged anesthesia, although others consider the use of a 2 per cent solution to be irrational.[5]

The surgeon must take care when applying sponges that have been soaked in lidocaine to the vascular orbicularis or mucous membranes, as systemic absorption is enhanced and toxic levels are more easily reached. Early signs of overdose are sleepiness, personality change, and nausea and vomiting. A drop in blood pressure and convulsions may soon follow.

Mepivacaine. Mepivacaine (Carbocaine) has gained popularity. It is essentially the equivalent of lidocaine in terms of available strengths, potency, dosage, and toxicity. Although I personally have had no experience with this agent in cosmetic eyelid surgery, I would consider using it in a patient who is allergic to lidocaine.

Bupivacaine. Bupivacaine (Marcaine) is available in solutions of 0.25, 0.5, and 0.75 per cent. It has the advantage of prolonged duration of anesthetic effect, obviating the need for repeated injections during lengthy procedures. It also aids in reducing pain postoperatively.

Its disadvantage is its prolonged onset of action. A rapid anesthetic effect, together with a prolonged duration (4–12 hours), may be obtained by mixing equal volumes of 0.75 per cent bupivacaine and 1 per cent lidocaine with epinephrine 1:100,000.

Epinephrine. As a vasoconstrictor, epinephrine slows the absorption of infiltrated anesthetic agents and thereby prolongs their effect. It also increases the maximum safe dosage and helps to provide hemostasis. There is no benefit to using concentrations greater than 1:100,000. At this concentration, injection should not exceed 10 ml in 10 minutes or 30 ml in 1 hour.[6]

Epinephrine should not be used in conjunction with general anesthetic agents that sensitize the myocardium. It should be avoided in patients with thyrotoxicosis and coronary artery disease.

table 8–1

Local Anesthetic Agents for Injection

Agent	Onset (minutes)	Duration (hours)	Maximum Dose (mg/kg)
Lidocaine (Xylocaine)	5	2–3	4–7
Mepivacaine (Carbocaine)	5	2–4	4–5
Bupivacaine (Marcaine)	10	6–24	3–5

From Epstein GA: Anesthesia in ophthalmic plastic surgery. In Hornblass A (ed): Oculoplastic, Orbital, and Reconstructive Surgery, vol 1: Eyelids, pp 42–51. Baltimore, Williams & Wilkins, 1988.

Combinations. My personal experience with a 50/50 mixture of 2 per cent lidocaine with epinephrine 1:100,000 mixed with 0.5 per cent bupivacaine with epinephrine 1:200,000 has been excellent. This mixture combines the benefits of the rapid onset of action of lidocaine, the long-acting postoperative analgesia of bupivacaine, and the hemostatic effects of epinephrine.

Hyaluronidase. Hyaluronidase (Wydase) is an enzyme that degrades polysaccharide hyaluronic acid, which exists in the interstitial spaces. Hyaluronidase may be added to local anesthetics to increase tissue permeability and enhance anesthetic diffusion. In cosmetic eyelid surgery, this action helps establish the plane between skin and orbicularis muscle and facilitates dissection. Its use is essential to the pinch technique of upper lid blepharoplasty. The increased tissue spread from hyaluronidase accelerates the onset of anesthetic effect and reduces the volume of anesthetic agent required; however, the duration of anesthetic effect is also decreased. Hyaluronidase is useful in obtaining adequate sensory anesthesia of the deep orbital fat.

Sodium Bicarbonate. Sodium bicarbonate has been recommended as an additive to adjust the acidic pH (2.74–3.91) of infiltration anesthetic agents containing epinephrine, thereby reducing the discomfort associated with infiltration. It is specifically designed to reduce the chemical irritation associated with low pH infiltration. There is some concern that permanent skin pigmentation may sometimes occur (Putterman AM: oral communication, 1991). I have no personal experience with this agent, and with timely intravenous sedation, its use is not necessary.

INJECTION TECHNIQUES

It is imperative that intravenous administration be avoided. This goal is best accomplished by repeated aspiration during injection or else by having the needle constantly moving during injection.

Local Infiltration

Local infiltration consists simply of injecting the agent into the surgical site. The discomfort associated with infiltration may be decreased by using a 27-gauge needle and by slowing the rate of injection. The premixed solutions of lidocaine containing epinephrine are more acidic than the plain solutions and therefore produce more patient discomfort when injected. The discomfort can be avoided by preparation of fresh solution in the operating room. Extreme care should be taken during preparation to avoid any miscalculation in amounts. The more neutral pH of fresh solution also enhances tissue penetration.

I find it useful to inject directly into the fat pockets of the lower eyelid to minimize the discomfort associated with manipulating and cauterizing the orbital fat (see Chapters 16–18).

Saline or Balanced Salt Solution

Tenzel and colleagues[7] have described a technique to reduce the discomfort of infiltration anesthesia with saline or balanced salt solution diluting the anesthetic. The initial injection is made with local anesthetic diluted 1:9 with balanced salt solution. After 3–10 minutes, the full-strength anesthetic may be injected without discomfort. This technique may be useful for office procedures when intravenous sedation is not available.

It has been suggested that the reduction in pain is due to the anesthetic effect of benzyl alcohol present in bacteriostatic saline.[8] However, this would not explain the decreased pain associated with dilution using balanced salt solution.

INTRAVENOUS ANESTHESIA, ANALGESIA, AND AMNESIA

The use of intravenous medications to induce marked analgesia and psychomotor retardation has been termed *neuroleptanalgesia*.[1] This state of consciousness may be obtained without hazardous alterations in cardiovascular and pulmonary function, obviating the need for endotracheal intubation. Under ideal control, the patient's cortical functions are left somewhat intact. It is in the capacity of "mental guru" to the iatrogenically intoxicated patient's psyche that the artistic anesthetist stands apart from his or her colleagues. With the use of drugs, positive suggestion, and the empathy of a held hand, the patient is assured of leaving the operating room emotionally unscathed.

I have found several agents to be effective in inducing neuroleptanalgesia. To help titrate these intravenous drugs, the anesthetist can dilute some agents from their stock concentrations to increase the volume of injection, thereby minimizing the effects of "dead space" in the syringe and intravenous tubing. Short-acting intravenous hypnotics are now widely used before any painful manipulation, specifically the infiltration of local anesthesia and the excision of orbital fat.

Propofol

Propofol (Diprivan) is an intravenous sedative-hypnotic agent. Because of low water solubility, it is formulated in a distinctive white oil-in-water emulsion, commonly called milk of amnesia. Rapid hypnosis is obtained usually within 40 seconds from the start of injection of this drug. The usual initial dose is 0.5 mg/kg via slow intravenous injection over 3–5 minutes.

A rapid onset of action and excellent depth of hypnosis, followed by rapid awakening, make this my preferred sedative agent before administration of local infiltration anesthesia. Administration of propofol with a continuous infusion pump is an excellent sedation technique for facelifts and other extended procedures.

Thiopental

Thiopental (Pentothal) is an excellent sedative with no analgesic effect. It is very short-acting, and no intubation is needed when the drug is given in small doses. I prefer to dilute it to a concentration of 25 mg/ml and to give an initial dose of 2 ml. It is especially useful when the anesthetist is faced with the problem of dealing with overly anxious patients who insist that the premedication has had no effect and are certain that their anxiety and discomfort will not be relieved. In such instances, the use of thiopental is extremely helpful. Before the surgeon's arrival, the anesthetist can give the patient a 25–50 mg bolus of this hypnotic. When full alertness is regained within 5–10 minutes, the patient's anxiety should be greatly reduced. This change in the patient's attitude serves to decrease the effective dose of subsequent medications.

Methohexital

Methohexital (Brevital) is a rapid, ultra-short-acting barbiturate anesthetic agent. It is twice as potent as thiopental, and its duration of action is about half as long. The cumulative effects are fewer, and recovery is more rapid with methohexital than with thiobarbiturates.

Methohexital should be administered intravenously in a concentration no greater than 1 per cent. The usual dosage is 50–70 mg by intermittent intravenous injection, providing anesthesia and amnesia for short periods, during which local eyelid blocks can be given. Additional injections can be given in anticipation of the discomfort associated with orbital fat excision.

Narcotics

Morphine, meperidine, fentanyl, and alfentanil may also be used intravenously to provide analgesia. A rapid onset of action, combined with a short half-life, makes alfentanil my preferred analgesic agent. Alfentanil is administered in increasing doses of 125–250 µg. The patient's response and tolerance are evaluated, and the dosage is adjusted accordingly. As the surgeon approaches a part of the procedure that is usually associated with patient discomfort, such as infiltration or fat excision, the anesthetist can be alerted and can give the patient an additional amount of analgesia 2–3 minutes before the procedure in order to minimize the discomfort.

Diazepam

Diazepam is an excellent tranquilizer that has the additional benefit of producing significant amnesia. It can be diluted to a concentration of 1 mg/ml, and the intravenous dose can be titrated, starting with 1–2 mg. It must not be diluted with solutions that contain dextrose because a precipitate will form. I have found that patients are extremely susceptible to hypnotic suggestion while under the effects of diazepam; it alters their memory perception and sometimes prevents the recollection of any discomfort from the procedure, although paradoxical agitation also occurs occasionally.

Because of the incidence of phlebitis that has been reported with use of diazepam, care should be taken to flush out the intravenous line after each administration. This potential complication, combined with the widely accepted usage of midazolam, has decreased the intraoperative use of diazepam.

Midazolam

Midazolam (Versed) is a short-acting, benzodiazepine, central nervous system depressant. When initially introduced, the drug was used in a concentration of 5 mg/ml, resulting in significant apnea. If it is given intravenously in slow incremental doses of 1 mg, a semiconscious deep sedation can safely be achieved.

Midazolam is specifically indicated to impair memory of perioperative events. Intravenous use is associated with a high incidence of partial or complete impairment of recall for the next several hours.[9] The drug is also very useful as an anxiolytic agent. I prefer midazolam to diazepam because of its shorter half-life and duration of action.

Ketamine

Ketamine is an anesthetic agent that produces a dissociated sleep. It is sometimes useful in children to avoid endotracheal intubation.

Serious side effects, however, are associated with this drug. Ketamine raises the blood pressure and heart rate and has been reported to produce seizures. In my experience, 50 per cent of patients experience an adverse psychological reaction to this drug. In addition, psychotic reactions have been reported after its use. I find that there is no place for ketamine in cosmetic eyelid surgery.

Synopsis of Preferred Intravenous Technique

My preferred technique for intravenous anesthesia, analgesia, and amnesia is as follows:

1. Premedicate with incremental doses of midazolam (0.5–2 mg).
2. Give intravenous propofol before local infiltration (0.5 mg/kg). For full facial procedures, continuous infusion of propofol is given.
3. Locally infiltrate the surgical area with a 50–50 mixture of 2 per cent lidocaine with epinephrine (1:100,000) mixed with 0.5 per cent bupivacaine (1:200,000). Alter the formula for a large-volume injection, such as during a coronal brow lift.
4. Supplement analgesia with incremental doses of fentanil (250–500 µg) before anticipated painful procedures or when the patient perceives pain.
5. Supplement intravenous sedation with midazolam as needed.

table 8-2
Subjective Symptoms of Nitrous Oxide–Oxygen Conscious Sedation

Stage I Anesthesia	Stages II–IV Anesthesia
Level 1	Unconscious
Feeling of relaxation	
Tingling sensation in fingers, lips, or tongue	
Feeling of warmth	
Level 2	
Humming, droning, buzzing sounds	
Lethargy	
Drowsiness	
Euphoria	
Analgesia	
Level 3	
Hallucination	
Dreams	
Fears (falling, dying)	
Nausea	

Adapted from Epstein GA: Anesthesia in ophthalmic plastic surgery. In Hornblass A (ed): Oculoplastic, Orbital, and Reconstructive Surgery, vol 1: Eyelids, pp 42–51. Baltimore, Williams & Wilkins, 1988.

NITROUS OXIDE–OXYGEN CONSCIOUS SEDATION

The use of a combination of nitrous oxide and oxygen as inhalation agents in subanesthetic doses has been termed nitrous oxide–oxygen conscious sedation.[10] The subanesthetic effects of N_2O-O_2 make it a useful, safe, and controllable tool for providing patient comfort during cosmetic oculoplastic surgery. Onset of action and recovery are rapid as a result of low blood gas solubility. The pharmacologic effects of N_2O vary with the concentration and are thus dose-related. N_2O-O_2 should be administered with an analgesic machine, a gas delivery system specifically designed for conscious sedation. This is not an anesthetic machine for delivery of general anesthesia.

The analgesic machine has safety features not found on an anesthetic machine, including:

- A minimum oxygen flow
- An automatic shutoff triggered by O_2 depletion
- A maximum N_2O concentration
- A flush valve that allows administration of 100 per cent O_2

These features, together with the administration of N_2O-O_2 through a nasal cannula, limit sedation analgesia to stage I, level 2 anesthesia (Tables 8–2 and 8–3). This is the deepest level of safe use of N_2O-O_2 sedation.

table 8-3
Objective Signs of Nitrous Oxide–Oxygen Conscious Sedation

Stage I Anesthesia

Level 1
Normal relaxed, fully conscious
Follows directions

Level 2
Relaxed, euphoric, less aware of surroundings
Follows directions but is slower

Level 3
Brow perspiration, body stiffening, claw hand, less aware of surroundings
Usually does not follow directions

Stage II Anesthesia
Rigid, active, unpredictable movements

Adapted from Epstein GA: Anesthesia in ophthalmic plastic surgery. In Hornblass A (ed): Oculoplastic, Orbital, and Reconstructive Surgery, vol 1: Eyelids, pp 42–51. Baltimore, Williams & Wilkins, 1988.

table 8–4

Contraindications to Nitrous Oxide–Oxygen Conscious Sedation

Nasal obstruction
    Acute rhinitis
    Nasal tumor
    Nasal deformity
Acute respiratory disease
    Pneumonia
    Tuberculosis
    Bronchitis, chronic obstructive lung disease
    Severe asthma
Psychiatric patients
Severe cardiac disease
    Congestive heart failure, pulmonary edema
    Severe angina
Pregnancy
Teratogenic effects of N_2O shown in rat embryo; no documentation in humans
No known effect on long-term exposure to N_2O during pregnancy

Adapted from Epstein GA: Anesthesia in ophthalmic plastic surgery. In Hornblass A (ed): Oculoplastic, Orbital, and Reconstructive Surgery, vol 1: Eyelids, pp 42–51. Baltimore, Williams & Wilkins, 1988.

The advantages of rapid onset and rapid recovery enable intermittent anesthesia for procedures in which patient cooperation may be necessary. N_2O-O_2 sedation can eliminate the need for intravenous sedation, which is useful in office-based procedures. When parenteral medications are avoided, so is the need for an anesthetist and recovery room personnel.

Safe administration of N_2O-O_2 sedation by the surgeon requires a working knowledge of the levels of anesthesia, inhalation equipment, and contraindications to N_2O-O_2 sedation (Table 8–4). Epstein[10] has provided an excellent, comprehensive description of N_2O-O_2 conscious sedation.

References

1. Lynch S: Hypnosis, amnesia, anesthesia. In Rees TD, Woodsmith D (eds): Cosmetic Facial Surgery, pp 34–43. Philadelphia, WB Saunders, 1973.
2. Ritchie JM, Cohen PJ: Cocaine, procaine and other synthetic local anesthetics. In Goodman LS, Gilman A (eds): The Pharmacological Basis of Therapeutics, 5th ed, pp 379–403. New York, Macmillan, 1975.
3. Boozan CW, Cohen PJ: Ophthaine: A new topical anesthetic for the eye. Am J Ophthalmol 1953; 36:1619.
4. Standards and guidelines for cardiopulmonary resuscitation and emergency cardiac care. JAMA 1980; 244:453–509.
5. Havener WH: Ocular Pharmacology, 4th ed, pp 68–113. St. Louis, CV Mosby, 1978.
6. Fehs JA, Silver B: Anesthesia in lid surgery. In Silver B (ed): Ophthalmic Plastic Surgery, 3rd ed, pp 53–62. Rochester, Minn, American Academy of Ophthalmology, 1977.
7. Tenzel RR, Hustead RF, Schietroma J, Hustead J: The best trick I learned this year. Presented at the Seventh Annual Scientific Symposium of the American Society of Plastic and Reconstructive Surgeons, New Orleans, November 8, 1986.
8. Dolman P, Yuen V-H: Comparison of full-strength, dilute, and buffered lidocaine with epinephrine for eyelid anesthesia. Presented at the 27th Annual Scientific Symposium of the American Society of Plastic and Reconstructive Surgeons, Chicago, October 26, 1996.
9. Baker TJ, Gordon HL: Midazolam (Versed) in ambulatory surgery. Plast Reconstr Surg 1988; 82:244.
10. Epstein GA: Anesthesia in ophthalmic plastic surgery. In Hornblass A (ed): Oculoplastic, Orbital, and Reconstructive Surgery, vol 1 (Eyelids), pp 42–51. Baltimore, William & Wilkins, 1988.

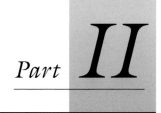

UPPER EYELID
TECHNIQUES

Allen M. Putterman

Chapter 9

Treatment of Upper Eyelid Dermatochalasis and Orbital Fat: Skin Flap Approach

Upper eyelid dermatochalasis and herniated orbital fat occasionally are treated by excision of the excess skin and prolapsed fat without excision of orbicularis oculi muscle and without reconstruction of the crease. This is especially useful in older individuals with skin hanging over their eyelid margins who seek a functional improvement in vision but do not have much concern for cosmesis.

In this chapter, I describe and illustrate the steps of the surgical techniques I use to remove redundant skin and herniated orbital fat. Additionally, the W-plasty and triangular skin excision techniques used to treat excess medial canthal and nasal upper eyelid skin are described and illustrated.

I have found that most of my patients have ill-defined, duplicated, or low upper eyelid creases. Therefore, I treat upper eyelid dermatochalasis and herniated fat in about 95 per cent of my patients by excising upper eyelid skin, orbicularis muscle, and herniated orbital fat and by reconstructing the upper eyelid crease (see Chapter 10). The skin flap approach described in this chapter is used in about 5 per cent of the upper blepharoplasties that I perform.

ALLEN M. PUTTERMAN

EXCISION OF UPPER EYELID SKIN AND ORBITAL FAT

Upper eyelid dermatochalasis (excess skin) and herniation of orbital fat are occasionally treated surgically without excision of orbicularis muscle and without crease reconstruction (Fig. 9–1*A*). This procedure is performed mainly for functional reasons to improve vision that is hindered by skin hooding the upper eyelid margin like an awning, but occasionally it is done to improve appearance. It is an easy technique for surgeons performing their first blepharoplasties.

Preparation for Surgery

The patient's entire face is prepared with povidone-iodine (Betadine) soap and paint. The patient is draped so that the entire face is exposed. Topical tetracaine is applied over each eye. A scleral contact lens is placed over the eye and under the eyelids to protect the eye from foreign objects, to prevent the operating lights from bothering the patient, and to avoid causing the patient distress from seeing the procedure being performed.

Skin Marking

The surgeon uses a marking pen to outline excess upper eyelid skin. If the lower eyelid is also being treated surgically, a lateral canthal line is drawn on the lower eyelid first to ensure at least 5 mm of skin between the

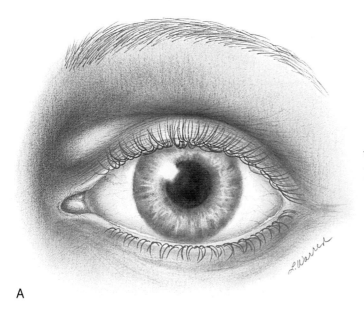

A, Upper eyelid with dermatochalasis (excess skin) and nasal herniated orbital fat before excision.

A

upper and lower lateral canthal incisions (Fig. 9–1*B*). This line starts about 2–3 mm temporal to the lateral canthus and travels in a horizontal but slightly downward direction for a total of 1–1.5 cm.

The upper lid fold is elevated with the surgeon's finger, and the patient is instructed to gaze slightly upward. A line is drawn where the lid creases with this maneuver (Figs. 9–1*C* and *D*). The line begins nasally above the upper punctum, extends to the lateral canthus, and then slopes slightly upward in one of the lateral canthal creases, about 1–1.5 cm beyond the lateral canthus.

A smooth forceps is placed horizontally to grasp the skin at the central aspect of the marked line and is applied to the skin superiorly. The forceps is closed at various levels until the amount of skin pinched together eliminates all excess eyelid skin, everts the lashes, and minimally elevates the upper lid from its apposition to

the lower lid (Fig. 9-1*E*). A mark is made at this superior site. The procedure is repeated nasally and temporally. The surgeon uses a marking pen to connect the central, nasal, and temporal superior lines with the nasal and temporal ends of the eyelid crease line (Fig. 9–1*F*).

The other upper eyelid is marked in a similar manner, and the amount of excess skin outlined is compared with that outlined on the first upper lid. Measurements are made from the upper eyelid margins to the lid crease lines and between the upper and lower marked lines. These measurements should be similar if the amounts of skin fold noted preoperatively were the same. Otherwise, differences in measurement should correspond to the preoperative asymmetry. For example, if the left upper eyelid fold is more redundant or the left eyebrow is more ptotic than the right, a slightly greater outlined ellipse of skin is expected on the left upper lid than the right.

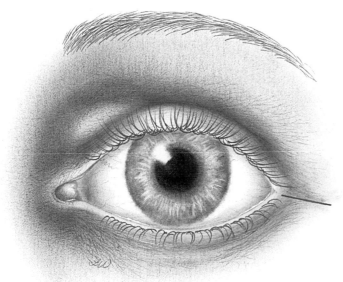

B, A line 1–1.5 cm is drawn with a marking pen over the lateral canthal lower eyelid incision site. The line begins 2–3 mm temporal to the lateral canthus and extends 1–1.5 cm in a horizontal but slightly downward direction.

B

C, The upper eyelid skin fold is elevated by raising the eyebrow and with a marking pen indicating the upper eyelid crease site. This begins above the punctum and extends 1–1.5 cm beyond the lateral canthus in one of the natural lateral canthal creases. The distance from the lower eyelid lateral canthal mark to the upper eyelid mark should be at least 5 mm.

5 mm

C

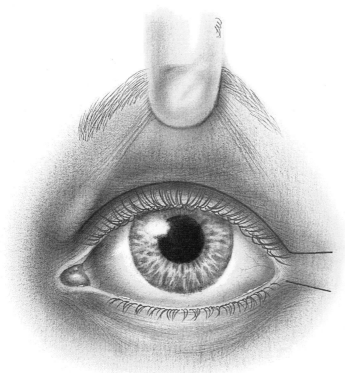

D, When the patient looks slightly upward, the marked line on the upper lid should fall into the upper eyelid crease that forms on slight up gaze.

D

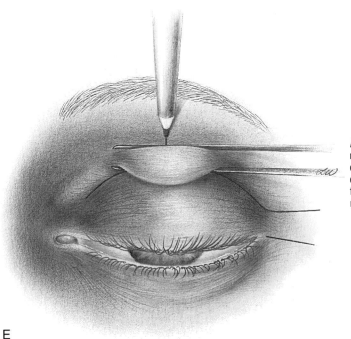

E, One blade of a smooth forceps is used to grasp the center marked line, and the other blade is used to grasp the skin superiorly. The forceps is reapplied until all redundant upper eyelid skin is eliminated, the lashes evert, and the upper eyelid is elevated slightly from its closed position when the forceps blades meet. A mark is made centrally at the site of the upper forceps blade in this position.

E

Skin Excision

Two per cent lidocaine with epinephrine, with or without hyaluronidase, is injected subcutaneously over the outlined upper eyelid and lateral canthus for anesthesia, hemostasis, and hydraulic dissection of skin from orbicularis muscle. A No. 15 Bard-Parker blade is used to incise along the upper eyelid marks in a nasal to temporal direction, first over the lower line and then over the upper line.

Next, the skin is severed from orbicularis muscle with Westcott scissors (Fig. 9–1*G*). The assistant puts the upper eyelid skin on stretch by pulling upward on the brow and downward on the upper lid margins. The surgeon finds the plane between skin and orbicularis muscle by observing the points of the scissors beneath the translucent skin. (The upper eyelid skin is the thinnest in the body, and the scissors blades should be easily seen beneath it. Also, the operating light shining through the thin skin should be readily seen and will facilitate the skin-orbicularis dissection.)

A disposable cautery (Solan Accu-Temp, Xomed Sur-

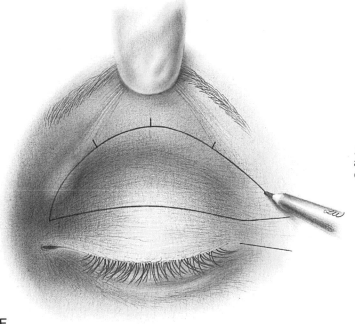

F, The central, temporal, and nasal superior marks are connected and then are extended to the nasal and temporal extremes of the eyelid crease line.

F

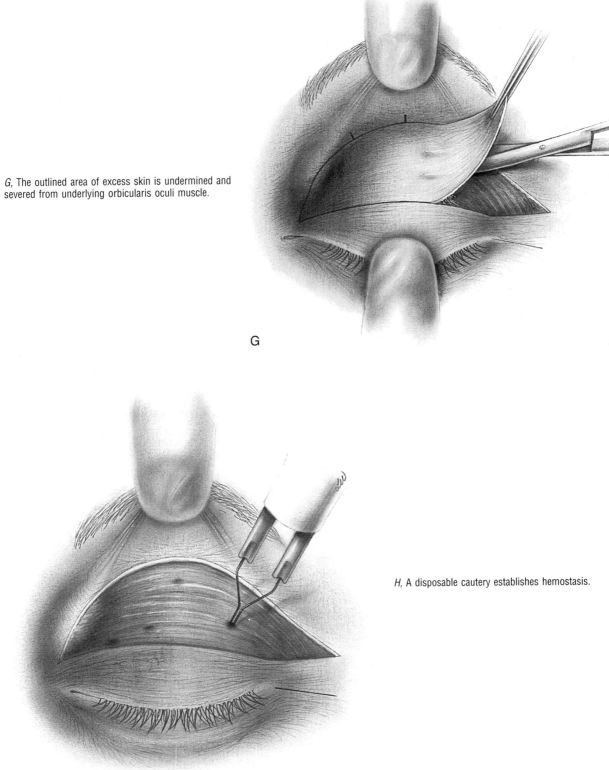

G, The outlined area of excess skin is undermined and severed from underlying orbicularis oculi muscle.

G

H, A disposable cautery establishes hemostasis.

H

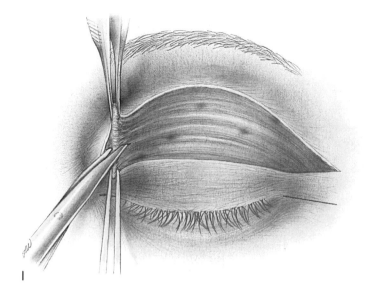

I, A forceps grasps the nasal orbicularis oculi muscle. As one forceps pulls the orbicularis directly downward, the superior forceps pulls upward and outward. The orbicularis muscle tented with this maneuver is cut with a Westcott scissors that is directed inward and slightly upward. This should allow entrance into space beneath the orbicularis muscle, where herniated orbital fat is located.

gical Products, Jacksonville, Fla.) is used to control bleeding (Fig. 9–1*H*) and can also be used for dissecting skin from orbicularis muscle.

Excision of Orbital Fat

Any herniated fat noted preoperatively is removed next. Usually, nasal orbital fat (which is white) is herniated; at times, however, the middle fat (which is yellow) is also displaced. (There is no temporal fat in the upper eyelid. A protrusion in this area is usually caused by a prolapsed lacrimal gland and should be handled as noted in Chapter 17.)

Slight pressure is applied to the globe, and the nasal

orbicularis muscle is observed for tenting by the herniated fat. The orbicularis muscle at this site is picked up with forceps and pulled upward and outward, away from the globe. Using forceps, the assistant grasps the muscle close to the crease incision and pulls the eyelid downward. The surgeon severs the orbicularis muscle between the two forceps with a Westcott scissors that is directed slightly upward and inward (Fig. 9–1*I*). This maneuver pulls the orbicularis away from the levator aponeurosis. Severing the orbicularis muscle in this manner creates a space between it and levator aponeurosis that should be easily seen at this time. Herniated orbital fat should be observed in this potential space.

Pressure is applied to the globe, and fat protruding through the opening in the orbicularis is noted. The fat

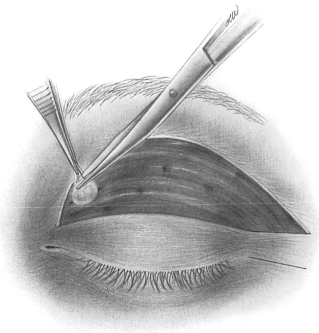

J, The nasal herniated orbital fat capsule is grasped with forceps and severed.

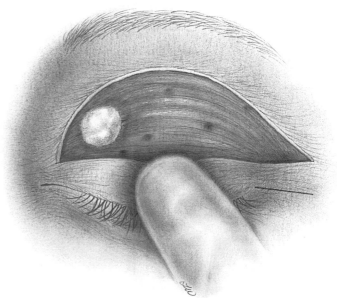

K, Pressure is applied to the globe through the upper eyelid to determine the amount of fat that herniates with gentle pressure.

K

capsule is grasped with forceps and severed (Fig. 9–1*J*). Pressure is again applied to the globe, and fat should now flow through the orbicularis opening (Fig. 9–1*K*). The fat that protrudes easily with gentle pressure on the globe is grasped with forceps and pulled outward from the wound. It is important not to pull too vigorously on the fat because the anterior nasal orbital fat communicates with the posterior orbital fat, through which the ophthalmic and ciliary arteries may pass. Undue tension on these vessels may lead to blindness.

The protruding fat is clamped with a straight hemostat and severed by slicing with a Bard-Parker blade against the hemostat (Fig. 9–1*L*). The surgeon should inspect the hemostat before applying it to make sure that the jaws meet completely when closed. If they do not, the fat can slip out of the hemostat, leading to

serious bleeding that is difficult to control and has the potential to cause blindness.

Hemostasis is achieved with a Bovie cautery applied to the hemostat. The surgeon chooses a medium setting on the Bovie cautery to cauterize adequately without charring the tissue. The hemostat is held away from other eyelid tissues with cotton-tipped applicators (Fig. 9–1*M*).

The fat beneath the hemostat is grasped with a forceps, and the hemostat is released. The surgeon inspects the severed fat for bleeding before allowing it to retract into the orbit (Fig. 9–1*N*). Any bleeding is treated with a disposable cautery (Solan Accu-Temp) applied to the severed end of the orbital fat until the bleeding is controlled.

Any herniated midorbital fat noted preoperatively is

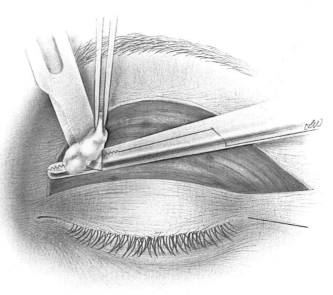

L, Nasal orbital fat that prolapses with gentle pressure is clamped with a hemostat and excised by running a No. 15 Bard-Parker blade along the edge of the hemostat.

L

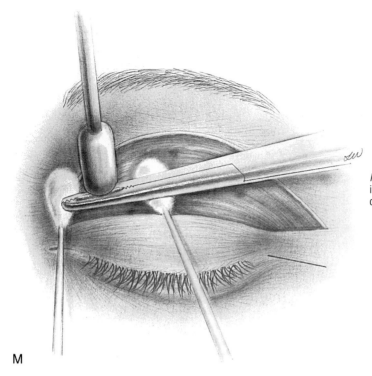

M, Cotton-tipped applicators separate the hemostat from underlying eyelid tissue, and a Bovie cautery is applied to the hemostat to cauterize the excised nasal orbital fat stump.

M

removed in a similar fashion through the same orbicularis opening. Occasionally, an orbicularis incision slightly temporal to the nasal site is necessary to isolate midorbital fat.

Care must be taken to avoid pulling the levator aponeurosis into the hemostat clamped with the orbital fat. The tissue beneath the hemostat should be inspected carefully to make sure that it is fat and not levator aponeurosis before it is severed.

The same procedure is followed for the other eyelid.

Skin Closure

The skin incisions are sutured closed with continuous 6-0 black silk in multiple close bites that are pulled

snugly during closure (Fig. 9–1*O*). Usually, I start this closure approximately 2 mm temporal to the nasal end of the incision to avoid nasal skin puckering. Also, I place 2–3 interrupted 6-0 polyglactin (Vicryl) sutures at intervals across the eyelids.

I prefer to use running continuous 6-0 black silk through the upper eyelid wound. This suture is easier to work with than the stiffer nylon or polypropylene (Prolene) sutures. However, suture cysts are a common complication that will require hydrolysis at a later date. These cysts presumably can be avoided if other sutures are used.

Alternative sutures include the continuous 6-0 polypropylene suture and a subcuticular suture of 6-0 nylon. However, I have found nylon sutures difficult to remove, and their difficult removal can cause wound de-

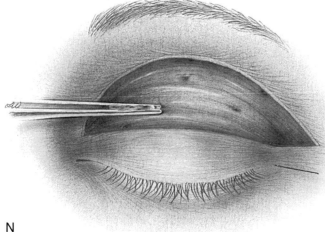

N, A forceps is used to hold the nasal herniated orbital fat stump after the release of the hemostat while the surgeon checks that hemostasis has been achieved before allowing the fat to slip back into the orbit.

N

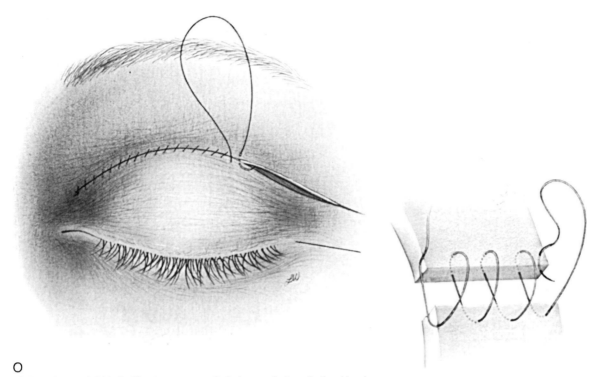

O

O, A continuous 6-0 black silk suture runs nasally to temporally to unite the skin edges.

hiscence, even 10–14 days postoperatively. Use of a 6-0 plain catgut fast-absorbing suture eliminates the discomfort of suture removal. The dissolution of this suture, however, is unpredictable, and I believe that it can cause more scarring than do the nonabsorbable sutures. Although polyglactin and 6-0 polyglycolic acid (Dexon) sutures also dissolve with minimum reaction, the process takes 4–6 weeks and a good deal of scarring can be created in that time.

Another alternative is to use interrupted 6-0 black silk or nylon sutures and remove them by pulling them out rather than by cutting them from the skin. This procedure prevents suture cysts and tunnels because the outer surface of any cyst or tunnel is pulled off with this technique. I find that this maneuver lacks surgical finesse, and I prefer to perform hydrolysis of the cysts postoperatively.

W-PLASTY AND TRIANGULAR EXCISION FOR MEDIAL DERMATOCHALASIS

If there is a moderate amount of medial canthal skin, a W-plasty is performed medially. Instead of ending in a point medially, the upper and lower lines are connected together as a W (Fig. 9–2*A*). When closed, the central triangle of the W is pulled temporally to eliminate nasal dermatochalasis (Fig. 9–2*B* and *C*).

Another technique for eliminating redundant medial canthal skin is to remove a triangle of tissue above the nasal skin resection site. I prefer this technique. It is especially useful if an ellipse of upper eyelid skin has already been removed, thereby making a W-plasty impossible.

In the nasal triangle technique, a superior nasal cut is made about 8–10 mm from the nasal skin resection ellipse (Fig. 9–3*A*). The skin nasal to this cut is undermined, and the flap is pulled temporally to create slight tension (Fig. 9–3*B*). The place where the overlapped flap meets the underlying skin edge determines the site at which this triangular skin flap is excised. Suturing this area together reduces excess medial canthal skin (Fig. 9–3*C*). It is unwise to create incisions nasal to the punctum to eliminate excess nasal skin because webs at the canthal folds and excessive scarring may be produced. I prefer the triangular skin resection to the W-plasty to reduce medial canthal skin.

POSTOPERATIVE CARE

No dressings are used after surgery. The patient is instructed to apply ice-cold compresses on the eyelids. Pads 4 × 4 inches, soaked in a bucket of saline and ice, are applied with slight pressure to the lids. When the pads become warm, they are dipped again into the saline and ice and reapplied. This process is repeated for 24 hours. The applications should be fairly constant for the first few postoperative hours. After that, the compresses are applied for about 20 minutes with 15-minute rest periods in between until bedtime. The applications are resumed on awakening.

To reduce edema postoperatively, the patient lies in bed with the head approximately 45 degrees higher than the rest of the body. Nurses should check for bleeding associated with proptosis, pain, or loss of vision every 15 minutes for the first 3 hours postoperatively or until the patient leaves the surgical facility. Every hour there-

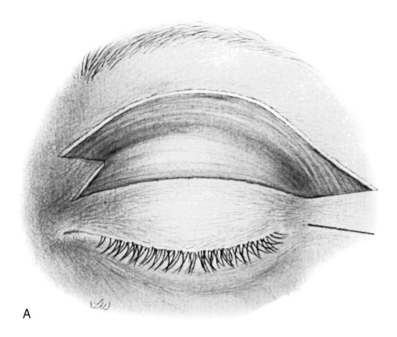

A

figure 9–2
Treatment of nasal upper eyelid excessive skin with W-plasty. *A,* A W-incision is made at the nasal aspect of the upper eyelid skin resection site.

B, A 6–0 black silk suture passes through skin edges approximately 5–8 mm temporal to the passage through the subcutaneous apex of the W-incision.

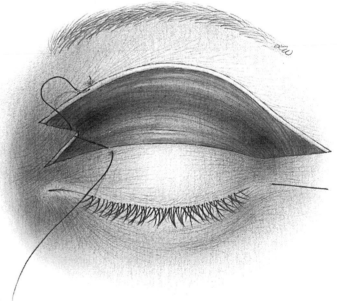

B

C, The 6–0 black silk suture depicted in *B* is tied so that the apex of the W is drawn temporally to reduce medial canthal skin. Several interrupted 6-0 black silk sutures are used to close the upper and lower limbs of the triangular incision sites.

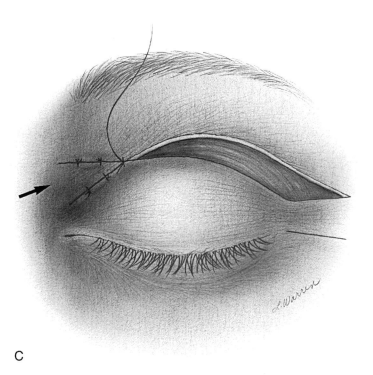

C

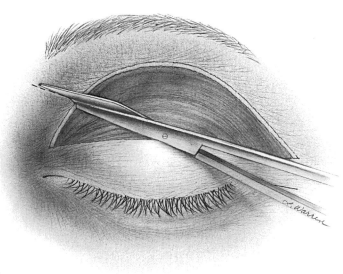

A

figure 9–3

Nasal triangle technique to treat upper eyelid nasal dermatochalasis. *A,* The scissors is used to sever the skin in a superonasal direction, approximately 8–10 mm from the nasal end of the upper eyelid skin resection site, for a distance of approximately 10 mm.

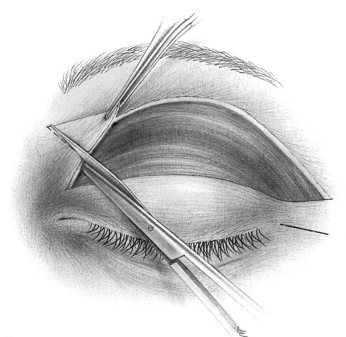

B, The skin flap is drawn temporally and superiorly in the area of excessive skin to the degree needed to reduce medial canthal dermatochalasis. The triangle overlapping the underlying skin incision site is excised.

B

C, Closure of the superonasal incision pulls the excess medial canthal skin temporally and eliminates it.

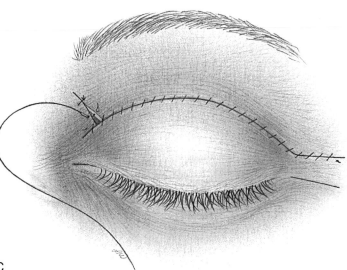

C

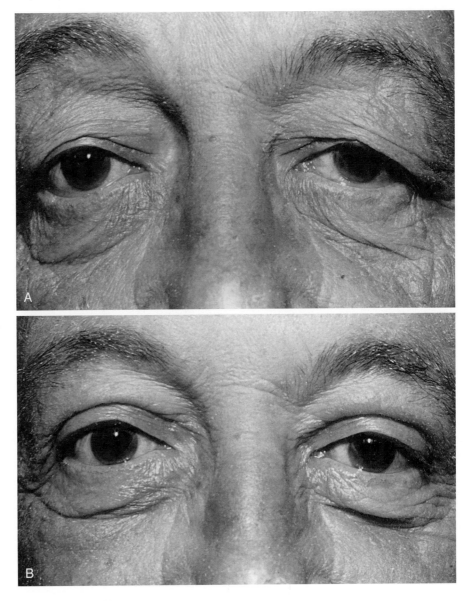

figure 9–4

A, Preoperative photograph of patient with dermatochalasis and herniated orbital fat of upper eyelids. *B*, Postoperative photograph of the same patient after excision of excess skin and herniated orbital fat.

after until bedtime, the family or patient should monitor the patient's ability to count fingers and should check for unusual proptosis and pain. If the patient cannot count fingers or has proptosis or pain, the family should take him or her to an emergency room. If loss of vision occurs secondary to retrobulbar hemorrhage, it can be detected quickly and treated by opening the incision involved.[1]

The 6-0 black silk skin sutures are removed 4 days postoperatively. The 6-0 polyglactin sutures are removed 3 weeks postoperatively if they have not dissolved. The incision is supported with ¼-inch sterile tape (Steri-strips) applied over weak areas, usually the lateral upper and lower canthal incision sites, for 3 more days.

COMPLICATIONS

In approximately 80 per cent of my patients, suture cysts have occurred, ranging from one to 15 per patient, with

an average of seven. These have been treated with light hydrolysis about 2 months postoperatively.

RESULTS

I have performed this procedure in more than 700 upper eyelids with satisfactory results (Fig. 9–4). It has been necessary to remove more skin in approximately 10 patients. No patient has experienced secondary ptosis or lagophthalmos.

Reference

1. Putterman AM: Temporary blindness after cosmetic blepharoplasty. Am J Ophthalmol 1975; 80:1081–1083.

Chapter 10

Treatment of Upper Eyelid Dermatochalasis with Reconstruction of Upper Eyelid Crease: Skin-Muscle Flap Approach

I treat only about 5 per cent of my patients with dermatochalasis (excess skin) and herniated orbital fat of the upper eyelid by performing an upper eyelid blepharoplasty with skin resection alone. In 95 per cent of patients, I perform a skin and orbicularis oculi muscle resection and reconstruction of the eyelid crease.

The skin-muscle resection with crease reconstruction allows less skin to be removed and thereby decreases lagophthalmos (incomplete eyelid closure), which is especially important in patients with low basic tear secretion. Also, I find that most patients with upper eyelid dermatochalasis have ill-defined eyelid creases and eyelash ptosis (inversion of lashes), and reconstructing the creases helps these problems also. This approach also allows for resection of orbicularis muscle, which might be redundant if skin is removed alone. Finally, it provides access for other procedures, such as redepositing a lacrimal gland, performing an internal brow lift, and performing levator aponeurosis resection-ptosis surgery.

ALLEN M. PUTTERMAN

There are three methods of removing upper eyelid skin and orbital fat:

The simplest upper blepharoplasty method involves removal of upper eyelid skin without the orbicularis muscle, with or without nasal herniated orbital fat (see Chapter 9). This procedure, however, neither alters the position of the eyelid crease nor tightens loose skin between the eyelid margin and eyelid crease. It also leaves redundant orbicularis muscle. The technique is most useful in patients who have a functional loss of vision as a result of extra skin hanging over the eyelid margins.

The second method consists of excising excess skin and orbicularis muscle of the upper eyelid, with or without orbital fat resection, but with no attempt at crease formation. This technique is useful in reducing the bulk of orbicularis muscle as well as excess skin. At times, this method also leads to the formation of an eyelid crease that is higher than before surgery and it may also tighten the skin between the eyelid margin and fold. This method is useful in patients with excess upper eyelid skin, orbicularis muscle, and orbital fat who have close-to-normal upper eyelid creases.

The third method consists of excising skin, orbicularis muscle, and herniated fat and reconstructing the upper eyelid crease. I believe that this method gives the best results in most patients. It also leads to the greatest reduction of the upper eyelid skin fold with the least amount of resection. Redeposition of the lacrimal gland, an internal brow lift, and a levator aponeurosis advancement or resection-ptosis procedure can be easily combined with this approach.

PREPARATION FOR SURGERY

The patient's entire face is prepared with povidone-iodine (Betadine) soap and paint. The patient is draped so that the entire face is exposed. Topical tetracaine is applied over each eye. A scleral contact lens is placed over the eye and under the eyelids.

SURGICAL TECHNIQUE

Skin Marking

A line is drawn with a methylene blue marking pen, beginning at the lateral canthus and extending in a horizontal direction of approximately 1 cm. This line marks the site of the lower lateral canthal incision. The site of the predetermined eyelid crease is then marked. When the surgeon is drawing the eyelid crease marks, the eyebrow must be elevated to reduce the excess upper eyelid skin fold and to make the upper eyelid skin taut and the lashes slightly everted. If this is not done, the crease may result in being much higher than desired because the skin is usually loose before it is marked.

The temporal, central, and nasal crease sites are marked by placing a millimeter ruler so that the zero line is at the eyelid margin. The distances above the eyelid margin can then be viewed and marked with a specially designed marking instrument. In women, the temporal mark usually is placed 10 mm above the upper eyelid margin; the central mark, 11 mm above the margin; and the nasal mark, 9 mm above the margin. In men, the marks are usually 9 mm temporally, 10 mm centrally, and 8 mm nasally.

The temporal, central, and nasal marks are then connected and are extended with a line, which begins at the punctum and ends at the lateral canthus (Fig. 10–1*A*). The line sweeps laterally approximately 1 cm temporal to the lateral canthus in a slightly upward direction. There should be at least 5 mm of skin between this line and the line placed for the lower lateral incision.

A smooth forceps is used to grasp the crease line at the center of the eyelid with one blade. The other blade is used to pinch upper eyelid skin at various positions until, when the forceps is closed, all the redundant upper eyelid skin is eliminated and there is no eversion of the lashes and no lifting of the eyelid from its apposition to the lower eyelid margin (Fig. 10–1*B*).

Once this position is determined, a dot is made with the marking pen at the top blade of the forceps. Similar marks are made nasally and temporally after the amounts of extra skin are determined in these positions. The three superior dots are connected and joined with the nasal and temporal ends of the eyelid crease line (Fig. 10–1*C*). The opposite eyelid is marked in the same manner. To ensure symmetry, the surgeon then com-

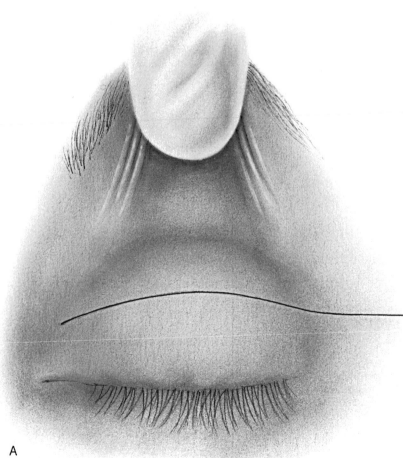

figure 10–1

A, A line is drawn on the eyelid at the level of the eyelid crease.

A

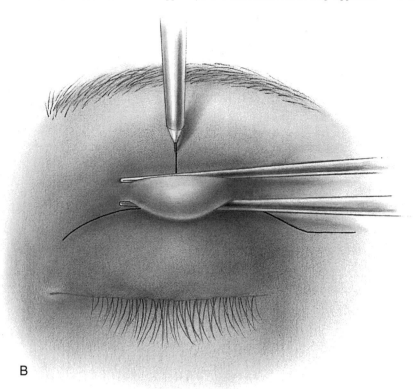

B, A smooth forceps is used to eliminate redundant upper eyelid skin and to slightly evert the eyelashes.

B

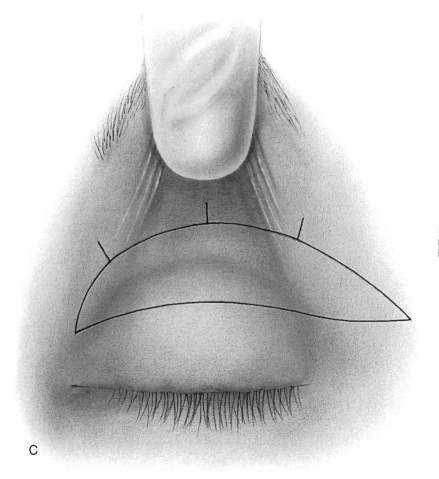

C, Connection of superiorly marked dots to the nasal and temporal ends of the eyelid crease incision line.

C

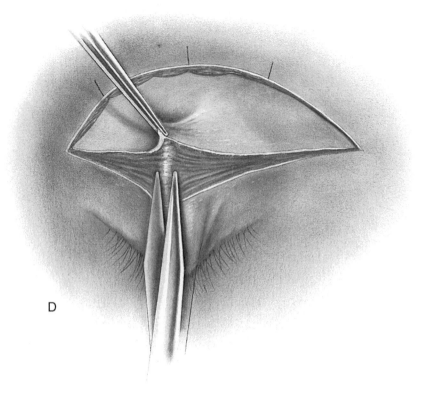

D

D, A blunt Westcott scissors is used to make a buttonhole incision in the orbicularis oculi muscle.

pares the measurements of the eyelid crease and the amount of skin to be excised temporally, nasally, and centrally in the two eyelids.

Skin-Muscle Excision

Several milliliters of 2 per cent lidocaine (Xylocaine) with epinephrine is injected subcutaneously in the areas of the marked ellipse as well as between the upper eyelid margin and eyelid crease across the eyelid.

A No. 15 Bard-Parker blade is used to make an incision through skin at the marked lines. A 4-0 black silk traction suture is placed through skin, orbicularis muscle, and superficial tarsus at the center of the upper eyelid just above the eyelid margin. Approximately 12.5 cm of suture is left on each arm, and a knot is tied at this end. The traction suture is used to pull the upper eyelid straight downward while a toothed forceps is used to grasp the upper eyelid centrally just above the crease incision and to pull upward and outward.

A blunt Westcott scissors is used to make a buttonhole incision in orbicularis muscle and to sever central orbicularis muscle at the skin crease level (Fig. 10–1*D*). With the scissors directed superiorly and inward, the orbicularis muscle can be penetrated and the suborbicularis space entered without injury to the levator aponeurosis and other important eyelid structures. This maneuver is possible because the orbicularis muscle is firmly attached to skin, whereas the orbital septum, levator aponeurosis, Müller's muscle, and conjunctiva stay deep surrounding the globe.

The orbicularis muscle is then undermined temporally and nasally at the site of the eyelid crease while the surgeon keeps the eyelid in the same position with the traction suture and forceps. The orbicularis muscle is severed along the incision site of the eyelid skin crease with the use of a disposable cautery (Fig. 10–1*E*), a Colorado needle, a sapphire-tipped scalpel neodymium:YAG (Nd:YAG), or a carbon dioxide (CO_2) ultrapulse laser. Each instrument coagulates blood vessels as it cuts through tissues (see Chapters 35 and 36).[1]

When this has been accomplished, the surgeon should be able to view the levator aponeurosis. At times, orbital septum is in the way and must be identified with the use of a forceps. The orbicularis muscle at the superior skin incision site is then severed with a disposable cautery (Fig. 10–1*F*), Colorado needle, or the Nd:YAG or CO_2 ultrapulse laser. Thereby, an ellipse of skin and orbicularis muscle is excised with simultaneous cauterization of blood vessels.

Isolation and Excision of Orbital Fat

The septum is pulled upward and outward. Then the Westcott scissors, a disposable cautery, Colorado needle, or Nd:YAG or CO_2 ultrapulse laser is used to penetrate orbital septum and suborbicularis tissue just beneath the orbital septal rim until herniated orbital fat is visible (Fig. 10–1*G*).

The orbital septum and suborbicularis fascia are opened from the nasal to temporal aspect of the eyelid; when this is accomplished, the surgeon should see nasal, central, and, at times, central-temporal herniated orbital fat pads. Usually, the nasal fat is white, whereas the central and central-temporal fat is yellow and very loose. Bleeding is controlled with the cautery.

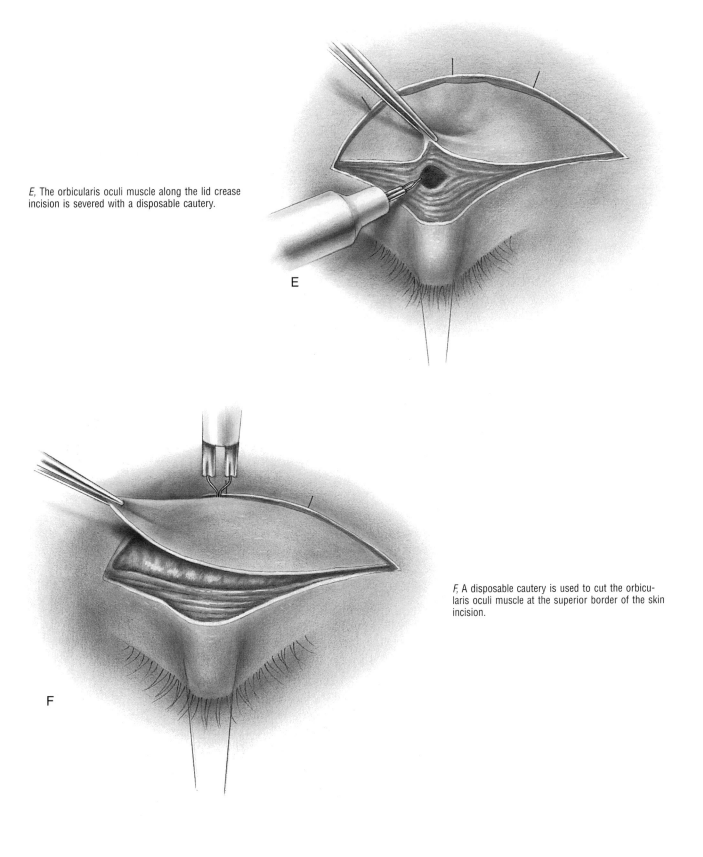

E, The orbicularis oculi muscle along the lid crease incision is severed with a disposable cautery.

F, A disposable cautery is used to cut the orbicularis oculi muscle at the superior border of the skin incision.

E

F

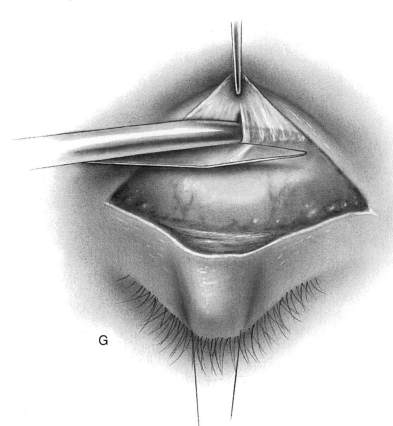

G, The orbital septum and suborbicularis tissue are penetrated with Westcott scissors just beneath the orbital septal rim until herniated orbital fat is visible.

G

H, The central fat pocket is removed.

H

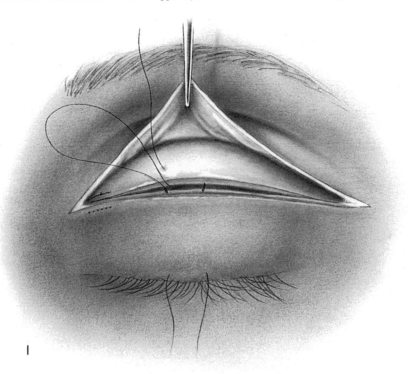

I, A 6-0 polyester fiber (Mersilene) suture enters the superior surface of the levator aponeurosis and exits through the inferior surface. Then the suture passes through the orbicularis oculi muscle.

I

The capsule over the nasal fat pad is then penetrated with Westcott scissors. The eye is pushed on through the upper eyelid, and the nasal fat that herniates upon gentle pressure applied to the eye is grasped with a straight forceps. With a No. 15 Bard-Parker blade, the surgeon severs the fat along the hemostat. Cotton-tipped applicators are placed under the hemostat, and a Bovie cautery is applied to the hemostat to coagulate any vessels with the fat pad. A forceps is used to grasp the fat beneath the hemostat as the hemostat is released. This gives the surgeon a chance to inspect the fat stump for any residual bleeding before it is allowed to retract into the orbit. An alternative is to remove the herniated orbital fat with a laser (see Chapters 35 and 36).

The central and central-temporal fat pads are removed in a similar manner (Fig. 10–1*H*). If an internal brow lift or levator aponeurosis advancement or resection is contemplated, it is performed at this time (see Chapters 12 and 13).

There is no fat at the temporal extreme of the upper eyelid. If the surgeon sees prolapse of tissue at this position, it is most likely a prolapsed lacrimal gland rather than orbital fat. If a prolapsed lacrimal gland is seen, it is treated by redepositing of the gland in the

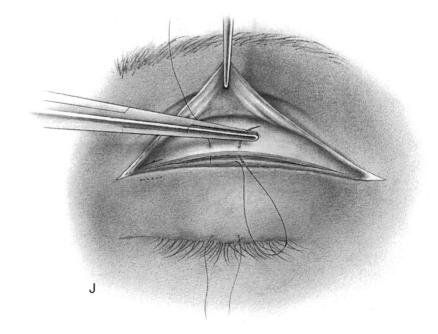

J, The 6-0 polyester fiber suture passes through the levator aponeurosis inferiorly to superiorly.

J

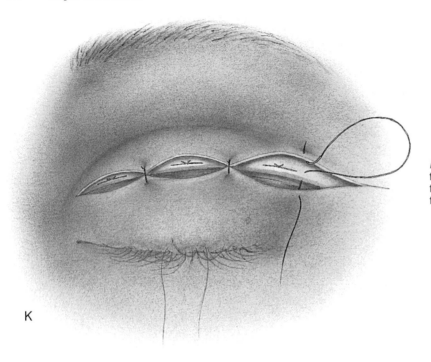

K

K, Three 6-0 polyglactin (Vicryl) sutures are passed through skin, levator aponeurosis, and skin centrally, temporally, and nasally to further establish the eyelid crease.

lacrimal fossa rather than by excision, which can cause a dry eye (see Chapter 17).

Reconstruction of Eyelid Crease

The upper eyelid crease is formed by placing four 6-0 white polyester fiber (Mersilene) sutures to connect orbicularis muscle with the levator aponeurosis. These are placed in the nasal, temporal, central temporal, and central nasal positions. Two toothed forceps are used to grasp the skin at the eyelid crease position, and the skin is pulled to the extent that skin between the lashes and

the crease is taut and the lashes are slightly everted. The surgeon notes the position at which the skin overlaps the levator aponeurosis. This determines the position to suture orbicularis muscle to the levator aponeurosis in order to form the eyelid crease. The 6-0 polyester fiber suture is first passed through the levator aponeurosis superiorly to inferiorly. The suture is then passed nasally to temporally through adjacent orbicularis muscle of the lower skin flap (Fig. 10–1*I*).

The suture is next passed through the levator aponeurosis inferiorly to superiorly (Fig. 10–1*J*). When the suture is drawn up and tied with four knots, the orbicularis muscle of the lower skin flap will unite with the

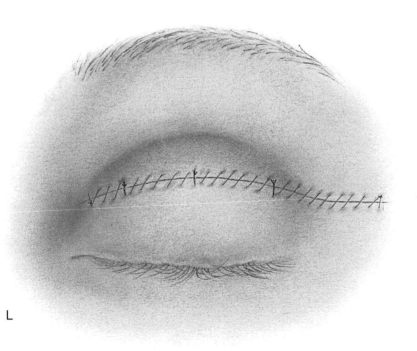

L

L, The eyelid skin is united with a continuous 6-0 black silk running suture, which is passed nasally to temporally.

levator aponeurosis to form a crease at this position. The surgeon should measure the distance between the eyelid margin and the site of the suture to make sure that it is at the desired level.

To further establish the eyelid crease (Fig. 10–1*K*), the surgeon then passes three 6-0 polyglactin (Vicryl) sutures through the skin, the levator aponeurosis, and the skin centrally, temporally, and nasally. Last, the skin is united with a continuous 6-0 black silk running suture, which is passed nasally to temporally (Fig. 10–1*L*).

POSTOPERATIVE CARE

For 3 hours postoperatively, the patient applies cold compresses to the eyelids. Ophthalmic signs are closely observed. The recovery room staff checks the patient every 15 minutes for the ability to count fingers and to make sure that there is no severe pain or proptosis. If the patient demonstrates either an inability to count fingers or proptosis or complains of severe pain, the surgeon is called immediately, because these problems may indicate a retrobulbar hemorrhage, which has the potential to cause blindness.

For 24 hours postoperatively, the patient or the patient's family continues to apply cold compresses to the eyelids and checks for the ability to count fingers every hour (other than during sleep). If the patient cannot count fingers or if there is severe pain or proptosis, he or she should immediately return to the surgical facility or other emergency facility for evaluation of a possible retrobulbar hemorrhage (see Chapters 37 and 38).

Four days postoperatively, the 6-0 black silk skin sutures are removed. The polyglactin sutures are usually removed 2–3 weeks postoperatively or are allowed to dissolve spontaneously.

SEQUELAE

Postoperative ecchymosis and edema of the eyelid are to be expected. Most patients think that their appearance is acceptable, and they are ready to go out in public a week after the procedure. When an upper eyelid crease has been formed, the patient experiences a slight amount of postoperative ptosis and has difficulty looking upward. These problems gradually resolve over the first 2 postoperative months. Some patients are emotionally depressed several weeks after surgery because their appearance is not back to normal, but this unhappiness commonly goes away at about 6 weeks after surgery. The appearance of the eyelids generally continues to improve over the course of 1 year after the operation.

Figure 10–2 shows the preoperative appearance and postoperative results in a patient who underwent upper eyelid surgery with the skin-muscle flap approach.

POSTOPERATIVE COMPLICATIONS

The main complication is asymmetry of the eyelid creases and folds. If this is noted postoperatively, the surgeon can make an adjustment by removing the polyglactin sutures from the eyelid in which the crease is too high. Slight asymmetry, however, usually resolves spontaneously over the first few months. If there are distinct differences between the eyes, further eyelid skin

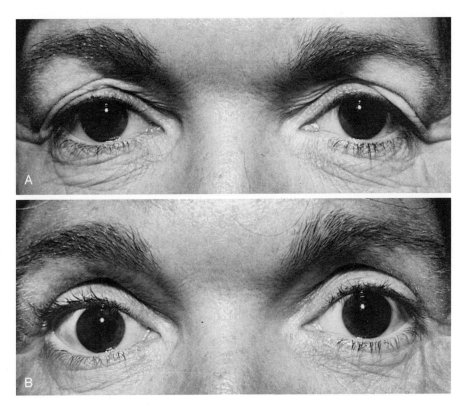

figure 10–2

A, Preoperative appearance of a patient with dermatochalasis (excess skin) of upper eyelid with ill-defined creases. *B,* Postoperative appearance after excision of upper eyelid skin, the orbicularis oculi muscle, and fat with crease reconstruction. The lower eyelids were also treated with external blepharoplasty.

can be removed or the crease can be placed at a higher level on the side that is too low (see Chapter 37).

Suture cysts are common and are believed to occur by healing beneath the skin where the sutures are in place. If these persist, they are removed 2 months postoperatively by light hydrolysis with a Birtcher hyfrecator.

Upper eyelid ptosis rarely occurs and can be treated by ptosis surgery.

A retrobulbar hemorrhage associated with loss of vision is treated by removal of the upper eyelid sutures and control of the hemorrhage.

RESULTS

I have performed upper eyelid blepharoplasty with crease reconstruction in more than 2000 patients, with a high rate of good results.

Reference

1. Putterman AM: Scalpel neodymium:YAG laser in oculoplastic surgery. Am J Ophthalmol 1990; 109:581–584.

William P. Chen

Chapter 11

Upper Blepharoplasty in the Asian Patient

Because the anatomy of the Asian eyelid differs from that of the Caucasian eyelid, I believe that a separate chapter emphasizing the difference is important. In the first edition, I showed how to westernize, or occidentalize, the Asian appearance by constructing an eyelid crease similar to the technique used in Caucasians. It later became apparent that most Asians would like to enhance their appearance by having a crease that conforms with Asian features, and this chapter was added to the second edition.

William Chen again describes the many variations in upper eyelid creases. He emphasizes that many Asians have what he refers to as a nasal tapering type of crease, in which the crease converges and tapers to the eyelid margin nasally, while other Asians possess a crease that is parallel to the eyelid margin. With a nasally tapered crease, it is important that the reconstructed upper eyelid crease extend to this inside nasal fold. Forming a parallel crease nasally in such a patient leads to a duplicated nasal crease and, frequently, to an unhappy patient.

Dr. Chen also emphasizes removal of a small amount of preaponeurotic fat and pretarsal tissue. He creates an eyelid crease by suturing skin to the levator aponeurosis along the superior tarsal border, at 6.5–8.5 mm above the eyelid margin (10–11 mm in a Caucasian). I vary my technique slightly by excising the superior pretarsal tissues and by passing sutures through tarsus and then the levator aponeurosis and skin. I also have the patient sit up on the operating table to make sure that the creases are forming in the desired positions.

ALLEN M. PUTTERMAN

A review of the medical literature published in English reveals more than 25 major articles describing upper eyelid surgery in Asians. Most of the articles describe the technique of construction of an upper eyelid crease in a patient without the crease. Authors of some of the earlier reports aimed to westernize the patient's appearance, whereas other authors insisted on creating a crease alone and preserving the Asian features.

In this chapter, before I review the steps of upper eyelid blepharoplasty in Asians, I explain the basic difference between Asians and Caucasians with respect to ethnic differences in eyelid creases, anatomy of the face and upper eyelids, and psychological and aesthetic needs of the patient.

ETHNIC DIFFERENCES

Depending on the study and the population sampled, approximately 50 per cent of the Asian population have upper eyelid creases (including Chinese, Koreans, and Japanese—all descendants of the Han race). The remaining 50 per cent are not born with an eyelid crease or may have only rudiments of a crease. Asians who do not have an eyelid crease have been described as having "single eyelids." Those with a distinctive crease ("double eyelids") appear to have two segments of eyelid skin between the eyebrow and the eyelashes. The upper eyelid crease seems to be present in most Caucasians. A person with an eyelid crease appears to have a wider palpebral fissure or a bigger eye than a person without an eyelid crease, even though the physical dimensions of the palpebral fissures are the same.

PSYCHOLOGICAL AND AESTHETIC NEEDS

The desire of some Asian women to have an eyelid crease surgically formed as a way to beautify themselves (i.e., to have "bigger" eyes) is sometimes perceived as an attempt to westernize (occidentalize) their appearance. In my opinion, most of the individuals who want to have an eyelid crease placed do not like the idea of appearing Caucasian, although they are well aware that western surgical techniques make this cosmetic change possible. Some people argue that because very few of these operations were performed until after World War II, it must be the influence of Westerners that catalyzed this enthusiasm for placement of an upper eyelid crease in Asians. From my extensive travels in Asia, it is my perception that the concept of beauty reaches even the most remote area and that the desire for "double eyelids" did not start just in the last 60 years. These patients need only to be aware that such surgical procedures are available without necessarily wanting to resemble Caucasians or even know what westernized means. Furthermore, I do not believe that Asian patients who live in the Western Hemisphere want to have the procedure so they can blend in with Caucasians.

ANATOMY

Upper Eyelids

The difference between the Asian and Caucasian eyelid lies at the lower point of fusion of the orbital septum with the levator aponeurosis.[1] In Caucasians (Fig. 11–1), the orbital septum fuses with the levator aponeurosis at approximately 8–10 mm above the superior tarsal border, limiting the downward extent of the preaponeurotic fat pads while allowing the terminal interdigitations of the aponeurosis to insert toward the subdermal surface of the pretarsal upper eyelid skin, starting along the superior tarsal border and heading inferiorly (see Chapter 7). As a result, when the levator muscle contracts and pulls the upper eyelid up, the skin forms a crease above the superior tarsal border and the skin above the crease forms the fold.

In Asians who do not have this crease (Fig. 11–2), as suggested by the anatomic studies of Doxanas and Anderson,[1] the point of attachment of the orbital septum to the levator aponeurosis is lower, frequently as low as the superior tarsal border. This position allows the preaponeurotic fat pads to be present at a lower point on the upper eyelid, giving it a fuller appearance, and prevents the terminal strands of the levator aponeurosis from attaching to the subdermal surface of the pretarsal upper eyelid skin. The result is an apparently puffier "single eyelid" without a crease (Fig. 11–3A).

In terms of fat distribution and compartments, Uchida[2] first described the presence of four areas of fat pads in Asian eyelids:

- Subcutaneous fat
- Pretarsal fat
- Central fat pads, which are more appropriately termed submuscular or preseptal fat pads
- Preaponeurotic fat pads, which he termed "orbital fat pads" (see Chapter 7)

Face

Onizuka and Iwanami[3] note that Asians, particularly Japanese, have a flat face and a head shape that is mesocephalic. The eyes tend not to be recessed deep in the orbit. These authors also find the lateral canthus to be 10 degrees superior to the medial canthus. They believe that creating an upper eyelid crease and removing any upper lid hooding would make the palpebral fissure appear wider and more open, which is aesthetically pleasing. I do not believe that all Asians have a lateral canthus 10 degrees above the medial canthus; however, certainly some of the other observations by these authors may be true.

Eyelid Crease

The configuration of the crease in the upper eyelids of Asians varies greatly. As I describe in other publications,[4–6] the crease may be absent in one eye (see Fig. 11–3A) and present in the other. It may be continuous (see Fig. 11–3B) or discontinuous (see Fig. 11–3C). The crease may be partial or incomplete (usually present from the medial canthal angle and then fading laterally) (see Fig. 11–3D), and there may be multiple creases on an eyelid (see Fig. 11–3E).

Individuals who have a continuously formed eyelid crease may have either the inside-fold (nasal tapering) type of crease (see Fig. 11–3F) or a crease that is more parallel to the ciliary margin from the medial canthus to the lateral canthus (see Fig. 11–3G). With the inside-fold type, the crease may start from the medial canthal angle and gently flare away from the eyelid margin as it reaches the lateral canthal region (lateral flare) (see Fig. 11–3F); less often, it may start in the medial canthal angle and run fairly parallel to the ciliary margin from the middle of the eyelid onward. Asians rarely have an eyelid crease with a semilunar shape, as in Caucasians, in whom either end of the crease is closer to the respective canthal angle than the central portion of the crease (see Fig. 11–3H).

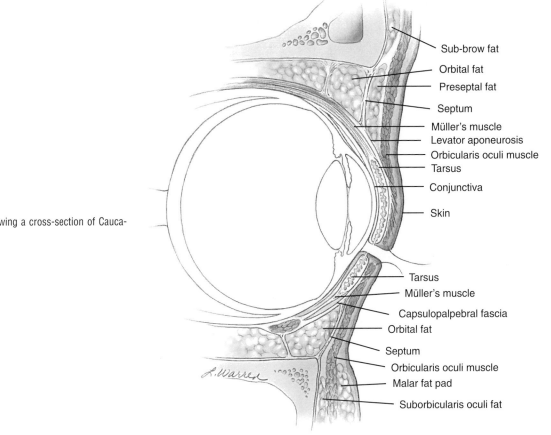

figure 11–1

Schematic drawing showing a cross-section of Caucasian upper eyelid.

Sub-brow fat
Orbital fat
Preseptal fat
Septum
Müller's muscle
Levator aponeurosis
Orbicularis oculi muscle
Tarsus
Conjunctiva
Skin

Tarsus
Müller's muscle
Capsulopalpebral fascia
Orbital fat
Septum
Orbicularis oculi muscle
Malar fat pad
Suborbicularis oculi fat

PREOPERATIVE COUNSELING

The shape of the crease is clearly an important factor for the surgeon to discuss with the patient before surgery. The patient will need to be informed of the desirability of either a nasally tapered crease or a parallel crease and the undesirability of a semilunar crease, which is truly a Caucasian crease and appears incongruous on the face of an Asian. The ultimate decision, of course, rests with the patient. None of my Asian patients, however, have chosen the semilunar crease after I explained to them the different crease configurations and their prevalence in Asians.

Most of the patients I encounter know what they want in terms of the crease configuration and its degree of prominence. They may be unaware, however, that swelling accompanies the procedure or that sutures are used. These are important points that need to be addressed with the patient preoperatively.[7]

SURGICAL TECHNIQUES

There are two approaches to the creation of an upper eyelid crease: (1) conjunctival suturing and (2) external incision. The champions of the conjunctival suturing technique include Mutou and Mutou,[8] Boo-Chai,[9] and some of the surgeons in Japan. The advantage is that it

is a relatively noninvasive technique. The major drawback is that the crease may disappear with time.

Early proponents of the external incision approach include Sayoc[10–15] and Fernandez.[16] This technique is preferred in the Western Hemisphere and is also practiced in Taiwan and Hong Kong.

Conjunctival Suturing

In the conjunctival suturing technique, the eyelid is first anesthetized with local infiltration of lidocaine (Xylocaine). The upper eyelid is everted, and three double-armed sutures are placed from the conjunctival side in a subconjunctival fashion above the superior tarsal border. Then *either* of the two following techniques is performed:

Alternative 1: Both ends of the suture pass through to the skin side; then one end is again passed subcutaneously to exit through the second needle's exit site on the skin. The two ends are tied and buried subcutaneously. (Or one end of the suture goes through the eyelid and exits through a stab skin incision; the other end goes through skin next to the stab incision and is repassed subcutaneously to join the first suture that exited through the stab incision. The two suture ends are tied in the stab incision and buried.) The suture knot encompasses Müller's muscle, levator apo-

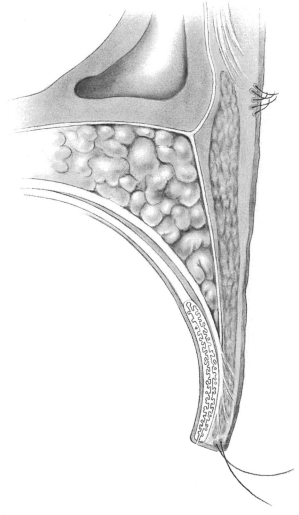

figure 11–2

A midsagittal section through an Asian upper eyelid without a crease. The orbital septum is usually seen fused to the levator aponeurosis along the superior tarsal border in an Asian without an upper eyelid crease. (Modified from Doxanas MT, Anderson RL: Oriental eyelids: an anatomic study. Arch Ophthalmol 1984; 102:1232–1235. Copyright 1984, American Medical Association.)

neurosis, and some pretarsal orbicularis muscle, creating a scarring process between the subdermal tissue along the superior tarsal border and the levator aponeurosis-Müller's muscle complex.

Alternative 2: Without piercing the skin, one end of the double-armed suture is passed through Müller's muscle and levator aponeurosis to the subcutaneous plane along the superior tarsal border. With the needle staying subcutaneously, the suture arm is passed back through the same tissue and exits conjunctivally. The two ends of the suture are knotted and buried within the conjunctiva above the superior tarsal border. The effect is the same as that of the first alternative.

I have seen quite a few Asian patients who underwent these procedures overseas and complained of corneal irritation.

External Incision

I favor the external incision technique and perform it as follows.

Premedication and Anesthetic Agents

The patient usually receives 10 mg of diazepam (Valium) and 5 mg of hydrocodone (Vicodin) by mouth 1 hour before the procedure. One drop of topical anesthetic, 0.5 per cent proparacaine (Ophthaine), is instilled on each cornea for comfort during surgical preparation. The upper eyelid receives a subcutaneous injection along the superior tarsal border, consisting of 0.25–0.5 ml of a mixture of 1 ml 2 per cent lidocaine with a 1:100,000 dilution of epinephrine diluted with 9 ml of injectable normal saline. During the next 5 minutes, one can see the vasoconstrictive effect of the mixture even though the epinephrine was diluted ten times (1:1,000,000). The purpose of this preinfiltration is to allow for a relatively painless injection because the pH of acidic 2 per cent lidocaine is restored closer to neutrality when it is diluted with the buffering action of injectable normal saline.

Then I inject 0.5–1 ml of the 2 per cent lidocaine with a 1:100,000 dilution of epinephrine (10 ml mixed with 150 units of hyaluronidase [Wydase]) in the suborbicularis plane along the superior tarsal border. The hyaluronidase promotes dispersion of the anesthetic and greatly reduces any tissue distortion. Rarely, when confronted with a patient with low tolerance to pain, I supplement the local field infiltration with a frontal nerve block.

The eyelids and face are then prepared in the usual fashion for ophthalmic surgery. The eyes are again given a drop of tetracaine for enduring corneal anesthesia. Corneal protectors are applied over each eye.

Marking the Eyelid Crease

With the eyelid everted, the vertical height of the tarsal plate over the central portion is measured with a caliper. In Asians, the vertical height of the tarsus is usually 6.5–8.5 mm. This measurement is then transcribed on the external skin surface on the central part of the upper eyelid using methylene blue on a fine point. This marking directly overlies the superior tarsal border centrally. If a crease is to be nasally tapered, I mark the medial third of the incision line to taper toward the medial canthal angle or to merge with the medial canthal fold. The lateral third is marked in either a leveled or a flared configuration. For the parallel crease, the measured height of the superior tarsal border is drawn on the skin surface across the eyelids.

To create adequate adhesions, it is necessary to remove some subdermal tissue. A strip of skin measuring approximately 2 mm is then marked above and parallel to this lower line of incision. Again, in the patient who desires a nasally tapered configuration, I taper this upper line of incision toward the medial canthal angle or merge

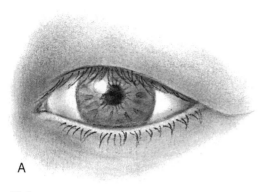

A

figure 11-3

Schematic diagrams *(A–G)* showing the different configurations of creases in the Asian upper eyelid. *A,* Absence of a lid crease and fullness of upper eyelid.

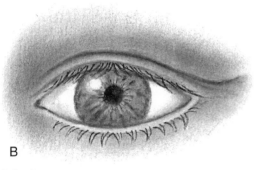

B

B, Continuous crease.

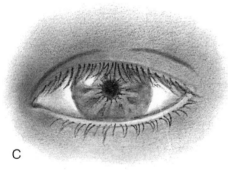

C

C, Discontinuous crease.

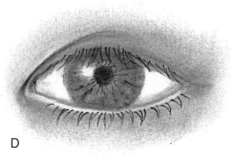

D

D, Incomplete crease.

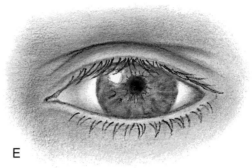

E

E, Multiple creases.

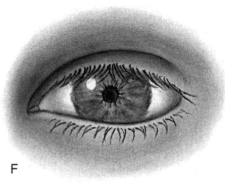

F

F, Inside fold with tapering of the eyelid crease toward the medial canthal angle and gentle lateral flare of the crease.

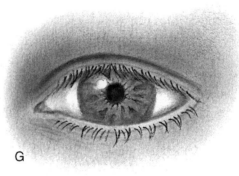

G

G, Parallel crease.

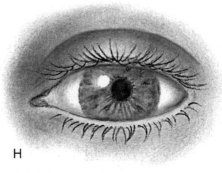

H

H, Typical Caucasian eyelid crease.

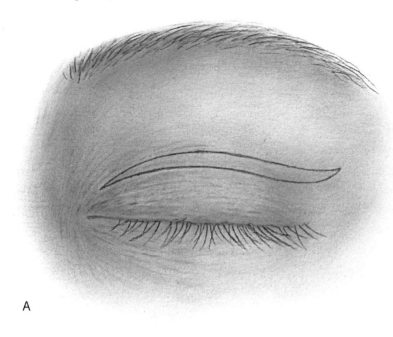

figure 11–4

A, The vertical height of the central portion of the upper tarsus is transcribed onto the skin surface centrally. This serves as the central point for the lower line of incision, with the overall line dictated by the shape of the crease desired. The upper line of incision usually includes 2 mm of skin.

A

it with any medial canthal fold that may be present (Fig. 11–4*A*).

Incision and Excision

An incision is then carried out using a No. 15 (Bard-Parker) surgical blade along the upper and lower lines, and I cut just below the subcutaneous plane. Fine capillary oozing is stopped with a delicate bipolar (wet-field) cautery. The strip of skin is excised with scissors. The superior tarsal border is still covered by pretarsal and preseptal orbicularis oculi muscle, the terminal portions of the septum orbitale, and the anteriorly directed terminal fibers of the levator aponeurosis behind the septum.

Then I retract the incision wound superiorly and use a fine-tipped monopolar cautery in the cutting mode to incise through the orbicularis muscle and orbital septum along the upper skin incision (see Fig. 11–4*B*).

In Asians, even though the orbital septum is now only 2–3 mm above the superior tarsal border, it is readily opened, and preaponeurotic fat pads can be seen bulging forward in most cases. The septum is opened horizontally (see Fig. 11–4*C*), and this strip of preseptal orbicularis muscle and orbital septum hinged along the superior tarsal border is then carefully excised. Depending on the degree of fullness of the upper eyelid, either none or a small amount of the preaponeurotic fat pad is excised with sharp scissors (see Fig. 11–4*D*). Any bleed-

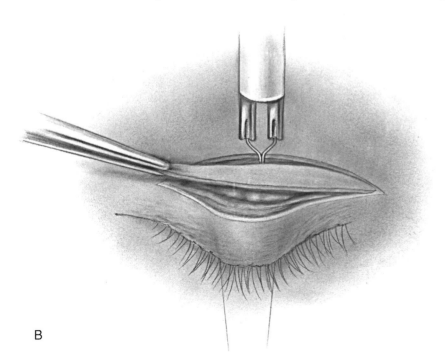

B, After the incisions are made, a wet-field cautery is applied for hemostasis and a surgical cautery is used to incise through the orbicularis oculi muscle along the superior incision site.

B

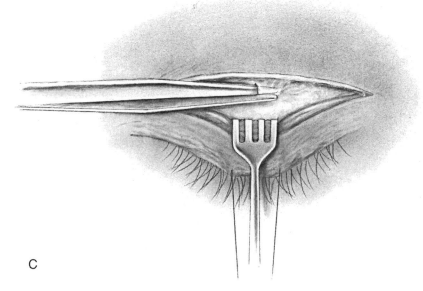

C, The orbital septum is first opened with a monopolar cautery along the upper line of incision. It is then extended horizontally with Westcott spring scissors.

C

ing points in the fat pads are controlled with light application of the wet-field cautery. The fat excision often requires a small local supplement of lidocaine in the space beneath the preaponeurotic fat pads. The terminal portion of the levator aponeurosis is now seen along the superior tarsal border. To facilitate the infolding of the surgically created crease, I further excise a 2–3-mm strip of pretarsal orbicularis muscle along the lower skin incision (see Fig. 11–4*E*).

Some authors routinely debulk the entire pretarsal tissue, believing that it is better to have only skin along the anterior surface of the tarsus. My experience has not been so, and I remove pretarsal tissue only if pretarsal fat is quite apparent and threatens the surgical formation of the desired upper eyelid crease. In the pretarsal plane of an Asian eyelid, there are very few, if any, terminal interdigitations of the levator aponeurosis to the dermis in a creaseless eyelid. I refrain from vigorous dissection along the pretarsal plane, as I believe that this creates long-term postoperative edema and increases the risk of the undesirable formation of more than one crease. Furthermore, Asians who have a natural eyelid crease often have some degree of pretarsal fullness along the area between the crease and the eyelashes.

Skin Closure

To create adequate adhesion between the terminal portions of the levator aponeurosis above the superior tarsal border to the crease incision lines, I use 6-0 nonabsorbable (silk or nylon) sutures to pick up the lower skin edge, the levator aponeurosis along the superior tarsal border, and the upper skin edge and then tie each of these as an interrupted suture (see Fig. 11–4*F*). Usually, besides the central stitch, two or three sutures are placed medially and two laterally. With these five or six crease-

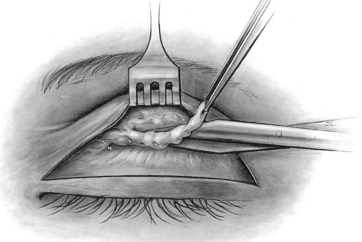

D, A small amount of the preaponeurotic fat pad is excised.

D

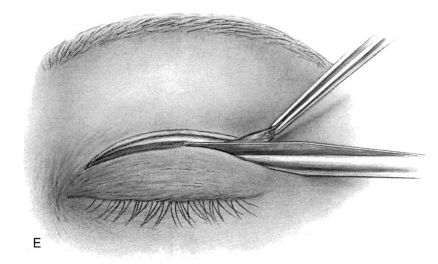

E, From 2–3 mm of the pretarsal orbicularis muscle is excised along the inferior edge of the skin wound.

E

F, Placement of an interrupted suture from the skin to the levator aponeurosis to the skin.

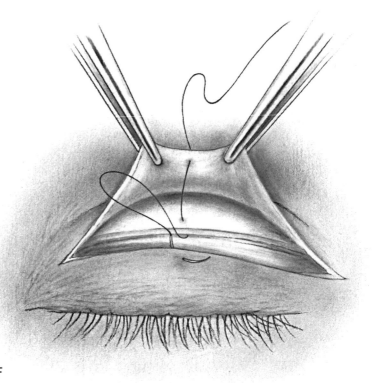

F

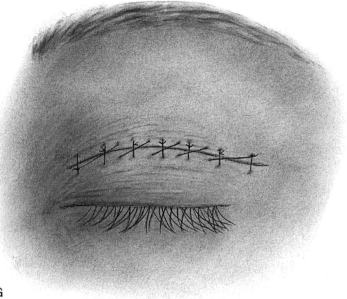

G, Skin closure using placement of five to six interrupted 6–0 sutures to form the crease and a continuous suture to approximate the edges of the wound.

G

forming sutures in place, the rest of the incision may be closed with 6-0 or 7-0 nylon in a continuous or subcuticular fashion (see Fig. 11–4*G*).

POSTOPERATIVE CARE

The wound is cleaned daily and covered with antibiotic ointment. Diuretics and steroids are not usually given. The sutures are removed in 5–7 days, depending on the suture material.

PATIENT PSYCHOLOGY: POSTOPERATIVE EXPECTATIONS

Postoperatively, the eyelid crease invariably appears high; the patient should again be reminded after the operation that this seeming "overcorrection" is from tissue swelling (Fig. 11–5). I usually inform my patients to expect a certain degree of postoperative edema to last for at least 4 months and that the crease configuration may vary from month to month and from one eyelid to the other. When the patients are instructed not to expect a stable and satisfactory appearance for 6 months, I find that they are much more accepting of the normal wound-healing process.

I also inform my patients to expect a 5 per cent chance of needing touch-up revisions if the creases are uneven. This is a realistic estimate in my practice, and most patients feel comfortable with it.

COMPLICATIONS

Complications are similar to those seen with any blepharoplasty operation and may include hemorrhage, grossly asymmetric creases, obliteration or fading of the crease, prolonged postoperative edema, hypertrophic scar formation, excessive fat removal with a hollowed eye appearance, and formation of multiple creases. The detailed description of correction of some of these problems is beyond the scope of this chapter. Interested readers may find helpful ideas in References 5 and 17.

I have seen other complications develop in two unusual cases. In one of my patients, the crease was obliterated after 6 months by proliferation of submuscular (preseptal) fat of the upper eyelid in conjunction with a 35 per cent weight gain during recovery from anorexia nervosa. Another patient had a low tolerance to pain and hardly moved her upper eyelids for 1 week postoperatively; the crease formed poorly in this patient. Since then, I have encouraged my patients to practice up gaze and down gaze after the first 48 hours to facilitate the formation of subdermal-levator aponeurosis adhesions.

EPICANTHAL FOLDS

Epicanthal folds, as found in Asians, present a challenging problem to cosmetic surgeons. The literature includes many articles dealing with this topic.[18–29] I tend to be conservative in my treatment and, with few exceptions, refrain from correcting epicanthal folds in Asians, for several reasons.

First, many Asians appear to have epicanthus palpebralis (a fold equally divided between the upper and lower eyelid) when they are young but then appear to have epicanthus tarsalis when they reach adulthood; one possible explanation is development of the nasal bridge.

Second, Asians tend to have more reactive skin and tend to have hypertrophic scarring in the thick medial canthal skin area.

Third, a nasally tapered crease that merges with the origin or a mild epicanthus tarsalis provides an aesthetically natural eyelid crease, as observed in Asians who have a crease.

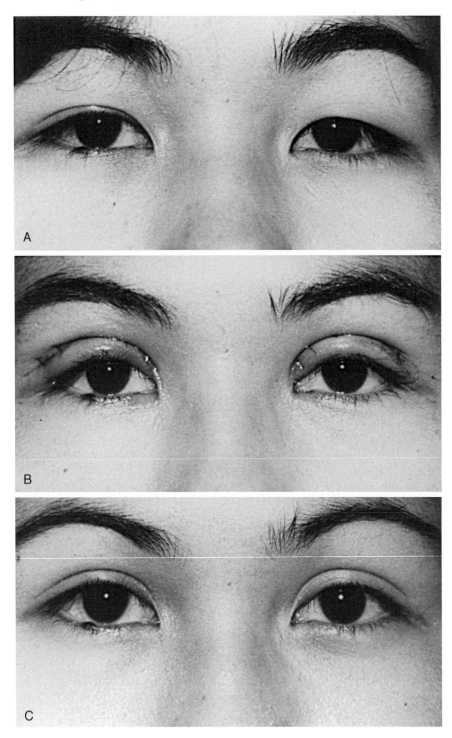

figure 11–5

A, Preoperative appearance. *B*, One week after upper blepharoplasty. *C*, Ten months after operation. (From Chen WP: Asian blepharoplasty. J Ophthalmol Plast Reconstr Surg 1987; 3:135–140.)

References

1. Doxanas MT, Anderson RL: Oriental eyelids: An anatomic study. Arch Ophthalmol 1984; 102:1232–1235.
2. Uchida J: A surgical procedure for blepharoptosis vera and for pseudo-blepharoptosis orientalis. Br J Plast Surg 1962; 15:271–276.
3. Onizuka T, Iwanami M: Blepharoplasty in Japan. Aesthetic Plast Surg 1984; 8:97–100.
4. Chen WP: Asian blepharoplasty. J Ophthalmic Plast Reconstr Surg 1987; 3:135–140.
5. Chen WPD: Asian Blepharoplasty: A Surgical Atlas. Boston, Butterworth Heinemann, 1995.
6. Chen WP: Concept of triangular, rectangular and trapezoidal debulking of eyelid tissues: Application in Asian blepharoplasty. Plast Reconstr Surg 1996; 97:212–218.
7. Chen WP: Insights from a series of Asian blepharoplasties. Presented at the 1990 meeting of the American Society of Ophthalmic Plastic and Reconstructive Surgery, Atlanta.
8. Mutou Y, Mutou H: Intradermal double eyelid operation and its follow-up results. Br J Plast Surg 1972; 25:285–291.
9. Boo-Chai K: Aesthetic surgery for the oriental. In Barron JN, Saed MN (eds): Operative Plastic and Reconstructive Surgery, vol 2, pp 761–773. New York, Churchill Livingstone, 1980.
10. Sayoc BT: Plastic reconstruction of the superior palpebral fold. Am J Ophthalmol 1954; 38:556–559.
11. Sayoc BT: Simultaneous construction of the superior palpebral

fold and ptosis operation. Am J Ophthalmol 1956; 41:1040–1043.

12. Sayoc BT: Absence of superior palpebral fold in slit eyes. Am J Ophthalmol 1956; 42:298–300.

13. Sayoc BT: Surgical management of unilateral almond eye. Am J Ophthalmol 1961; 52:122.

14. Sayoc BT: Anatomic considerations in the plastic construction of a palpebral fold in the full upper eyelid. Am J Ophthalmol 1967; 63:155–158.

15. Sayoc BT: Surgery of the oriental eyelid. Clin Plast Surg 1974; 1:157–171.

16. Fernandez LR: Double eyelid operation in the oriental in Hawaii. Plast Reconstr Surg 1960; 25:257–264.

17. Weng CJ, Nordhoff MS: Complication of oriental blepharoplasty. Plast Reconstr Surg 1989; 83:622–628.

18. Johnson CC: Epicanthus. Am J Ophthalmol 1968; 66:939–946.

19. Verwey A: Der Maskenhafte Antlitz und seine Behandlung. Z Augenheilkd 1909; 22:241.

20. Lessa S, Sebastia R: Epicanthoplasty. Aesthetic Plast Surg 1984; 8:159–163.

21. Von Ammon FA: Klinische Darstellungen der Krankheit des Auges und Augenlider. Berlin, G Reimer, 1841.

22. Von Arlt CF: Erweiterung der Bidspalte Kantoplastik. In Graef-Saemisch Handbuch des Augenheilkunde, vol 3, p. 443. Leipzig, Wilhelm Engelmann, 1874.

23. Berger E, Loewy R: Nouveau procédé opératoire pour l'épicanthus. Arch Ophthalmol 1889; 18:453.

24. Mustarde JC: The treatment of ptosis in epicanthal folds. Br J Plast Surg 1959; 12:252.

25. Converse JM, Smith B: Naso-orbital fractures and traumatic deformities of the medial canthus. Plast Reconstr Surg 1966; 38:147.

26. Spaeth EB: Further considerations on the surgical corrections of blepharophimosis (epicanthus). Am J Ophthalmol 1956; 41:61.

27. Spaeth EB: Further considerations on the surgical correction of blepharophimosis and ptosis. Arch Ophthalmol 1964; 71:510.

28. Blair VP, Brown JP, Hamm WG: Correction of ptosis in epicanthus. Arch Ophthalmol 1932; 7:831.

29. Matsunaga RS: Westernization of the Asian eyelid. Arch Otolaryngol 1985; 111:149–153.

C. Bradley Bowman
Myron Tanenbaum
Clinton D. McCord, Jr.

Internal Brow Lift: Browplasty and Browpexy

An internal brow lift offers the patient a method of raising the eyebrow without any additional incisions or scars; however, it is useful only for mild brow ptosis that is confined to the central and temporal aspect of the eyebrow. This technique does not lift the nasal brow, reduce excessive tissue above the nose, or treat overaction of the corrugator or procerus muscle. Nonetheless, I have been using this technique for several years and find it invaluable in many cases.

The authors point out the usefulness of the internal brow lift in many patients who do not demonstrate significant brow ptosis preoperatively. Before blepharoplasty, many patients keep their brows lifted almost constantly to reduce excessive upper eyelid skin folds. After upper blepharoplasty, these patients no longer have to lift their brows to be able to see better and, therefore, seem to have ptotic brows. The internal brow lift is thus advantageous in this group of patients as well. The surgeon can identify such a patient by evaluating brow levels with the patient's forehead muscles in repose.

Myron Tanenbaum and colleagues have demonstrated that some cases of upper eyelid "fullness" are due to brow fat. In this group of patients, excision of the brow fat through a browplasty significantly improves the effect of the traditional blepharoplasty. I have also found this technique of value in patients with this condition who were unhappy after traditional blepharoplasty.

One complication of internal brow lifts is dimpling of the skin in the area of the sutures if they pass too close to the skin. Most of the time, this problem can be determined during the surgical procedure and replacement of the suture can avoid the complication. If dimpling is noted, massaging the area frequently resolves the problem.

In a few patients in whom I have performed the internal brow lift according to the technique described in this chapter, a high upper eyelid crease was created that made it difficult for the patients to look upward. The patients found this crease objectionable. One possible cause of this complication is that the orbital septum and suborbicularis fascia slid upward with the brow elevation. This allowed the orbicularis oculi muscle to fuse to levator aponeurosis at a high level.

To help prevent this complication, I perform the browplasty and browpexy without penetrating the orbital septum and suborbicularis fascia. Then I penetrate orbital septum and suborbicularis fascia, excise herniated orbital fat, and perform eyelid crease reconstruction. I then incorporate the inferior edge of the orbital septum–suborbicularis fascia flap to the inferior edge of the levator aponeurosis and to each edge of the skin wound.

This procedure enhances the crease and forms a barrier between the orbicularis muscle and the levator aponeurosis. I believe that this modification decreases the potential complication of a high upper eyelid crease, which would cause the patient difficulty in looking upward. At the end of this chapter, I describe my modification.

ALLEN M. PUTTERMAN

Many patients who request cosmetic upper eyelid surgery have ptotic or drooping eyebrows that accentuate their upper eyelid abnormalities. In addition, patients often are most concerned about changing a "fullness" in the lateral brow area (Fig. 12–1). This fullness represents an increased thickness in the sub-brow fat pad. Failure to recognize and treat mild forms of brow ptosis and sub-brow fat pad thickening can yield a suboptimal blepharoplasty result.

The browplasty and browpexy techniques are important adjunctive procedures in selected blepharoplasty patients.[1-3]

ANATOMIC CONSIDERATIONS

The eyebrow and its surrounding soft tissues represent a specialized anatomic region of the face and the superficial sliding muscle plane of the forehead. Cadaveric studies by Lemke and Stasior[4] have helped to define the brow-eyelid anatomic unit and its importance in repair of brow ptosis and dermatochalasis.

A fat pad exists beneath the eyebrow, from which dense attachments secure the brow to the supraorbital ridge. This fat pad enhances eyebrow motility, especially laterally, where it is most pronounced (Fig. 12–2*A*). The brow fat pad often extends inferiorly into the suborbicularis fascia–preseptal plane in the upper eyelid and can be mistaken for orbital fat by the novice blepharoplasty surgeon (Fig. 12–2*B*).

Both the size and position of the brow fat pad contribute to gender differences in eyebrow appearance, which the surgeon must take into consideration. In women, the brow is generally arched and above the level of the supraorbital rim; in men, it is flatter and positioned at the level of the supraorbital rim. The fat pad in men is more prominent, producing a fuller appearance in the lateral brow area. Surgical manipulation of the size and position of the fat pad should respect these variations in men and women so that a natural and aesthetically pleasing result is obtained.

Early ptosis of the brow occurs most commonly over the lateral brow. The firm attachments of the brow fat pad to the supraorbital rim periosteum extend only over the medial one half to two thirds of the orbit around the supraorbital ridge prominence. Laterally, the attachments are weaker.

In addition, the frontalis muscle of the forehead supports the medial two thirds of the eyebrow and interdigitates with the orbicularis muscle. However, because the frontalis muscle fibers do not extend as far laterally as the lateral brow, frontalis muscle contraction cannot effectively prevent lateral eyebrow ptosis.

The supraorbital artery and nerve emanate from the supraorbital notch and pass superiorly within the medial portion of the eyebrow fat pad. For this reason, fat pad debulking should involve only tissue lateral to the supraorbital notch, so that damage to sensory nerves of the forehead is avoided.

INDICATIONS

Dermatochalasis (excessive skin) can often be dramatically improved with simple upper lid blepharoplasty alone. When ptotic eyebrows accompany dermatochalasis, however, they often accentuate the upper eyelid abnormality and should be taken into consideration during surgery. Debulking of the sub-brow fat pad via the blepharoplasty incision is an effective way to reduce the

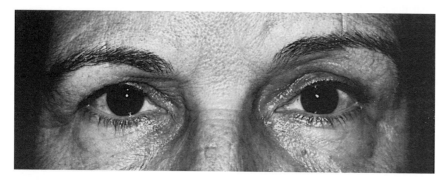

figure 12–1

A "fullness" in the lateral brow area is caused by a thickened and ptotic sub-brow fat pad, not by excess upper eyelid skin.

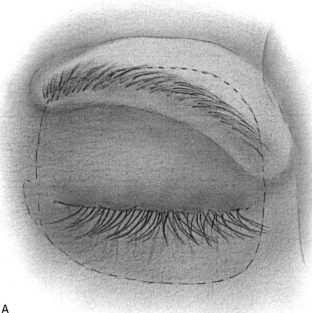

figure 12–2

A, Frontal illustration of a ptotic left brow. The brow and the sub-brow fat pad extend below the orbital rim *(dotted line),* and brow ptosis is more prominent temporally.

A

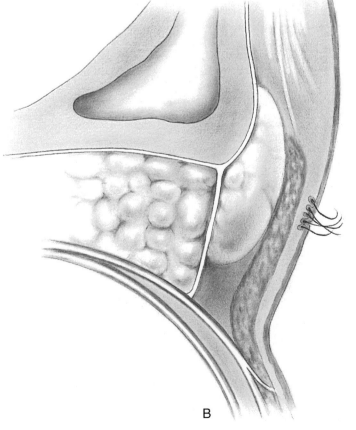

B, Midsagittal illustration of the ptotic brow with inferior extension of the sub-brow fat pad anterior to the orbital septum. Note the relation of the thick ptotic sub-brow fat pad anterior to the orbital septum and orbital fat.

B

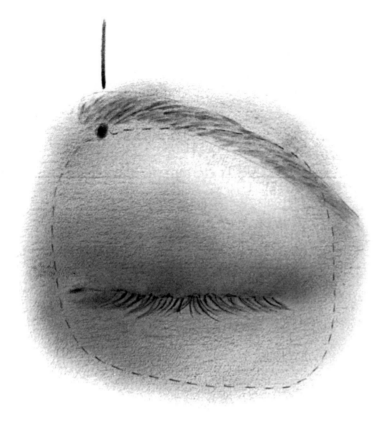

figure 12–3

The supraorbital notch is marked, and a line is made above the brow to indicate the location of the supraorbital nerve.

fullness often present in the lateral brow and can produce a more aesthetic overall result. This browplasty procedure is particularly important in women, in whom a thickened sub-brow fat pad can create a masculine appearance.

In patients with mild to moderate brow ptosis, plication of the brow at or above the supraorbital rim through the blepharoplasty incision can reduce the brow component of the upper lid dermatochalasis. This restores the natural height and curvature of the brow, thus enhancing the result of blepharoplasty.

Although the coronal forehead lift procedures provide the most pronounced correction of forehead and glabella laxity, these techniques may be more extensive than the patient or the surgeon desires. It should be emphasized that the internal browpexy procedure does not replace conventional brow lifts and should not be done in patients with severe brow ptosis (see Chapters 27 and 28).

The browpexy and browplasty procedures described later can be used together or separately as an adjunct to standard blepharoplasty in carefully selected patients. The browplasty technique can be used alone in selected patients with "fullness" of the lateral brow in whom there is no significant element of brow ptosis. Many patients have mild to moderate brow ptosis without a significant thickening of the sub-brow fat pad. Although the debulking aspect of the browplasty procedure is not necessary in these patients, some amount of sub-brow fat needs to be removed so that periosteum for the browpexy can be exposed.

SURGICAL TECHNIQUE

The amount of brow lift desired is determined while the patient is seated on the operating table. The site of the blepharoplasty is marked in the upper lid crease, and the supraorbital notch is palpated and marked to localize the supraorbital nerve and vessels (Fig. 12–3). The patient can then be reclined, and the upper eyelid and brow infiltrated with 2 per cent lidocaine with epinephrine.

Browplasty

After the standard blepharoplasty excision of skin and orbicularis muscle, the dissection is extended superiorly toward the brow in the submuscular plane in the postorbicularis fascia (Fig. 12–4*A* and *B*) (see also Chapter 10). Dissection should extend approximately 1–1.5 cm above the superior and lateral orbital rim. The brow fat pad can then be identified overlying the lateral orbital margin. As has been emphasized, excision of the fat pad should be confined to the lateral aspect of the brow to avoid injury to the medial supraorbital neurovascular complex.

Following identification and exposure of the brow fat pad, an elliptical section measuring 1–1.5 cm vertically and tapering nasally and temporally can be marked with methylene blue (Fig. 12–5*A*). The fat pad is then removed en bloc from the central third of the superior orbital margin laterally as far as the frontozygomatic

figure 12–4

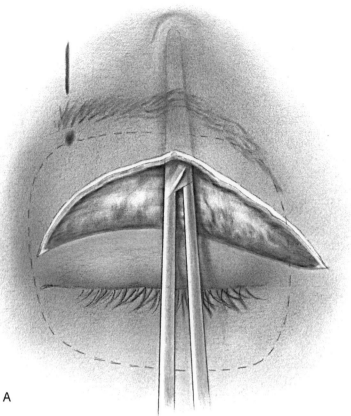

A, Frontal illustration of browplasty. A skin-muscle eyelid crease approach is used to expose the sub-brow fat pad. The plane of dissection is in the submuscular postorbicularis fascia.

A

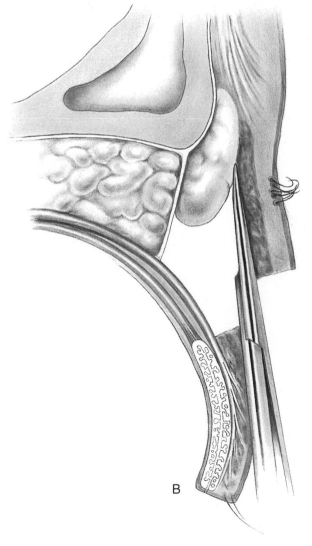

B, Midsagittal illustration of browplasty.

B

117

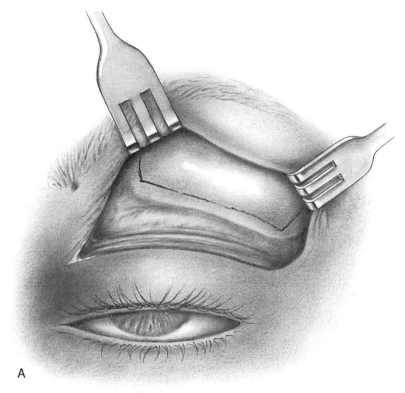

A

figure 12–5

Illustrations of browplasty technique. *A*, After an eyelid crease incision is made, the upper eyelid skin is retracted superiorly. The thick sub-brow fat pad is exposed and marked with methylene blue.

B, The surgeon uses the cutting-cautery unit to resect the sub-brow fat pad, leaving the periosteum intact.

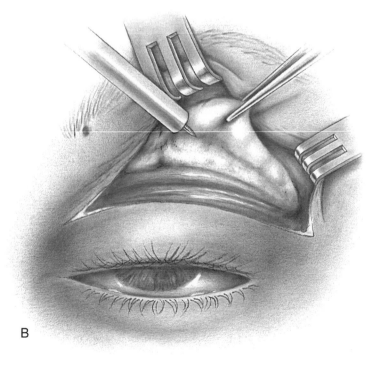

B

suture (Fig. 12–5*B*). The fat pad should be removed down to, but not including, the periosteum. The periosteum should remain intact so that adhesions can be avoided in an area designed for motility. If brow fixation or elevation is not desired, the blepharoplasty can then be completed.

Browpexy

Fixation or plication of the brow to the supraorbital rim periosteum can provide elevation of the ptotic or lax brow. One to three 4-0 polypropylene (Prolene) sutures are passed transcutaneously from the lower edge of the brow hairs into the previously dissected sub-brow space approximately 1 cm apart (Fig. 12–6A). This transcutaneous introduction of the sutures allows the surgeon to mark the position of the brow hairs while working underneath the dissected flap.

Each suture is then passed through periosteum approximately 1–1.5 cm above the supraorbital rim (Fig. 12–6B). At this stage of the procedure, the height and curvature of the brow can be adjusted according to the patient's gender. Placing the more central suture slightly higher allows the characteristic arch of the female brow to be restored or preserved.

The sutures are then passed again into the sub-brow muscular tissue at the level of the original transcutaneously passed marking suture (Fig. 12–6C). It is important to engage firm subcutaneous tissue so that the polypropylene browpexy sutures have the desired effect. The surgeon must, however, avoid suturing into the

figure 12–6

Illustrations of internal browpexy technique. *A*, A 4-0 polypropylene (Prolene) suture is passed transcutaneously from the lower edge of the brow hairs into the previously dissected sub-brow space.

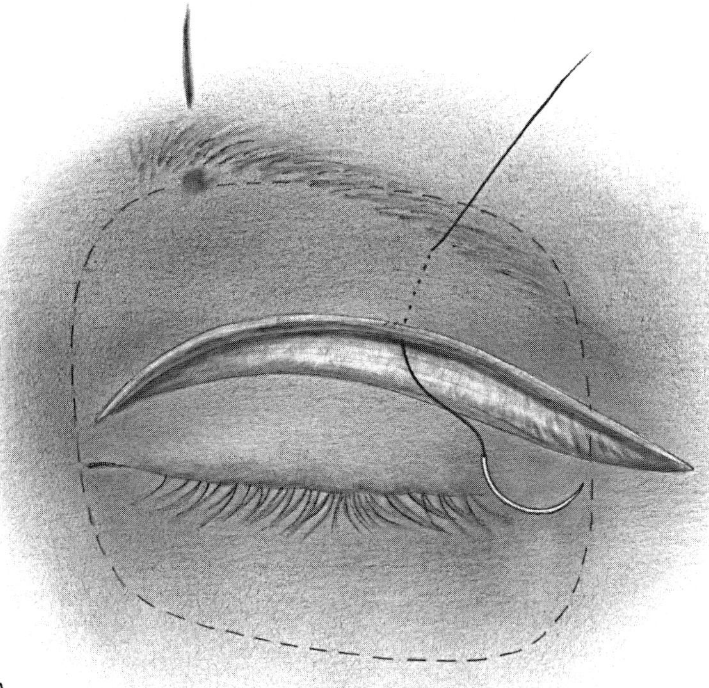

A

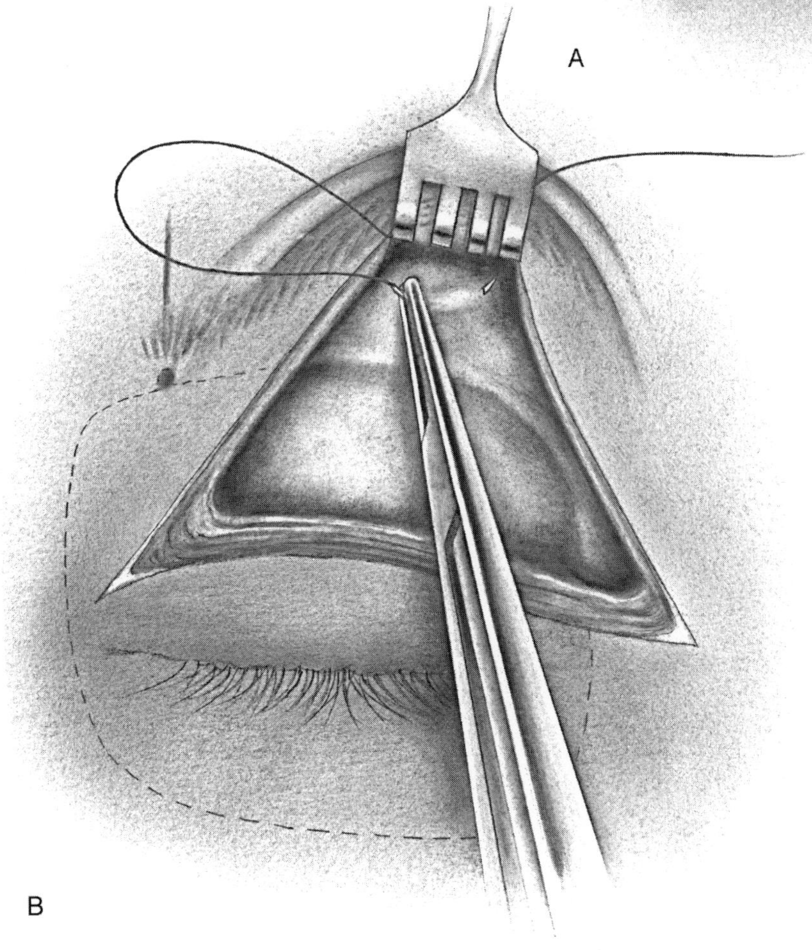

B, A 4-0 polypropylene suture is sewn through the sub-brow tissue and through the periosteum above the orbital rim.

B

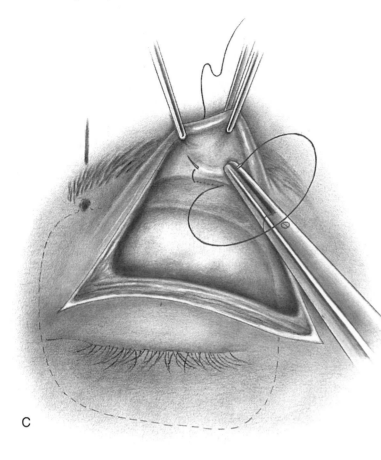

C

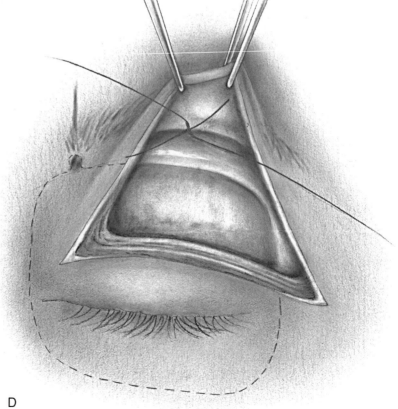

D

C, The suture is then passed again into the sub-brow muscular tissue at the level of the original, transcutaneously passed marking suture. The transcutaneous suture is removed.

D, The surgeon ties the suture in a loop over a 4-0 silk knot, releasing the suture if adjustment is necessary. Care is taken to avoid overtightening the suture once adequate placement is achieved, which may immobilize the brow.

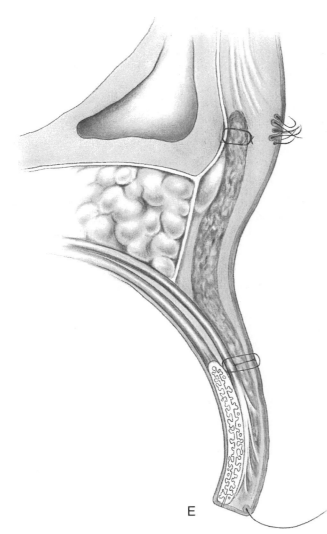

E, Midsagittal section of completed browpexy.

very superficial sub-brow tissues. This can lead to a dimpling of the skin as well as erosion of superficial tissues over the sutures and exposure of the sutures.

The original transcutaneous suture ends are then pulled through the skin under the flap. The sutures are tied carefully in an attempt to avoid overtightening the 4-0 polypropylene loop (Fig. 12–6D). Ideally, these subcutaneous sutures should provide a mild brow-lifting effect and still allow the brow a good range of mobility (Fig. 12–6E). Placement and tightening of the 4-0 polypropylene sutures may require more than one attempt before the surgeon is satisfied with the position and symmetry of the eyebrows. The upper lid blepharoplasty can then be completed (see Chapter 10).

COMPLICATIONS

Complications of the browpexy and browplasty procedures, as with routine blepharoplasty, are few but notable. During exposure and debulking of the sub-brow fat pad, the surgeon may notice a significant venous plexus lying below and within the fat pad. Appropriate cautery

may be necessary to obtain adequate hemostasis and prevent postoperative hematoma. In addition, removal or disruption of this venous network may contribute to prolonged postoperative eyelid edema. In our experience, edema usually resolves in 2–4 weeks. Although a small amount of brow asymmetry may be unavoidable and acceptable, occasionally the extent of asymmetry may be unacceptable. This complication may be due to unilateral failure of the browpexy secondary to "cheesewiring" of the suture through subcutaneous tissue. It can usually be avoided if the subcutaneous suture is passed into the sub-brow muscular tissue.

As stated previously, the internal browpexy procedure works well for mild to moderate brow ptosis and as an adjunct to blepharoplasty in selected patients. This procedure in patients with severe brow laxity commonly yields unsatisfactory results.

RESULTS

We have used the browplasty and/or browpexy procedures over the past decade in more than 1000 selected patients undergoing upper lid blepharoplasty and have had good results (Figs. 12–7 and 12–8).

The browplasty fat removal technique has been uniformly successful in predictably debulking the thick, full lateral brow fat pad in selected patients. Most patients tolerate the somewhat prolonged postoperative edema and the transient lateral brow numbness quite well.

Similarly, the internal browpexy procedure yields good results once the surgeon gains adequate experience with the technique. Single-suture browpexy for correction of mild lateral brow ptosis has consistently yielded excellent results in our patients. Occasionally, brow asymmetry has been encountered in patients with more marked brow ptosis in whom the browpexy procedure required more than two fixation sutures. Recurrent brow ptosis does often occur, at least partially, within 12 months of the internal suture browpexy procedure.

PUTTERMAN MODIFICATION OF INTERNAL BROW LIFT

Allen M. Putterman

As mentioned in my introduction to this chapter, when I used the technique described here for elevating eyebrows, several of my patients developed a high upper eyelid crease and had difficulty elevating their eyelids on up gaze. Therefore, I modified this procedure and now perform the internal brow lift with the septum still covering the levator aponeurosis. Once the brow is placed in the proper position, I penetrate the orbital septum and suborbicularis fascia and then excise herniated orbital fat. When I form a lid crease by suturing skin to levator aponeurosis, I also include the inferior edge of the orbital septum-suborbicularis fascia.

This technique provides a layer between skin and levator aponeurosis and avoids the complications of a crease that is too high and an eyelid that will not elevate properly.

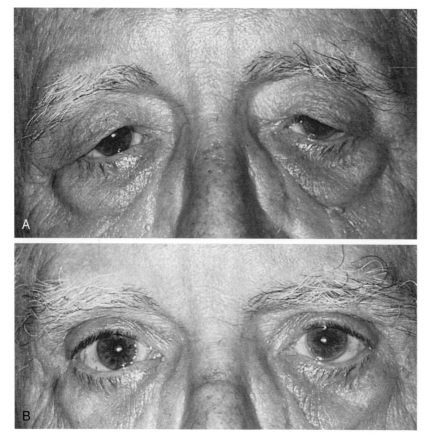

figure 12–7

A, A man with significant dermatochalasis (excessive skin) also has a thickening of the sub-brow fat pad that produces a "fullness" in the lateral brow. *B,* Same patient 6 weeks after bilateral upper eyelid blepharoplasty and browplasty.

figure 12–8

A, "Droopy eyelids" manifest in a woman with lateral brow ptosis and dermatochalasis. *B,* Same patient 6 weeks after bilateral upper eyelid blepharoplasty and internal browpexy.

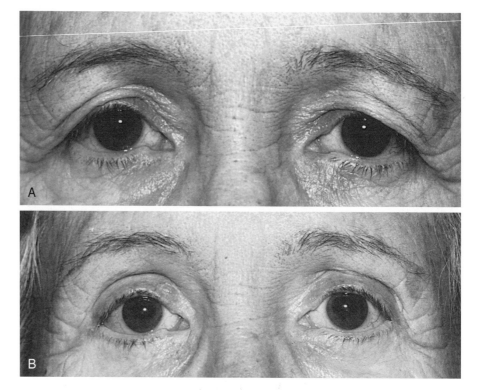

Surgical Technique

The surgeon marks the upper eyelid skin resection site, and the assistant holds the eyebrow upward at the desired position. Only skin and orbicularis muscle are removed over the outlined area of excessive skin. The surgeon should avoid any penetration into the orbital septum or suborbicularis fascia. To enter the sub-brow plane, the surgeon carries out dissection between orbicularis muscle and orbital septum to the superior orbital rim, then between the orbicularis muscle and sub-brow fat above the superior orbital rim. The excision of sub-brow fat and attachment of the orbicularis muscle to the periosteum are carried out, as described earlier in this chapter.

After this procedure, the patient should be seated up on the operating table so that the surgeon can judge the position and arch of the eyebrow. Suture placement should be altered until the surgeon obtains the desired level and arch.

Once the brow is set in the proper position, the surgeon penetrates the orbital septum and suborbicularis fascia. This is achieved by pulling the upper lid downward with a 4-0 silk traction suture that has been placed through central skin orbicularis and superficial tarsus.

The orbital septum and suborbicularis fascia are picked up with toothed forceps and pulled upward and outward. The tented inferior aspect of the septum and suborbicularis fascia is penetrated with Westcott scissors until the subseptal space can be seen (Fig. 12–9A). The area then is widened by spreading the scissors blades.

With the eyelid still kept in this position with a traction suture and forceps, one blade of the Westcott scissors is used to penetrate the central opening in orbital septum–suborbicularis fascia and is slid across the temporal eyelid. Cutting with the Westcott scissors proceeds anteriorly, and the septum–suborbicularis fascia is cut at its inferior aspect (Fig. 12–9A).

The maneuver is repeated over the nasal half of the orbital septum–suborbicularis fascia. This maneuver creates a flap of septum–suborbicularis fascia that has an inferior edge close to the superior tarsal border (Figs. 12–9B and C).

An eyelid crease is formed by attaching four 6–0 white polyester fiber (Mersilene) sutures from the orbicularis muscle of the lower skin flap to levator aponeurosis (see Chapter 10, Fig. 10–1I–K). Next, three 6-0 white polyglactin (Vicryl) sutures are sewn to connect skin to levator aponeurosis to the inferior edge of the septum–suborbicularis fascia flap (Figs. 12–9D and E). One of these sutures is placed centrally, and one is placed nasally

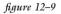

figure 12–9

A, The brow has been elevated through internal fixation sutures, as described in Figure 12–4. The suborbicularis fascia–septal layer is entered at its inferior position and is severed temporally and nasally. This is facilitated by pulling the upper eyelid downward with a traction suture while lifting the central suborbicularis fascia–septal tissue upward and outward with a forceps.

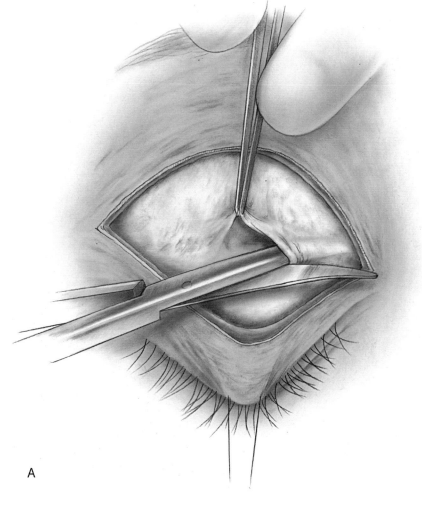

A

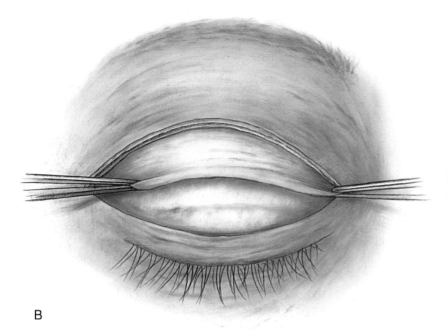

B, Two toothed forceps grasp the inferior edge of the suborbicularis fascia–septal tissue after it has been severed from its inferior attachment slightly above the superior tarsal border.

B

C, The surgeon uses the two toothed forceps to lift the suborbicularis fascia–septal layer upward and outward, thereby exposing the orbital fat and levator aponeurosis.

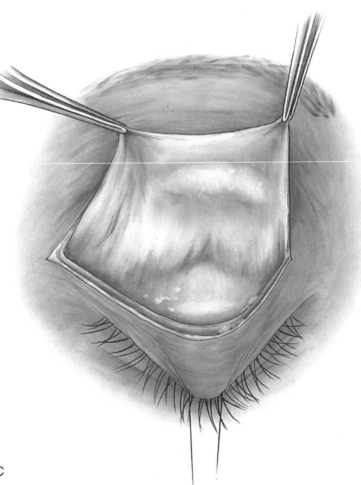

C

D, Orbital fat is excised, and the levator aponeurosis is attached to suborbicularis fascia, as described in Figures 10–1H–J. Then 6-0 polyglactin (Vicryl) sutures pass through the inferior skin edge, levator aponeurosis, and inferior edge of the suborbicularis fascia–septal layer and exit through the superior skin edge. Three sutures are placed to add to formation of the crease and to ensure that the suborbicularis fascia–septal layer covers the levator aponeurosis.

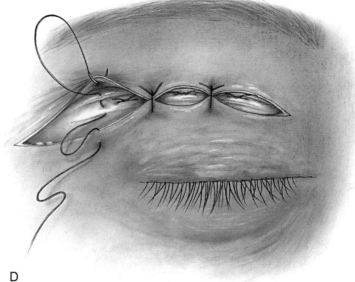

D

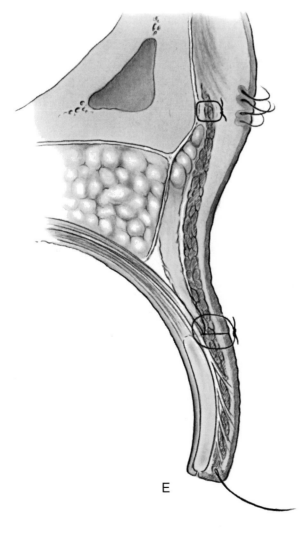

E

E, Cross-section of eyelid and eyebrow, as depicted in Fig. 12–9D.

and temporally. The skin is closed with a 6-0 black silk suture run continuously.

Results

Since I have added the above modification to the internal brow lift, no patient undergoing this procedure has developed an undesirable upper eyelid crease or has experienced any difficulty in looking upward.

References

1. McCord CD, Doxanas MT: Browplasty and browpexy: An adjunct to blepharoplasty. Plast Reconstr Surg 1990; 86:248–254.
2. May JW, Fearon J, Zingarelli P: Retro-orbicularis oculus fat (ROOF) resection in aesthetic blepharoplasty: A 6-year study in 63 patients. Plast Reconstr Surg 1990; 86:682–689.
3. Stasior OG, Lemke BN: The posterior eyebrow fixation. Adv Ophthalmic Plast Reconstr Surg 1983; 2:193–197.
4. Lemke BN, Stasior OG: The anatomy of eyebrow ptosis. Arch Ophthalmol 1982; 100:981–986.

William M. McLeish
Richard L. Anderson

Chapter **13**

Upper Blepharoplasty Combined with Levator Aponeurosis Repair

In this chapter, William McLeish and Rick Anderson demonstrate how to treat an acquired ptosis of the upper eyelids by levator aponeurosis surgery combined with removal of excess skin and herniated orbital fat. Two techniques are presented for two different situations. One consists of a true levator disinsertion, in which the ptosis is repaired by advancing the recessed levator aponeurosis to the superior tarsal border. The second is an attenuation of the levator aponeurosis, in which the levator aponeurosis is tucked or resected.

For the most part, I continue to obtain superior results by performing the Müller's muscle–conjunctival resection–ptosis procedure in combination with excision of excess skin and orbital fat in patients whose upper eyelids elevate to a normal level with phenylephrine. I reserve the levator aponeurosis procedure for those patients who do not experience a response to phenylephrine. These generally are the patients who have severe attenuation or a large disinsertion of the levator aponeurosis.

The authors advocate reconstructing the temporal crease 5–6 mm above the lid margin. I prefer reconstruction 9–10 mm above the lid margin. They also excise the central orbital fat pad without clamping and cauterization. I believe this practice carries a small risk of retrobulbar hemorrhage. The authors use mild intravenous sedation during the procedure. I prefer to use no sedation until I achieve the desired eyelid level because I am concerned that sedation may alter it. Finally, I dissect the levator aponeurosis from Müller's muscle and excise and advance the levator aponeurosis in all cases of levator aponeurosis attenuation, whereas Drs. McLeish and Anderson do this only for large advancements.

ALLEN M. PUTTERMAN

Disinsertion of the levator aponeurosis is the most common cause of blepharoptosis seen in patients seeking cosmetic eyelid surgery. Upper eyelid blepharoplasty lends itself well to simultaneous correction of ptosis via repair of an aponeurotic disinsertion. There are several advantages to the use of this combined procedure:

1. Both procedures can be addressed with the use of a single incision.
2. Both procedures directly address and correct anatomic defects responsible for dermatochalasis and ptosis.
3. The conjunctival surface is left undisturbed, leading

to less postoperative edema, discomfort, and corneal irritation.

The fact that none of the elements responsible for production of the trilaminar tear film are removed decreases the potential for postoperative tear film dysfunction. The technique of combined blepharoplasty with aponeurotic ptosis repair has proved tremendously successful and is applicable for almost every patient seeking cosmetic eyelid surgery.

EVALUATION

Preoperative recognition of ptosis is extremely important because postoperative eyelid height asymmetry will not go unnoticed by the scrutinizing patient. A systematic preoperative evaluation of all patients desiring cosmetic eyelid surgery identifies the presence of ptosis as well as other eyelid and upper facial maladies. The examination should also serve to thoroughly educate the patient and engender an amicable and trusting relationship between the patient and physician.

The preoperative examination entails a thorough review of the physical relationships of the patient's entire upper face. The heights and contours of the upper eyelids are noted with the forehead and eyebrows in a relaxed, natural position. An asymmetric or heavily furrowed brow often masks the presence of ptosis. Frequently, redundant upper eyelid skin must be gently elevated out of the way to visualize the lid margin and the natural eyelid crease, which is typically elevated by an aponeurosis disinsertion.

The amount of levator function present should be recorded. Levator aponeurosis disinsertion results in ptosis with normal levator function. If the levator function measures less than 12 mm, the cause should be sought. The eyelid skin should be examined for scars from previous surgery or trauma. Any lagophthalmos should be noted, as its presence may help to identify a previously uncorrected congenital ptosis or the presence of significant internal scar tissue or symblepharon. Bilateral ptosis with poor levator function may be the only feature of a systemic condition such as chronic progressive external ophthalmoplegia. Variable ptosis and levator function are classically associated with myasthenia gravis. In general, conditions associated with levator function of less than 12 mm require specialized care, and affected patients may not be candidates for a combined blepharoplasty and aponeurotic ptosis repair.

UPPER EYELID CREASE

Symmetry between the two upper eyelids is of paramount importance in achieving the desired cosmetic result. Correct placement of the eyelid crease incision, therefore, is one of the most important steps in the combined blepharoplasty and aponeurotic ptosis repair procedure. The central eyelid crease height should be 9–12 mm above the lid margin. It should taper temporally to a height of 5–6 mm above the lateral canthus

and medially to 6–7 mm above the punctum. The configuration of this incision roughly corresponds to the superior border of the tarsal plate, the level at which the levator aponeurosis normally sends fibers through the orbicularis oculi muscle to the skin.

The incision continues temporally approximately 1 cm beyond the lateral canthus in a natural skin crease. One should avoid the temptation to extend the incision beyond this point in an attempt to incorporate temporal crow's feet (rhytids) into the excision. The skin beyond the lateral orbital rim is thicker and less forgiving than eyelid skin, and the incision scar in this area may be visible for months after surgery. Rhytids in the temporal region are best addressed by an upper facial rhytidectomy and not through an "extended blepharoplasty" procedure (see Chapter 29). Alternatively, carbon dioxide (CO_2) laser resurfacing has proved quite effective in the treatment of temporal rhytids and is an excellent treatment option for individuals who do not require extensive skin excision (see Chapter 31).

During simultaneous aponeurotic ptosis repair, there is a tendency for the eyelid crease to establish itself lower than the originally desired height. This occurs when the surgeon must expose the superior border of the tarsal plate to facilitate placement of tarsal sutures. If desired, the surgeon can counter this tendency by minimizing the dissection along the superior border of the tarsal plate, by not excising any pretarsal orbicularis muscle, and by marking the eyelid crease skin incision 1 mm higher than the intended postoperative height.

SURGICAL TECHNIQUE

The skin incision is carried superiorly to circumscribe redundant skin and orbicularis muscle tissue. The surgeon establishes the proper amount of skin and muscle that can be safely excised by placing one blade of a smooth forceps on the marked eyelid crease incision and gently pinching sufficient redundant tissue between it and the second blade of the forceps to cause the lid margin to just begin to evert. This maneuver is repeated along the length of the eyelid crease incision, and the superior extent of the incision is marked with a pen at each location (Fig. 13–1*A*). As a general guide, the superior limb of the incision should be 12–15 mm below the inferior margin of the eyebrow at the midpupillary position; this ensures that adequate anterior lamella remains to allow for complete eyelid closure and to prevent iatrogenic brow ptosis.

After the skin markings have been completed, the tissues are infiltrated with 2 per cent lidocaine with 1:100,000 epinephrine to facilitate hemostasis. No hyaluronidase is used, as it would enhance deep penetration of the local anesthetic, which may result in diminished levator function and subsequent difficulty adjusting the eyelid to the proper height. For similar reasons, minimal intravenous sedation is used.

After anesthesia is obtained, a 4-0 silk traction suture is passed through the upper lid margin and secured to the drape below. The skin incision is made with a No. 15 Bard-Parker blade. The skin-muscle flap is then ex-

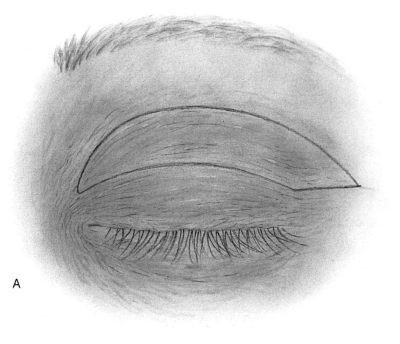

figure 13–1

A, Ellipse of upper eyelid skin to be removed is outlined.

A

cised as a single unit with tenotomy scissors or a cutting cautery unit. Elevation of the skin-muscle flap exposes the plane between the suborbicular fascia and the orbital septum, greatly speeding the dissection and protecting the levator aponeurosis from iatrogenic damage (Fig. 13–1*B*). Hemostasis is controlled with either a monopolar or bipolar cautery.

Novice surgeons may be unsure whether they are viewing the orbital septum or the aponeurosis at this point. By grasping the structure with a forceps and pulling inferiorly, the surgeon can immediately make the correct identification. The orbital septum fuses with the arcus marginalis at the orbital rim and is immobile. In contrast, the levator aponeurosis travels inferiorly with little resistance.

Once identified, the septum is incised medially, where it is frequently rarefied. The septum is opened approximately 1 cm above the tarsal plate, where the preaponeurotic fat protects the underlying aponeurosis from accidental injury. The opening in the septum is then extended the length of the eyelid incision. The central preaponeurotic fat compartment is bluntly teased into view. This fat is yellow and generally contains few vessels. The redundant fat is grasped with forceps and sharply

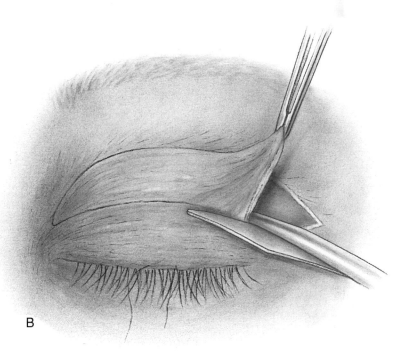

B, Elevation of the skin and orbicularis oculi muscle flap facilitates dissection just deep to the suborbicular fascial plane, thus helping to prevent iatrogenic damage to the levator aponeurosis.

B

excised with tenotomy scissors. We have found that clamping the fat before excision is not required, provided that the bleeding vessels are meticulously cauterized before allowing the stump to retract back into the orbit. Surgeons uncomfortable with this approach may wish to clamp the fat in standard fashion before its removal. The fat is generally trimmed to a level just inside the orbital rim.

The medial fat pocket is more extensive than the central pocket. It can be discerned from the medial compartment by its whiter coloration, thicker or denser consistency, and greater vascularity. Frequently, sharp lysis of normally occurring fibrous septa is required before the fat in this compartment presents itself. Gentle retropulsion of the globe further enhances delivery of the fat. Hemostasis is particularly important in this region because the medial fat pad contains terminal branches of the ophthalmic artery and multiple large-caliber veins. Bleeding from these vessels can be significant and, if inadequately controlled, can result in vision-threatening orbital hemorrhage.[1] Furthermore, blind cautery in this area can lead to damage to the trochlea and to subsequent diplopia.[2] For these reasons, we advocate clamping the fat in this region before excision (Fig. 13–1*C*). Care should be taken not to excise too much fat from the medial fat pockets because this can create a depression, which in some individuals creates a hollowed appearance. Aggressive inferior dissection in this area can damage the medial horn of the levator aponeurosis, aggravating ptosis and "lateralization" of the tarsal plate, as described by Shore and McCord.[3]

Temporally, the position of the lacrimal gland should be noted. A prolapsing lacrimal gland creates fullness in this area, which can masquerade as fat prolapse and even temporal brow ptosis.[4] A prolapsed lacrimal gland needs

to be repositioned within the lacrimal gland fossa (see Chapter 17). One should avoid the temptation to "shrink" the gland back with cautery or excise it, since either maneuver may result in diminished aqueous tear production and dry eye symptoms.

With the appropriate preaponeurotic fat now removed, the underlying aponeurosis is visualized. Frequently, a distinct disinsertion between the tarsus and the leading edge of the aponeurosis is encountered (Fig. 13–1*D*). This is easily recognized because the peripheral arcade running through Müller's muscle just above the superior border of the tarsal plate is clearly visible. Alternatively, a rarefied but intact aponeurosis or an aponeurosis with extensive fatty infiltration is found (Fig. 13–1*E*).

At this point, a single-armed 5-0 polyglactin (Vicryl) suture on a spatula needle is passed vertically in a partial-thickness fashion through the superior border of the tarsal plate just medial to the pupil. The suture position corresponds to the highest point of the natural eyelid contour. We have found that *vertical* suture passes produce a smoother eyelid contour and less tendency to cause eversion of the lid margin than the more frequently described *horizontal* mattress suture techniques. It is imperative that the suture bites be placed at the superior border of the tarsal plate to avoid creating an ectropion of the upper eyelid.

The needle is then regrasped and passed through the disinserted edge of the levator aponeurosis (see Fig. 13–1*D*). No attempt is made to dissect the strongly adherent and vascular Müller's muscle off the undersurface of the aponeurosis. Any bleeding is immediately controlled with a bipolar cautery to avoid creating a hematoma in Müller's muscle, which can complicate adjustment of the eyelid height and contour. The suture

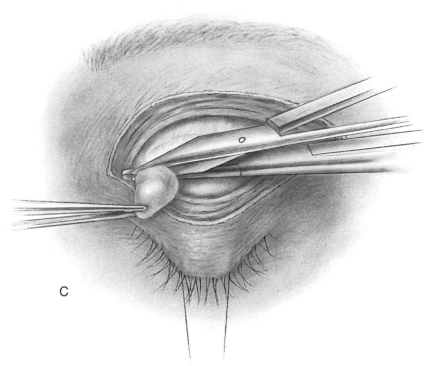

C, The medial fat pad is clamped, and the redundant fat is excised with tenotomy scissors.

C

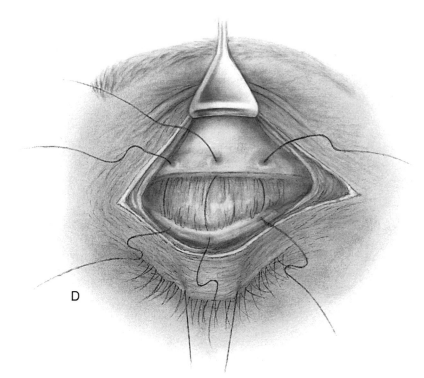

D, **Alternative 1:** The spontaneously disinserted edge of the levator aponeurosis is identified. The 5-0 polyglactin (Vicryl) sutures are passed vertically through the superior border of the tarsal plate and then passed through the disinserted edge of the levator aponeurosis.

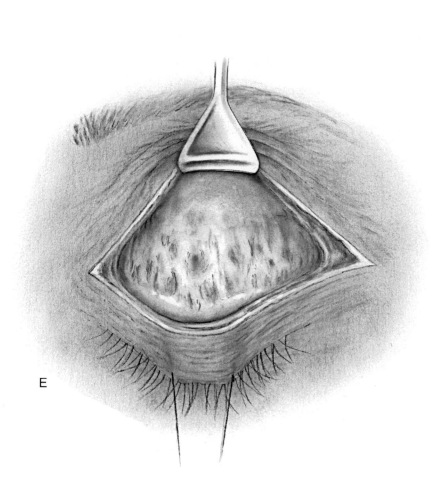

E, **Alternative 2:** Fatty infiltration of the levator aponeurosis. No distinct disinsertion is noted.

is permanently tied. All subsequent suture passes between the aponeurosis and the tarsus will also be permanently secured at the time of the procedure. Other surgeons have advocated the use of temporarily tied, adjustable aponeurotic sutures, which can be manipulated during the perioperative period to alter the eyelid height as needed.[5] We have found these sutures to be awkward to use; more importantly, they have not improved our results.

With the central suture permanently set, the patient is asked to open his or her eyes, and the height of the eyelid is examined with reference to the superior limbus and the height of the contralateral eyelid. If the height of the lid margin appears appropriate, the patient is placed in the sitting position and the lid height is reconfirmed. A lid height 1–2 mm higher than the intended final position is usually ideal because the eyelid will settle as swelling and the effects of the epinephrine dissipate. If the eyelid is undercorrected, the suture is removed and repositioned higher on the aponeurosis.

Once the desired height is achieved, the patient is placed back in the recumbent position and additional sutures are passed in an identical manner at the temporal and nasal limbal positions (see Fig. 13–1*D*). Again, the height and contour of the eyelid are reassessed with the patient in both reclining and sitting positions.

When an attenuated aponeurosis is still attached to the tarsus, a thin strip of pretarsal orbicularis muscle is excised along the superior border of the tarsal plate (Fig. 13–1*F*). This maneuver bares the superior border of the tarsal plate of the soft tissue and the aponeurotic adhesions and freshens the edge of the aponeurosis, which will ensure solid refixation. This step also results in the lowering of the eyelid crease already discussed. The 5-0 polyglactin sutures are passed through the tarsal plate in the manner previously described and are then passed through and above the leading edge of the aponeurosis. The amount of levator advancement and resection is determined empirically; typically, the range is between 3 and 10 mm.

If more than 4 mm of aponeurotic advancement is required, the aponeurosis is sharply dissected off the underlying Müller's muscle to the desired level, and the redundant aponeurosis is excised (Fig. 13–1*G–I*). No attempt is made to resect Müller's muscle. The lid height is again checked with the patient in both the reclining and sitting positions. If there is any question about the desired height of the eyelid, it is always safest to err on the side of overcorrection, as this can easily be corrected postoperatively. Once the appropriate lid height is reached, the temporal and nasal sutures are placed like the suture used to set the lid contour (Fig. 13–1*H–J*).

The blepharoplasty incision is closed with 6-0 fast-absorbing plain gut sutures (Fig. 13–1*K*). These sutures dissolve in 4–7 days, eliminating the need for suture removal. Interrupted sutures are preferred because they produce better wound apposition. Only the skin layer is closed. The septum should never be incorporated into the closure because doing so could result in postoperative lagophthalmos. A redundant medial skin fold or dog ear can be excised in a triangular fashion. Because the orbital septum is fully opened and the redundant preaponeurotic fat is sharply excised in addition to removal of a strip of pretarsal orbicularis muscle, a strong eyelid crease is achieved without the need for supratarsal

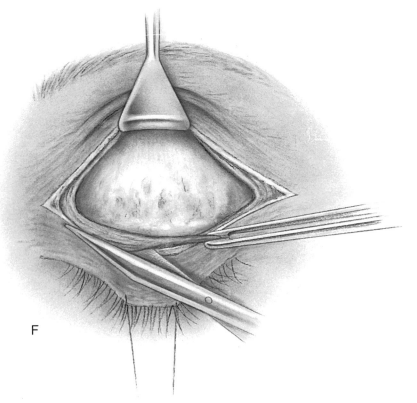

F, **Alternative 2:** Excision of the pretarsal orbicularis muscle bares the superior aspect of the tarsal plate.

F

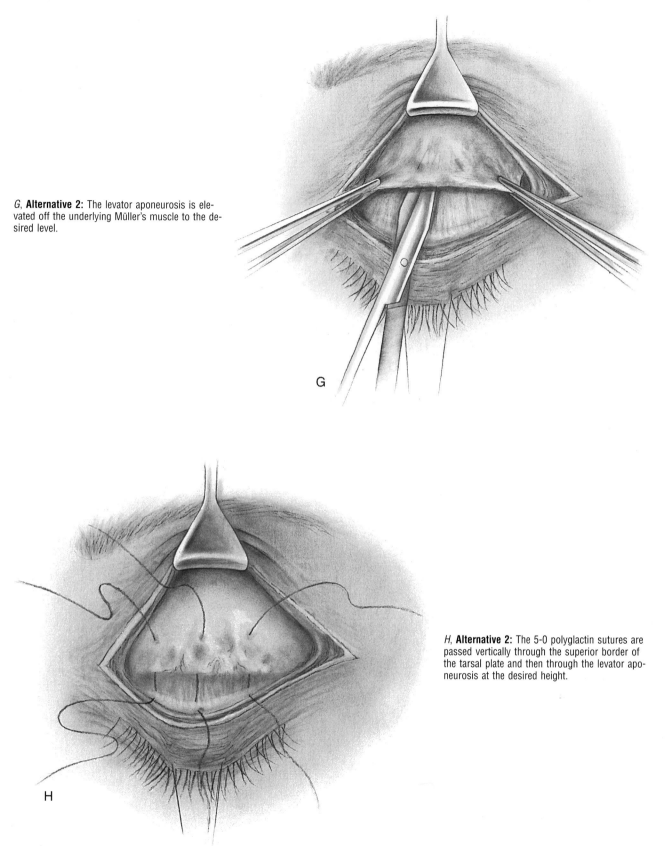

G, **Alternative 2:** The levator aponeurosis is elevated off the underlying Müller's muscle to the desired level.

H, **Alternative 2:** The 5-0 polyglactin sutures are passed vertically through the superior border of the tarsal plate and then through the levator aponeurosis at the desired height.

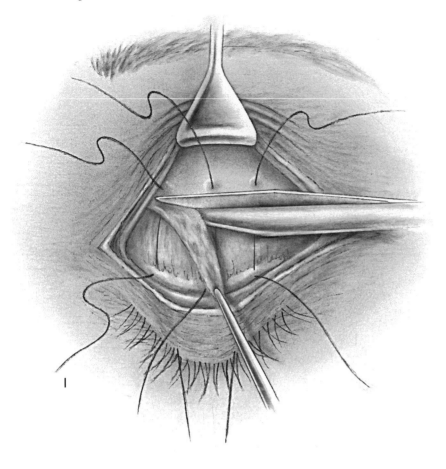

I, **Alternative 2:** The redundant levator aponeurosis is excised.

J, The 5-0 polyglactin sutures are secured.

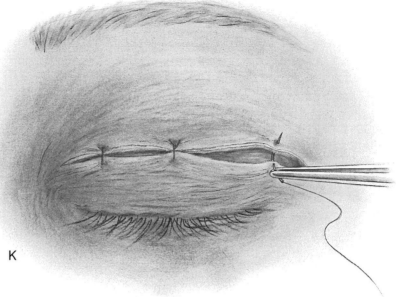

K, Skin closure with interrupted 6-0 plain gut sutures.

K

fixation sutures. We generally avoid the use of supratarsal fixation sutures, as they have been associated with recurrent ptosis, epithelial inclusion cysts, suture abscesses, and asymmetric eyelid creases.

POSTOPERATIVE CARE

Postoperatively, the patient is instructed to apply cold compresses to the eyelids for several days and to place lubricating drops and ointment in the eyes for several weeks until the incisions begin to relax and eyelid closure becomes complete. A mild to moderate amount of temporary lagophthalmos is expected postoperatively. Postoperative edema completely clears in 2–4 weeks.

Patients should refrain from taking aspirin-containing products for several weeks. They also should limit sun exposure so as to avoid skin and wound discoloration.

COMPLICATIONS

The most common postoperative complications are mild lagophthalmos and exposure keratitis. In almost every case, these complications are self-limiting and respond to topical lubricants and eyelid massage. Other complications include occurrences of wound dehiscence, wound infection, temporary eyelash eversion, rare epithelial suture cysts, and allergic dermatologic and conjunctival reactions from antibiotic ointments.

TREATMENT OF OVERCORRECTION AND UNDERCORRECTION

Overcorrection

Postoperative management of lid height asymmetry is relatively simple with the external aponeurotic ptosis

repair and can usually be performed in the office.[6] Small overcorrections generally respond to gentle massage of the eyelid for 5–10 minutes four times a day. To accomplish this, we have the patient hold his or her eyebrow up with one hand while pushing the eyelid both down and in with the index finger of the other hand. This massage can begin as soon as the skin incisions have healed.

Significant overcorrections noted in the first 10 days after the procedure can be corrected by opening a portion of the wound and removing one or more of the 5-0 polyglactin sutures suspending the aponeurosis to the tarsal plate. The area surrounding the eyelid crease incision is usually relatively free of sensation during the first few days postoperatively, and typically, minimal local anesthesia is required for this procedure. After the lid height is corrected, the wound is closed with one or two 6-0 fast-absorbing plain gut sutures.

Undercorrection

Significant undercorrections are much more difficult to deal with. To repass sutures through the tarsal plate and aponeurosis, almost the entire length of the skin incision must be reopened. Once the height of the eyelid is reset, the contour must be readjusted. In effect, the entire procedure must be repeated to correct an undercorrection. For this reason, it is always best to achieve a slight overcorrection rather than an undercorrection in an aponeurotic ptosis repair.

If an obvious undercorrection (>2 mm) needs to be repaired, it is best to do so within the first postoperative week to take advantage of the relative ease of dissection afforded by the original procedure. If the undercorrection is minimal (1 mm), we advocate observation of the eyelid until the postoperative edema has cleared before any additional intervention is pursued.

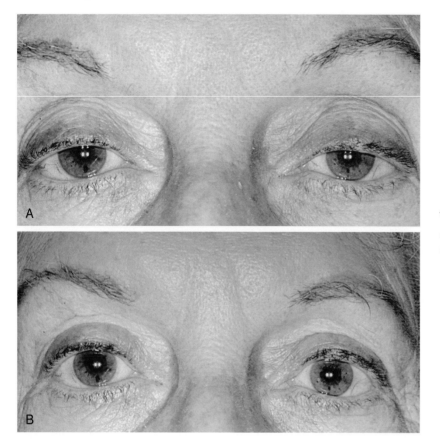

figure 13-2

Preoperative *(A)* and postoperative *(B)* appearance following combined upper eyelid blepharoplasty and aponeurotic ptosis repair.

RESULTS

The combined upper eyelid blepharoplasty and external levator aponeurotic ptosis repair procedure has been performed in more than 1600 patients over the past two decades (Fig. 13–2*A* and *B*). Good to excellent results, as determined by symmetric lid contour and central lid height within 1.5 mm of the desired position, were achieved with a single procedure in approximately 95 per cent of patients.

Primary overcorrections requiring removal of aponeurotic sutures in the office occurred in 3 per cent of patients; all instances were successfully corrected. Primary undercorrections were noted in fewer than 1 per cent of patients. These patients required a second procedure with more aggressive aponeurotic advancement. Late ptosis recurrence (occurring more than 6 months following the initial procedure) was seen in 1–2 per cent of patients. Most of these recurrences were in patients noted to have fatty infiltration of the aponeurosis at the initial procedure. At the time of the second operation, most of these patients were found to have attenuation of the aponeurosis immediately above the tarsal plate. Very few true disinsertions were encountered. Presum-ably, the levator aponeurosis in this group of patients is inherently weak and prone to stretching.

The technique of combined blepharoplasty with aponeurotic ptosis repair has proved tremendously success-ful. With a thorough knowledge of eyelid anatomy, proper suture placement, appropriate depth of anesthe-sia, and careful intraoperative assessment of eyelid heights and contours, the surgeon can accurately correct dermatochalasis and blepharoptosis using this technique in almost every patient seeking cosmetic eyelid surgery.

References

1. Anderson RL, Edwards JJ, Wood JR: Bilateral visual loss after blepharoplasty. Ann Plast Surg 1980; 5:288–292.
2. Wesley RE, Pollard ZF, McCord CD: Superior oblique palsy after blepharoplasty. Plast Reconstr Surg 1980; 66:283–287.
3. Shore JW, McCord CD: Anatomic changes in involutional blepharoptosis. Am J Ophthalmol 1984; 98:211–227.
4. Smith B, Petrelli R: Surgical repair of prolapsed lacrimal glands. Arch Ophthalmol 1978; 96:113–114.
5. Collins JR, O'Donnell BA: Adjustable sutures in eyelid surgery for ptosis and lid retraction. Br J Ophthalmol 1994; 78:167–174.
6. Jordan DR, Anderson RL: A simple procedure for adjusting eyelid position after aponeurotic ptosis surgery. Arch Ophthalmol 1987; 105:1288–1291.

Allen M. Putterman

Müller's Muscle–Conjunctival Resection–Ptosis Procedure Combined with Upper Blepharoplasty

It is possible to combine an upper lid blepharoplasty with ptosis surgery. Although this technique is commonly performed through an external approach with levator aponeurosis resection, many cosmetic surgeons do not appreciate the possibility of combining an internal Müller's muscle–conjunctival resection with an external upper blepharoplasty, especially when the skin and orbicularis oculi muscle are excised and an eyelid crease is reconstructed.

This chapter demonstrates how to combine a Müller's muscle resection with an upper lid blepharoplasty, a procedure I have performed for years. I find that this combined procedure gives me better results than the levator aponeurosis procedure with upper blepharoplasty in patients whose upper eyelids elevate to normal levels after administration of phenylephrine. The phenylephrine test also can be helpful in identifying candidates for this combined procedure.

ALLEN M. PUTTERMAN

The Müller's muscle–conjunctival resection–ptosis procedure, described in 1975 by Putterman and Urist, is a technique in which Müller's muscle in the upper eyelid is partially resected and advanced.[1] The procedure is used to treat upper eyelid ptosis and can be combined with an upper eyelid blepharoplasty with or without crease reconstruction. The operation has the advantage of preserving tarsus, which creates less risk of suture-induced keratopathy. There also is rarely a need for additional surgery to treat residual ptosis.

DIAGNOSIS AND PREOPERATIVE EVALUATION

Two tests are done preoperatively to determine candidates for the Müller's muscle–conjunctival resection procedure:

- Margin reflex distance-1 (MRD_1) measurement
- Phenylephrine test

MRD$_1$ Test

The MRD_1 measurement is used to assess the upper eyelid levels (see Chapter 2, Fig. 2–8). It should be performed both before and during the phenylephrine test.

The difference in MRD_1 between the normal and ptotic sides indicates the degree of ptosis. The normal MRD_1 is approximately 4.5 mm, and this value is used as a reference in bilateral cases. The MRD_1 measurement has the advantage of being able to quantify the ptosis alone without the palpebral fissure width. This is preferred because there is a Müller's muscle in the lower eyelid that can also respond to phenylephrine. Measuring the palpebral fissure width would lead to an erroneous interpretation of the upper eyelid level after instillation of phenylephrine.

Phenylephrine Test

The MRD_1 is again measured, this time after instillation of 2.5 per cent or 10 per cent phenylephrine drops. The patient's head is tilted backward, the upper eyelid is lifted, and the patient is instructed to gaze downward. Several drops of phenylephrine are dripped between the upper eyelid and the globe. To minimize the excretion of phenylephrine into the nasal cavity and the potential side effects of systemic absorption, the examiner uses the finger to compress the canaliculi for 10 seconds. This step is repeated immediately two more times. One minute later, two additional drops are applied. Three to 5 minutes after instillation of the phenylephrine, the MRD_1 is measured.

Side effects, such as myocardial infarction and hypertension, have been reported after instillation of phenylephrine drops.[3] Therefore, it is important to make sure that the patient does not have a cardiac problem before the phenylephrine test is performed.

Glatt and colleagues[2] have compared test results using 2.5 per cent and 10 per cent phenylephrine. It appears that both solutions are effective in determining candidates for the Müller's muscle–conjunctival resection procedure but that the 2.5 per cent solution may result in

fewer complications. My experience has been primarily with the 10 per cent solution.

INDICATIONS

The procedure is used to treat blepharoptosis in patients whose upper eyelids elevate to a normal level when phenylephrine drops are applied to the upper ocular fornix. Candidates for this procedure usually have minimal congenital ptosis and varying degrees of acquired ptosis.

GOAL OF THE OPERATION

The procedure should result in cosmetically acceptable upper eyelid levels on both sides and improvement of vision, especially on down gaze during reading.

SURGICAL TECHNIQUE

Anesthesia

Local anesthesia is preferred in adults. The upper eyelid skin to be removed is marked according to the technique for upper blepharoplasty with crease reconstruction (see Chapter 10) or without crease reconstruction (see Chap-

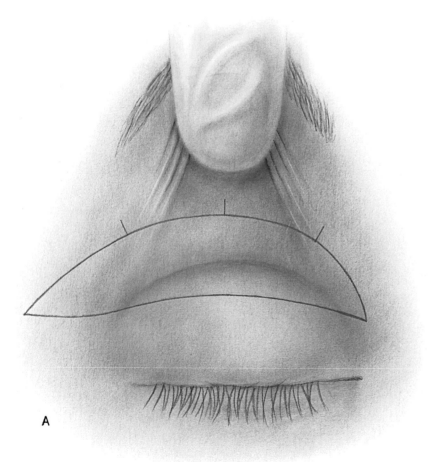

A

figure 14–1

A, Outline of skin or skin and orbicularis oculi muscle to be excised.

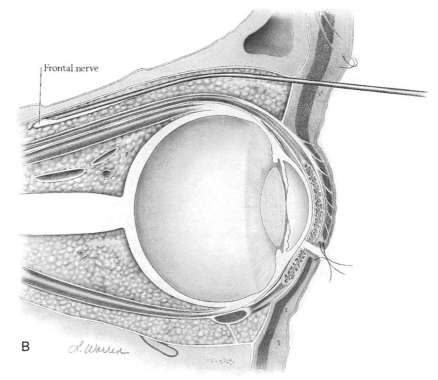

B, Administration of anesthesia before the Müller's muscle–conjunctival resection. A 4-cm, 23-gauge retrobulbar needle is inserted along the central orbital roof to its full length. An injection of 1.5 ml of 2 per cent lidocaine with epinephrine achieves a frontal nerve block and avoids infiltration of the eyelid.

ter 9) (Fig. 14–1A). A frontal nerve block is used with local anesthesia to avoid swelling of the upper eyelid by local infiltration, which would make the operation more difficult and inexact.[4]

A 23-gauge retrobulbar needle is inserted into the superior orbit, entering just under the midsuperior orbital rim (Fig. 14–1B). The needle hugs the roof of the orbit during insertion until a depth of 4 cm is reached; then 1.5 ml of 2 per cent lidocaine (Xylocaine) with epinephrine is injected. Another 0.5 ml of 2 per cent lidocaine with epinephrine is injected subcutaneously over the central upper eyelid just above the lid margin, and a small amount is injected under the lines marked on the upper eyelid (Fig. 14–1C).

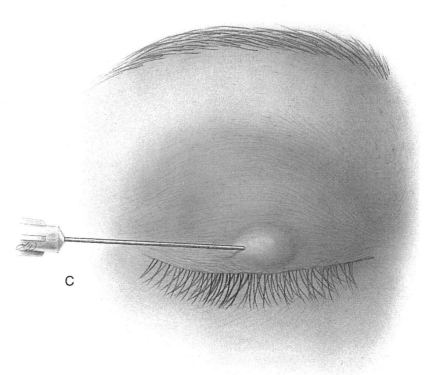

C, A second injection of 0.5 ml of 2 per cent lidocaine with epinephrine is given subcutaneously over the central upper eyelid above the lashes.

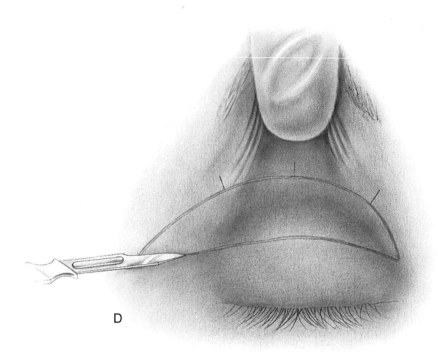

D, Scratch incision over marked upper eyelid.

D

E, The upper eyelid is everted over a Desmarres retractor, and a 6-0 black silk marking suture is placed through conjunctiva 6.5–9.5 mm above the superior tarsal border. One suture bite is taken centrally, and one bite is made 7 mm nasal and temporal to the central bite.

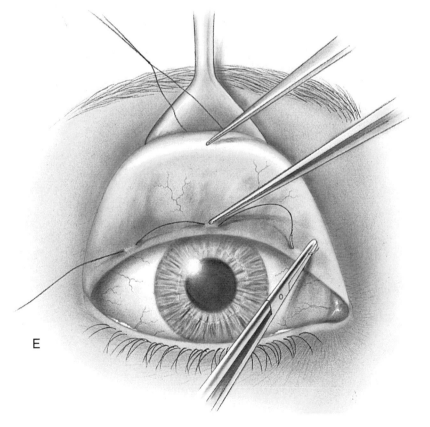

E

Marking Areas of Excision and Resection

A scratch incision is made over the marked upper eyelid lines (Fig. 14–1*D*). A 4-0 black silk traction suture is inserted through skin, orbicularis muscle, and superficial tarsus 2 mm above the lashes at the center of the upper eyelid. A medium-sized Desmarres lid retractor is used to evert the upper eyelid and to expose the palpebral conjunctiva from the superior tarsal border to the superior fornix. Topical tetracaine drops are then applied over the upper palpebral conjunctiva.

A caliper set at 8.5 mm, with one arm at the superior tarsal border, facilitates insertion of a 6-0 black silk suture through the conjunctiva 8.5 mm above the superior tarsal border (Fig. 14–1*E*). One suture bite centrally and two others approximately 7 mm nasal and temporal to the center mark the site. The preferred placement of the 6-0 black silk marking suture is 8.5 mm above the superior tarsal border, but the suture may be placed 6.5–9.5 mm above the border if the response of the upper eyelid level to the phenylephrine test is slightly greater or less than desired.

Separation of Müller's Muscle from the Levator Aponeurosis

A toothed forceps is used to grasp conjunctiva and Müller's muscle between the superior tarsal border and the marking suture and to separate Müller's muscle from its loose attachment to the levator aponeurosis (Fig. 14–1*F*). This maneuver is possible because Müller's muscle is firmly attached to conjunctiva but only loosely attached to the levator aponeurosis (see Chapter 7, Fig. 7–1).

Clamp Application

One blade of a specially designed Müller's muscle–conjunctival resection–ptosis clamp (Karl Ilg & Co., St. Charles, Ill.) should be placed at the level of the marking suture. Each tooth of this blade engages each suture bite that passes through the palpebral conjunctiva (Fig. 14–1*G*).

The Desmarres retractor is then slowly released as the other blade of the clamp engages conjunctiva and Müller's muscle adjacent to the superior tarsal border (Fig. 14–1*H*).

Any entrapped tarsus is pulled out of the clamp with the surgeon's finger (Fig. 14–*I*). The clamp is compressed, and the handle is locked. This leads to the incorporation of conjunctiva and Müller's muscle between the superior tarsal border and the marking suture.

The upper eyelid skin is pulled in one direction while the clamp is pulled simultaneously in the opposite direction (Fig. 14–1*J*). During this maneuver, the surgeon may feel a sense of attachment between the skin and the clamp. If this occurs, the levator aponeurosis has been inadvertently trapped in the clamp. In this situation, the clamp should be released and reapplied in its proper

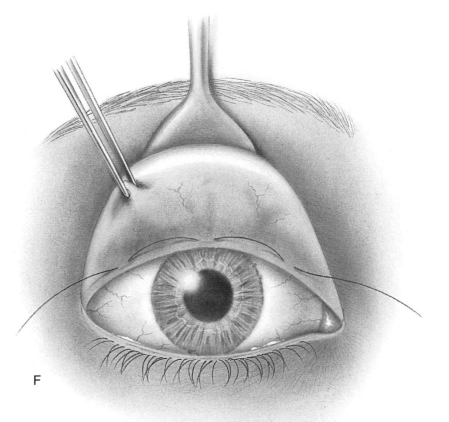

F, A toothed forceps is used to separate the conjunctiva and Müller's muscle from its loose attachment to the levator aponeurosis at various sites between the upper tarsal border and the marking suture.

F

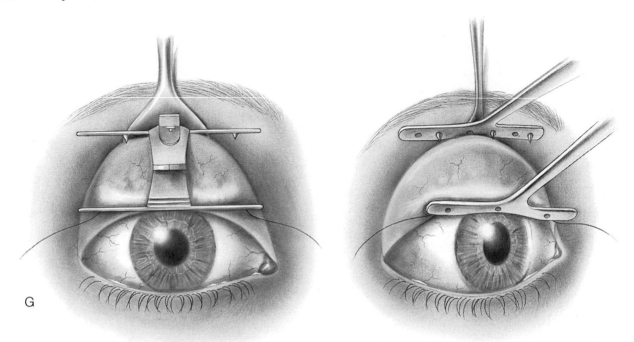

G, A clamp is positioned so that each tooth of one blade engages each site of the marking suture; the other blade is above the superior tarsal border.

position. This maneuver is possible because the levator aponeurosis sends extensions to orbicularis muscle and skin to form the lid crease (see Fig. 7–1).

Suturing and Resection of Conjunctiva and Müller's Muscle

With the clamp held straight up, a 5-0 double-armed plain catgut mattress suture is run 1.5 mm below the clamp along its entire width in a temporal to nasal direction, through the upper margin of the tarsus on one side and through Müller's muscle and conjunctiva on the other side, and vice versa (Fig. 14–1*K* and *L*). The sutures are placed approximately 2–3 mm from each other. The surgeon uses a No. 15 surgical blade to excise the tissues held in the clamp by cutting between the sutures and the clamp. The knife blade is rotated slightly, with its sharp edge hugging the clamp.

As the tissues are sliced from the clamp, the surgeon

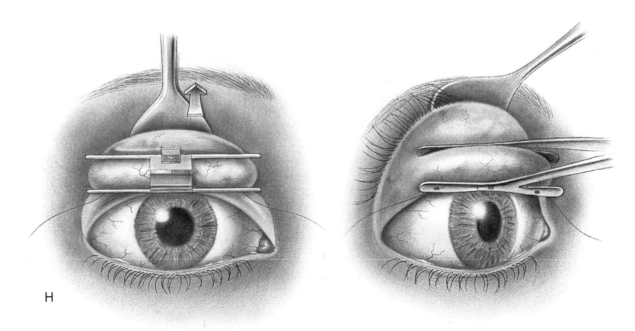

H, As the Desmarres retractor is gradually released through rotation, the other clamp blade slides over tarsus as its teeth engage conjunctiva and Müller's muscle above the superior tarsal border.

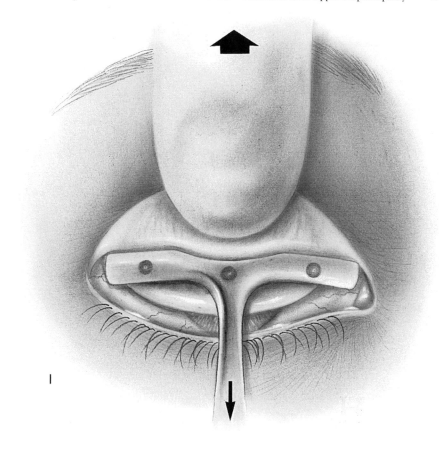

I, Before locking the clamp, the surgeon slides out any entrapped tarsus.

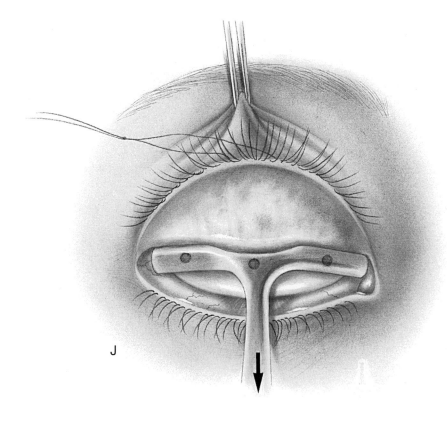

J, The closed clamp includes 6.5–9.5 mm of conjunctiva and Müller's muscle just above the superior tarsal border. Clamp and skin are pulled in opposite directions to ensure that the levator aponeurosis is not caught in the clamp.

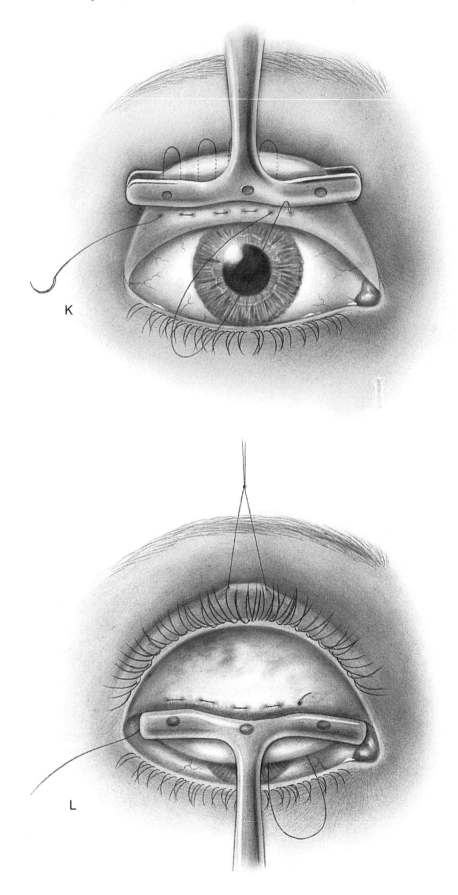

K and L, A 5-0 plain catgut mattress suture runs in a temporal to nasal direction about 1.5 mm distal to the clamp; each suture bite includes upper tarsus, Müller's muscle, and conjunctiva.

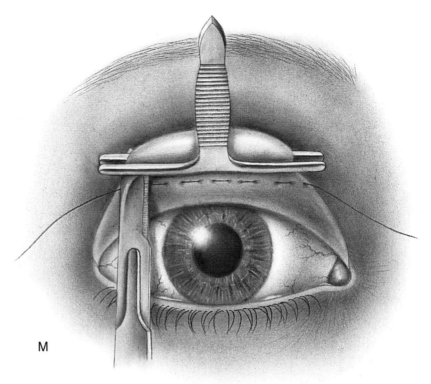

M, Conjunctiva–Müller's muscle is excised by running a No. 15 surgical blade against the edge of the clamp.

M

and the assistant watch to ensure that the sutures on each side are not cut (Fig. 14–1*M*).

The Desmarres retractor again is used to evert the eyelid while gentle traction is applied to the 4-0 black silk centering suture. The nasal end of the suture is then run continuously in a temporal direction; the stitches should be about 2 mm apart through the edge of superior tarsal border, Müller's muscle, and conjunctiva (Fig. 14–1 *N*). Commonly, this suture just connects the edges of conjunctiva.

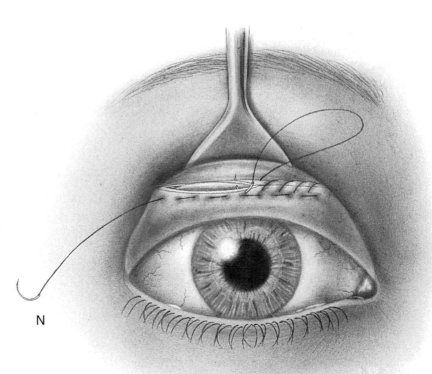

N, The nasal suture arm runs continuously in a nasal to temporal direction through the edges of conjunctiva, Müller's muscle, and tarsus.

N

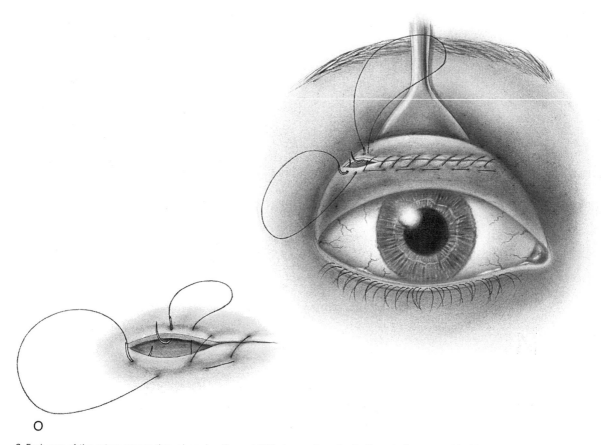

O, Each arm of the suture passes through conjunctiva and Müller's muscle and exits through the temporal incision; the suture arms are tied.

During continuous closure with the 5-0 plain catgut suture, the surgeon must be careful to avoid cutting the original mattress suture. This is facilitated by the surgeon's using a small suture needle (S-14 Spatula, Ethicon) in addition to observing the mattress suture position during each suture bite and by the assistant's applying continuous suction along the incision edges. The 5-0 plain catgut suture ends are passed through each side of the conjunctiva and Müller's muscle before they exit through the temporal end of the incision (Fig. 14–1*O*). Once each arm of the suture reaches the temporal end of the eyelid, the suture ends are connected with a serrefine clamp.

Upper Blepharoplasty

Several milliliters of 2 per cent lidocaine (Xylocaine) with epinephrine is injected subcutaneously over the upper eyelids. Then an upper eyelid blepharoplasty is performed (as described in Chapters 9 and 10) through the steps of skin or skin and orbicularis muscle resection, excision of fat, and completion of hemostasis (Fig. 14–1*P*). The eyelid is again everted with a Desmarres retractor, the 5-0 plain catgut suture arms are tied with 4–5 knots, and the ends are cut close to the knot. In this way, the knot can be buried subconjunctivally, lessening postoperative keratopathy.

After this step, the crease sutures are placed and the skin is closed (see Chapter 10) (Fig. 14–1*Q*). If no crease is reconstructed, the skin is sutured at this time, as described in Chapter 9.

POSTOPERATIVE CARE

Patients are observed for several hours postoperatively to make sure that there is no retrobulbar hemorrhage, which has the potential for causing blindness. The patient applies cold compresses to the eyelids for the first 24 hours postoperatively. A topical antibiotic such as gentamicin (Garamycin) ophthalmic ointment on the eye is used twice a day for the first week and then once a day for another week. The patient also uses a sterile eyewash applied to cotton pads to wipe over the eyelids twice a day for 2 weeks after surgery. Patients are instructed for the first 2 weeks after surgery to bathe or shower only from the neck down and to wash their hair so as to avoid contact of soap and water with the eyes.

RESULTS

The average follow-up is 3.3 months but varies from 2 weeks to 7 years. Follow-up generally lasts until the patient's eyelids cease to change. The MRD$_1$ at stabilization of lid levels is considered the final result.

In most patients with acquired ptosis (90 per cent in

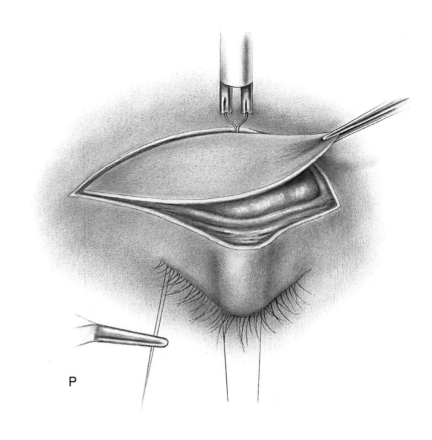

P, Excision of outline ellipse of skin and orbicularis muscle with a disposable cautery.

P

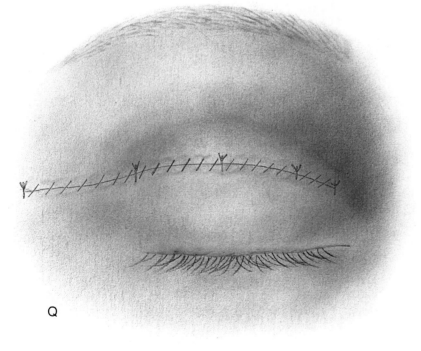

Q, Placement of three 6-0 polyglactin (Vicryl) sutures uniting skin and levator aponeurosis. A 6-0 continuous silk suture closes the skin. (Parts *B, C,* and *E–O,* From Putterman AM, Fett DR: Müller's muscle in the treatment of upper eyelid ptosis: A ten-year study. Ophthalmic Surg 1986; 17:354–356. With permission.)

Q

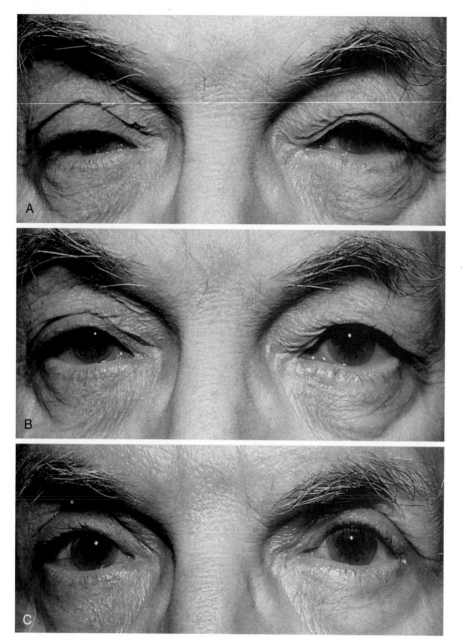

figure 14–2

A, Preoperative appearance of a patient with bilateral upper eyelid ptosis associated with dermatochalasis (excessive skin) and herniated orbital fat of all four eyelids. *B*, After instillation of phenylephrine in both upper fornices with elevation of both upper eyelids. *C*, After a bilateral Müller's muscle–conjunctival resection–ptosis procedure and excision of skin, orbicularis muscle, and orbital fat from both upper eyelids with eyelid crease reconstruction.

my experience), the final eyelid level after treatment is within 2 mm of the opposite eyelid. In 88 per cent of these treated eyelids, an MRD_1 of 1.5–5 mm is achieved.[5]

Patients with congenital ptosis have a final eyelid level after treatment within 1.5 mm of the opposite eyelid. In 84 per cent of these treated eyelids, an MRD_1 of 2.5–5 mm is achieved.

Rarely, in less than 2 per cent of patients, additional surgery may be required to treat residual ptosis. This is achieved with a levator aponeurosis procedure (see Chapter 13).

Occasionally, the upper eyelid is too high. If this elevation occurs, the patient massages the upper eyelid downward while simultaneously fixating the brow 2–4 times each day for 1–4 weeks. If massage is ineffective, a simplified levator recession is performed.[6]

ALTERNATIVE TECHNIQUES

The Müller's muscle–conjunctival resection procedure has an advantage over the Fasanella procedure because it allows the tarsus to be preserved.[7, 8] This carries less risk of suture keratopathy because the sutures are at the superior tarsal border instead of 3–4 mm closer to the eyelid margins, as in the Fasanella procedure. This operation also is also superior to the levator aponeurosis advancement and tuck procedure because results are much more predictable and there is less need for subsequent surgery.[8, 9]

I have performed this procedure on more than 1000 upper eyelids. In a report of results in 232 of the treated lids, 230 lids had levels that were considered cosmetically acceptable (Figs. 14–2 and 14–3).[5]

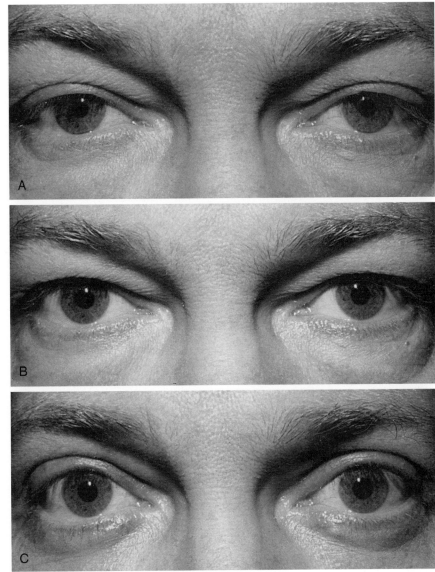

figure 14–3

A, Preoperative appearance of a patient with upper eyelid ptosis associated with dermatochalasis and herniated orbital fat of all four eyelids. *B*, After instillation of phenylephrine in both upper fornices with elevation of eyelids to normal levels. *C*, After bilateral Müller's muscle–conjunctival resection–ptosis procedure with excision of skin, orbicularis oculi muscle, and orbital fat from the upper eyelids and eyelid crease reconstruction. A lower eyelid external blepharoplasty using a skin–muscle flap approach (see Chapter 19) was performed simultaneously.

References

1. Putterman AM, Urist MJ: Müller's muscle–conjunctival resection: Technique for treatment of blepharoptosis. Arch Ophthalmol 1975; 93:619.
2. Glatt HJ, Fett DR, Putterman AM: Comparison of 2.5% and 10% phenylephrine in the elevation of upper eyelids with ptosis. Ophthalmic Surg 1990; 21:173.
3. Fraunfelder FT, Scafidi A: Possible adverse effect from topical ocular 10% phenylephrine. Am J Ophthalmol 1978; 85:447–453.
4. Hildreth HR, Silver B: Sensory block of the upper eyelid. Arch Ophthalmol 1976; 77:202–231.
5. Putterman AM, Fett DR: Müller's muscle in the treatment of upper eyelid ptosis: A ten-year study. Ophthalmic Surg 1986; 17:354–356.
6. Putterman AM, Urist MJ: A simplified levator palpebrae superioris muscle recession to treat overcorrected blepharoptosis. Am J Ophthalmol 1974; 77:358–366.
7. Fasanella RM, Servat J: Levator resection for minimal ptosis: Another simplified operation. Arch Ophthalmol 1961; 65:493–496.
8. Putterman AM, Urist MJ: Müller's muscle–conjunctival resection-ptosis procedure. Ophthalmic Surg 1978; 9:27–32.
9. Jones LT, Quickert MH, Wobig JL: The cure of ptosis by aponeurotic repair. Arch Ophthalmol 1975; 93:629–634.

J. Justin Older

Chapter 15

Treatment of Upper Eyelid Retraction: External Approach

Upper eyelid retraction secondary to thyroid ophthalmopathy is treated by release of the upper eyelid retractors (the levator aponeurosis and Müller's muscle). I commonly treat this condition through an internal eyelid approach, which is described in Chapter 16. However, a successful alternative way to treat upper eyelid retraction is through an external approach.

J. Justin Older beautifully describes the release of the levator aponeurosis and Müller's muscle through an external blepharoplasty approach. An advantage of this approach, compared with the internal one, is that it allows the excision of skin, orbicularis oculi muscle, and orbital fat to be performed through the same incision from which Müller's muscle and levator aponeurosis are released. Even though an upper blepharoplasty can be combined with an internal approach, when only Müller's muscle is excised, I have found that if there is extensive levator recession, an upper blepharoplasty is usually best treated secondarily to avoid an overcorrection or undercorrection. Performing the procedure primarily from an external approach avoids this secondary surgery, which is at times required with the use of the internal approach.

Another advantage of Dr. Older's approach is that it easily allows for redeposition of prolapsed lacrimal glands and removal of sub-brow fat, which often is advantageous in patients with thyroid ophthalmopathy.

ALLEN M. PUTTERMAN

The goal in the treatment of eyelid retraction secondary to thyroid eye disease is to weaken Müller's muscle and, in many cases, the levator palpebra superioris. To achieve this goal, numerous approaches have been advocated. Many of these approaches have been successful, which suggests that there is no one perfect way to correct eyelid retraction. The choice of procedure is usually determined by the surgeon's experience and comfort zone.

There have been two basic approaches: (1) the *internal* approach through the conjunctiva and (2) the *external* approach through a skin incision. Spacers have also been used to keep the recessed Müller's muscle and levator aponeurosis from reattaching to the tarsus. Eye bank sclera, fascia lata, and other substances have been used as spacers, which can be placed in the eyelid through either the conjunctival or skin approach.

One advantage of a skin approach is that the anatomy is more straightforward compared with the everted eyelid in the conjunctival approach. In an effort to achieve the best possible results, surgeons have developed many types of transcutaneous procedures. These include:

1. A müllerectomy and recession of the levator aponeurosis combined with medial transposition of the lateral horn of the levator aponeurosis.[1]
2. Myectomy of the levator muscle.[2, 3]
3. Levator aponeurotic Müller's muscle recession with maintenance of the normal attachment of the orbital septum to levator aponeurosis.[4]

4. Use of exteriorized adjustable sutures that fasten the levator aponeurosis to the superior tarsus.[5]

In the technique described in this chapter, the orbital septum is not violated unless fat is to be removed as part of the procedure and the orbital septum and levator aponeurosis are recessed as one block of tissue. Müller's muscle is usually dissected separately, since the aponeurosis comes away from Müller's muscle easily, but Müller's muscle is closely adherent to the conjunctiva. In other skin approach techniques, Müller's muscle may be completely extirpated or may be recessed. In many of the other techniques in which levator aponeurosis and Müller's muscle are recessed, the edges are tied to either the underlying conjunctiva or the orbicularis muscle and skin combination. In some cases, a loose suture is placed between the recessed levator aponeurosis and the superior border of the tarsus.

In the technique I describe here, no sutures are used to hold the recessed levator–Müller's muscle complex in position. The assumption is that the eyelid swelling will cause the recessed structures to stay in position. A small amount of return to the original position is expected; therefore, a 1–2 mm overcorrection is usually planned.

In some techniques, the upper eyelid is taped to the lower eyelid during the healing phase. I have not done that, but I have been told that when it is done, there is a tendency toward an overcorrection. The only sutures used in this procedure are for skin closure.

PATIENT SELECTION

Patients with thyroid eye disease who have not shown progression of any ocular changes for at least 6 months are candidates for this operation. If Graves' disease is not under control or if the eyelid has been retracted for

only a few months, there still might be eyelid position changes.

Therefore, it is best to wait at least 6 months from the time the eyelids become stable. Patients must be able to cooperate during surgery because they must sit up and perform various eye movements during the procedure. Bilateral or unilateral procedures can be done. Cosmetic blepharoplasty with or without fat removal can also be performed with this procedure.

SURGICAL TECHNIQUE

For a unilateral procedure, a line is drawn in the upper eyelid crease in an effort to match the eyelid crease on the opposite side (Fig. 15–1A). The anesthetic agent used throughout the procedure is 2 per cent lidocaine with epinephrine. This is mixed 50:50 with 0.5 per cent bupivacaine with epinephrine and then mixed 20:1 with sodium bicarbonate (a buffered agent causes less pain when injected). The anesthetic is given in the pretarsal area under the skin and in the preseptal area of the orbicularis muscle. Injections may also be given through the conjunctiva above the tarsus.

If a blepharoplasty is performed, the appropriate blepharoplasty lines are drawn before injection. The incisions are made so that the skin and underlying orbicularis muscle are removed together. Preaponeurotic fat and fat in the medial fat pockets can also be removed before recession of Müller's muscle and the levator aponeurosis. Dissection is then continued to expose the levator aponeurosis as it attaches to the upper border of the tarsus.

If a blepharoplasty is not performed, an eyelid crease incision is made and dissection must be carried laterally to the lateral part of the tarsus. The levator aponeurosis is identified, and the attachments of the aponeurosis to

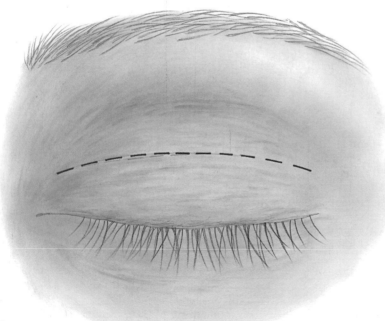

figure 15–1

A, A line is drawn at the proposed site of the skin incision.

A

the tarsus are released (Fig. 15–1*B* and *C*). Once all of the levator aponeurosis is detached from the superior border of the tarsus, the patient is asked to sit up to evaluate the amount of the correction.

Releasing the levator aponeurosis yields only a small amount of correction for eyelid retraction. In most cases, recession of Müller's muscle is necessary. Müller's muscle is very vascular, and cautery must be used constantly during this procedure. Release of the fibers of Müller's muscle can be achieved with a scissors or a light cauterizing instrument, such as a disposable cautery (Fig. 15–1*D* and *E*). The tarsus is held inferiorly, usually by the assistant, and with downward pressure on the tarsus, slips of Müller's muscle are grasped with a fine forceps and cut with a scissors, hot cautery, or an electric knife on a low power setting. Dissection must be carried laterally to the lateral part of the tarsus (Fig. 15–1*F* and *G*). Lacrimal gland tissue may be encountered in this area. I have never seen any symptomatic dry eyes result from this procedure.

Another maneuver that I find helpful for pulling Müller's muscle away from the tarsus is to grasp Müller's muscle fibers with a forceps and pull superiorly while pressing the tarsus down with a cotton-tipped applicator.

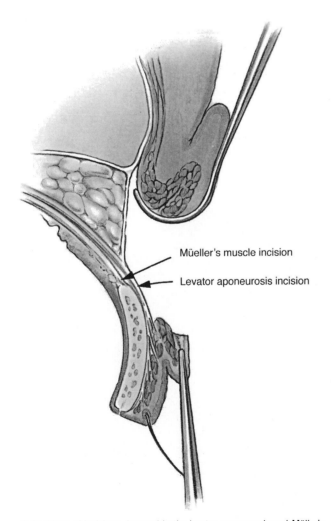

Müeller's muscle incision

Levator aponeurosis incision

B, Positions of incisions *(arrows)* in the levator aponeurosis and Müller's muscle.

At this point, there is only conjunctiva covering the cornea; therefore, very careful dissection must be done. I have never used a corneal protector, but the decision whether to use such a device is up to the operating surgeon. If a protector is used, I suggest removing it each time the patient is asked to sit up for evaluation of the eyelid height.

For an eyelid retraction of 2–3 mm, I often find that most of Müller's muscle is recessed about 7–8 mm above the tarsus, so that most of the cornea is showing through the conjunctiva. Usually, a few fibers of Müller's muscle are still attached to the tarsus. The curve must be natural, and this can be manipulated by performing further recession of Müller's muscle and levator laterally to allow the eyelid to drop in the lateral area. If the eyelid drops too far, some of the slips of fibrous tissue connecting with Müller's muscle can be reattached to the superior tarsus, or a flap made up of Müller's muscle and fibrous tissue can be created as a rotation flap and brought down to the superior border of the tarsus. It is then sutured to the tarsus. The patient is asked to look up, and this flap can be lengthened or shortened, as necessary, to get the eyelid to the correct height. This type of flap can also be used to lift the center of the eyelid if the eyelid curvature seems too flat.

Surgical judgment is extremely important in deciding exactly where to set the eyelid height. For bilateral surgery in a young or middle-aged person, I try to set the lid margin about 2 mm below the upper limbus, anticipating 1–2 mm of lift postoperatively. For the older patient who normally has a smaller palpebral fissure, the eyelid can be set a bit lower. For unilateral surgery, I try to set the involved eyelid about 1–2 mm below the opposite eyelid, again because I anticipate a 1–2 mm lift during the postoperative period.

If swelling occurs during surgery, this has to be factored into the equation. Generally, however, the amount of swelling that occurs intraoperatively is usually not enough to affect the decision regarding placement of the eyelid.

If a buttonhole in the conjunctiva is created during the surgical procedure, I repair it with a 7-0 chromic suture with the knot away from the cornea. When the correct height is achieved and all bleeding is controlled, I repair the skin incision with a running 6-0 or 7-0 polypropylene (Prolene) suture. No deep sutures for positioning the levator aponeurosis or Müller's muscle are used.

In some patients, there is a great deal of lateral lift. To release this lift, the surgeon would have to perform a fair amount of dissection through the lacrimal tissue. To avoid the potential for a dry eye, I limit my dissection through lacrimal tissue and correct the lateral lift by performing a lateral tarsorrhaphy (see Chapter 26). This technique also helps pull the lower eyelid up a small amount, which may be desirable.

POSTOPERATIVE CARE

After surgery, an antibiotic ointment and a cold compress are placed on the eye. The patient remains in the

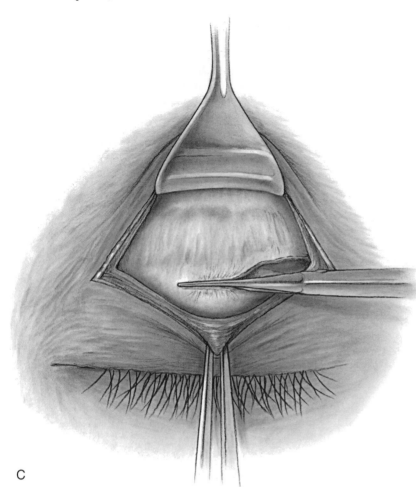

C

C, Release of the levator aponeurosis from the superior tarsal border.

D, Undermining of Müller's muscle.

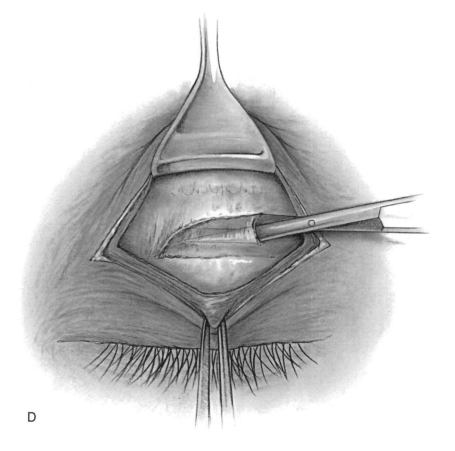

D

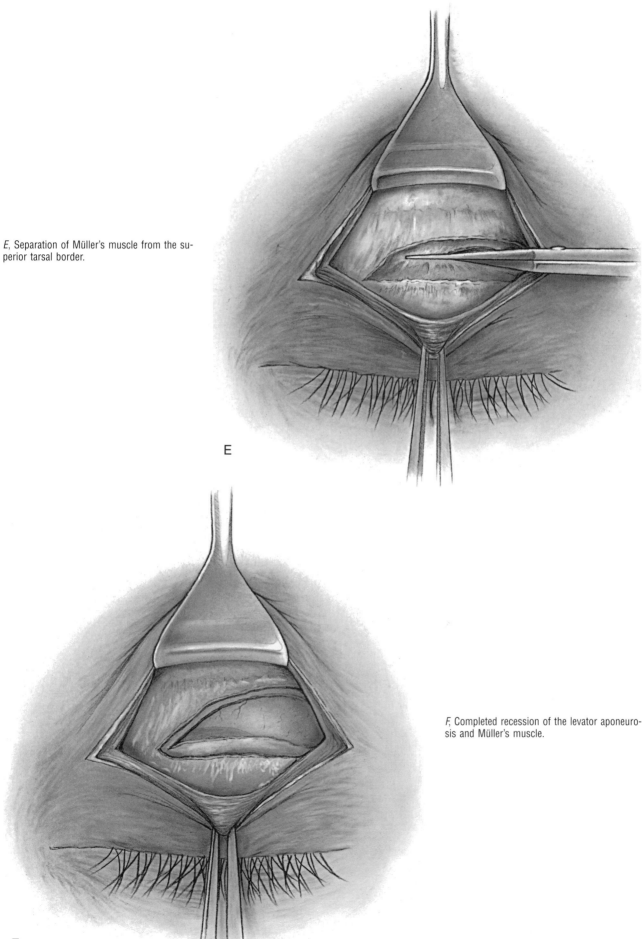

E, Separation of Müller's muscle from the superior tarsal border.

E

F, Completed recession of the levator aponeurosis and Müller's muscle.

F

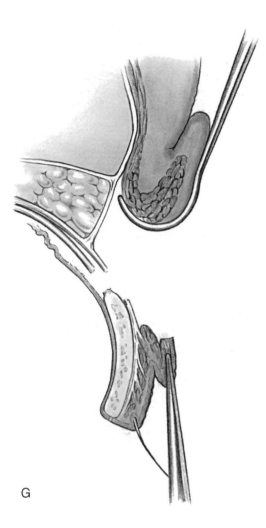

G

G, Appearance of tissue layers before skin closure. (*C–G,* Modified from Older JJ: Surgical treatment of eyelid retraction associated with thyroid eye disease. Ophthalmic Surg 1991; 22(6):318–322. With permission.)

figure 15–2

A, A 33-year-old woman with right upper eyelid retraction secondary to thyroid eye disease. *B,* Same patient 1 month after levator aponeurosis and Müller's muscle recession and lateral tarsorrhaphy of the right eye.

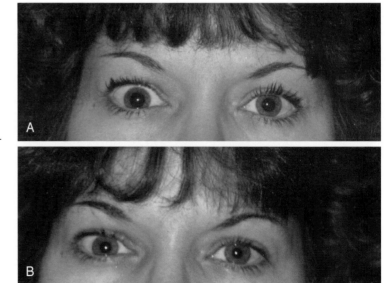

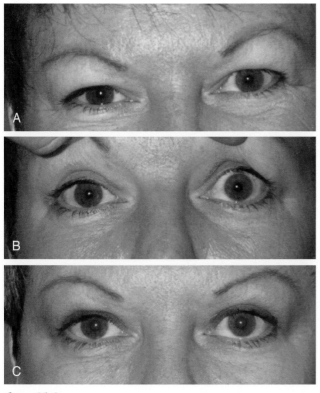

figure 15–3

A and *B*, A 44-year-old woman with left upper eyelid retraction secondary to thyroid eye disease and bilateral dermatochalasis (excessive skin). *C*, Same patient 8 months after levator aponeurosis and Müller's muscle recession in the left upper eyelid combined with bilateral upper eyelid blepharoplasties.

recovery area for approximately 1 hour before being allowed to go home.

On the first postoperative day, one can expect significant swelling. The eyelid is usually 2–4 mm below the opposite eyelid. If the eyelid seems too high, I sometimes grab the eyelashes and pull the eyelid down with the patient looking up. This breaks some of the fibers that are beginning to form and cause a tendency toward return of the eyelid retraction. In most cases, however, the eyelid is more ptotic than would be desired in the postoperative period, and the patient must be reassured that 1–2 mm of lift is expected during the first 6 weeks after surgery (Figs. 15–2 and 15–3).

COMMENT

The question often arises as to why this technique is repeatable, since neither the levator aponeurosis nor Müller's muscle is sutured to any other structures. I believe that the epinephrine in the anesthetic agent causes some eyelid retraction. Therefore, when the epinephrine wears off, the eyelid will be 1–2 mm lower than where I set it at surgery. I expect that some retraction will occur, but I think that the swelling present in the eyelid helps to keep the levator and Müller's muscle separated from the upper border of the tarsus during healing. By setting the eyelid approximately 1 mm below the intended final result, I am actually overcorrecting the eyelid position by about 3 mm, since if epinephrine were not used, the eyelids would be lower at the end of surgery. If epinephrine is not used, however, the surgical field is much more edematous and hemorrhagic, and dissection is more difficult.

Judging the lid position in the very swollen eyelid when epinephrine is not used is quite difficult. Therefore, I think that epinephrine should be used and taken into consideration when the final eyelid position is being set. Regardless of the mechanism, however, I have found that the results are excellent with this technique.

COMPLICATIONS

Although residual ptosis has not occurred in any of my patients, I would treat this complication as a new ptosis. If the levator function were reasonable, I would perform levator aponeurosis surgery. If the ptosis were severe with minimal levator function, I would consider using a sling. However, I think this complication would be very unlikely.[6–8]

RESULTS

Of 102 patients treated with this technique, 64 had unilateral procedures and 38 underwent bilateral surgery. No patient had residual ptosis requiring surgery. Only two eyelids had residual retraction, and these were corrected by repeating the operation. If there seems to be a tendency toward slight (1 mm) residual retraction, I pull on the eyelid in the office and have the patient look up.

References

1. Ceisler EJ, Bilyk JR, Rubin PA, et al: Results of Müllerotomy and levator aponeurosis transposition for the correction of upper eyelid retraction in Graves' disease. Ophthalmology 1995; 102:483–492.
2. Grove AS: Eyelid retraction treated by levator marginal myotomy. Ophthalmology 1980; 87:1013–1018.
3. Grove AS: Levator lengthening by marginal myotomy. Arch Ophthalmol 1980; 98:1433–1438.
4. Levine MR, Chu A: Surgical treatment of thyroid-related lid retraction: A new variation. Ophthalmic Surg 1991; 22:90–94.
5. Collin JR, O'Donnell BA: Adjustable sutures in eyelid surgery for ptosis and lid retraction. Br J Ophthalmol 1994; 78:167–174.
6. Anderson RL: Commentary. Ophthalmic Surg 1991; 22:322–323.
7. Harvey JT, Corin S, Nixon D, et al: Modified levator aponeurosis recession for upper eyelid retraction in Graves' disease. Ophthalmic Surg 1991; 22:313–317.
8. Older JJ: Surgical treatment of eyelid retraction associated with thyroid eye disease. Ophthalmic Surg 1991; 22:318–322.

Allen M. Putterman

Chapter 16

Treatment of Upper Eyelid Retraction: Internal Approach

For more than 25 years, I have preferred treating upper eyelid retraction secondary to thyroid ophthalmopathy with an internal rather than external approach. Excellent results, high patient satisfaction, and minimal need for secondary surgery lead to my bias toward this approach.

The main disadvantage of treating upper eyelid retraction from an internal approach is that the procedure is slightly more cumbersome if an external blepharoplasty is needed simultaneously. It requires the surgeon to perform the retraction surgery from an internal approach and the blepharoplasty from an external approach.

I perform the external blepharoplasty along with internal retraction surgery only if I need to excise Müller's muscle without performing a levator recession. If I excise Müller's muscle and recess the levator aponeurosis from an internal approach and then perform an external blepharoplasty, I am concerned that I might interfere with the results of the upper eyelid retraction procedure.

Many patients require only excision of Müller's muscle to obtain a satisfactory upper eyelid level. In these patients I am more aggressive in performing an excision of skin, orbicularis oculi muscle, and orbital fat and sometimes sub-brow fat, along with reconstruction of the upper eyelid crease.

I recommend that surgeons experiment with both the external approach described by J. Older in Chapter 15 and the one I describe in this chapter to determine which gives them the best results.

ALLEN M. PUTTERMAN

Upper eyelid retraction, a manifestation of thyroid ophthalmopathy, often continues after the underlying systemic disease has been successfully treated. Upper eyelid retraction not only is cosmetically deforming because the amount of exophthalmos is exaggerated but also contributes to corneal and conjunctival exposure and to ocular irritation.

Upper eyelid retraction surgery occasionally is combined with retraction surgery of the lower eyelid, with or without lateral tarsorrhaphies (see Chapters 25 and 26). If there is minimal upper eyelid retraction, the surgery can be combined with an upper eyelid skin-muscle-fat excision and eyelid reconstruction; if the retraction is moderate or severe, the external tissue excision is deferred to a second surgical sitting.

Upper eyelid retraction can be performed in patients who do not require orbital decompression or strabismus surgery. If exophthalmos or strabismus surgery is required, this eye muscle surgery is performed first. Usually, thyroid surgery is considered once the eyelid retraction, ocular proptosis, and strabismus are stable for at least 6 months.

The external approach to treating upper eyelid retraction is described in Chapter 15. In this chapter, I describe a technique that Urist and I reported on in 1972, in which Müller's muscle is excised and the levator aponeurosis is recessed from an internal approach.[1] The procedure is performed with sensory but not motor anesthesia. The eyelid level is controlled intraoperatively while the patient is seated up on the operating table.

Treatment of upper eyelid retraction not only places the upper eyelid in a more normal position but also decreases the exophthalmic appearance and relieves ocular irritation and keratopathy.

ANATOMY

Müller's muscle in the upper eyelid originates from the levator aponeurosis approximately 15 mm above the superior tarsal border (see Chapter 7, Figs. 7–1 and 7–7) and inserts onto the superior tarsal border. This muscle spans the horizontal dimension of the eyelid, is firmly attached to conjunctiva on its posterior surface, and is loosely attached to the levator aponeurosis on its anterior surface. Müller's muscle resembles other smooth muscle tissue and is approximately 1 mm thick.

MARGIN REFLEX DISTANCE-1

It is important to assess the upper eyelid levels with the margin reflex distance-1 (MRD_1) measurement (see Chapter 2, Fig. 2–8).

SURGICAL TECHNIQUE

Anesthesia

In this procedure, only local anesthesia is used. Anesthesia given in this manner maintains the eyelid level at its preoperative position while providing an absence of lid sensation. The patient is given no preoperative medication. Lidocaine hydrochloride (0.25 ml of a 2 per cent concentration) with epinephrine is injected subcutaneously into the center of the upper eyelid just above the lid margin.

A 4-0 silk suture is placed in the center of the upper eyelid 2 mm above the eyelash line, through the skin, orbicularis muscle, and anterior tarsus (Fig. 16–1A). Topical 0.5 per cent tetracaine drops are applied to the eye, and a scleral lens is placed over the globe to protect it during surgery.

Conjunctival Dissection

With a Desmarres retractor, the surgeon everts the upper eyelid to expose the superior palpebral conjunctiva. The upper palpebral conjunctiva is flooded with 0.5 per cent tetracaine drops. Cotton-tipped applicators saturated with tetracaine also are rolled over the conjunctiva. Then, 0.25–0.5 ml of 2 per cent lidocaine with epinephrine is injected subconjunctivally adjacent to the superior tarsal border over the entire width of the eyelid (Fig. 16–1B).

The conjunctiva is grasped just over the superior tarsal border at the temporal aspect of the eyelid and is severed with Westcott scissors. The surgeon inserts straight, sharp-pointed iris scissors between the conjunctiva and Müller's muscle and spreads the scissors blades to separate conjunctiva from the muscle (Fig. 16–1C).

Conjunctiva is severed from the superior tarsal border (Fig. 16–1D). The surgeon further dissects conjunctiva from the muscle by spreading the scissors blades between the two tissues to the superior fornix (Fig. 16–1E). The surgeon can facilitate this dissection by observing the points of the blades through the translucent conjunctiva. Sharp dissection with the iris scissors releases any remaining attachments between conjunctiva and Müller's muscle.

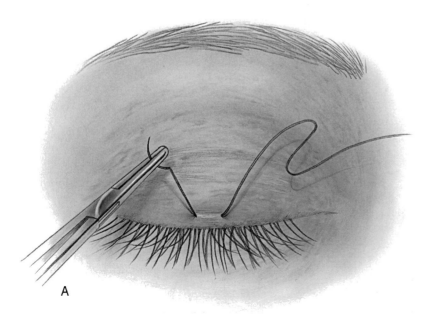

figure 16–1
A, Placement of traction suture.

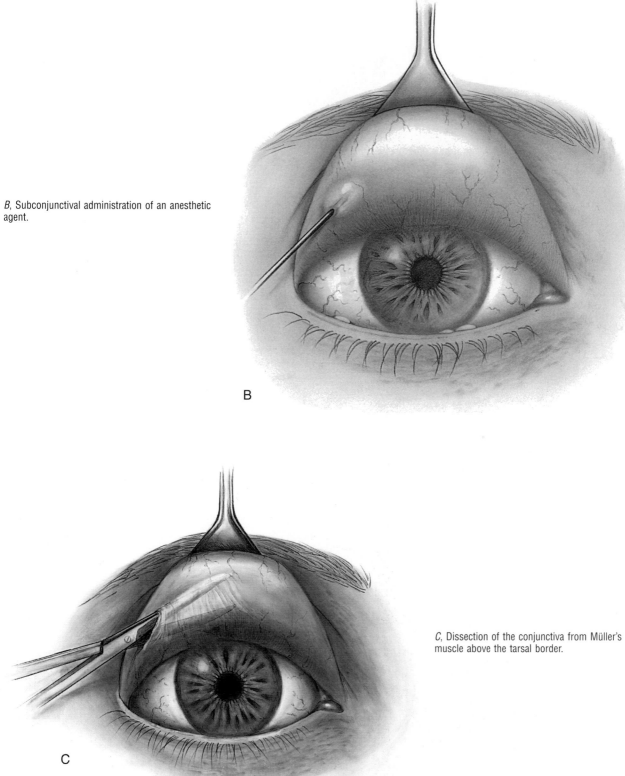

B, Subconjunctival administration of an anesthetic agent.

B

C, Dissection of the conjunctiva from Müller's muscle above the tarsal border.

C

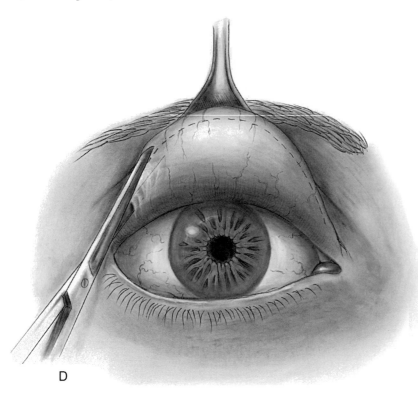

D, Severing of the conjunctiva from the superior tarsal border.

D

Müller's Muscle Dissection

The surgeon grasps Müller's muscle with a toothed forceps at the temporal aspect of the eyelid just above the superior tarsal border. The muscle is pulled outward, and the Desmarres retractor is pulled simultaneously in the opposite direction. Müller's muscle is cut from the tarsus temporally (Fig. 16–1*F*).

Müller's muscle is then undermined from the levator aponeurosis at the level of the superior tarsal border (Fig. 16–1*G*). Müller's muscle, which is all the tissue attached to the top of the tarsus, is severed over the temporal two thirds of the eyelid (Fig. 16–1*H*).

Wet cotton-tipped applicators are used to dissect Müller's muscle bluntly from its loose attachment to the levator aponeurosis. This dissection is performed

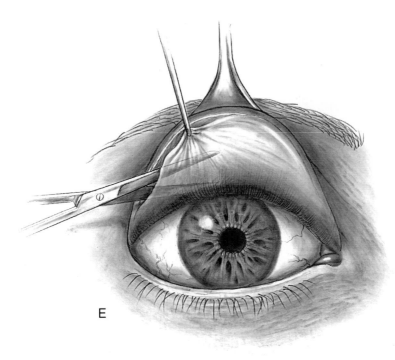

E, Further dissection of the conjunctiva from Müller's muscle.

E

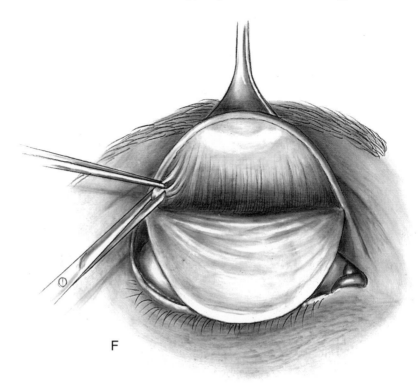

F, Severing of temporal Müller's muscle.

F

approximately 10–12 mm above the superior tarsal border over the temporal one half to two thirds of the eyelid (Fig. 16–1*I*).

The scleral lens is removed, and the patient is brought to a sitting position by raising the head of the operating table. The levels of the upper eyelids are evaluated while the patient looks in the primary and up and down positions of gaze and widely opens his or her eyelids.

If the upper eyelid is at a satisfactory position, the head of the operating table is lowered and the patient lies down. The section of Müller's muscle that has been detached is clamped with a straight hemostat at its base and is excised. Bleeding from the stump of Müller's muscle is carefully controlled with a disposable cautery. If there is residual retraction, Müller's muscle is released to 10–15 mm above the tarsus over the temporal two

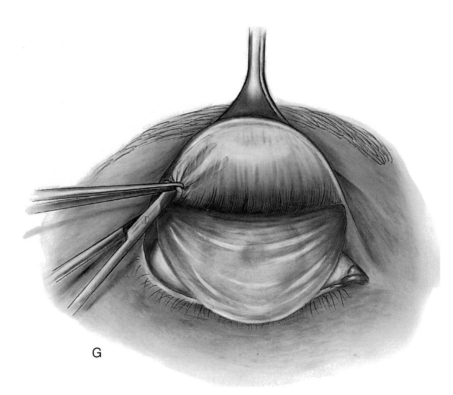

G, Dissection of Müller's muscle from levator aponeurosis. A Desmarres retractor and West-cott scissors are pulled away from each other.

G

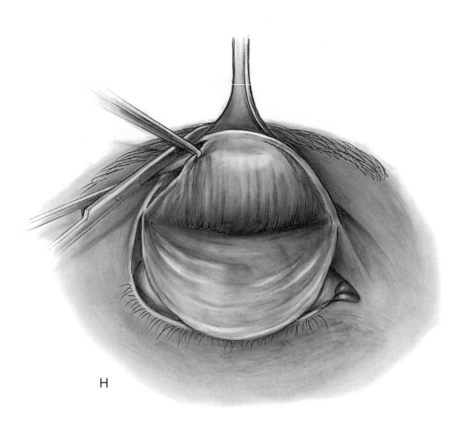

H, Severing of Müller's muscle from the superior tarsal border.

H

I, Blunt dissection with a cotton-tipped applicator separates Müller's muscle from loose attachment to the levator aponeurosis.

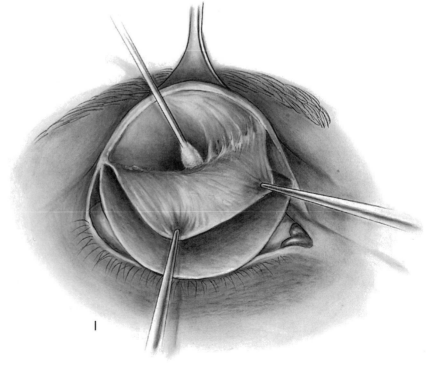

I

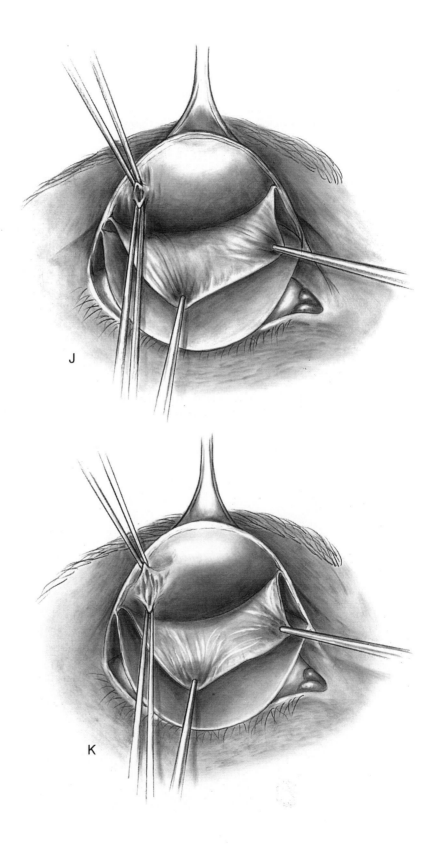

J and *K*, Stripping of the levator aponeurosis.

thirds to three fourths of the eyelid. It is better to be conservative in releasing Müller's muscle nasally because a nasal ptosis can easily occur.

Levator Stripping

Again, the patient is brought to a sitting position and the eyelid levels are evaluated. If the eyelid is still retracted, overaction of the levator muscle is implicated and this muscle must be released. The patient lies down, and the scleral lens and Desmarres retractor are reapplied. With the eyelid everted, the fibers of the levator aponeurosis that pass over the anterior surface of the tarsus are exposed. Using two toothed forceps, the surgeon grasps the superficial layers of the levator aponeurosis at the level of the superior tarsus. The levator aponeurosis layers are stripped vertically, layer by layer, along the sections of the eyelid that remain retracted (Fig. 16–1*J* and *K*).

The patient is brought to a sitting position at various times during the levator aponeurosis stripping procedure until a desirable end point is reached. This gradual, step-by-step lengthening of the levator aponeurosis allows the retraction of the eyelid to be corrected slowly and precisely.

Müller's Muscle Excision

The detached part of Müller's muscle is then clamped with a straight hemostat at its base and is excised (Fig.

16–1*L*). Pulling the conjunctival flap downward with a cotton-tipped applicator brings the stump of Müller's muscle into view and facilitates cauterization of any bleeding areas.

Conjunctival Reattachment

When a desired eyelid level is achieved, either by excision of Müller's muscle alone or in conjunction with the stripping of the levator aponeurosis, the conjunctiva is sutured to the superior tarsal border with a continuous 6-0 plain catgut suture (Fig. 16–1*M*).

In most cases, I remove the 4-0 black silk traction suture placed in the upper eyelid at the beginning of the procedure. However, if I have performed a significant amount of levator recession, I tape the 4-0 black silk traction suture to the patient's cheek to put a small amount of stretch on the upper eyelid and then apply a light pressure dressing. This traction suture is removed on the first postoperative day.

The upper eyelid should be at approximately the mid-pupil on the first postoperative day. If it appears too high on the first postoperative day or starts retracting during the first postoperative weeks, the patient is instructed to massage the eyelid downward while raising the eyebrow upward.

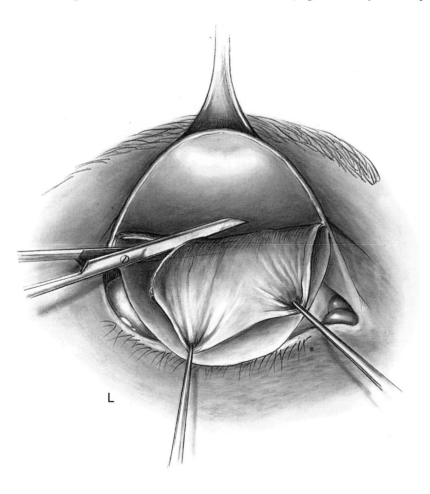

L, Excision of Müller's muscle and recession of the levator aponeurosis.

L

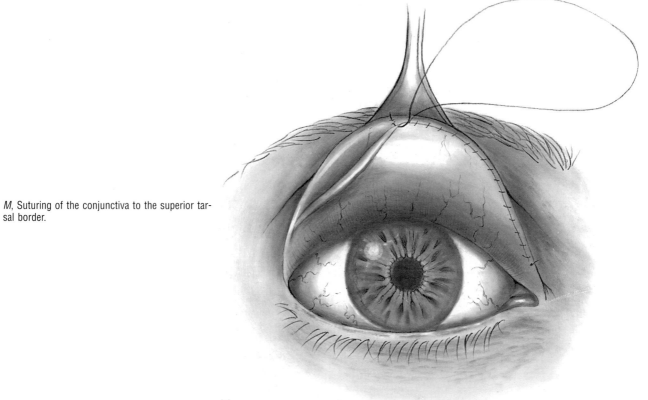

M, Suturing of the conjunctiva to the superior tarsal border.

M

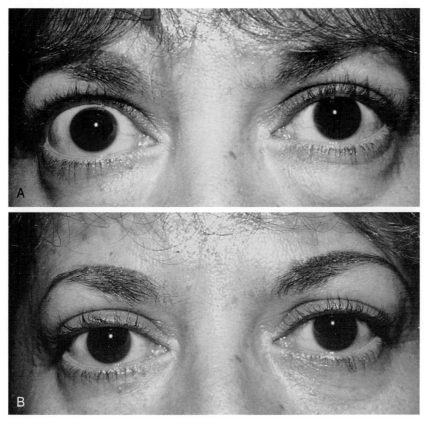

figure 16–2

Bilateral upper eyelid retraction secondary to thyroid ophthalmopathy before *(A)* and after *(B)* excision of Müller's muscle and recession of the levator aponeurosis through an internal approach. The herniated orbital fat in both lower eyelids was removed through an internal approach simultaneously.

COMMENTS

The excision of Müller's muscle and levator aponeurosis in the manner described is a highly successful technique for treating thyroid-related retraction of the upper eyelid (Fig. 16–2). The procedure is based on the theory of the physiologic and anatomic origin of the condition. It is a relatively simple technique that does not alter the major anatomic relationship in the eyelid by the implantation of a foreign body or by distortion of the tissues.

With the patient sitting up at various times during the procedure, the surgeon can make adjustments by progressively recessing Müller's muscle and levator aponeurosis until the desired eyelid level and arch are achieved. Overcorrection can be recognized during the surgery and dealt with by reattaching the recessed tissues to tarsus or skin.

The levator muscle obeys *Hering's law* of equal upper eyelid innervation. I therefore believe that during surgery on a patient with unilateral retraction the affected eyelid should be placed at a slightly higher level than that of the unaffected eyelid to ensure symmetry postoperatively. During bilateral surgery, the more retracted eyelid is operated on first and is placed at an acceptable level. This eyelid commonly becomes ptotic, probably secondary to edema or innervation changes when the second eyelid is being operated on. To avoid a postoperative ptosis of the second eyelid, one should place it at the same level the first eyelid was originally placed rather than matching it to the position that the first eyelid obtains at this point in the procedure.

RESULTS

I have performed this procedure on close to 1000 upper eyelids. The results have been studied in several pre-viously reported publications.[1-4] The success rate of bringing the upper eyelid close to a normal level is approximately 90 per cent.

In approximately 10 per cent of cases, the eyelid is retracted or ptotic and requires secondary surgery. If the eyelid continues to be retracted, secondary treatment with a simplified levator recession[5] is recommended. If the eyelid is ptotic, I perform an internal vertical eyelid shortening operation[6] over the ptotic area or I employ an external approach and perform a levator aponeurosis advancement technique similar to that described in Chapter 13.

References

1. Putterman AM, Urist M: Surgical treatment of upper eyelid retraction. Arch Ophthalmol 1972; 87:401–405.
2. Chalfin J, Putterman AM: Müller's muscle excision and levator recession in upper lid: Treatment of thyroid-related retraction. Arch Ophthalmol 1979; 97:1487–1491.
3. Putterman AM: Surgical treatment of thyroid-related upper eyelid retraction. Trans Am Acad Ophthalmol Otolaryngol 1981; 88:507–512.
4. Putterman AM, Fett DR: Müller's muscle in the treatment of upper eyelid retraction: A 12-year study. Ophthalmic Surg 1986; 17:361–367.
5. Putterman AM, Urist MJ: A simplified levator palpebrae superioris muscle recession to treat overcorrected blepharoptosis. Am J Ophthalmol 1974; 77:358–366.
6. Putterman AM: Internal vertical eyelid shortening to treat surgically induced segmental blepharoptosis. Am J Ophthalmol 1976; 82:1232–1238.

Charles R. Leone, Jr.

Chapter 17

Treatment of a Prolapsed Lacrimal Gland

Prolapse of the lacrimal gland is an important consideration in the cosmetic oculoplastic surgery patient because it can be easily confused with herniation of orbital fat. Charles Leone tells us how to differentiate these two entities so that we can avoid the serious complication of lacrimal gland excision and a secondary dry eye. He also details the technique to treat the prolapsed lacrimal gland by redepositing it into the lacrimal fossa.

I have found that prolapsed lacrimal glands occur relatively commonly in patients with baggy upper eyelids. At times it can be diagnosed preoperatively, and at other times it is found only during the surgical procedure. If the approach to the upper eyelid skin fold excision consists of excising skin and orbicularis oculi muscle and herniated orbital fat, the prolapsed lacrimal gland will sometimes be seen during this approach. If the lacrimal gland is prolapsed, it is routinely corrected in order to avoid a postoperative fullness in the temporal upper lid.

ALLEN M. PUTTERMAN

When the suspensory ligaments of the orbital septum of the lacrimal gland loosen, the gland can prolapse forward and produce a noticeable bulge in the eyelid.[1, 2] If there is a significant amount of herniated orbital fat, the gland may not be evident externally but the patient may complain of a movable "knot" in the eyelid. As a rule, this happens in older people; however, it may occur in younger people who have experienced trauma, repeated bouts of orbital edema, or true blepharochalasis.[3]

Palpation of the gland reveals a sharp-bordered, easily reducible mass (Figs. 17–1 and 17–2). This mass must be differentiated from a lacrimal gland tumor and an inflammatory process.[4] A tumor or inflammatory pseudotumor is not easily reducible and is usually larger in bulk; with an inflammatory process, the gland may be tender. Occasionally, in cases of marked herniated orbital fat, the prolapsed gland may not be discovered until surgery is performed.

ANATOMY

The lacrimal gland is divided by the levator aponeurosis into two lobes, orbital and palpebral.[5] The larger, orbital portion is almond-shaped and lies within the lacrimal gland fossa of the frontal bone (see Chapter 7). The sharp anterior border is usually behind the superior rim; hence, it is not ordinarily palpable. Suspensory ligaments keep the gland in place and are attached to the fossa superiorly, the zygomatic bone inferiorly, and the periorbita posteriorly, where the lacrimal nerve and vessels enter the gland. The orbital lobe is contiguous with the lateral aspect of the preaponeurotic fat.

The palpebral lobe is about one third the size of the orbital portion and lies beneath the levator aponeurosis and within the lateral aspect of the superior fornix. The lacrimal gland is innervated by the fifth cranial nerve and is responsible for reflex tear secretion. Thus, removal of any part of the gland will reduce reflex tear secretion and may result in keratitis sicca.[6]

TECHNIQUE

An incision is made in the upper eyelid crease from the level of the upper punctum to the lateral canthus. If a blepharoplasty is being done as well, the eyelid is marked and redundant skin is excised (Fig. 17–3A). The orbicu-

Text continued on page 174

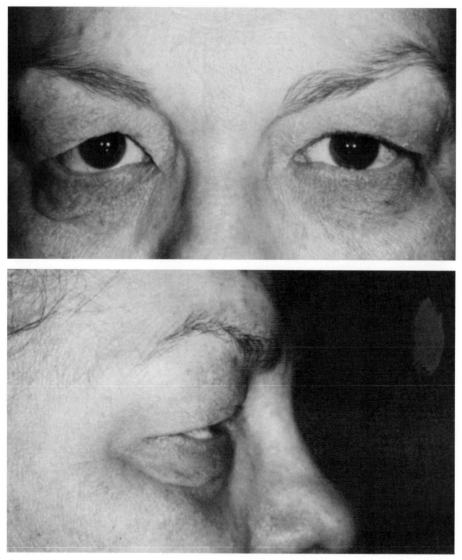

figure 17–1

Preoperative appearance of a woman with moderately severe herniated orbital fat and a prolapsed lacrimal gland. The prolapsed gland is not evident externally, but it can be palpated.

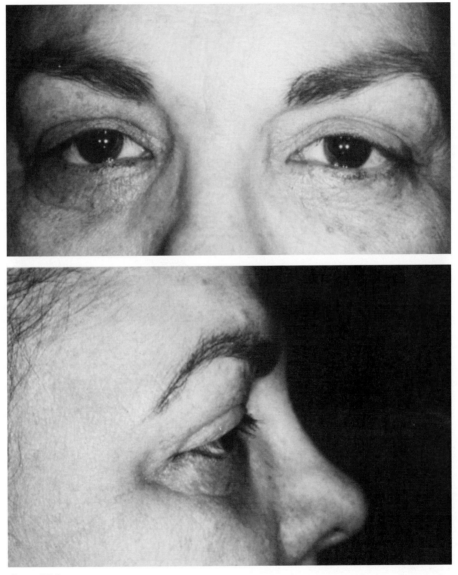

figure 17–2

Postoperative appearance of the same patient shown in Figure 17–1 following blepharoplasty and repositioning of the prolapsed lacrimal gland.

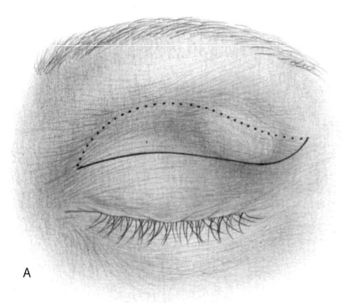

A

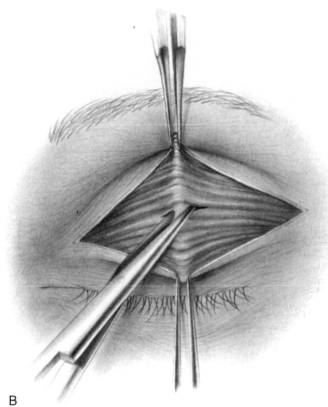

B

figure 17–3

Surgical technique to treat a prolapsed lacrimal gland. *A*, An incision is made in the upper eyelid crease from the level of the upper punctum to the lateral canthus. If a blepharoplasty is to be done concomitantly, the dotted line represents the superior incision to complete the ellipse of skin to be removed. *B*, The orbicularis oculi muscle is severed.

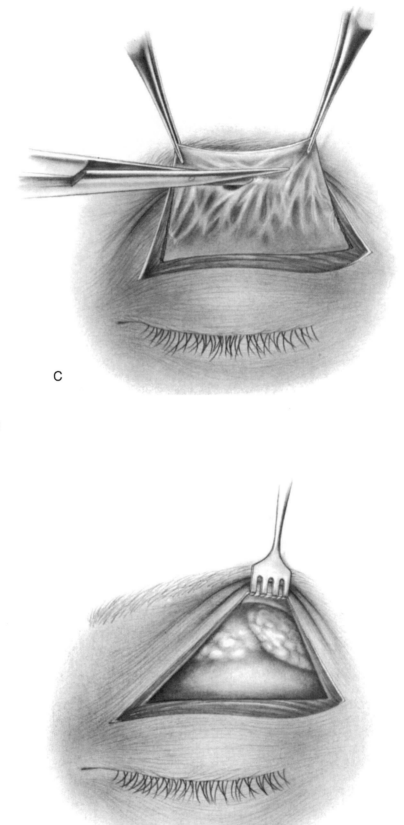

C, The septum is incised across the eyelid, exposing the preaponeurotic fat. *D*, The prolapsed gland will appear as a pinkish tan structure that is firm and lobulated, with a sharp anterior border, in contrast to the soft, yellow preaponeurotic fat.

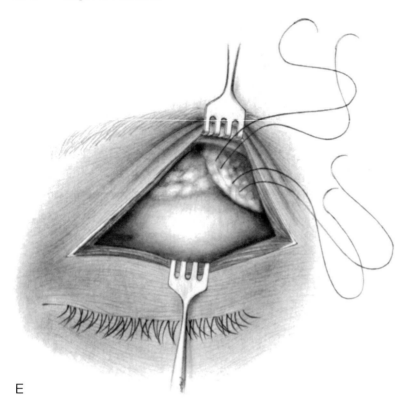

E, One or two double-armed sutures of 5-0 polypropylene (Prolene) are placed through the leading edge of the gland.

E

laris muscle is severed with scissors, and the orbital septum is identified (Fig. 17–3*B*). The septum is cut from the medial to the lateral extent to expose the preaponeurotic fat (Fig. 17–3*C*). If the gland is prolapsed, a pinkish tan structure that is firm and lobulated with a sharp anterior border will be found in the lateral third of the upper eyelid (Fig. 17–3*D*). This is in contrast to the soft, yellow preaponeurotic fat. The gland should be fairly easily reduced to its normal position inside the superior rim within the lacrimal gland fossa. Therefore, if there is any question of whether the mass is a pseudotumor or neoplasm, the gland should be sampled for biopsy or excised.

One or two double-armed sutures of 5-0 polypropylene (Prolene) are placed through the leading edge of the gland (Fig. 17–3*E*), then through the periosteum posterior to the superior rim (Fig. 17–3*F* and *G*). When these are tied, the gland should be securely returned to the lacrimal gland fossa (Fig. 17–3*H*). The preaponeurotic fat can be removed if a blepharoplasty is being done concomitantly. The orbital septum is left unsutured, and the skin is closed with continuous or interrupted 6-0 polypropylene sutures (Fig. 17–3*I*). Antibiotic ointment is placed across the incision, and wet saline-soaked eye pads are loosely taped over the eyelids. The sutures are removed in 1 week.

DISCUSSION

Excision of a prolapsed lacrimal gland for cosmetic reasons or for epiphora should be condemned because of the threat of keratitis sicca.[6, 7] Scherz and Dohlman[6] reported a case of persistent unilateral keratoconjuncti-

vitis sicca that developed immediately following a palpebral dacryoadenectomy in a healthy 43-year-old woman who had normal tear function before the operation. In a review of eight previously reported cases, the authors determined that the main lacrimal gland is indispensable in maintaining normal wetting of the eye.

Repositioning a prolapsed lacrimal gland does not disturb its function; rather, it merely restores the gland to its normal position and eliminates either a palpable or noticeable bulge in the eyelid. One must exercise caution to avoid mistaking a prolapsed gland for orbital fat; however, attention to the position, color, consistency, and shape of the mass should preclude this mistake.

The lacrimal gland is located in the lateral third of the upper eyelid, is pinkish tan, has a sharp anterior border, and is firm. Any patient with a bulge or mass in the orbit, particularly if it is of recent onset, should be examined with the intention of ruling out a neoplasm or pseudotumor. Any mass that is more than just barely palpable, not easily reducible, or tender warrants further orbital evaluation, including computed tomographic (CT) scanning. This should eliminate the necessity of biopsy of a prolapsed lacrimal gland, except in the most unusual circumstances.

Prolapse of the lacrimal gland is actually a relatively rare condition. Occasionally, a small prolapse that is insignificant and not worthy of repair is seen at the time of blepharoplasty; if the gland is protruding 1 cm beyond the rim, it should probably be repaired in order to prevent further progression. Rarely, a patient presents with noticeable prolapsed lacrimal glands without accompanying herniated orbital fat. In patients in whom I have performed this repair, there has not been a recur-

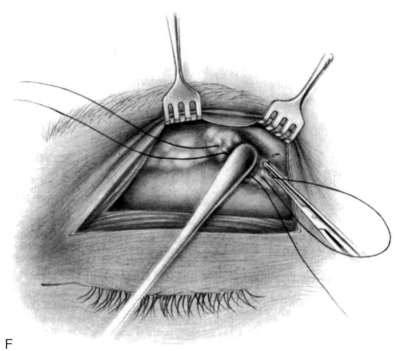

F

F and *G*, The double-armed sutures are then passed
through the periosteum of the superior rim.

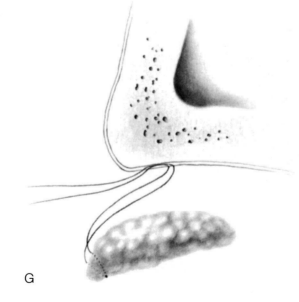

G

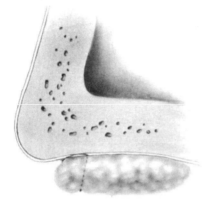

H

H, When the sutures are tied, the gland should return to the lacrimal gland fossa. *I,* The orbital septum is left unsutured, and the skin is sutured with 6-0 polypropylene.

I

rence over a 10-year period. There was no change in the postoperative results of Schirmer's No. 1 secretion test from preoperative values in these patients.

References

1. Smith B, Petrelli R: Surgical repair of prolapsed lacrimal glands. Arch Ophthalmol 1978; 96:113–114.
2. Horton CE, Carraway JH, Potenza AD: Treatment of a lacrimal bulge in blepharoplasty by repositioning the gland. Plast Reconstr Surg 1978; 61:701–702.
3. Duke-Elder S: The ocular adnexa: Disease of the eyelids. In Duke-Elder S (ed): System of Ophthalmology, vol 13, p 350. St. Louis, CV Mosby, 1975.
4. Jones IS, Jakobiec FA: Diseases of the Orbit, pp 335–370. Hagerstown, Md, Harper & Row, 1979.
5. Wolff E: Anatomy of the Eye and Orbit, 5th ed, p 199. Philadelphia, WB Saunders, 1961.
6. Scherz W, Dohlman CH: Is the lacrimal gland dispensable? Keratoconjunctivitis sicca after lacrimal gland removal. Arch Ophthalmol 1975; 93:281–283.
7. Amdur J: Excision of palpebral lacrimal gland for epiphora. Arch Ophthalmol 1964; 71:71–72.

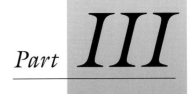

Part III

LOWER EYELID TECHNIQUES

Allen M. Putterman

Treatment of Lower Eyelid Dermatochalasis, Herniated Orbital Fat, Abnormal-Appearing Skin, and Hypertrophic Orbicularis Oculi Muscle: Skin Flap Approach

Three approaches are used to excise excess skin and herniated orbital fat in the lower eyelid: (1) a skin flap approach, (2) a skin-muscle flap approach, and (3) an internal approach.

In this chapter, I describe and illustrate the skin flap method. I frequently use this technique in patients with markedly excessive lower eyelid skin. Removal of skin nasally rather than temporally is also highlighted as a method to decrease pigmented or crinkly, abnormal-appearing eyelid skin.

Last, I describe a technique to excise hypertrophic lower eyelid orbicularis muscle, which some patients find cosmetically undesirable when they smile.

ALLEN M. PUTTERMAN

Baggy lower eyelids are usually the result of herniated orbital fat or dermatochalasis (excess skin). At times, a hypertrophic orbicularis muscle adds to the cosmetic disfigurement. The surgical treatment consists of excision of excess skin, herniated orbital fat, and a hypertrophic orbicularis muscle. Surgery is performed mainly to improve the patient's appearance.

The skin flap approach is used when markedly excessive lower lid skin needs to be removed. I rarely use this technique to treat baggy lower eyelids. The skin-orbicularis flap method is used when there is herniated orbital fat and minimally to moderately excessive lower lid skin (see Chapter 19). The internal approach to resect herniated orbital fat is usually used in patients without excess skin and in patients with thyroid disease who require simultaneous hard-palate grafting to correct lower lid retraction (see Chapters 20 and 25). The internal approach can also be used in patients who have minimal amounts of excess skin if the technique is combined with plication sutures, skin peeling, or laser resurfacing (see Chapters 22, 30, and 31).

Baggy lower eyelids are frequently associated with baggy upper eyelids. If all four eyelids are treated surgically at the same time, the skin and fat of the upper eyelids are excised and all incisions closed before the lower eyelids are operated on (see Chapters 9 and 10). Occasionally, the lower eyelids are treated alone. The following technique is the skin flap approach to baggy eyelids.

EXCISION OF EXCESS SKIN AND HERNIATED ORBITAL FAT

Topical tetracaine drops are instilled over the eye. A tinted scleral lens is slid under the upper eyelid as the

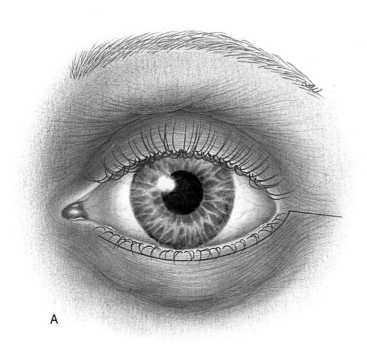

A

figure 18–1

A, A lateral canthal line is drawn, beginning 2–3 mm temporal to the lateral canthus and extending for 1–1.5 cm in a horizontal, but slightly downward, direction. Another line in the lower eyelid, 1.5–2 mm beneath the lashes, indicates the site of the lower eyelid incision. (This line is usually not drawn.)

B, An incision is made in the lower eyelid 1.5–2 mm beneath the eyelashes, beginning at the punctum and extending to 2 mm beyond the lateral canthus. The incision is then extended in the marked lateral canthal line.

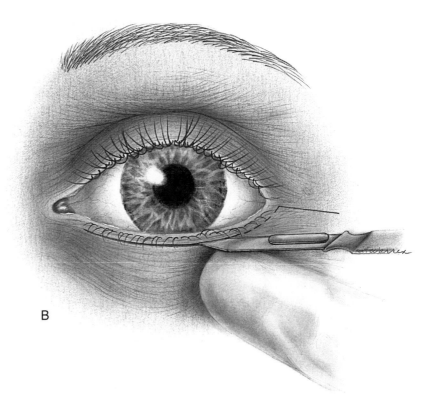

B

patient looks downward and then under the lower eyelid as the patient looks upward. This protects the eye from injury during surgery and lessens the patient's photophobia from the operating room lights. It also prevents the patient from needing to view the surgery.

Lid Marking

A line, 1–1.5 cm, is drawn, beginning 2–3 mm temporal to the lateral canthus and extending slightly downward but almost horizontally in one of the laugh lines (Fig. 18–1A). A longer incision is used if more excess skin needs to be excised. If the upper eyelid is also treated, this line should be at least 5 mm from the temporal incision in the upper eyelid (see Chapter 9, Fig. 9–3). Leaving skin between these two incisions lessens the risk of complications of lateral canthal webbing and eyelid lymphedema postoperatively.

Skin Dissection

Lidocaine 2 per cent with 1:100,000 epinephrine is injected subcutaneously over the lower eyelid. With a No. 15 Bard-Parker blade, the skin is incised about 2 mm below the cilia, beginning 1–2 mm temporal to the punctum and extending across the horizontal length of the eyelid to 2–3 mm lateral to the lateral canthus (Fig. 18–1B). The incision is extended temporally over the line previously drawn in the temporal laugh line.

The skin is dissected from orbicularis muscle with Westcott scissors (Fig. 18–1C). The correct subcutaneous plane is judged by observing the spread scissors

blades through the translucent skin. With one blade of the scissors placed beneath the skin and the other at the skin edge, the subcutaneous attachments are severed. The skin usually is undermined from the orbicularis muscle to the level of the inferior orbital rim. If there is marked dermatochalasis, the dissection can be carried out as far as 10 mm below the inferior orbital rim and the lateral canthal incision can be extended to 2 cm beyond the lateral canthus.

Bleeding is controlled with a disposable cautery (Solan Accu-Temp, Xomed Surgical Products, Jacksonville, Fla.) (Fig. 18–1D).

Excision of Orbital Fat

Next to be removed is any herniated orbital fat observed preoperatively. The orbicularis muscle is severed with Westcott scissors, just above the orbital rim level, across the entire horizontal dimension of the eyelid. For a procedure on the right lower eyelid, the assistant grasps the internal surface of the skin flap in the lower lid with forceps and pulls it downward and outward. The surgeon picks up central-superior orbicularis muscle and pulls it upward and outward. (In the left lower lid, the assistant and surgeon reverse the positions of their forceps.) This maneuver pulls muscle away from underlying capsulopalpebral fascia, septum, and orbital fat and creates a space between orbicularis muscle and capsulopalpebral fascia.

The central orbicularis muscle is severed just above the inferior orbital rim with Westcott scissors directed downward and slightly inward between these two forceps (Fig. 18–1E). The potential space beneath the or-

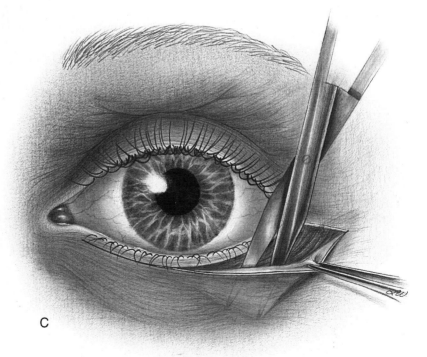

C, Skin is undermined from the orbicularis oculi muscle, usually to the level of the inferior orbital rim.

C

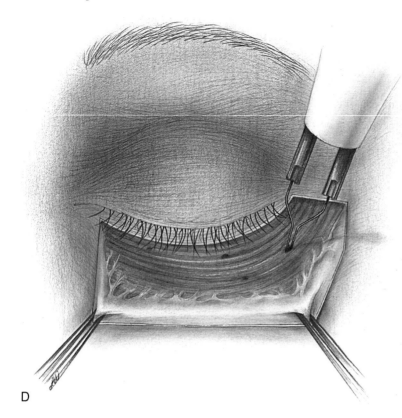

D, Bleeding is controlled with a disposable cautery.

D

E, The central orbicularis muscle beneath the central eyelashes is drawn upward as the skin flap is simultaneously pulled downward and outward with forceps. The orbicularis muscle tented with this maneuver is severed with Westcott scissors directed inward and slightly downward.

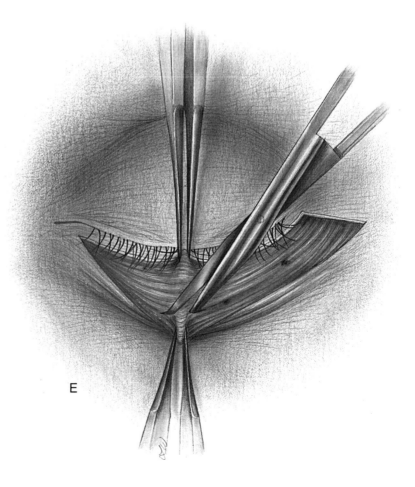

E

bicularis muscle should now be seen. Then the orbicularis muscle is cut just above the junction of skin and orbicularis muscle to the temporal end of the lid (Fig. 18–1F). With the scissors reversed, the incision is carried out to the nasal extreme of the eyelid. Bleeding is controlled with Solan Accu-Temp disposable and Bovie cauteries.

An alternative method of isolating the orbital fat pockets is to make three openings in the orbicularis muscle over each of the three fat pads. This is accomplished in a manner similar to that previously described for finding herniated nasal orbital fat in the upper eyelid (see Chapter 9). The technique is also similar to the one described in the preceding paragraph for opening the central orbicularis muscle. Instead of cutting the orbicularis muscle all the way across the eyelid, the surgeon repeats the maneuver over the nasal and temporal fat pockets to create three small orbital openings. I prefer to open the orbicularis muscle all the way across the eyelid because at times it is difficult to isolate the herniated fat with the small openings.

If the orbital fat was noted preoperatively to be herniated in all three pockets, the temporal pad is removed first. If the nasal and middle pads are removed first, it is more difficult to prolapse the temporal fat, which may then be resected inadequately. The temporal fat is prolapsed by applying gentle pressure to the globe (Fig. 18–1G). The fat capsule is grasped with forceps and severed (Fig. 18–1H).

The fat that protrudes when gentle pressure is applied to the globe is clamped with a hemostat and severed with a Bard-Parker blade that the surgeon slides over the hemostat (Fig. 18–1I). The surgeon should inspect the hemostat first to make sure that the jaws meet completely before applying it to the fat. If the fat slips out of the hemostat after being cut, uncontrollable bleeding has the potential to cause blindness.[1]

The Bovie cautery is adjusted to a setting that adequately cauterizes without producing charred tissue and is applied to the hemostat; cotton-tipped applicators are used to separate the hemostat from the underlying lid (Fig. 18–1J). The fat is grasped below the hemostat with forceps, and the hemostat is released. The severed edge of fat is inspected for hemostasis (Fig. 18–1K).

Once bleeding is controlled with the disposable cautery, the fat is allowed to retract into the orbit. The same technique is used to remove orbital fat in the middle and nasal lower eyelid until fat fails to protrude from the opening in the orbicularis muscle when gentle pressure is applied to the globe.

In most cases, I have noted a second temporal orbital fat pad, which accounts for four rather than three fat pads in the lower eyelid.[2] This second temporal pad is not appreciated until the first temporal pad is excised. Pushing on the globe after excising the first temporal pad leads to herniation of the second pad (Fig. 18–1L). This pad is excised in the same manner as the first until fat fails to prolapse when gentle pressure is applied to the globe. Residual temporal fat observed postoperatively in several patients probably has been due to

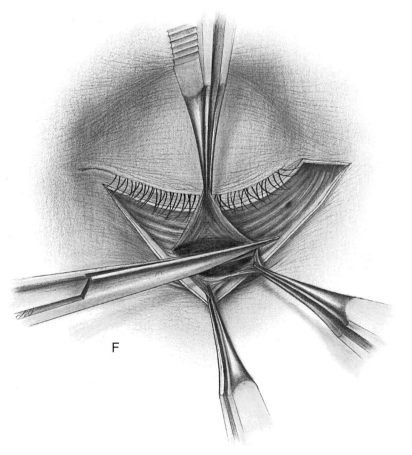

F, The space created by the severing of orbicularis muscle is entered with Westcott scissors. The scissors is used to cut the orbicularis muscle from the central opening to the temporal end of the eyelid several millimeters above the inferior orbital rim. (The surgeon continues to pull the lid upward and the skin flap downward and outward during this maneuver in order to pull the orbicularis muscle away from the orbital septum, capsulopalpebral fascia, and Müller's muscle.)

F

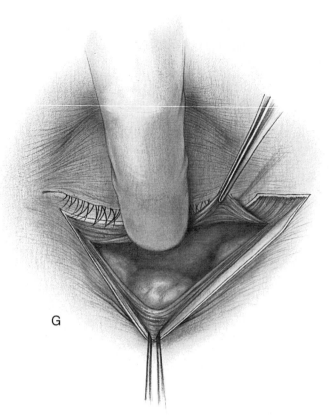

G, Pressure on the eye through the lower eyelid prolapses herniated orbital fat.

H, The temporal orbital fat capsule is severed with scissors.

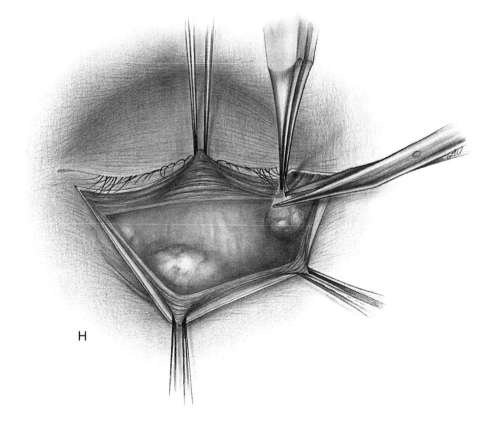

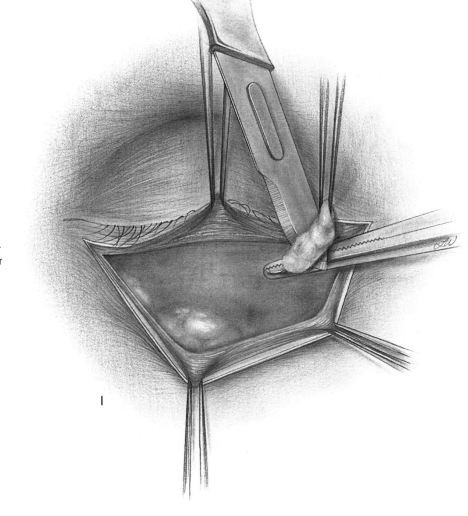

I, Temporal orbital fat that prolapses with gentle pressure is clamped with a hemostat and is excised by slicing over the hemostat with a No. 15 Bard-Parker blade.

I

the nondetection or nonappreciation of this second temporal fat pad.[2]

Skin Excision

The skin flap is draped over the lower eyelid incision, and the patient is instructed to look upward if local anesthesia is used, or pressure is applied to the globe through the upper eyelid if general anesthesia is used (Fig. 18–1*M*). Both maneuvers place the lower eyelid in the position it assumes on up gaze and help to prevent excessive resection of skin, which can result in cicatricial ectropion. The skin that drapes the incision is excised with a small vertical triangle above the inferior lash line and a large lateral triangle temporal to the lateral canthus. To avoid an ectropion, it is better to tighten the lower eyelid skin with the lateral triangle than the vertical one. It is rarely necessary to remove more than 3–5 mm of vertical skin.

The eyelid skin flap is elevated and placed on the orbicularis muscle several times to make sure that it is not sticking to the muscle at an abnormal position. A Westcott scissors is then used to excise the skin above the inferior eyelash incision site in a temporal to nasal direction with the patient gazing upward or with pressure applied to the globe (Fig. 18–1*N*). It is better to err on the conservative side by cutting just above the infralash incision edge rather than directly on it.

The temporal aspect of the skin flap is pulled outward and upward with slight tension, and the skin overlapping the temporal incision is then excised. A small cut is first made where the infralash incision meets the lateral incision, about 2–3 mm temporal to the lateral canthus. The scissors is used to connect the most temporal aspect of the skin flap to this cut (Fig. 18–1*O*). The flap is again reflected downward, and any residual bleeding is controlled with the disposable cautery.

Skin Closure

The skin is sutured with a 6-0 black silk suture initially run continuously from lateral canthus to the temporal wound edge (Fig. 18–1*P*). Another continuous 6-0 black silk suture is run continuously across the eyelid in a nasal to temporal direction with fewer bites because this incision site is under minimal tension. A 6-0 poly-

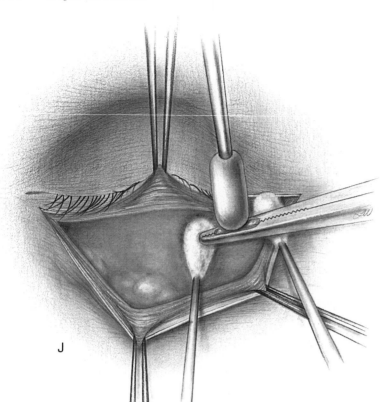

J, Cotton-tipped applicators separate the hemostat from underlying tissues, and a Bovie cautery is applied to the hemostat to provide hemostasis of the temporal fat stump.

K, With a forceps, the surgeon continues to grasp the temporal orbital fat stump after the release of the hemostat while checking for hemostasis before allowing the fat to retract into the orbit.

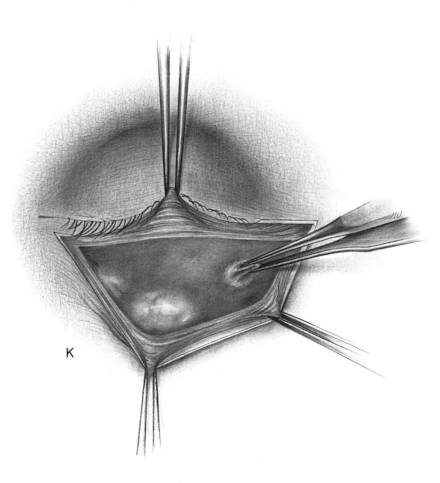

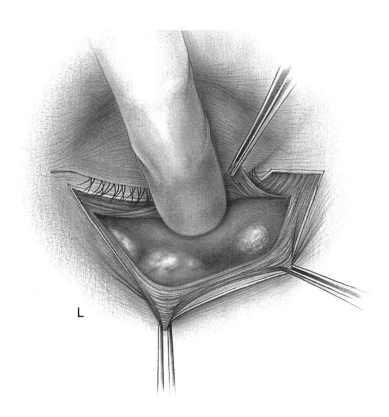

L, A second temporal fat pocket frequently prolapses after the removal of the first temporal fat pocket.

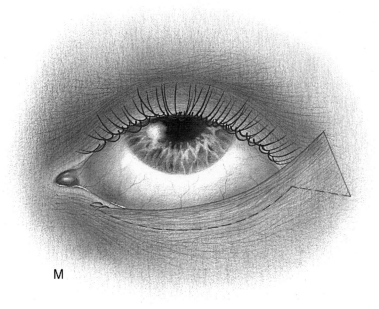

M, The lower eyelid skin flap drapes the incision site as the patient gazes upward.

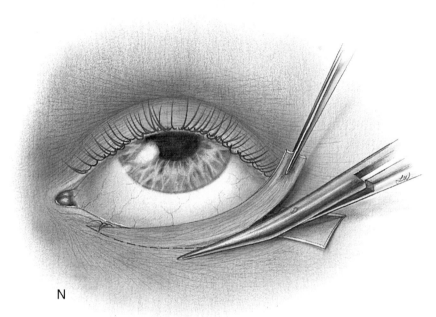

N, Vertical skin draping the lower eyelid incision site is excised conservatively.

N

O, The skin flap is pulled temporally, and the temporal extreme of the skin incision site is connected to a small cut made in the skin flap where the lower eyelid incision meets the lateral canthal incision.

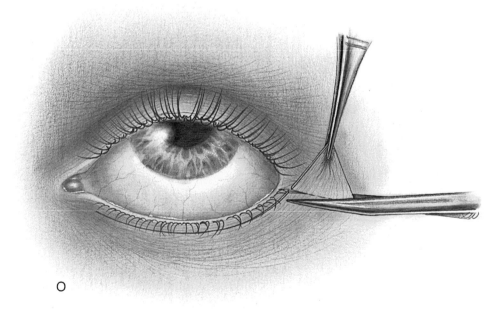

O

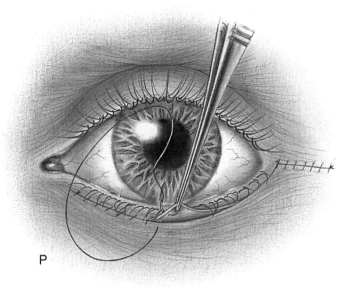

P, The lateral canthal incision site is closed with a continuous 6-0 black silk suture run from the lateral canthus to the temporal extreme of the eyelid. Another 6-0 black silk suture is run continuously in a nasal to temporal direction.

propylene (Prolene), 5-0 plain catgut, or 6-0 nylon suture, run continuously, in an interrupted fashion, or in a subcuticular manner, can also be used to close the lower eyelid skin. I prefer the silk suture because it is less stiff, its removal is easy, and scarring is minimal.

TREATMENT OF ABNORMAL-APPEARING OR PIGMENTED NASAL LOWER EYELID SKIN

Rarely, patients present with abnormal-appearing crinkly or pigmented skin over the nasal section of the lower eyelid. Treating these problems with a standard skin or skin-muscle flap technique, in which the skin is pulled and tightened temporally, often makes the conditions worse by leaving all the abnormal-appearing skin and also diffusing it more temporally.

In 1983, I described a technique to treat lower eyelid dermatochalasis and abnormal-appearing skin simultaneously.[3] This modification of the skin, or skin-muscle flap approach, is accomplished by extending the infraciliary incision to the nasal end of the eyelid and extending it inferiorly in a temporal-oblique direction for another 1–1.5 cm (Fig. 18–2*A*).

After undermining the skin or skin-muscle flap and removing herniated orbital fat, the surgeon draws the flap nasally and superiorly (Fig. 18–2*B*). Skin overlapping the incision site is removed with a triangle of nasal skin as well as a triangle of skin that overlaps the infraciliary incision (Fig. 18–2*C* and *D*). One should appreciate, when draping the skin flap over the incision site, that the eyelid skin rests in a slight concavity; therefore, the surgeon should be conservative in the resection of the nasal triangle of skin. The nasal vertical incision is closed with a 6-0 continuous black silk suture. The

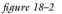

figure 18–2

A, Following an infraciliary and a lateral canthal incision, an incision is made at the nasal aspect of the first incision in a temporal inferior oblique direction. The skin or skin-muscle flap is undermined.

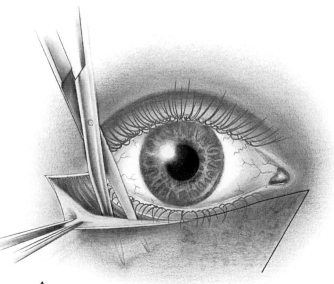

A

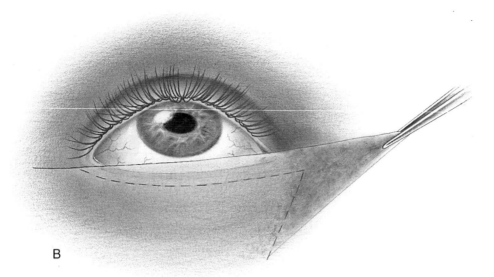

B, The skin or skin-muscle flap is draped over the incision site.

C, The skin or skin-muscle flap that drapes over the infraciliary and lateral canthal incision sites is excised.

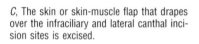

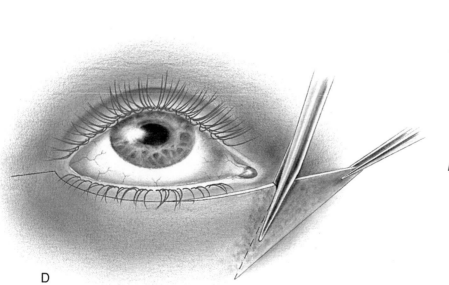

D, Excision of a triangle of nasal skin.

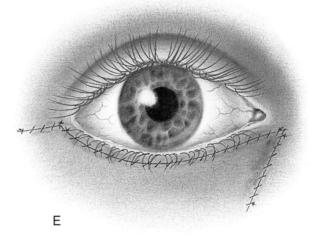

E

E, The nasal vertical incision is closed with a continuous 6-0 black silk suture. Another suture closes the infraciliary and lateral canthal incision. (*A–E,* From Putterman AM: Simultaneous treatment of lower eyelid dermatochalasis and abnormal-appearing skin. Am J Ophthalmol 1983; 96:6–9. With permission from The American Journal of Ophthalmology. Copyright by the Ophthalmic Publishing Company.)

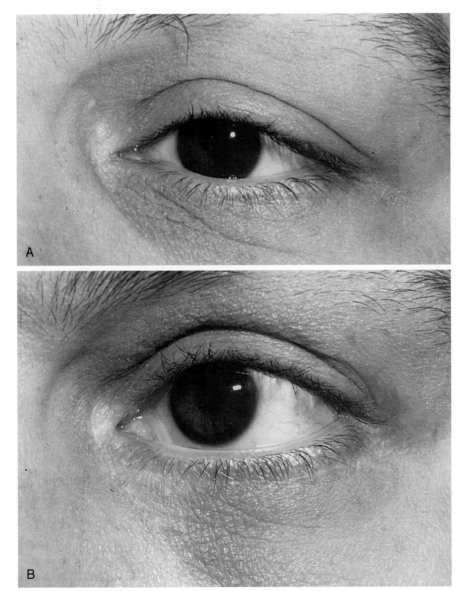

figure 18–3

A, Preoperative photograph shows abnormal-appearing, crinkly, pigmented nasal skin. *B,* Appearance after lower eyelid skin flap procedure with resection of the nasal triangle.

infraciliary skin is then closed using another 6-0 silk suture run continuously nasally to temporally (Fig. 18–2*E*).

This technique allows part of the abnormal-appearing nasal skin to be removed and diffuses the more normal temporal skin into the eyelid. The procedure has improved the appearance of the lower eyelid in more than 15 of my patients with abnormal-appearing pigmented or crinkly skin (Fig. 18–3). There have been no complications.

EXCISION OF HYPERTROPHIC ORBICULARIS MUSCLE

Any orbicularis muscle hypertrophy noted preoperatively, especially when the patient smiles and looks upward, is removed. This is performed after the skin of the lower eyelid is dissected from the orbicularis muscle and before the fat is resected.

The hypertrophic muscle usually consists of a ridge about 5 mm wide that starts about 3–5 mm below the eyelash line. It may extend all the way across the eyelid or may be segmental. The site is carefully noted preoperatively because the muscle may not be seen when the skin flap is reflected during surgery. A Westcott scissors, directed horizontally and placed parallel to the muscle, is used to excise the superficial aspect of the muscle in a temporal to nasal direction (Fig. 18–4).

POSTOPERATIVE CARE

No dressings are used. The patient is instructed to apply ice-cold compresses to the eyelids. Pads (4 × 4 inches) soaked in a bucket of saline and ice are wrung out and applied with slight pressure directly and slightly upward to the lids. Pulling the lower lid upward also allows the orbital septum to reattach to the capsulopalpebral fascia in a more inferior position, which reduces postoperative eyelid retraction. When the pads become warm, they are dipped again into the saline and ice and are reapplied.

This process is continued for 24 hours. The applications should be constant for the first 2 postoperative hours. After that, the compresses are applied for about 20 minutes with 10- to 15-minute rest periods in between until bedtime. The applications are resumed after the patient awakens.

To reduce postoperative edema, the patient lies in bed with the head of the bed about 45 degrees higher than the rest of the body. Nurses should check for bleeding associated with proptosis, pain, or loss of vision every 15 minutes for the first 3 hours after surgery.[1] If loss of vision secondary to retrobulbar hemorrhage occurs, it can be detected and treated quickly by opening the involved incision sites.

The black silk 6-0 sutures are removed 4 days postoperatively. Weak areas of the incisions are supported with ¼-inch sterile tape (Steri-strips), usually at the lateral canthus, for another 3 days.

COMPLICATIONS

One to three suture cysts, especially in the temporal end of the incision, developed in approximately 10 per cent of the eyelids I have treated with the skin flap technique. The cysts were easily removed 2 months postoperatively with hydrolysis. Retrobulbar hemorrhage occurred with temporary loss of vision in one patient and with a resid-

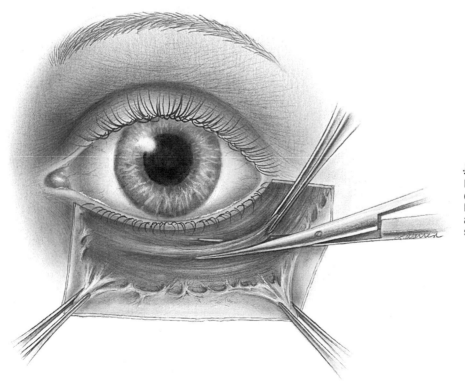

figure 18–4

Excision of hypertrophic orbicularis muscle. The area of thickened, elevated orbicularis muscle is picked up with a forceps and is excised until a smooth orbicularis surface is produced.

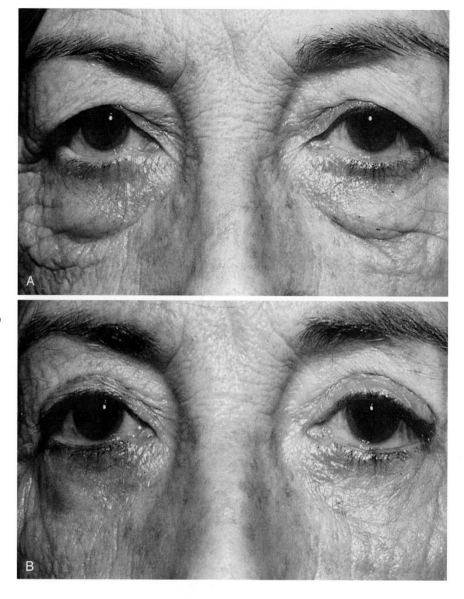

figure 18–5

A, Preoperative appearance: dermatochalasis (excess skin) and herniated orbital fat of all four eyelids associated with moderate nasal upper eyelid skin. B, Appearance after resection of excess skin and herniated orbital fat through both upper and lower eyelid skin flap techniques. The nasal upper eyelid skin was treated with a bilateral W-plasty (see Chapter 9).

ual scotoma in another patient.[1] No unusual complications were noted in any other patient, and no cicatricial ectropion was observed postoperatively.

RESULTS

This skin flap technique of lower blepharoplasty has been performed in more than 600 lower eyelids with satisfactory results (Fig. 18–5).

References

1. Putterman AM: Temporary blindness after cosmetic blepharoplasty. Am J Ophthalmol 1975; 80:1081–1083.
2. Putterman AM: The mysterious second temporal fat pad. Ophthalmic Plast Reconstr Surg 1985; 1:83–86.
3. Putterman AM: Simultaneous treatment of lower eyelid dermatochalasis and abnormal-appearing skin. Am J Ophthalmol 1983; 96:6–9.

Allen M. Putterman

Treatment of Lower Eyelid Dermatochalasis, Herniated Orbital Fat, and Hypertrophic Orbicularis Muscle: Skin-Muscle Flap Approach

A skin-muscle flap approach is advantageous, and the technique I commonly use, in patients with lower eyelid herniated orbital fat and dermatochalasis (excess skin). I still prefer a skin flap approach in patients with markedly excessive lower lid skin, whereas I use an internal approach for patients with slightly excessive skin.

In this chapter, I outline the technique I use to excise herniated orbital fat through a skin-muscle flap approach. The advantage of this procedure is the easy isolation of the orbital fat. Its disadvantage is the difficulty in eliminating marked dermatochalasis.

ALLEN M. PUTTERMAN

There are three methods of performing a lower blepharoplasty. In the most commonly used method, the excess skin and herniated orbital fat are removed from the lower eyelid through a skin–orbicularis oculi muscle flap approach. Hypertrophic orbicularis muscle can easily be removed by this approach also. This technique carries the advantage of using a relatively avascular plane, the suborbicularis space.

The two other techniques are the skin flap and internal approaches. The skin flap procedure is indicated probably only if the patient has marked excess skin or xanthelasma tumors (see Chapter 18).

The internal approach is useful when the procedure is being performed along with correction of thyroid ophthalmopathy, with either orbital decompression or hard-palate grafting (see Chapter 25). It is also useful in the patient who has minimal excess skin or orbicularis muscle or who has a tendency to keloid formation (a rare condition in the lower eyelids) (see Chapter 20).

PREPARATION FOR SURGERY

The patient is prepared for surgery in the same manner as for an upper blepharoplasty (see Chapters 9 and 10).

SURGICAL TECHNIQUE

A line is drawn beginning at the lateral canthus and extending approximately 1 cm in an almost horizontal direction. Several milliliters of 2 per cent lidocaine with epinephrine is subcutaneously injected diffusely across the lower eyelid. Also, a 25-gauge, 1.5-cm needle is passed through the nasal lower lid skin just above the skin of the inferior orbital rim and then over the inferior orbital rim in a slightly downward direction to avoid penetrating the eye. The needle is inserted for approximately 1 cm, and 0.5–1 ml of 2 per cent lidocaine with epinephrine is injected. This is repeated centrally and temporally.

A No. 15 Bard-Parker blade is used to make a skin incision 1.5 mm beneath the lower lid lashes (Fig. 19–1*A*). The incision begins below the punctum and extends temporally for a distance of 2–3 mm temporal to the lateral canthus. The incision is extended for another 1 cm in an almost horizontal direction.

A 4-0 black silk traction suture is placed through skin, orbicularis muscle, and superficial tarsus of the central lower eyelid and is used to pull the lower eyelid upward.

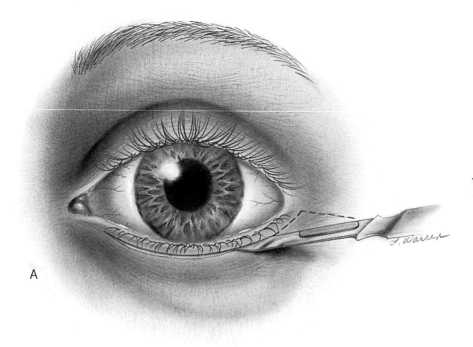

figure 19–1

A, Incision of infralash and lateral canthal skin.

A

With a toothed forceps, the surgeon grasps the central lower lid at the skin incision site and pulls the eyelid downward and outward. A Westcott scissors is used to penetrate the central orbicularis muscle, with the scissors tips pointed inward and downward (Fig. 19–1B). The suborbicularis space should be seen. The Westcott scissors is inserted into the space, and its blades are spread to elongate this dissection.

The traction suture and forceps are kept in the same position as the orbicularis muscle is severed along the incision site with Westcott scissors (Fig. 19–1C) or other suitable instrument. A disposable cautery (Solan Accu-Temp, Xomed Surgical Products, Jacksonville, Fla.), Colorado needle, sapphire-tipped scalpel neodymium:YAG laser, or carbon dioxide laser (see Chapters 35 and 36) also can be used.[1] These four instruments

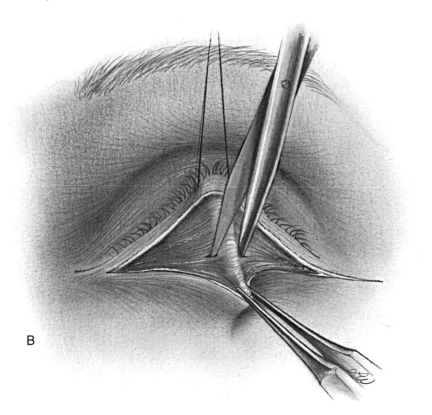

B, Westcott scissors are used to penetrate the central orbicularis oculi muscle, with the scissors tips pointed inward and downward.

B

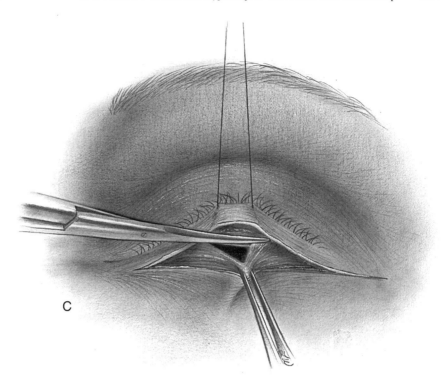

C, The orbicularis oculi muscle is severed along the skin incision site with Westcott scissors.

C

coagulate blood vessels while they simultaneously cut the orbicularis muscle.

Blunt dissection with a cotton-tipped applicator or Westcott scissors is applied under the orbicularis muscle (Fig. 19–1*D*). This step should allow visualization of the nasal, central, and temporal herniated orbital fat pads (Fig. 19–1*E*).

A 4-0 black silk traction suture is placed through the orbital septum and is used to pull the lower lid skin flap downward. It is secured to the drape with a hemostat. The lower eyelid is pulled upward with the central traction suture, which is attached to the superior drape. Any remaining bleeding vessels are coagulated with a disposable cautery.

A Westcott scissors is used to make a small opening in the temporal orbital fat capsule. The surgeon pushes on the eye, the fat that prolapses with gentle pressure applied to the eye is clamped with a hemostat, and the tissues above the hemostat are cut with a No. 15 Bard-Parker blade that is slid over the hemostat (Fig. 19–1*F*). Cotton-tipped applicators are applied under the hemostat, and a Bovie cautery is used to coagulate the fat stump. Before releasing the hemostat, the surgeon grasps the orbital fat beneath the hemostat with a forceps. The fat is inspected for bleeding before it is allowed to retract into the orbit. Bleeding can lead to retrobulbar hemorrhage and the potential for blindness.[2]

After the temporal orbital fat pad is removed, the surgeon pushes on the eye again to ensure that the entire pad has been removed. Commonly, after removal of the temporal orbital fat pad, a second temporal fat pad appears when the surgeon pushes on the eye. This may be a second temporal fat pad that is not apparent

until the first pad is removed, or it may be a deeper portion of the temporal fat that becomes visible after the anterior part is removed.[3] In either case, the surgeon must remove the second pad in order to prevent postoperative fullness in the temporal aspect of the eyelid. Once the temporal fat is completely removed, the central and nasal fat pads are removed in a similar manner. The central and nasal fat pads are separated by the inferior oblique muscle, and the nasal fat pad is white.

The patient is then asked to look upward while the lower lid skin-muscle flap is draped over the incision site (Fig. 19–1*G*). The skin and orbicularis muscle that drape over the incision site are excised with Westcott scissors. This excision is performed temporally over the lateral canthal incision site and then horizontally over the incision site of the lower lid skin from lateral canthus to punctum.

With two toothed forceps, the surgeon grasps the skin-muscle flap nasally and temporally and pulls it downward. A strip of orbicularis muscle is routinely excised over the superior skin-muscle flap temporally to nasally for a distance of 4–5 mm beneath the flap (Fig. 19–1*H*). (This prevents postoperative fullness in that area.) If orbicularis muscle is noted to be hypertrophic preoperatively, it is now excised over the sites noted preoperatively in the same manner as the strip that is routinely taken. Bleeding is controlled with a disposable cautery.

The surgeon sutures the skin by running a 6-0 black silk suture continuously from the lateral canthus to the temporal end of the incision site. A second 6-0 black silk suture is run continuously from the nasal end of the incision to the lateral canthus (Fig. 19–1*I*).

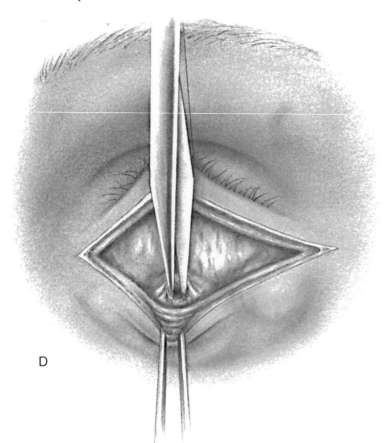

D, Blunt dissection with Westcott scissors is applied under the orbicularis muscle.

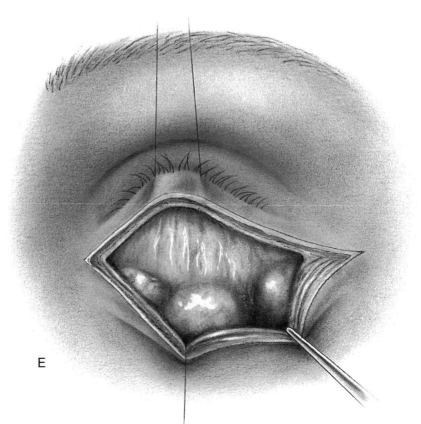

E, The nasal, central, and temporal herniated orbital fat pads are now visible.

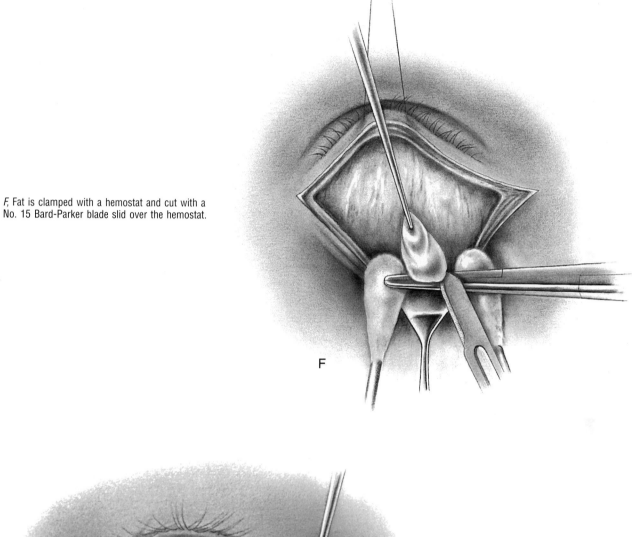

F, Fat is clamped with a hemostat and cut with a No. 15 Bard-Parker blade slid over the hemostat.

F

G, The skin and orbicularis muscle are draped over the incision site and are excised.

G

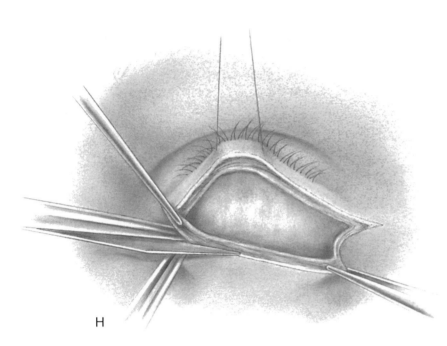

H, A strip of orbicularis muscle is routinely excised over the superior skin muscle flap, temporally to nasally, for a distance 4–5 mm beneath the flap.

H

I, A 6-0 black silk suture is run continuously from the lateral canthus to the temporal end of the incision. A second 6-0 black silk suture is run continuously from the nasal end of the incision to the lateral canthus.

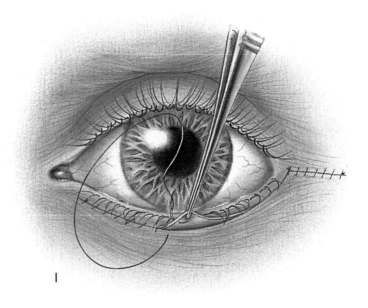

I

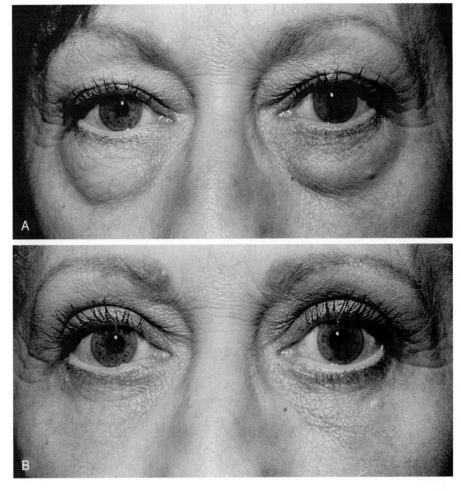

figure 19–2

Before *(A)* and after *(B)* skin-muscle flap treatment of lower eyelid dermatochalasis (excess skin) and herniated orbital flap. The patient's upper eyelids were treated simultaneously with a skin-muscle resection and crease reconstruction (see Chapter 10).

POSTOPERATIVE CARE

Postoperative treatment is the same as described for upper blepharoplasty (see Chapters 9 and 10), with the exception that there are no polyglactin (Vicryl) sutures to remove.

POSTOPERATIVE COMPLICATIONS

Lower eyelid ectropion and retraction are possible complications from lower blepharoplasty. Usually, these complications can be prevented by careful preoperative assessment of patients with horizontal eyelid laxity who have the potential for development of these problems and by a simultaneous tarsal strip procedure in these patients (see Chapter 21). Should these complications occur, however, they can be treated with a tarsal strip postoperatively (see Chapter 38).

If too much skin is removed, a cicatricial ectropion can occur. If this happens, skin grafting, in addition to the tarsal strip procedure, is needed (see Chapter 38).

Another complication is loss of eyelashes. This can be prevented if the incision is placed 1.5 mm beneath the lash line, with minimal cauterization of the areas from which the eyelash follicles emanate. There is no satisfactory treatment of loss of eyelashes.

Suture cysts are possible postoperatively. They can be treated by light hydrolysis 2 months postoperatively with a Birtcher hyfrecator.

If a retrobulbar hemorrhage occurs, the sutures of the lower lid should be removed immediately and bleeding controlled.

RESULTS

More than 1500 patients have been treated with this technique with excellent results (Fig. 19–2).

References

1. Putterman AM: Scalpel neodymium:YAG laser in oculoplastic surgery. Am J Ophthalmol 1990; 109:581–584.
2. Putterman AM: Temporary blindness after cosmetic blepharoplasty. Am J Ophthalmol 1975; 80:1081–1083.
3. Putterman AM: The mysterious second temporal fat pad. Ophthalmic Plast Reconstr Surg 1985; 1:83–86.

Allen M. Putterman

Chapter 20

Transconjunctival Approach to Resection of Lower Eyelid Herniated Orbital Fat

I use the transconjunctival approach in patients who have herniated orbital fat with minimal or no excessive lower eyelid skin. Many patients want to have this approach done because it eliminates external scarring and produces less ecchymosis; however, it has been my experience that many patients develop conjunctival chemosis and slight redundancy and wrinkling of the skin compared with those who were treated with the external approach. Therefore, I find that more frequently I am combining this approach with laser resurfacing of the lower eyelid skin and with plication sutures.

The technique described in this chapter can be modified for patients with thyroid ophthalmopathy and lower lid retraction by the addition of the recession of conjunctiva and lower eyelid retractors with hard-palate grafting (see Chapter 25).

ALLEN M. PUTTERMAN

The transconjunctival approach to removal of herniated orbital fat is the preferred method of treatment in patients who have only herniated orbital fat with minimal evidence of dermatochalasis (excess skin) and no hypertrophic orbicularis oculi muscle. This technique is also especially advantageous for:

- Younger patients
- Patients who have had previous blepharoplasties in whom an external approach might lead to eyelid retraction or ectropion
- Patients with lower eyelid retraction secondary to thyroid disease in whom hard-palate grafts are required
- Patients with wrinkled or minimally excessive lower eyelid skin in whom plication of the lateral canthi or laser resurfacing of lower eyelid skin is useful (see Chapters 22 and 31)

If there is horizontal lower eyelid laxity, this procedure can be easily combined with a horizontal eyelid tightening through a tarsal strip procedure (see Chapter 21).

SURGICAL TECHNIQUE

The transconjunctival procedure is performed with the patient under local anesthesia. Two per cent lidocaine (Xylocaine) with 1:100,000 epinephrine is injected subcutaneously at the center of the lower eyelid just beneath the lashes. An additional anesthetic agent is injected under the orbicularis muscle diffusely across the eyelid and into each fat pad. To inject the anesthetic agent into the nasal, central, and temporal fat pad, the surgeon inserts a 25-gauge, 0.8-cm needle just above the inferior orbital rim and is directs it downward slightly until it penetrates its entire length (0.8 cm). The barrel of the syringe is withdrawn to make sure that no blood vessel has been entered, and approximately 0.5 ml of the agent is injected into each of the three fat pads.

A 4-0 black silk traction suture is placed through skin, orbicularis muscle, and superficial tarsus at the center of the eyelid. The surgeon pulls the eyelid downward with the traction suture to expose the inferior palpebral conjunctiva. Additional anesthetic is injected subconjunctivally over the inferior palpebral conjunctiva across the eyelid. Topical tetracaine is instilled over the eye, and a scleral lens is placed over the eye to protect it. Two per cent lidocaine with epinephrine is also injected subcutaneously over the center of the upper eyelid, and a 4-0 black silk traction suture is placed through skin, orbicularis muscle, and superficial tarsus to pull the upper eyelid upward.

203

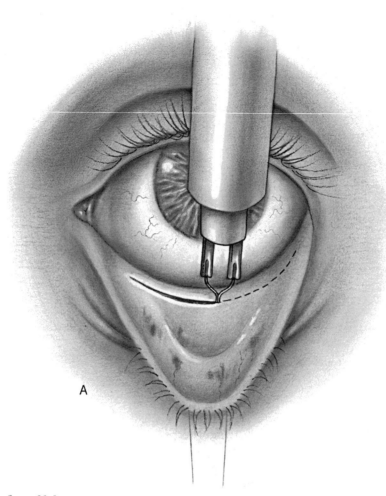

figure 20–1

A, A disposable cautery is applied to the inferior palpebral conjunctiva just above the fornix and is used to cut the conjunctiva from the medial to temporal end of the eyelid.

A disposable cautery (Solan Accu-Temp, Xomed Surgical Products, Jacksonville, Fla.), a sapphire-tipped neodymium:YAG (Nd:YAG) laser, or a carbon dioxide ultrapulse laser is applied to the inferior palpebral conjunctiva just above the fornix. The cautery or laser is used to cut conjunctiva from the medial to temporal end of the eyelid (Fig. 20–1*A*). The surgeon grasps the inferior edge of the severed palpebral conjunctiva while the assistant grasps the adjacent, more superior edge with another forceps (Fig. 20–1*B*). The two forceps are pulled apart. Further dissection with the disposable cautery, Nd:YAG or carbon dioxide ultrapulse laser, or a Colorado needle is carried out through Müller's muscle and capsulopalpebral fascia until fat is seen (see Chapters 35 and 36).

A 4-0 black silk suture is placed through the inferior edge of conjunctiva, Müller's muscle, and capsulopalpebral fascia and then through the gray line of the upper eyelid, exiting through orbicularis muscle and skin (Fig. 20–1*C*). The contact lens is removed, and the suture is drawn up and tied with a shoelace tie. The 4-0 silk suture through the upper eyelid is pulled upward and clamped to the drape with a hemostat. This maneuver protects the eye with the upper eyelid and the internal lamellae of the lower eyelid.

A Desmarres retractor is placed over the lower eyelid and is pulled downward and outward to expose the orbital fat. With the use of cotton-tipped applicators and Westcott scissors, blunt dissection is carried out to isolate the three orbital fat pads. The central and nasal fat pads are divided by the inferior oblique muscle, which can be easily seen through the internal approach and should be identified to avoid injury to this structure. Also, the nasal and central fat pads are found in a slightly more temporal position than when they are isolated through an external approach.

The temporal herniated orbital fat is isolated, and the fat that prolapses with gentle pressure on the eye is clamped with a hemostat and cut along the hemostat blade with a No. 15 Bard-Parker blade. Then cotton-tipped applicators are placed underneath the hemostat as a Bovie cautery is applied over the fat stump. The surgeon grasps the fat with a forceps before it is allowed to slide back into the orbit to make sure that there is no residual bleeding that might cause a retrobulbar hemorrhage.

After the first temporal fat pad is removed, the surgeon applies additional pressure to the eye to determine whether there is a second temporal fat pad. The central and nasal fat pads are then removed in a similar manner

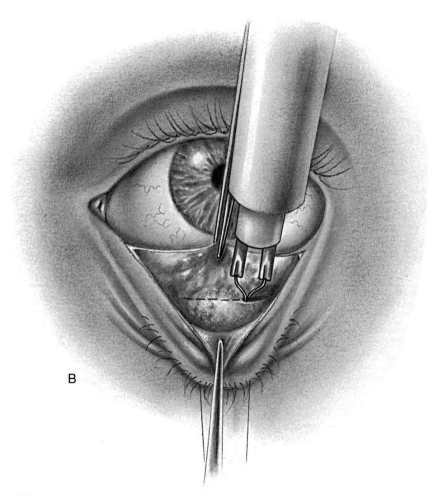

B, With forceps, the surgeon and surgeon's assistant grasp the inferior and superior edges, respectively, of the severed palpebral conjunctiva to facilitate dissection of Müller's muscle and capsulopalpebral fascia.

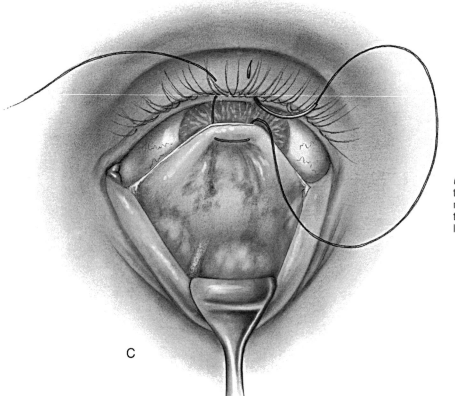

C, A 4-0 black silk suture is placed through the inferior edge of the conjunctiva, Müller's muscle, and the capsulopalpebral fascia and then through the gray line of the upper eyelid, exiting through orbicularis and skin.

C

D, The surgeon removes the temporal, central, and nasal orbital fat pads by cutting along the hemostat blade with a No. 15 Bard-Parker blade and then applying a Bovie cautery over the fat stump.

D

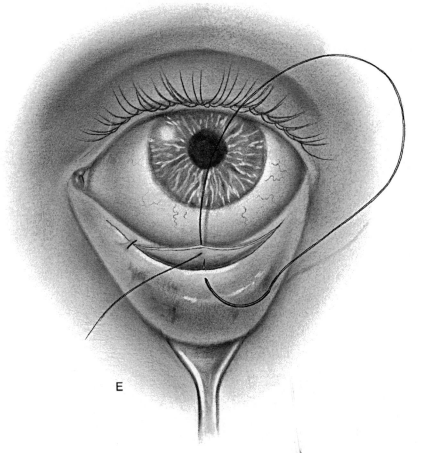

E, The conjunctiva is reapproximated with three 6-0 plain catgut buried sutures.

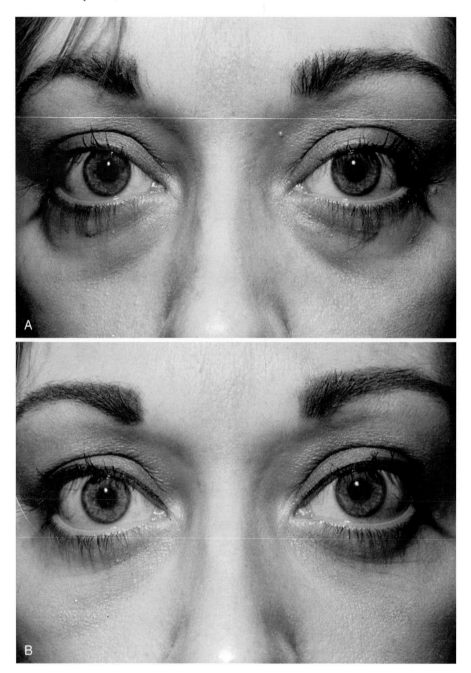

A

B

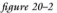

figure 20–2

A, Preoperative appearance of a patient with herniated orbital fat of both lower eyelids with no significant dermatochalasis (excess skin). *B,* Postoperative appearance after resection of orbital fat using the transconjunctival approach.

(Fig. 20–1*D*). If the Nd:YAG or carbon dioxide ultrapulse laser is used, the fat is prolapsed and severed with the sapphire tip at its base without being clamped with a hemostat (see Chapters 35 and 36.)

The 4-0 silk suture that attaches conjunctiva, Müller's muscle, and capsulopalpebral fascia to the upper eyelid is then severed. The contact lens is replaced over the eye. Conjunctiva is reapproximated with three 6-0 plain catgut buried sutures (Fig. 20–1*E*). Gentamicin (Garamycin) is applied over the eye.

POSTOPERATIVE CARE

The patient is instructed to apply cold compresses for the next 24 hours. Other postoperative care is similar

to that described for upper and lower blepharoplasties performed with other approaches (see Chapters 9, 10, 18, and 19).

COMPLICATIONS

Several patients in whom I performed the transconjunctival approach had postoperative residual dermatochalasis, which needed to be removed through an external approach or laser skin resurfacing. Better patient selection or combining the initial procedure with laser resurfacing could have prevented this problem.

Although this procedure has not caused any motility problems, in two patients in whom this procedure was combined with a tarsal strip procedure, ocular motility restriction and diplopia occurred, presumably secondary to scar tissue that developed between the globe and the temporal inferior orbital wall.

RESULTS

I have performed the transconjunctival approach in more than 1000 patients (Fig. 20–2). The procedure has the advantage of causing less eyelid retraction or ectropion than with the skin flap or skin-muscle flap approaches because the external lamellae are not manipulated. I believe that there is less ecchymosis because the orbicularis muscle and skin are not severed. There tends to be more conjunctival chemosis immediately postoperatively with this technique than with the external technique.

Because the procedure is more difficult to master than the external approach, a surgeon should not perform this procedure without prior exposure to it.

Allen M. Putterman

Chapter 21

Tarsal Strip Procedure Combined with Lower Blepharoplasty

An ectropion of the lower eyelid can occur after excision of skin, orbicularis oculi muscle, and orbital fat in patients with horizontally lax lower eyelids. This complication of cosmetic blepharoplasty can happen even with minimal lower eyelid vertical skin resection. The cause is usually redundant lower eyelid tissues or attenuation of the lateral canthal tendon.

In this chapter, I outline the steps of a tarsal strip procedure that can be combined with excision of lower eyelid skin, orbicularis muscle, and orbital fat through a skin-muscle flap approach to prevent a postoperative lower eyelid ectropion. A similar technique can be used in patients with horizontally lax or retracted lower eyelids when an internal transconjunctival blepharoplasty is performed.

Although I continue to perform the tarsal strip procedure in most patients with horizontal laxity or temporal retraction of the lower eyelid, I am beginning to perform a full-thickness resection in some patients. I describe this technique in the chapter on cheek and midface lifts (see Chapter 24).

ALLEN M. PUTTERMAN

The tarsal strip procedure was first described by Tenzel as a method of treating acquired ectropion.[1] Many cases of acquired ectropion result from both horizontal laxity of the eyelid and attenuation of the lateral canthal tendon. The tarsal strip procedure not only ensures a normal horizontal length of the eyelid but also corrects the attenuated lateral canthal tendon. Use of the procedure has now expanded to the treatment of lower eyelid retraction following cosmetic blepharoplasty.[2]

A similar technique can be used in horizontally lax or temporally retracted lower eyelids treated with an internal transconjunctival approach to blepharoplasty. After reviewing this chapter and Chapter 38, the reader should be able to understand this approach. At present, I also treat some patients with horizontal laxity or temporal retraction of the lower eyelids with a full-thickness temporal eyelid resection (see Chapter 24).

SURGICAL TECHNIQUE

A skin or a skin-muscle flap approach to lower blepharoplasty is carried out up to the steps of creating the flaps and excising herniated orbital fat (see Chapters 18 and 19). If an internal blepharoplasty is performed, a lateral canthotomy and lower cantholysis are done and the procedure is then carried out to the steps of removing fat and closing the conjunctiva (see Chapter 20).

Anesthesia

Several milliliters of 2 per cent lidocaine (Xylocaine) with 1:100,000 epinephrine is injected subcutaneously over the temporal upper and lower eyelids and lateral canthus. The needle is also inserted along the lateral orbital wall to a depth of 0.5 cm, and another milliliter of lidocaine with epinephrine is injected.

Lateral Canthotomy

After injecting the anesthetic agent, the surgeon performs a lateral canthotomy by cutting from the lateral canthus to the lateral orbital wall with Westcott scissors (Figs. 21–1*A* and *B*). The scissors is then used to dissect conjunctiva from the posterior surface of the lower limb of the lateral canthal tendon (Fig. 21–1*C*). The orbicularis muscle is then undermined from the anterior surface of this tendon limb. A forceps is used to grasp the lower eyelid and to pull it nasally.

Using the Westcott scissors, the surgeon palpates the taut lower lateral canthal tendon limb by strumming over the tendon with the points of the scissors. Once the tendon is identified, it is severed from its attachment to the lateral orbital wall (Fig. 21–1*D*). The surgeon will know that this tendon has been successfully severed after feeling a sudden nasal migration of the lower eyelid. If this is not achieved, the surgeon should again palpate the tendon with Westcott scissors and sever any remaining attachments. The surgeon should be careful not to be overzealous in the severing of lateral canthal attachments because doing this may cause scar tissue between the globe and lateral orbital wall with secondary restrictive ocular motility and diplopia.

Forceps and small rakes are used to retract the lateral canthal tissues. A disposable surgical cautery (Solan Accu-Temp, Xomed Surgical Products, Jacksonville, Fla.) is applied to control bleeding.

Formation of Tarsal Strip

The protective scleral contact lens is removed. A forceps is used to grasp the temporal aspect of the lower eyelid

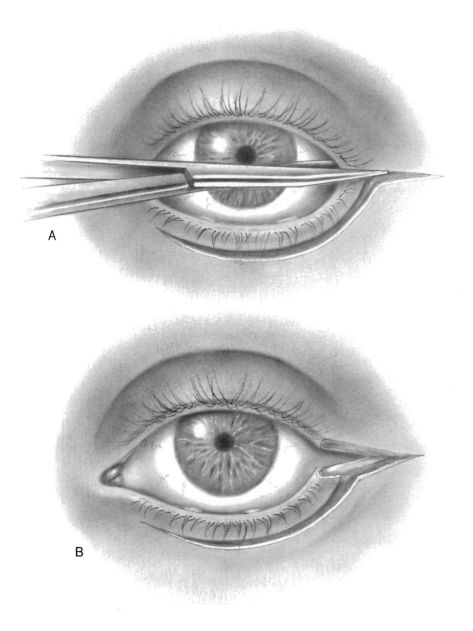

figure 21–1

A and *B*, The surgeon performs a lateral canthotomy by cutting from the lateral canthus to the lateral orbital wall with Westcott scissors.

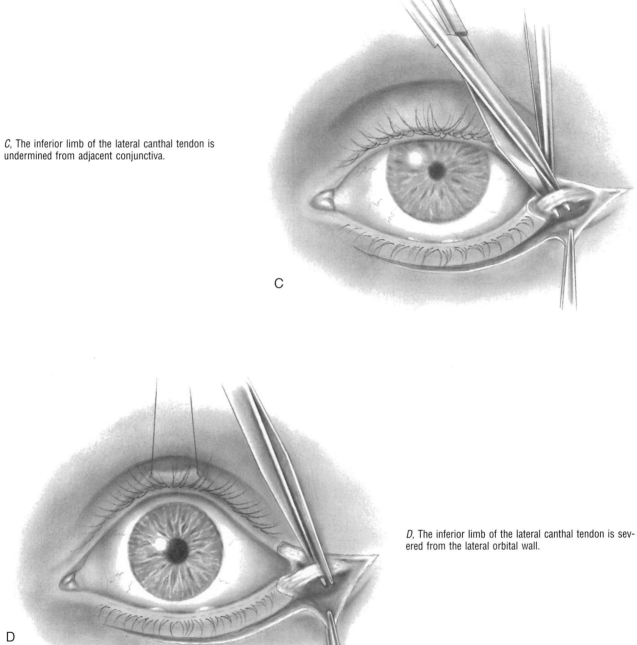

C, The inferior limb of the lateral canthal tendon is undermined from adjacent conjunctiva.

C

D, The inferior limb of the lateral canthal tendon is severed from the lateral orbital wall.

D

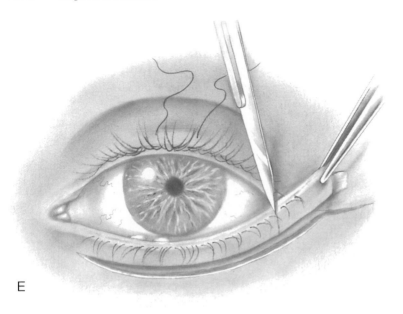

E, A scratch incision is made on the lower eyelid margin at the nasal end of the tarsal strip.

E

and to pull it temporally and slightly superiorly until slight tension of the eyelid is achieved. A scratch incision is made with a No. 11 Bard-Parker blade at the aspect of the lower eyelid margin that is now adjacent to the temporal cut edge of the upper eyelid margin (Fig. 21–1*E*). A measurement is made with a ruler from the temporal cut end of the lower eyelid to the scratch incision, which determines the length of the tarsal strip.

The surgeon then divides the eyelid into two lamellae by cutting with a Westcott scissors along the gray line from the temporal end of the eyelid to the scratch incision site (Fig. 21–1*F*). The Westcott scissors is used to remove skin and orbicularis muscle from the anterior surface of tarsus of this eyelid segment (Fig. 21–1*G*). Conjunctiva is then cut from the inferior tarsal edge (Fig. 21–1*H*). Bleeding is again controlled with the disposable cautery. Next, the surgeon scrapes off the

conjunctival epithelium on the posterior surface of the tarsus with a No. 15 Bard-Parker blade to prevent epithelial inclusion cysts (Fig. 21–1*I*).

Attachment of Tarsal Strip

Each arm of a 4-0 polypropylene (Prolene) double-armed suture is passed internally to externally through the tarsal strip at the junction of the strip and eyelid (Fig. 21–1*J*). The strip is pulled temporally until the area of the polypropylene sutures is adjacent to the lateral orbital wall. The strip is drawn superiorly and internally until it seems to be at an acceptable position. The temporal lower eyelid should also be in contact with the eye, not displaced anterior to the eye. If the patient's eye is proptotic, as in thyroid disease, the tarsal

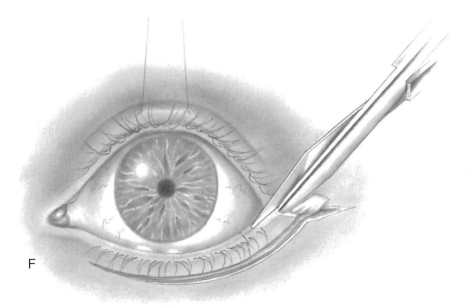

F, The surgeon divides the eyelid into two lamellae by cutting along the gray line from the temporal end of the eyelid to the scratch incision site.

F

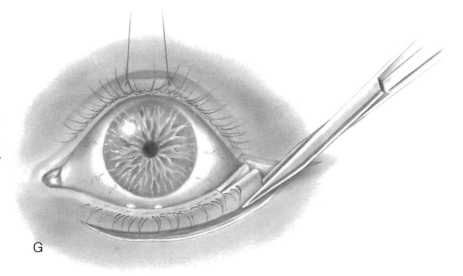

G, The orbicularis oculi muscle is severed below the skin of the planned tarsal strip in patients with a skin flap approach. The skin and orbicularis muscle are removed from the anterior surface of the eyelid margin.

G

strip should be placed much more anteriorly than for a recessed or enophthalmic eye. Once the desired lateral position is determined, each arm of the 4-0 polypropylene suture is passed internally to externally through the lateral orbital periosteum or through the upper limb of the lateral canthal tendon at this position (Fig. 21–1*K*).

The suture is tied with the first tie of the surgeon's knot over a 4-0 black silk knot-releasing suture. (The piece of silk is approximately 5 cm long and does not have a needle attached to it.) It is important, in placement of the tarsal strip, that the lower eyelid not retract further from the inferior corneal limbus and pull behind and under the eye. Excessive tension on the eyelid can lead to lower eyelid retraction. If the procedure is being performed bilaterally, the opposite side is treated up to this step of the procedure.

The patient is seated up on the operating table, and the position of the lateral canthus is compared with the other side. The top of a metal ruler is aligned with each

medial canthus, and the level at which the ruler bisects each lateral canthus is noted. The position of the lower eyelid adjacent to the eyes is also judged. If the lateral canthus is too high or low or too anterior or posterior, the knot-releasing suture is grasped with a forceps at each end of the suture and is pulled outward to release the knot. The suture arms are removed from the lateral wall periosteum or upper lateral canthal tendon and placed in a new position. This procedure is repeated until the desired position of the lateral canthus and lower eyelid is achieved. When this is accomplished, the polypropylene sutures are tied with approximately four knots.

A 4-0 polyglactin (Vicryl) suture is passed through periosteum adjacent and temporal to the polypropylene knot (Fig. 21–1*L*). It is passed through the tarsal strip internally to externally and then externally to internally. After being drawn up and tied, this suture further secures the tarsal strip to periosteum and buries the poly-

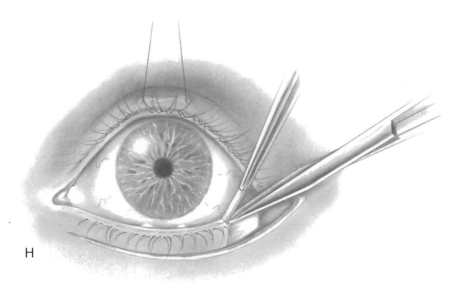

H, The posterior superior edge of the eyelid margin is excised.

H

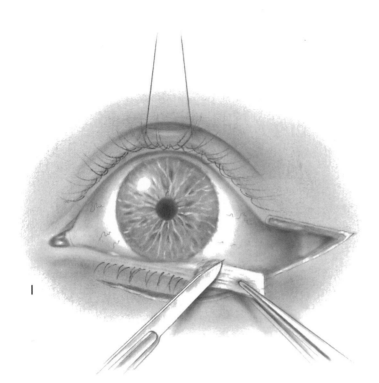

I, The conjunctival epithelium and the posterior surface of the tarsus are scraped off.

J, Each arm of the 4-0 polypropylene (Prolene) double-armed suture is then passed internally to externally through the tarsal strip at the junction of the strip and eyelid.

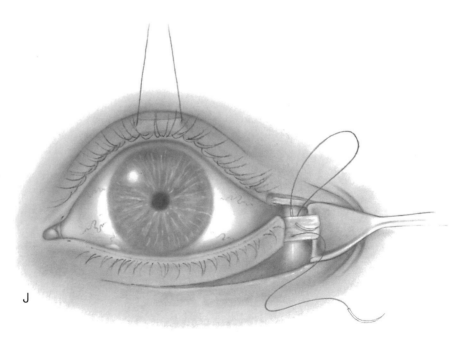

K, The polypropylene suture is passed internally to externally through the lateral orbital periosteum.

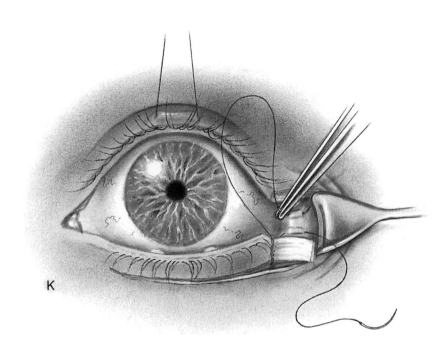

K

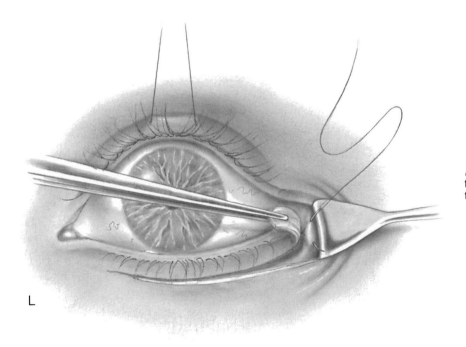

L

L, A 4-0 polyglactin (Vicryl) suture is passed through the periosteum adjacent and temporal to the polypropylene knot.

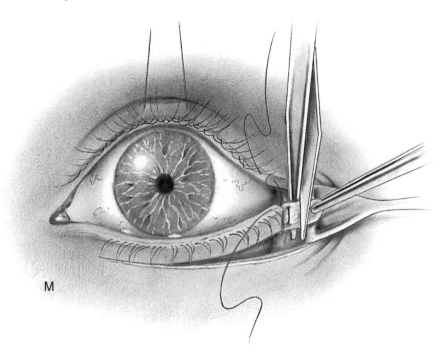

M, A 6-0 black silk suture is passed through the corner of each temporal upper and lower eyelid, and excess tarsal strip is excised.

propylene suture. The tarsal strip temporal to the polyglactin suture is then severed (Fig. 21–1*M*).

A 6-0 black silk suture is placed through the corner of each temporal upper and lower eyelid (see Fig. 21–1*M*). The 6-0 black silk sutures are drawn up and tied, forming the lateral canthal angle. The suture ends are left long and are eventually tied over the 6-0 silk sutures in the lateral canthal skin so that the knot can be easily found and so that the ends do not drag over the eye.

Because the 6-0 silk lateral canthal angle suture is difficult to remove without causing the patient pain, I now more frequently use a 5-0 chromic catgut buried suture. Each arm of this suture enters the gray line of the upper and lower eyelids about 2 mm nasal to the temporal end of each eyelid. The suture then passes through temporal upper and lower eyelids and exits the cut edges of the temporal eyelids. When the suture is

tied, it unites the temporal eyelids and creates the lateral canthal angle, and the suture knot is buried (see Fig. 21–1*M*).

Skin-Muscle Excision

While the patient gazes upward and the lower skin and the orbicularis muscle are draped over the lid margin and lateral canthus, any excess tissue is trimmed, as described in Chapter 19 (Fig. 21–1*N*). If the lower eyelid does not move up as the patient gazes upward, the surgeon pushes on the scleral contact lens covering the eye. This elevates the lower eyelid to a position similar to the level it will reach when the patient looks upward.

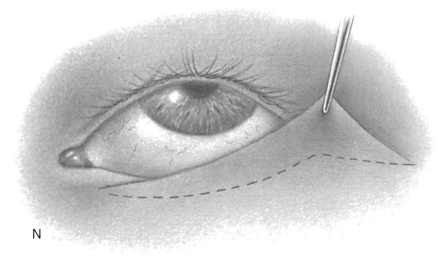

N, The skin-muscle flap is draped over the incision site, and excess skin–muscle is excised.

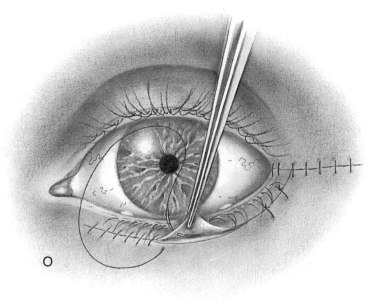

O, Skin incisions are closed with a continuous 6-0 black silk suture.

O

The orbicularis muscle temporal to the lateral canthus is then closed with 5-0 polyglactin interrupted sutures with deep placement of the knots. One or two additional 6-0 polyglactin interrupted sutures pass through the skin edges and inferior tarsal border at the temporal end of the eyelid. Finally, skin incisions are closed with a continuous 6-0 black silk suture (Fig. 21–1*O*).

POSTOPERATIVE CARE

Topical gentamicin sulfate (Garamycin) is applied over the sutures, and the patient places cold compresses on the eyelids for 24 hours postoperatively. The patient is observed for the first few postoperative hours to make sure that there is no retrobulbar hemorrhage, a complication that potentially can cause loss of vision.[3] The patient is checked every 15 minutes for 2 hours to ensure that there is neither a decrease in visual acuity to finger counting nor presence of pain and proptosis. If these findings exist, the surgeon should be called immediately and the sutures released in order to prevent permanent loss of vision due to a retrobulbar hemorrhage.

The skin sutures are removed 5–6 days postoperatively.

COMPLICATIONS

An occasional complication after the tarsal strip procedure is a granulomatous cyst around the polypropylene suture. Treatment involves severing the lateral canthal skin and removing the cyst and polypropylene suture. Most often, this complication occurs several months postoperatively, at which time the polypropylene suture is no longer needed, as scar tissue has united the temporal eyelid to the lateral canthus. If the lateral canthus migrates nasally on removal of this suture, however, a

5-0 or 6-0 polyglactin suture can be used to unite the temporal tarsus to the lateral orbital wall.

Another occasional complication is nasal migration of the lateral canthal angle. The surgeon can easily rectify this event by performing a lateral canthotomy and suturing the temporal edge of upper and lower eyelid conjunctiva to skin, which increases the horizontal length of the eyelid and makes it equal to the opposite side.

In two of my patients, restrictive ocular motility and diplopia developed after a lower blepharoplasty combined with a tarsal strip procedure. In a survey among oculoplastic surgeons, another 10 or so cases of this complication were discovered (unpublished data). I believe that this complication may have resulted from scar tissue that developed between the globe and inferior temporal orbital wall. For this reason, I recommend conservative or no release of inferior temporal lateral canthal attachments during the tarsal strip procedure. Should this complication occur, I recommend injection of about 0.5 ml of 40 mg/ml of triamcinolone (Kenalog) into the temporal inferior anterior orbit. Release of this scar tissue with and without conjunctival grafts was successful in some of the cases reported in the aforementioned survey.

RESULTS

I have combined a tarsal strip procedure with lower blepharoplasty in more than 1000 patients with good results (Fig. 21–2).

ALTERNATIVE TECHNIQUES

It is possible to shorten the lower eyelid horizontally by taking a full-thickness wedge resection from the eyelid (see Chapter 24). If there is a lax lateral canthal tendon, however, the lateral canthus will be drawn medially, which is undesirable.

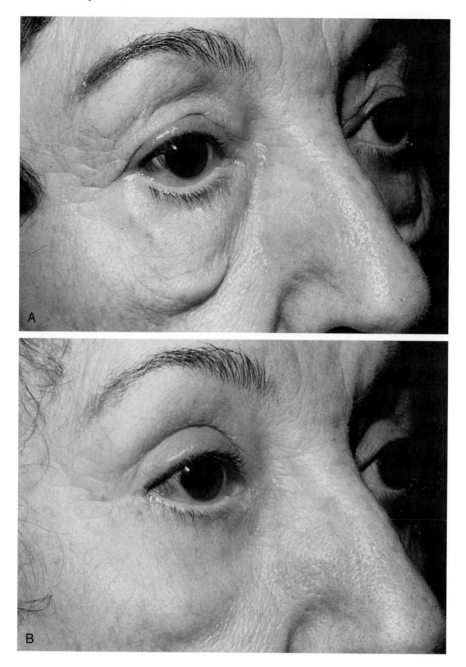

figure 21–2

A, Preoperative appearance of patient with dermatochalasis (excess skin) and herniated fat of all four eyelids associated with lower eyelid laxity and "cheek bags" (festoons). *B,* Postoperative appearance after excision of excess skin and fat of all four eyelids through skin-muscle flap approaches. Bilateral tarsal strip procedures were performed simultaneously.

References

1. Tenzel RR: Treatment of lagophthalmos of the lower eyelid. Arch Ophthalmol 1969; 81:366–368.

2. Hamako CH, Baylis HI: Lower eyelid retraction after blepharoplasty. Am J Ophthalmol 1980; 89:517–521.

3. Putterman AM: Temporary blindness after cosmetic blepharoplasty. Am J Ophthalmol 1985; 80:1081–1083.

Allen M. Putterman

Chapter 22

Lateral Canthal Plication

The lateral canthal plication technique is described here in its own chapter instead of being combined with the tarsal strip procedure, as in the second edition of this text. Although I believe that plication suturing has great merit, I rarely perform this technique with a tarsal strip procedure. Therefore, I think that readers will find this new organization more helpful, especially if they use this book to show patients illustrations of the various procedures that will be performed.

In my experience, plication of the temporal orbicularis oculi muscle to periosteum of the lateral orbital wall leads to a tighter and smoother lower eyelid. It also minimizes cheek bags (festoons) and fullness. In most patients for whom I perform a lower blepharoplasty through a skin-muscle flap approach, I also plicate the temporal orbicularis muscle to the periosteum. I find that the procedure is very useful in patients undergoing an internal transconjunctival blepharoplasty who also have slightly excessive skin or cheek fullness. In many of these cases, I also add laser surgery to the transconjunctival lower blepharoplasty and lateral canthal plication.

Additionally, lateral canthal plication enhances the results of the tarsal strip procedure, especially when it is done through a lower skin-muscle flap approach.

ALLEN M. PUTTERMAN

In the previous edition of *Cosmetic Oculoplastic Surgery,* I described plication sutures as an adjunct to the skin-muscle flap lower blepharoplasty and I repeat this information here. I also describe the use of plication sutures with horizontal lid shortening through either a tarsal strip or full-thickness temporal lower eyelid resection with a transconjunctival blepharoplasty approach (see Chapters 21 and 24). Other portions of this chapter describe plication sutures alone or combined with a transconjunctival blepharoplasty without a tarsal strip or full-thickness eyelid resection.

The lateral canthal incision of the lower blepharoplasty procedure is usually connected by just suturing skin. Since skin attached to skin does not tighten the orbicularis muscle of the lower eyelid, it is beneficial in many cases to attach orbicularis muscle to the periosteum at the lateral canthus. This technique tightens the lower eyelid and smooths the lower eyelid skin better than a skin closure alone would; it also decreases lower eyelid wrinkles and folds.

SURGICAL TECHNIQUES

Plication Sutures Combined with Skin-Muscle Flap Lower Blepharoplasty

A skin-muscle flap lower blepharoplasty is carried out through the excision of herniated orbital fat, skin, and orbicularis muscle, as described in Chapter 19. A 6-0 black silk suture then connects the skin of the lower eyelid flap, lateral canthal tendon, and superior skin approximately 2 mm temporal to the lateral canthus. It is tied with a surgeon's knot, and one end of the suture with the needle attached to it is left long.

Next, two 5-0 polyglycolic acid (Dexon) sutures are placed through orbicularis muscle of the lateral skin-muscle flap (Fig. 22–1). The sutures are then brought to the orbicularis muscle and periosteum over the lateral orbital wall between the previously placed 6-0 silk suture and the temporal end of the incision.

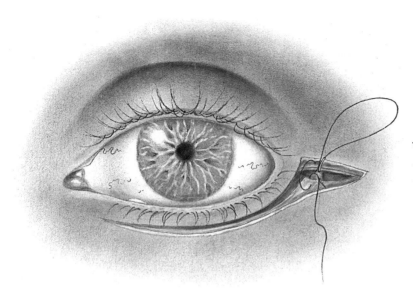

figure 22–1

Plication sutures of 5-0 polyglycolic acid (Dexon) unite the temporal lower eyelid orbicularis muscle to the lateral orbital rim orbicularis muscle and periosteum.

figure 22–2

A, Patient with dermatochalasis (excess skin) and herniated orbital fat of both lower eyelids associated with marked festoons ("cheek bags"). *B,* Same patient after a bilateral lower eyelid skin-muscle flap blepharoplasty with plication sutures. Cheek bags are persistent but smaller.

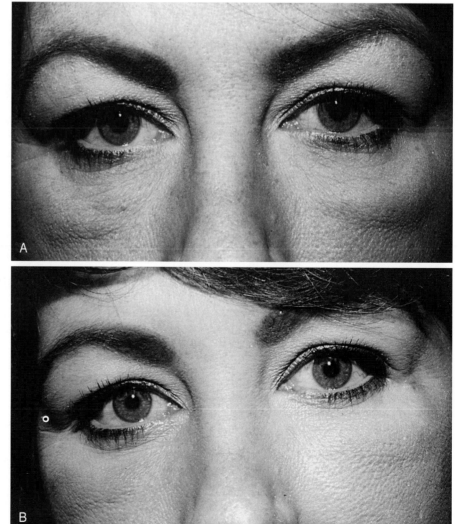

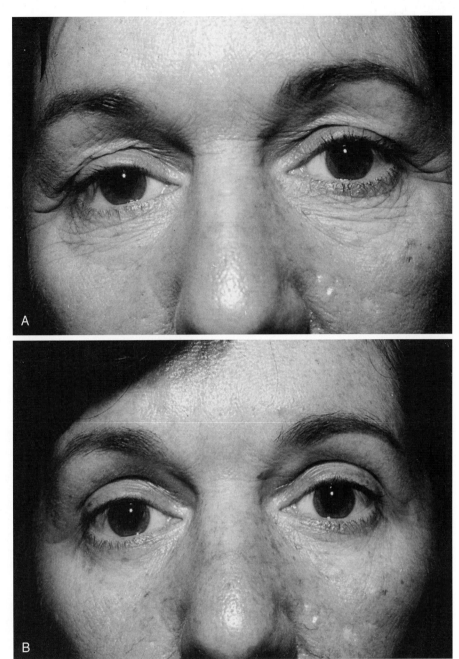

figure 22–3

A, Patient with dermatochalasis and herniated orbital fat of all four eyelids associated with marked lower eyelid skin wrinkling. *B,* Same patient after an external lower eyelid skin-muscle flap blepharoplasty along with plication sutures. There is marked reduction in lower eyelid wrinkling without having to perform laser resurfacing, which would be an alternative way to treat this patient. The upper eyelid excess skin and fat were removed simultaneously, and eyelid crease reconstruction was performed, according to the technique described in Chapter 10.

One arm of the suture passes through the deep orbicularis muscle of the lower skin-muscle flap and exits at the superficial edge of the orbicularis muscle. The suture then passes through the superficial orbicularis muscle at the superior aspect of the incision site, enters the periosteum over the anterior lateral orbital wall, and exits more deeply. When the suture needle is passed through the orbicularis muscle and lateral orbital periosteum, the surgeon should be able to pull on the needle and feel the inability to pull it away from the wound as a result of its sturdy attachment to periosteum.

When the suture ends are drawn up and tied, the knot falls deeply and the orbicularis muscle will be united and connected to periosteum. This causes the lower eyelid skin to become taut and smooth, with reduced furrows and wrinkles (Figs. 22–2 and 22–3).

The long end of the 6-0 silk suture initially placed at the lateral canthal angle is then run continuously to connect the skin from the lateral canthus to the temporal end of the incision site. Occasionally, it is necessary to place one or two 6-0 interrupted polyglactin (Vicryl) sutures through the skin if the 6-0 silk skin closure does not result in a smooth surface.

Plication Sutures Combined with Tarsal Strip Procedure and Lower Lid Skin Blepharoplasty

The lower lid skin-muscle blepharoplasty and the tarsal strip procedure are carried out to the steps involving removal of skin and herniated orbital fat and connection

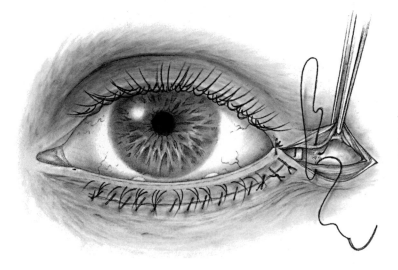

figure 22–4

A tarsal strip procedure is performed simultaneously with an external lower blepharoplasty to shorten both lower eyelids and to connect them to the lateral orbital wall. Plication sutures are also placed, as described in Figure 22–1.

figure 22–5

A, Patient with dermatochalasis and herniated orbital fat of all four eyelids associated with lower eyelid horizontal laxity. *B,* Same patient after removal of the herniated orbital fat and excess skin and muscle through a skin-muscle flap lower blepharoplasty and plication.

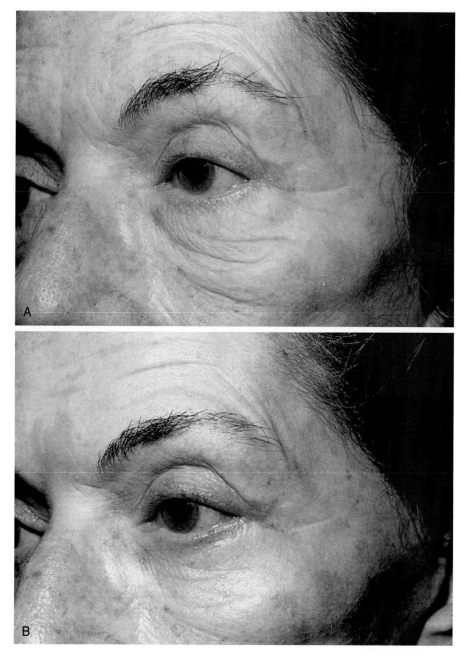

of the tarsal strip to the lateral orbital wall (see Chapter 21). Two 5-0 polyglycolic acid sutures are placed through the orbicularis muscle of the lateral skin-muscle flap and then to the orbicularis muscle and periosteum of the lateral orbital wall (Fig. 22–4), as described earlier. The results are shown in one patient (Fig. 22–5).

Plication Sutures Alone

Occasionally, plication of the orbicularis muscle to periosteum is performed alone. This is usually done to decrease loose lower eyelid skin that persists after a blepharoplasty. At times, this technique is performed just to smooth out the lower eyelid skin or to reduce wrinkles and furrows. The surgeon can determine whether plication sutures would have merit simply by pulling the temporal lower eyelid laterally and noting the improvement in the appearance of the lower eyelid.

A skin incision is made with a No. 15 Bard-Parker blade, beginning 2 mm temporal to the lateral canthus and extending 1–1.5 cm temporally in an almost horizontal direction. The orbicularis muscle is severed with Westcott scissors along the incision site and is undermined from suborbicularis fascia for approximately 1 cm inferiorly (Fig. 22–6A). The lower skin-muscle tissue is then pulled upward, and the part that overlaps the incision site is excised (Fig. 22–6B). Bleeding is controlled with a disposable cautery (Solan Accu-Temp, Xomed Surgical Products, Jacksonville, Fla.).

Two 5-0 polyglycolic acid sutures are then placed through the orbicularis muscle of the lower skin-muscle

figure 22–6

Plication sutures are performed as a sole procedure or with excision of herniated orbital fat through a transconjunctival approach, with or without laser resurfacing. An incision is made starting at the lateral canthus and extending approximately 1.5 cm laterally in almost a horizontal direction. *A,* Skin and orbicularis are undermined.

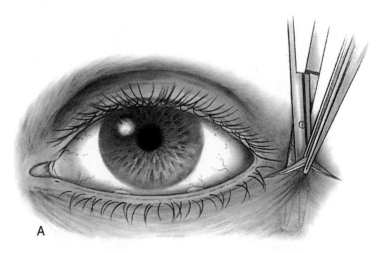

A

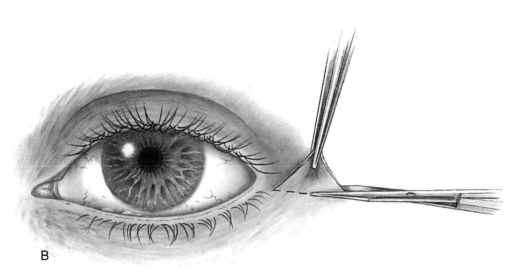

B

B, An ellipse of skin and orbicularis is removed.

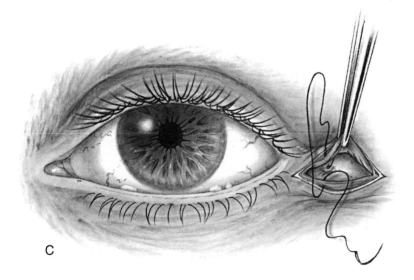

C

C, The plication sutures are placed as described in Figure 22–1.

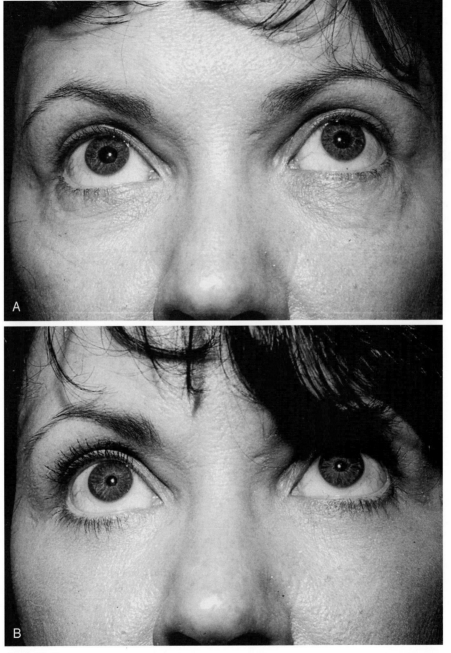

figure 22–7

A, Patient with dermatochalasis and herniated orbital fat of the eyelids associated with lower eyelid wrinkling. *B,* Same patient after plication sutures and removal of herniated orbital fat through an internal approach and laser resurfacing of the lower eyelids.

flap and through the orbicularis muscle and periosteum of the superior tissue (Fig. 22–6C), as already described in this chapter. A 6-0 silk suture is run continuously from one end of the incision to the other.

Plication Sutures Combined with Transconjunctival Blepharoplasty

The surgeon can perform the procedure described in the preceding section after a transconjunctival lower blepharoplasty to tighten and smooth the skin without resorting to a skin-muscle flap approach.

Plication Sutures Combined with Laser Resurfacing with or without Transconjunctival Blepharoplasty

Plication suturing can be performed along with laser resurfacing, as described in Chapter 31, with or without a transconjunctival blepharoplasty. If blepharoplasty is to be done, the internal blepharoplasty is performed first, followed by the plication sutures and ending with the laser resurfacing (Fig. 22–7). The surgeon should

avoid laser resurfacing within 3 mm of the plication incision site to prevent extensive lateral canthal scarring.

POSTOPERATIVE CARE

The wound is cared for in the same manner as described for the skin-muscle blepharoplasty approach in Chapter 10.

COMPLICATIONS

At times, immediately postoperatively there can be a slight dimple at the site that the 5-0 polyglycolic acid suture passes close to the undersurface of the skin. This dimple invariably resolves spontaneously when the suture dissolves, which can be as long as 4–8 weeks after surgery.

RESULTS

I have performed the lateral canthal plication technique more than 500 times without any major problems.

Allen M. Putterman

Chapter 23

Treatment of Eyelid Varicose Veins with Blepharoplasty

Treatment of eyelid varicose veins with blepharoplasty is a new chapter in this text. Although varicose veins occur only occasionally in the eyelids, they create a cosmetic disturbance that some patients desire to have eliminated.

For the treatment of small superficial veins, I use hyfrecation or laser. For deeper veins, however, it is usually necessary to isolate and obliterate the veins. I do this according to the technique described by Kersten and Kulwin. The procedure can easily be combined with a lower blepharoplasty, either through an external or internal approach. It has a high rate of success in eliminating deep, large, cosmetically unacceptable varicose veins.

Another technique that I am experimenting with consists of a skin flap to isolate the varicose veins that exist between internal skin and orbicularis oculi muscle. The veins are isolated under direct visualization and are directly cauterized. Lower blepharoplasty is then performed.

ALLEN M. PUTTERMAN

Varicose veins occasionally occur in the eyelids and in some patients produce a cosmetically unacceptable appearance. At times, they occur in association with dermatochalasis (excess skin) and herniated orbital fat of the eyelids; at other times, they present as the sole problem of the eyelids. The presentation of varicose veins varies from superficial and very small to deep and large.

Treatment is dictated by the patient's desire to have these varicose veins eliminated. Hyfrecation[1] or laser can be used for elimination of small superficial veins. For deeper veins, I have used the technique described by Kersten and Kulwin,[1] in which segments of the vein are isolated and obliterated.

Still another technique that can be used in combination with blepharoplasty in the lower eyelid is a skin flap approach. This approach allows for the removal of the skin and herniated orbital fat, exposes the veins on the inner aspect of the eyelid skin, and allows them to be treated by direct cauterization (see Chapter 18).

SURGICAL TECHNIQUE

Treatment of Superficial, Small Varicose Veins

I have used a Birtcher hyfrecator to treat small superficial veins of the eyelid. Usually, I perform this procedure without local anesthesia, since local anesthesia given subcutaneously can make varicose veins difficult to visualize. EMLA anesthesia (2.5 per cent lidocaine and 2.5 per cent prilocaine) plus a transparent dressing (Tegaderm) can also be used to minimize discomfort, although most patients tolerate this treatment without anesthesia.

The Birtcher hyfrecator is connected to the low setting. The amount of voltage varies among various hyfrecators, and the surgeon will have to determine the energy that produces the desired effect. A small tip is used for treatment. The surgeon uses either the foot pedal or hand control to initiate the flow of energy into the metal tip of the instrument as the tip is applied to the sites of the veins. The surgeon should be able to visualize the obliteration of the veins during application.

The same technique is possible with the carbon dioxide pulse laser that is used for skin resurfacing (see Chapter 31). I do not have experience using laser for treatment of varicose veins and therefore cannot comment on it here.

Treatment of Deep, Large Varicose Veins

Most of my experience in the treatment of varicose veins of the eyelid has involved the technique popularized by Kersten and Kulwin.[1] At times, I do this as a sole procedure. In most cases, however, I combine this with the excision of skin, orbicularis muscle, and herniated orbital fat through a skin-muscle flap of the lower eyelid or a skin-muscle-fat excision and reconstruction of the crease of the upper eyelid (see Chapters 10 and 19). I treat the varicose veins before excising skin, orbicularis muscle, and fat.

After the usual preparation and draping of the face (see Chapter 10), topical tetracaine is applied to the eyes and a scleral lens is applied over the eyes to protect them. A methylene blue marking pen is used to draw the site of the varicose veins on the eyelid skin. If the veins cannot be easily visualized, the patient is placed in a reverse Trendelenburg position. This position can increase the patient's venous pressure and can make these veins distend. The methylene blue marking pen also is used to draw 2–3 mm lines perpendicular to the marked varicose vein course, at 10–12 mm segments of the vein. These lines are first drawn approximately 10 mm from the beginning and end of the varicose vein, and then at 10–12 mm segments in between.

Two per cent lidocaine (Xylocaine) with epinephrine is injected subcutaneously throughout the eyelid. A No. 15 Bard-Parker blade is used to make incisions through the skin at the marked 2–3-mm lines that are perpendicular to the varicose vein (Fig. 23–1A).

A Westcott scissors is used to separate the subcutaneous tissues and to expose the varicose veins. Care must be taken during this dissection, since superficial veins can be penetrated by the scissors. Use of a forceps to pull the skin outward can facilitate this dissection. Also, blunt dissection with cotton-tipped applicators can be used to isolate the vein within these incision sites.

Once the vein is isolated in two adjacent incision sites, the blood within the vein is removed. The surgeon can accomplish this by pushing on the vein between the incision sites with cotton-tipped applicators.

A bipolar cautery, in which the tips are covered with tape except for approximately 2 mm at their ends, is used to cauterize and thereby obliterate the varicose vein. This is done at each site of the isolated segment of the vein, accompanied by compression of the vein segment with the cotton-tipped applicators (Fig. 23–1B). The tips of the bipolar cautery are applied to each side of the vein. As the tips are closed gently (see Fig. 23–1B), the surgeon initiates the bipolar cautery current by pressing on the foot pedal of the unit. This maneuver of vein compression and obliteration is repeated at each isolated vein segment. By obliterating the vein with pressure between the isolated segments and then occluding the vein at the isolated segments, the surgeon stops the vein from carrying blood. The veins thus cannot be seen through the skin.

Finally, each incision site is closed with several 6-0 black silk interrupted sutures (Fig. 23–1C).

Treatment of Varicose Veins Through Skin Flap Approach with Lower Blepharoplasty

In a few patients, I have approached both superficial and deep eyelid varicose veins through a lower blepharoplasty skin flap approach (see Chapter 18). At times, I have initially treated the veins according to the technique previously described in this chapter and then used the skin flap to take care of some of the remaining veins that I was not able to capture with this technique. At other times, I have used this technique as the sole treatment of the veins.

A line is drawn with a methylene blue marking pen at the lateral canthus, beginning 2–3 mm temporal to the lateral canthal angle and then extending for approxi-

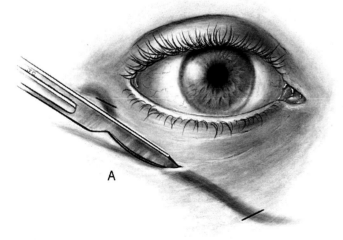

figure 23–1

A, An incision 2–3 mm long is made through skin at various segments of a varicose vein in the eyelid.

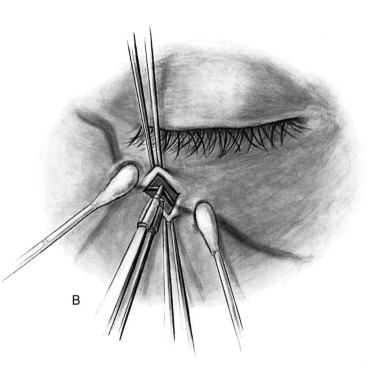

B, The blood within each segment of the varicose vein is decreased with cotton-tipped applicators while an insulated bipolar cautery is used to cauterize the narrowed varicose vein at each incision site.

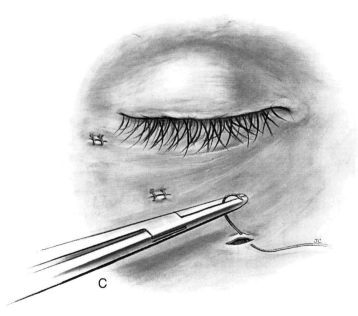

C, An incision site is closed with several 6-0 black silk interrupted sutures.

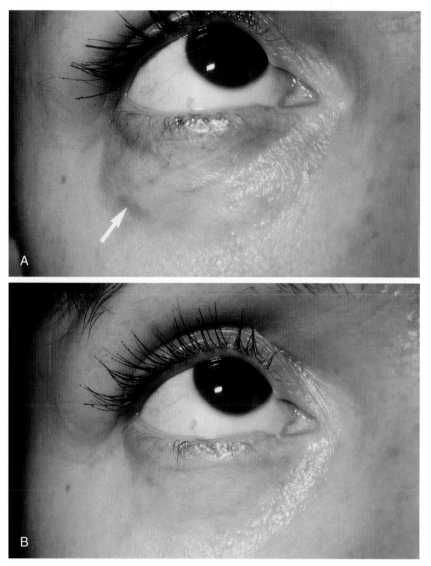

figure 23–2

A, Preoperative appearance of a patient with multiple superficial varicose veins and a prominent larger vein *(arrow).* B, Appearance after coagulation with the procedure described in text; see Surgical Technique.

mately 1–1.5 cm temporally in an almost horizontal direction. The areas of the varicose veins are drawn with the marking pen over the skin.

Two per cent lidocaine with epinephrine is then injected subcutaneously throughout the lower eyelid. A No. 15 Bard-Parker blade is used to make an incision in the lower eyelid, 1–1.5 mm beneath the eyelashes. The incision begins at the punctum site and extends temporally for a distance 2–3 mm temporal to the lateral canthus. The incision is then extended along the previously marked methylene blue line in the lateral canthus.

A Westcott scissors is then used to dissect skin from the orbicularis muscle throughout the eyelid. The dissection is facilitated by placing a 4-0 black silk suture through skin, orbicularis muscle, and superficial tarsus at the center of the eyelid, just beneath the eyelashes. This suture is pulled upward while the skin of the lower eyelid is dissected from the orbicularis muscle. The skin flap is carried out to the level of the inferior orbital rim. Once the skin flap is pulled downward, the varicose veins on the undersurface of the skin or over the outer surface of the orbicularis muscle can be visualized.

When the scissors have penetrated the veins during the dissection, the veins can be easily obliterated by cauterization of the bleeding sites with a disposable cautery (Solan Accu-Temp, Xomed Surgical Products, Jacksonville, Fla.). For those veins that have not been penetrated, the disposable cautery, Colorado needle, or neodymium:YAG or carbon dioxide pulse lasers can be used to obliterate the remaining veins (see Chapters 35 and 36). All of these modalities become effective simply by applying the energy source directly over the veins until they are flattened and obliterated. This can be seen under direct visualization.

Excision of herniated orbital fat and skin is then carried out, as described in Chapter 18.

POSTOPERATIVE CARE

Gentamicin (Garamycin) ophthalmic ointment is applied to the incision sites twice a day for approximately 1 week postoperatively.

COMPLICATIONS

The main complication of the Kersten-Kulwin technique is that incisions result within the eyelid and remain red for 4–6 weeks after surgery. These lines are not in natural creases, since most varicose veins do not follow natural crease lines. Therefore, patients should be warned that they will have these marks for several months and will have to apply makeup to cover them. Areas of cauterization and red lines also appear when the hyfrecator is used to treat superficial veins. These lines, too, can take several weeks to resolve.

RESULTS

I have used the techniques described in this chapter to treat varicose veins in more than 50 patients. Results in one patient are shown in Figure 23–2. My main experience has been using the Kersten-Kulwin[1] technique, and I have rarely encountered a recurrence of varicose veins. In using the Birtcher hyfrecator to treat superficial veins, I have sometimes had to give further treatment; for the most part, however, this has been an effective technique.

Although I have used the skin flap approach only in a few recent cases, I have been impressed with the results and believe that the technique has good potential in the treatment of eyelid varicose veins.

Reference

1. Kersten RC, Kulwin DR: Management of cosmetically objectionable veins in the lower eyelids. Arch Ophthalmol 1989; 107:278–280.

Allen M. Putterman

Cheek and Midface Lift Combined with Full-Thickness Temporal Lower Eyelid Resection

The topic of cheek and midface lifting is new to this textbook. This is a relatively new technique that I find useful in patients who have cheek ptosis or bags, prominent nasolabial folds, hollowing over the inferior orbital rim, nasal inferior orbital rim depressions, and cicatricial ectropion or retraction.

The cheek and midface lift is usually performed through an external lower eyelid skin-muscle flap approach. Periosteum is released from the cheekbone, then cut at the inferior end of the dissection and reflected upward. Suturing the internal cheek tissue to periosteum over the lateral orbital wall elevates the midface and places the cheek tissue in a more normal position. This maneuver also tightens the cheek tissue and thereby eliminates bagginess. The technique also adds extra skin, which is useful if a patient has cicatricial ectropion, and lifts cheek fat upward, which minimizes malar and inferior orbital rim depressions. In addition, when the cheek tissue is pulled upward, the nasolabial fold is lessened and softened.

If a cheek and midface lift is performed alone, the lower eyelid is commonly unstable and a secondary ectropion can result. Therefore, the lower eyelid is horizontally shortened through a tarsal strip procedure or, more commonly, by a full-thickness temporal resection. Therefore, in this chapter I describe this full-thickness temporal resection horizontal shortening procedure as an alternative to the tarsal strip procedure.

ALLEN M. PUTTERMAN

With age, the cheek migrates inferiorly and nasally (Fig. 24–1*A*). This contributes to cheek bags (festoons) and a nasolabial fold with depression. Conventional treatment for these problems has consisted of face lifts, excision of cheek bags, and cheek implants.

Hester and McCord[1] have popularized a cheek and midface lift through an external lower blepharoplasty approach. The procedure places the prolapsed cheek in a more normal position, relieves cheek bags, softens nasolabial fold depression, and minimizes depression over the nasal inferior orbital rim area. It also gives the effect of cheek implantation, adds skin to the lower eyelids in the treatment of cicatricial ectropion, and reduces hollowing of the lower eyelid that sometimes occurs secondary to overzealous fat removal in lower blepharoplasty.

Possible complications of the cheek and midface lift are lower eyelid retraction and ectropion. McCord[2] has recommended horizontal tightening of the lower eyelid through a full-thickness resection to stabilize the eyelid

235

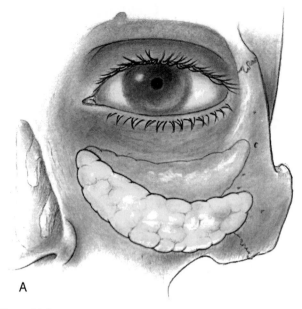

A

figure 24–1

A, Inferior and nasal descent of the cheek fat that occurs with aging. The more superior outlined area depicts the normal position of the cheek fat.

and to avoid a possible postoperative ectropion. A tarsal strip procedure can also be used to accomplish the same results (see Chapter 21).

SURGICAL TECHNIQUE

Patients are prepared for surgery in the same manner as for an upper blepharoplasty (see Chapters 9 and 10).

A mixture of 40 ml of 0.5 per cent lidocaine (Xylocaine) with 1:200,000 epinephrine, 150 units of hyaluronidase (Wydase), and 4 ml of 0.5 per cent plain bupivacaine (Marcaine) is prepared. Several milliliters of this mixture is injected subcutaneously and diffusely across the lower lids.

A 25-gauge, 1.5-cm needle is passed through the nasal lower eyelid skin, just above the inferior orbital rim and then over the inferior orbital rim in a slightly downward direction to avoid penetrating the eye. The needle is inserted for approximately 1 cm, and 0.5–1 ml of the anesthetic mixture is injected. This is repeated centrally and temporally.

A mark is applied with a methylene blue marking pen to the area of the infraorbital foramen, and several milliliters of the same anesthetic mixture is injected around the exit of the infraorbital nerve. Approximately 20 ml of the solution is injected subperiosteally over the cheek down to the upper gum and nasolabial fold areas.

The initial part of the technique is similar to that described for surgical treatment of lower eyelid dermatochalasis (excess skin), herniated orbital fat, and hypertrophic orbicularis oculi muscle, through a skin-muscle flap approach (see Chapter 19). The procedure is slightly modified, in that the lateral canthal incision extends 1.5–2 cm temporal to the lateral canthus rather than 1–1.5 cm (Fig. 24–1*B*). The procedure is carried out through the step of removing the herniated orbital fat.

Desmarres or smooth-tipped rake retractors are used to pull the skin-muscle flap downward to expose the tissues over the inferior orbital rim (Fig. 24–1*C*). An incision is made with a Bard-Parker blade through periosteum several millimeters beneath the inferior orbital rim from the lateral canthus to the nasal end of the inferior orbit (see Fig. 24–1*C*).

The sharp end of a Tenzel periosteal elevator is used to reflect periosteum from this incision site in a down-

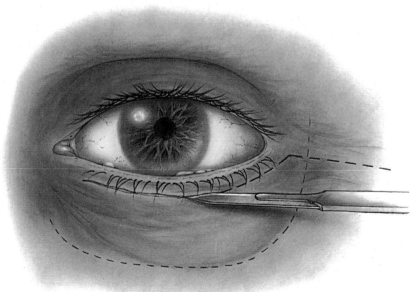

B, An infralash incision is made 1.5 mm beneath the lashes beginning at the level of the punctum and then sweeping throughout the eyelid to an area 2 mm temporal to the lateral canthus. At this position, a temporal horizontal incision is carried for a distance of approximately 1.5 cm.

B

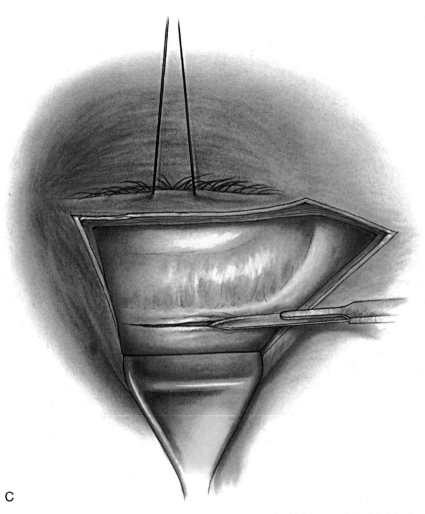

C

C, After dissection of a skin-muscle flap and removal of herniated orbital fat, a periosteal incision is made several millimeters beneath the inferior orbital rim throughout the extent of the rim. Dissection is then carried out over the inferior lateral orbital rim.

ward direction over the cheekbone (Fig. 24–1*D*). The surgeon should take care to avoid the area of the infraorbital foramen and nerve by palpating the infraorbital foramen, which was previously marked with a marking pen, and by dissecting inferior to this position.

Most of the time, it is unnecessary to dissect periosteum nasal to the infraorbital nerve canal; leaving periosteum nasal to the infraorbital nerve canal allows the nasal area to act as a fulcrum for the cheek lift. However, if the purpose of the surgery is to add skin to the lower eyelid in the treatment of cicatricial ectropion or to add tissue diffusely across the lower lid to correct hollowing of the lower eyelid, dissection nasal to the infraorbital nerve is performed.

Periosteum is dissected inferiorly to the level where the cheekbone ends and dips inward, which should be close to the upper gum (Figs. 24–1*E* and *F*). Nasally and inferiorly, the periosteal dissection extends into the nasolabial fold, with the surgeon taking care not to penetrate into the nasal cavity. Palpation of the periosteal elevator through the external skin and internal nares facilitates the dissection of the nasolabial fold. Also, the dissection in the nasolabial fold area is more superficial

to decrease the furrow in the nasolabial fold. The use of an Army-Navy retractor to lift the dissected cheek tissue outward and downward aids in the visualization of the dissection site.

A No. 11 Bard-Parker blade is used to incise the periosteum at the inferior aspect of the dissection, which should be at the area where the cheekbone depresses inward (Fig. 24–1*G*). The surgeon should be careful to penetrate only the periosteum and not any of the more superficial tissues. This incision can be facilitated with scissors similar to those used for endoscopic brow lifts (see Chapter 28). Once the periosteum has been incised over the entire horizontal dimension of the inferior aspect of the flap, the periosteum is reflected superiorly for approximately 1 cm with the Ramirez endoforehead periosteal spreader (Snowden-Pencer 88-5080, No. 7) to sweep the periosteum upward (Fig. 24–1*H*).

When this is accomplished, the surgeon places his or her index finger into the subperiosteal space, engages the area of the periosteal incision site, and lifts periosteum upward and outward (Fig. 24–1*I*). With this maneuver, the surgeon should feel a release of tissue that allows the patient's cheek to move upward and outward.

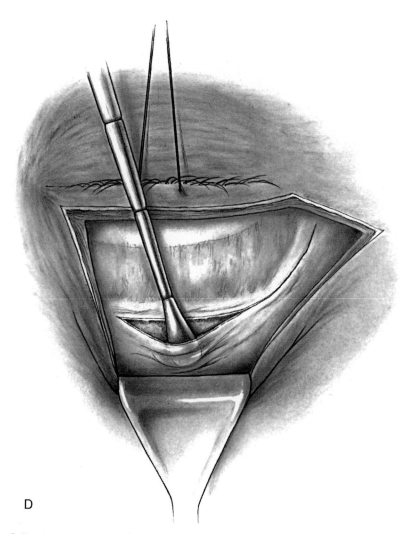

D, The sharp edge of a Tenzel periosteal elevator is used to reflect periosteum from the inferior and lateral orbital rim.

Horizontal Shortening of the Lower Eyelid Through Full-Thickness Resection or Tarsal Strip Procedure

At this point in the procedure, the lower eyelid is horizontally shortened and temporally elevated. This is accomplished through either a tarsal strip procedure or the full-thickness resection technique popularized by McCord,[2] which is similar to a Bick procedure. The purpose of this step is to stabilize the lower eyelid and prevent a postoperative ectropion. A lateral canthotomy and inferior cantholysis are performed as described in Chapter 21.

The lower eyelid is then pulled temporally and slightly upward, and the area where the lower lid margin meets the temporal cut end of the upper lid margin is marked with a scratch incision. This creates the site for either formation of a tarsal strip or removal of a full-thickness section of the eyelid. (The tarsal strip procedure is described in Chapter 21.)

A full-thickness wedge resection of the lower eyelid is done from the marked scratch incision to the temporal end of the lower eyelid (Fig. 24–1*J*). A 4-0 polypropylene (Prolene) suture with a half-circle needle or a double-armed spatula OPS-5 needle (both special-ordered from Ethicon) is then passed through the temporal end of the tarsus of the lower eyelid inferiorly to superiorly (Fig. 24–1*K*). It is important for the surgeon to engage a good bite of tarsus with this needle passage and to avoid passage through conjunctiva.

The temporal lower eyelid is then pulled temporally and upward with toothed forceps, and a position is determined that places the lower eyelid in the desired position. Once this site is noted, the needle on the superior end of the polypropylene suture is passed through the site internally to externally. This site is usually lateral orbital periosteum, but at times it is the upper lateral canthal tendon or upper eyelid temporal tarsus. The same suture arm is then passed externally to internally through the same tissues slightly below the area through which the needle first passed (see Fig. 24–1*K*). The suture is tied with the first two throws of a surgeon's knot placed over a small piece of a 4-0 black silk knot releasing suture.

The procedure is repeated on the opposite side to this

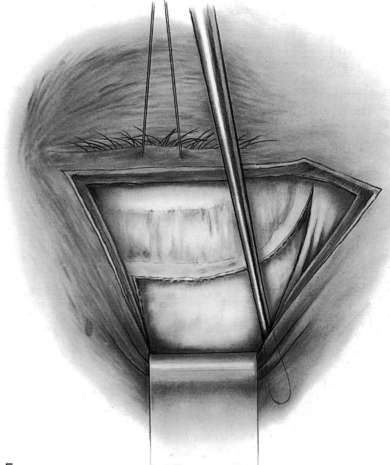

E, The dull edge of the Tenzel periosteal elevator is used to dissect periosteum from the cheekbone.

E

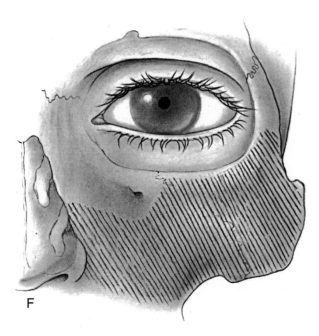

F

F, Diagonal lines indicate the area of periosteal dissection, which is under the infraorbital canal and extends to the nasolabial fold area as well as the upper gum.

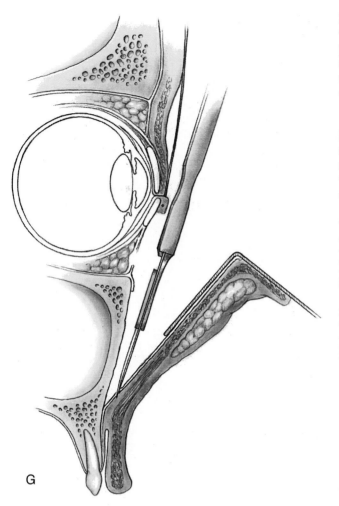

G, A No. 11 Bard-Parker blade is used to incise periosteum at the inferior edge of the periosteal flap.

step. The patient is seated up on the operating table so that the surgeon can observe the position of the lateral canthi. A millimeter ruler is passed through each medial canthus, and the site at which the ruler bisects the new lateral canthi is judged.

If one lateral canthus is higher or lower or more inward or outward than the other, the surgeon releases the suture tie by pulling the 4-0 black silk against the polypropylene knot. The polypropylene suture is then replaced until the desired position is achieved. When this is accomplished, the 4-0 black silk knot releasing suture is removed and the suture is secured with multiple ties.

Attachment of Cheek Tissues to Lateral Wall Periosteum

A large-toothed forceps is used to grasp the fibrous tissue beneath the temporal superior cheek fat. This tissue is commonly referred to as the SOOF (suborbicularis oculi fat pad) and is thought to be similar to the SMAS (superficial musculoaponeurotic system). This firm tissue is pulled upward and outward toward the

lateral canthal tendon attachment to the lateral orbital wall to the extent that the cheek is in a more normal position, the nasolabial fold is flattened, and the cheek skin is taut. When this position is found, the needle on a 4-0 polypropylene suture is passed inferiorly to superiorly through the tissues held by the forceps (Fig. 24–1*L*).

The same suture arm is then passed superiorly to inferiorly through the taut, firm temporal fascia over the superior lateral wall in the area temporal to the lateral canthal tendon (see Fig. 24–1*L*). The suture is then tied with the first tie (two throws) of a surgeon's knot over a small piece of a 4-0 black silk knot releasing suture.

The procedure is repeated on the opposite side, and the patient is seated up on the operating table. If the cheeks are not in proper position, the surgeon releases the polypropylene suture tie by pulling up on the 4-0 knot releasing suture and the polypropylene suture is replaced until the desired effect is achieved.

Once this is accomplished, the 4-0 black silk knot releasing suture is removed and the polypropylene suture is tied with several knots. An additional 4-0 polypropylene suture is passed through similar tissues slightly nasal to the first placement to further secure the attach-

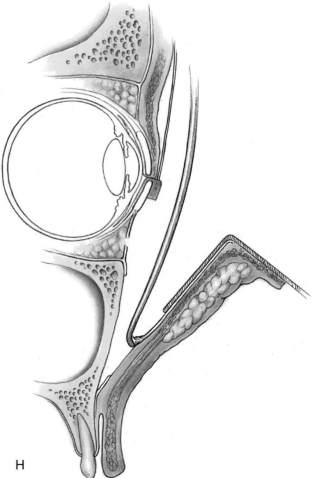

H, A Ramirez endoforehead periosteal spreader is used to sweep the incised periosteum upward and to reflect it from the subperiosteal tissues.

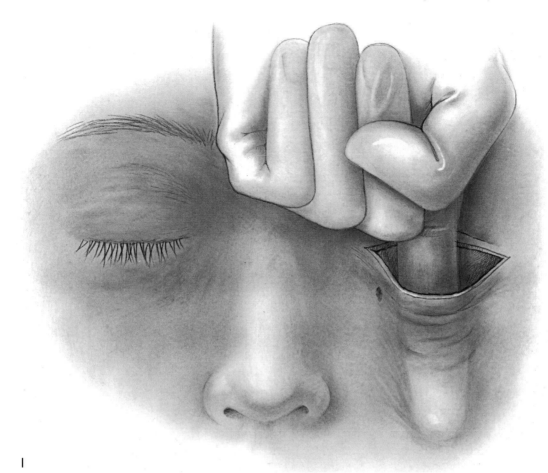

I

I, The surgeon places his or her finger under the skin-muscle-periosteal flap and palpates the dissected and reflected periosteum. If any attachments are inhibiting upward movement of the cheek flap, they are dissected, with the surgeon's finger in a sweeping motion that releases periosteum upward.

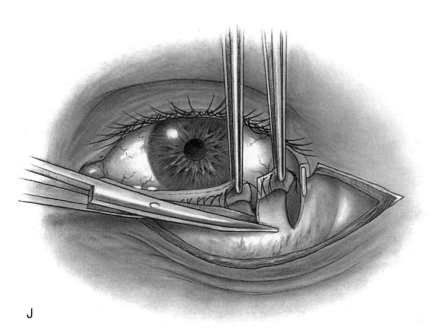

J, A full-thickness resection of the temporal lower eyelid is excised under the skin-muscle flap.

J

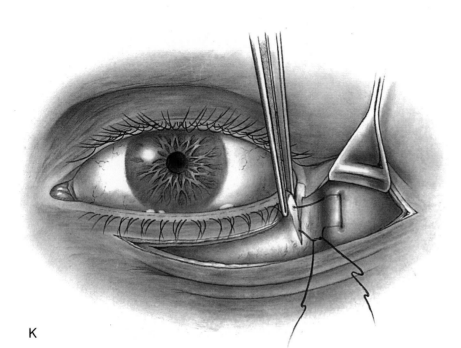

K, A 4-0 polypropylene (Prolene) suture unites the temporal tarsus of the lower eyelid to the periosteum over the lateral orbital rim and wall.

L, Two 4-0 polypropylene sutures unite the temporal suborbicularis oculi fat pad and fibrous tissue to the temporal fascia over the lateral orbital wall.

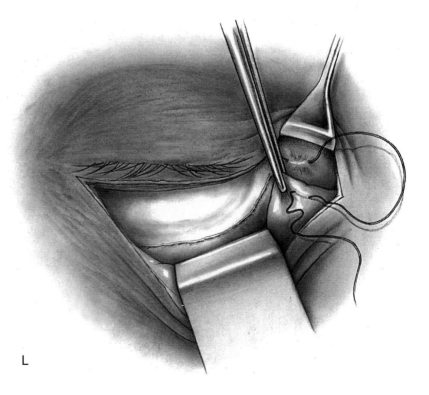

M, When the two 4-0 polypropylene sutures are tied, the cheek fat and sub-orbicularis oculi fat (SOOF) pad are elevated to a more superior temporal position. The inferior outlined area indicates the original downward displaced position of the SOOF, and the superior outline indicates the corrected position.

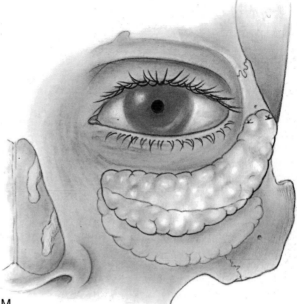

M

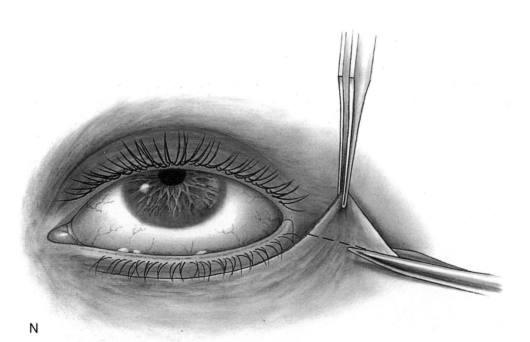

N

N, The skin and muscle that overlap the incision site when the patient looks upward and pressure is applied to the eye, when the surgeon pushes on the scleral lens, are excised.

ment of soft cheek tissue to periosteum (Fig. 24–1*M*). If a significant dimple appears in the skin in the vicinity of these sutures, the sutures are removed and replaced until the skin is minimally dimpled or smooth.

Excision of Skin or Orbicularis Muscle

The patient is asked to look upward while the lower lid skin-muscle flap is draped over the incision site. Because the horizontal shortening commonly inhibits the upward movement of the lower eyelid, a cotton-tipped applicator is pushed on the contact lens and thereby the eye. This maneuver lifts the lower eyelid to a position that is similar to its level on up gaze. The skin and orbicularis muscle that drape over the incision site are excised with Westcott scissors, first temporally over the lateral canthal incision site and then horizontally over the incision site of the lower eyelid skin from the lateral canthus to the punctum (Fig. 24–1*N*).

With two toothed forceps, the assistant grasps the skin-muscle flap nasally and temporally and pulls it downward. A strip of orbicularis muscle is routinely excised over the superior skin-muscle flap temporally to nasally for a distance of 4–5 mm beneath the flap. This prevents postoperative fullness in this area. If there is any excessive orbicularis muscle noted over the temporal end of the flap, it also is excised to reduce bulging of the tissues in the lateral canthus. Bleeding is controlled with a disposable cautery.

A 6-0 black silk, double-armed suture is then passed through the temporal upper and lower eyelid, entering the internal end of each eyelid and exiting through the gray line of the eyelid margin. Tying this suture reforms the angle of the eyelid. An alternative, consisting of 5-0 chromic double-armed catgut sutures, is to place each suture arm through the temporal upper and lower eyelid gray line and to exit through the cut ends of the temporal upper and lower eyelids. Tying this catgut suture also

reforms the lateral canthal angle and avoids the need for removal of the canthal angle suture.

Another 6-0 black silk suture is passed through skin adjacent to the lateral canthus. This suture is tied, and one arm is left long. This suture is also tied over the long ends of the 6-0 angle silk suture ends so that angle suture ends do not rub on the eye. Several 6-0 polyglactin (Vicryl) sutures are passed through skin–orbicularis muscle temporal to the lateral canthus to unite and smooth out the lateral canthus. Another 6-0 polyglactin suture is passed through the skin edges and inferior tarsal border, several millimeters medial to the lateral canthus. The 6-0 black silk suture at the lateral canthus is then run continuously from the lateral canthus to the most temporal aspect of the incision site. Another 6-0 black silk suture runs continuously nasally to temporally to unite the lower eyelid incision (Fig. 24–1*O*).

Gentamicin (Garamycin) ophthalmic ointment is applied to the sutures.

POSTOPERATIVE CARE

The patient is instructed to apply cold compresses for 24 hours after surgery. Postoperative treatment is the same as described for upper blepharoplasty (see Chapters 9 and 10).

COMPLICATIONS

Patients should be aware that they will have an Asian appearance for the first month or two after the procedure. They should also be told that they will have puckering and a possible dimple at the site of the polypropylene cheek sutures.

This dimple invariably resolves 2–3 months after surgery. If the pucker or dimple persists after 3 months

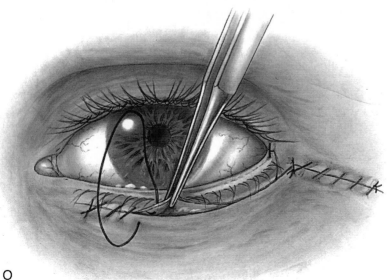

O, Skin is sutured together from the nasal to temporal aspect of the lower eyelid and from the lateral canthus to the temporal end of the incision.

O

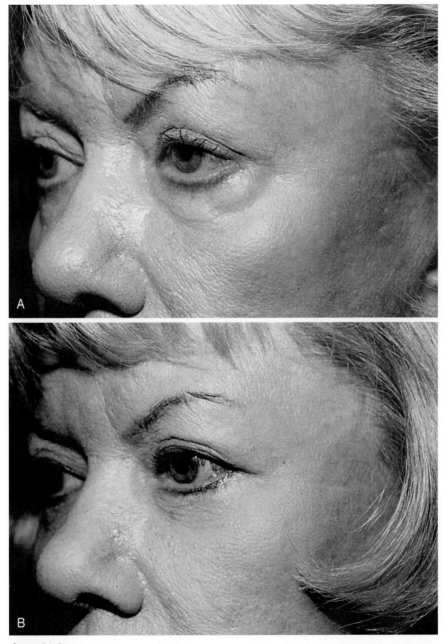

figure 24–2

A, Preoperative photograph of a patient with cheek depression and hollowing over the inferior orbital rim as well as upper eyelid ptosis. She had previously undergone a facelift and four-lid blepharoplasty, performed by another surgeon. *B,* Same patient after a cheek and midface lift. The cheek is in a higher, more temporal, normal position, simulating a cheek implant. In addition, the hollowing over the inferior orbital rim is decreased and the nasolabial fold depression is softened. A bilateral upper and lower blepharoplasty and a bilateral upper lid Müller's muscle–conjunctival resection–ptosis procedure were performed simultaneously.

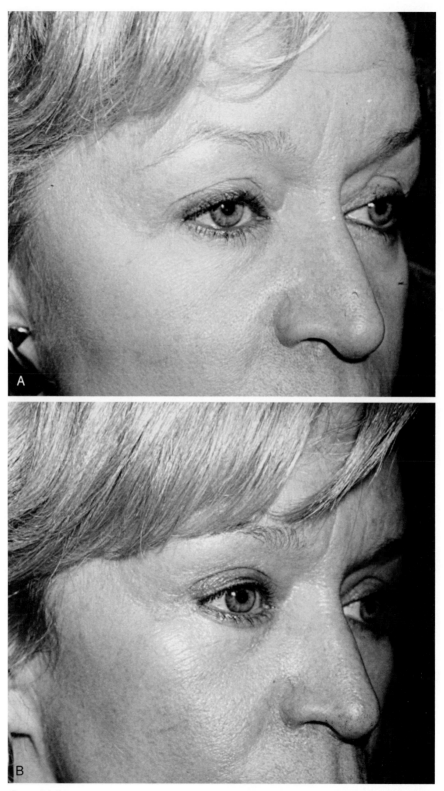

figure 24–3

A, Patient with sagging of the midface preoperatively. *B,* Same patient after a cheek and midface lift, which restored her cheeks to more normal positions, giving the appearance of cheek implants. An upper and lower blepharoplasty and a Müller's muscle resection–ptosis procedure also were performed.

postoperatively, the patient can massage and pull the puckered skin outward several times each day. The puckered tissues can also be excised and reunited if needed. If this procedure is anticipated, a temporal brow lift or facelift can be combined with the cheek and midface lift to tighten the lateral canthal skin.

Another complication is a postoperative ectropion or retraction. The surgeon can prevent this result by horizontally tightening the eyelid and by avoiding excessive skin muscle resection. Should these problems occur, further horizontal shortening, cheek lifting, or skin grafting can be done.

In the procedures I have performed, I have not noted any long-term complications.

RESULTS

More than 20 patients have been treated with excellent results (Figs. 24–2 and 24–3). The rate of patient satisfaction has been high. The main complaint has been the 2–3 months of cheek puckering.

References

1. Hester TR Jr, Codner MA, McCord CD Jr: Subperiosteal malar cheek lift with lower lid blepharoplasty. In McCord CD Jr (ed): Eyelid Surgery: Principles and Techniques, pp 210–215. Philadelphia, Lippincott-Raven, 1995.
2. McCord CD Jr: Lower lid blepharoplasty. In McCord CD Jr (ed): Eyelid Surgery: Principles and Techniques, pp 196–209. Philadelphia, Lippincott-Raven, 1995.

Chapter 25

Treatment of Lower Eyelid Retraction with Recession of Lower Lid Retractors and Hard-Palate Grafting

In the first edition of *Cosmetic Oculoplastic Surgery,* a chapter was devoted to treatment of lower eyelid retraction combined with an internal lower blepharoplasty. The second edition contained no discussions of thyroid ophthalmopathy. In this edition, I have, for the sake of completeness, once again included this material.

Treatment of lower eyelid retraction is common in patients with thyroid ophthalmopathy. It may also occur as a complication of previous blepharoplasty procedures, both cosmetic and functional. Treatment consists of recessing the lower lid retractors and placing a spacer between them and the inferior tarsal border. At present, I prefer hard-palate grafting for the spacer because (1) it provides a mucous membrane lining to the internal lower lid, (2) it is rigid and flat, and (3) it is autogenous.

A lower eyelid internal blepharoplasty along with lower retraction surgery is commonly performed. This approach differs slightly from the transconjunctival approach to resection of lower eyelid herniated orbital fat (see Chapter 20), in that the retractor incision is made at the inferior tarsal border rather than 5–6 mm inferior to the inferior tarsal border.

ALLEN M. PUTTERMAN

Lower eyelid retraction frequently occurs in patients with thyroid ophthalmopathy. At times, it is associated with exophthalmos. At other times, it is an entity in itself, presumably secondary to contracture of the inferior rectus muscle, which then lowers the eyelid through its attachment to the capsulopalpebral fascia and the capsulopalpebral fascia attachment to the tarsus. This not only creates a cosmetic disturbance but also leads to ocular irritation and keratopathy.

Frequently, lower eyelid retraction is minimal and can be ignored. If the patient undergoes an orbital decompression for treatment of exophthalmos, the eye will commonly descend, thus making the lower eyelid retraction less apparent. If the retraction is moderate to severe and a decompression is not in the picture, the lower eyelid retraction should be treated.

Lower eyelid retraction is measured by determining the distance from the lower eyelid to the inferior limbus of the eye in the primary position of gaze. This measurement is made not only centrally but also nasally and temporally.

Another method involves measuring the distance from a light reflex that is made to shine on the cornea to the lower lid as both patient and examiner look in the primary position of gaze, that is, the margin reflex distance–2 (MRD_2) (see Chapter 2, Fig. 2–9).[1] Normally, the lower eyelid rests at the inferior limbus. Measurements of retraction greater than 2 mm are common enough to warrant retraction surgery.

I prefer to treat lower eyelid retraction secondary to thyroid disease by recessing the lower lid retractors and placing a hard-palate graft between the recessed retractors and the inferior tarsal border. An alternative is to use donor sclera from an eye bank or the patient's ear cartilage. However, the use of donor sclera carries a small risk of transmission of infectious diseases, such as hepatitis or human immunodeficiency virus (HIV), and ear cartilage does not have a flat surface in many patients.

The hard-palate graft presents a surface that is not only flat and rigid but also lined by oral mucous membrane, which simulates the conjunctiva. The treatment of lower eyelid retraction by recession of the lower lid retractors and placement of a hard-palate graft is frequently performed in conjunction with excision of herniated orbital fat through an internal lower eyelid approach.

The procedure for recession of lower eyelid retractors and placement of a hard-palate graft, with excision of herniated orbital fat, is described under the topic Surgical Technique.

PREPARATION FOR SURGERY

Before surgery, a dentist makes a plastic plate that will fit onto the roof of the patient's mouth.[2, 3] This plate is

attached to several teeth with extensions that come off the plastic plate. After retrieval of the hard-palate grafts and the placement of an absorbable gelatin sponge (Gelfoam) to the donor site, the plastic plate is inserted onto the roof of the mouth. The plate provides comfort and maintains hemostasis.

SURGICAL TECHNIQUE

Local anesthesia with intravenous sedation is usually used (see Chapter 8). Topical tetracaine is applied over the eye. A scleral contact lens is placed over the eye and under the upper and lower eyelids to protect the eye and minimize the patient's discomfort from the operating lights. The patient is prepared and draped in the usual fashion, similar to that used for upper or lower blepharoplasty (see Chapter 10). The mouth is prepared with povidone-iodine (Betadine) sponges rubbed over the teeth, hard palate, and tongue surface.

Two per cent lidocaine (Xylocaine) with epinephrine is injected subcutaneously and diffusely throughout the lower eyelid. Injections of 2 per cent lidocaine with epinephrine (~0.5 ml) also are given into each fat pad. This is done via a 25-gauge needle inserted over

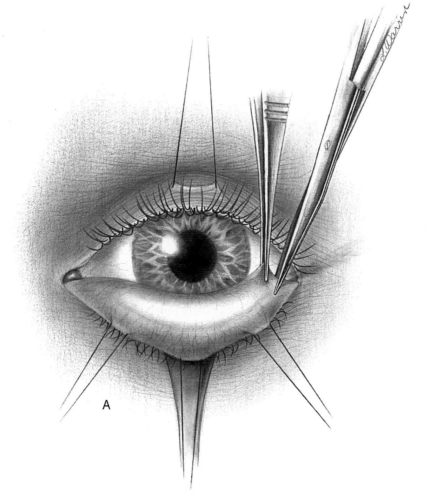

figure 25–1

A, A scissor is used to sever the conjunctiva, Müller's muscle, and the capsulopalpebral fascia at the temporal end of the lower eyelid, just below the inferior tarsal border.

the temporal, central, and nasal inferior orbital rim, for a distance of 1 cm, and aimed downward during each insertion. Additional 2 per cent lidocaine with 1:100,000 epinephrine is injected into the central aspect of the upper eyelid just above the eyelashes.

A 4-0 black silk suture is placed through skin, orbicularis oculi muscle, and superficial tarsus at the center of the upper eyelid. The suture is used to pull the upper eyelid upward. Another 4-0 black silk suture is placed through skin, orbicularis muscle, and superficial tarsus at the center of the lower eyelid to evert the eyelid over a Desmarres retractor. Two per cent lidocaine with epinephrine is injected subconjunctivally inferior to the inferior tarsal border and diffusely across the eyelid.

Recessing the Lower Eyelid Retractors

A toothed forceps grasps the conjunctiva, Müller's muscle, and the capsulopalpebral fascia at the temporal aspect of the eyelid, just beneath the inferior tarsal border (Fig. 25–1A). With a Westcott scissors, the surgeon penetrates this tissue and severs it from the inferior tarsal border. The Westcott scissors enters this opening and passes between capsulopalpebral fascia and orbicularis muscle across the eyelid (Fig. 25–1B). The surgeon

facilitates this maneuver by separating the Westcott scissors blades during the passage and by pulling the scissors upward toward the conjunctival surface. At the same time, the surgeon's assistant is releasing the Desmarres retractor slightly or pulling the skin surface outward. Because skin is firmly attached to the orbicularis muscle and the conjunctiva is firmly attached to Müller's muscle and capsulopalpebral fascia, the two lamellae separate in opposite directions during this maneuver.

While the eyelid structures are kept in these positions, the Westcott scissors is withdrawn and one blade is reinserted into the separated plane. Using the scissors, the surgeon severs the conjunctiva, Müller's muscle, and the capsulopalpebral fascia just beneath the inferior tarsal border (Fig. 25–1C to 1E). During this step, the surgeon must be careful to avoid cutting orbicularis muscle; cutting the muscle can interfere with the vascular supply to the eyelid margin and cilia, which might result in the loss of eyelashes. When first learning this technique, the surgeon should sever the conjunctiva and Müller's muscle in one step and the capsulopalpebral fascia in another step.

A toothed forceps is used to grasp the central conjunctiva, Müller's muscle, and the capsulopalpebral fascia. The surgeon pulls these tissues in a direction toward the eye while the assistant pulls the skin and orbicularis muscle away from the eye with the 4-0 black

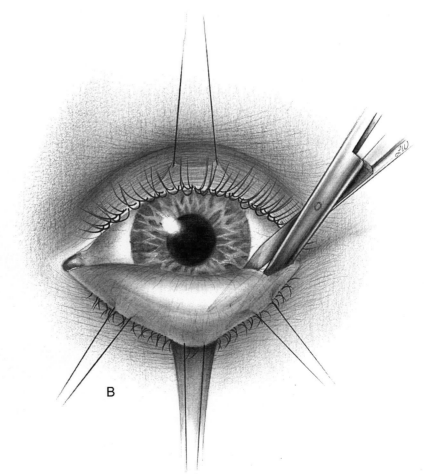

B, The scissors passes anterior to the tarsus in order to enter the space between the capsulopalpebral fascia and the orbicularis muscle.

B

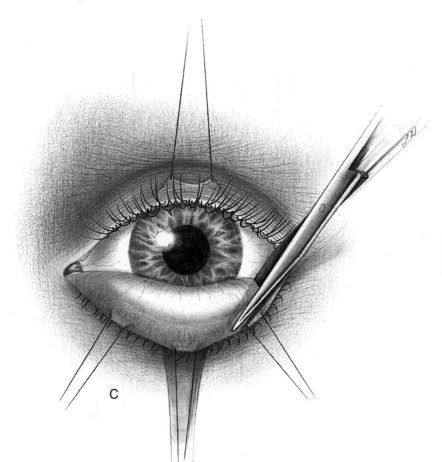

C, One blade of the scissors passes anterior to the tarsus until its tip is adjacent to the eyelid margin. The other blade of the scissors is external to the inside of the eyelid.

D, The scissors is rotated below the tarsal border.

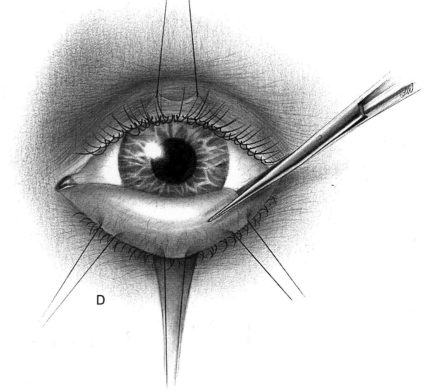

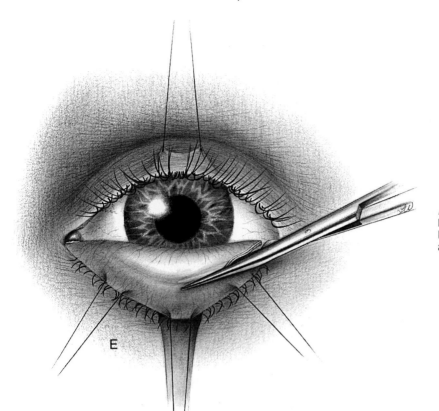

E, A Desmarres retractor pulls the skin and orbicularis muscle downward while the conjunctiva, Müller's muscle, and the capsulopalpebral fascia are cut adjacent to the tarsal border.

F, A Desmarres retractor pulls the skin and orbicularis muscle downward while the conjunctiva, Müller's muscle, and the edge of the capsulopalpebral fascia are pulled upward and outward with forceps. A Westcott scissors separates loose connective tissue between the orbicularis muscle and the capsulopalpebral fascia to enter the orbicularis space.

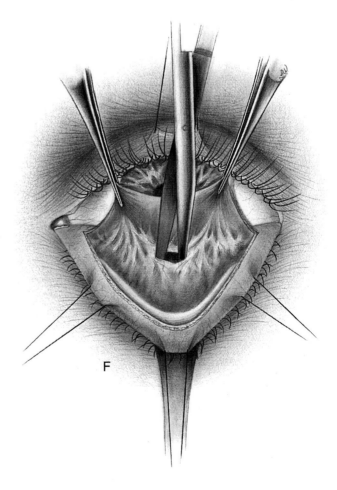

silk suture attached to the lower eyelid or with the eyelid everted over a Desmarres retractor. A Westcott scissors is used to penetrate the area between these retracted lamellae (Fig. 25–1*F*). The scissors should fall into the suborbicularis space. At this step, the surgeon should be able to visualize the white capsulopalpebral fascia surface on the internal surface and the reddish orbicularis muscle on the outer surface.

While still keeping the eyelid structures pulled in these directions, the surgeon uses the Westcott scissors to separate the remaining nasal and temporal tissues (Fig. 25–1*G*). (The Westcott scissors should hug the capsulopalpebral fascia surface rather than the orbicularis muscle surface.) Alternatively, this separation can be accomplished with a Colorado needle, a laser, or a disposable surgical cautery (Solan Accu-Temp, Xomed Surgical Products, Jacksonville, Fla.). Bleeding is controlled with a disposable cautery.

A 4-0 black silk, double-armed suture is then placed through the conjunctiva, Müller's muscle, and the capsulopalpebral fascia at the center of the lower eyelid. The suture is passed through the gray line of the central upper eyelid and exits through the orbicularis muscle and skin. The surgeon ties the suture with one tie of a surgeon's knot and then a shoelace tie. The suture in the upper eyelid is pulled upward and attached to the drape with a hemostat. This causes the eye to be covered and also places tension on the lower lid retractors and the graft.

Excision of Herniated Orbital Fat

A small Desmarres retractor is used to evert the lower eyelid and pull skin and the orbicularis muscle outward away from the eye. With the use of cotton-tipped applicators, the temporal, central, and nasal orbital fat pads are isolated and the inferior oblique muscle is identified (Fig. 25–1*H*). The capsule of the fat pads is then opened.

Fat that prolapses with general pressure is clamped with a hemostat, and the tissues held in the hemostat are cut free by running a No. 15 Bard-Parker blade over them (Fig. 25–1*I*). Cotton-tipped applicators are applied under the hemostat, and a Bovie cautery is applied to the fat stump. As the hemostat is released, the surgeon grasps and inspects the fat stump to make sure that there is no bleeding before allowing the fat pad to retract into the orbit. This maneuver is continued temporally, centrally, and nasally until fat no longer prolapses with general pressure applied on the eye.

The 4-0 silk suture that is connecting the retractors of the lower eyelid to the upper eyelid is then released. The lower eyelid is then placed in normal position, and the contact lens is removed.

At this point, the lower eyelid margin should rest at a normal position at the inferior limbus and should be easily pulled upward. If not, it may be necessary to further recess the lower lid retractors. Once the desired position is achieved, the surgeon flips the eyelid over

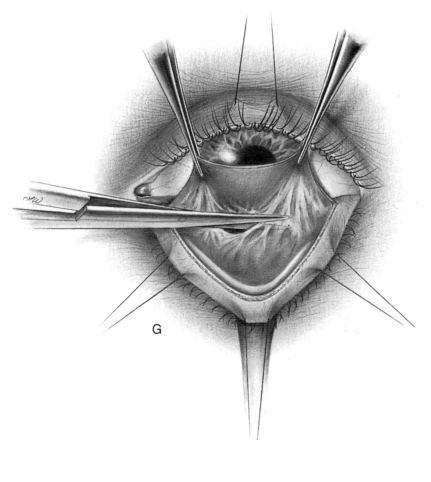

G, Loose connective tissue is then severed temporally from the central opening of the suborbicularis space.

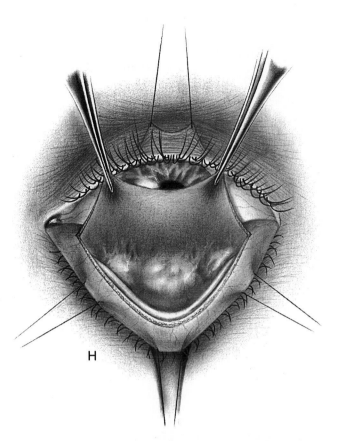

H, Herniated orbital fat is exposed between the capsulopalpebral fascia and the septum.

and measures the distance between the recessed lower lid retractors and the inferior tarsal border centrally, nasally, and temporally. This distance is approximately the vertical dimension of the hard-palate graft.

Obtaining the Hard-Palate Graft

A Jennings oral retractor is used to open the patient's mouth. A tongue blade is used to depress the tongue downward. The hard palate is then dried with a 4 × 4 gauze pad.

A methylene blue marking pen is used to draw the dimensions of the hard-palate graft. Commonly, this begins just posterior to the furrows that separate the hard-palate graft from the upper gum. The temporal aspect of the graft is usually the temporal aspect of the hard palate, and the central aspect is several millimeters temporal from the center of the hard palate. The posterior aspect is commonly at the junction where hard palate meets soft palate. Usually, two hard-palate grafts are taken, one for each lower eyelid. Each of these areas is marked on the hard palate at the same time.

Two per cent lidocaine with epinephrine is injected submucosally surrounding the areas marked on the hard palate. I usually give this injection about 10 minutes before I am ready to take the hard-palate graft so that hemostasis from the epinephrine has time to take place.

A No. 15 Bard-Parker blade is used to incise the

outlined areas of the hard-palate donor site (Fig. 25–1*J*). The Bard-Parker blade and a No. 66 Beaver blade are used to remove the hard-palate graft. The assistant pushes the tongue downward and suctions blood from the graft site during this step. Suction must also be maintained in the posterior pharynx to prevent the patient from swallowing any blood or saliva.

Bleeding is controlled with an absorbable gelatin sponge applied to the graft site. Occasionally, one must use microfibrillar collagen hemostat powder (Avitene). The gelatin sponge is pushed up against the hard palate with a tongue blade or the surgeon's finger for several seconds, and the mouth retractor is removed. Then a preoperatively made hard-palate prosthesis is applied over the roof of the mouth.[2, 3]

The graft is trimmed on its internal surface to free any excessive tissue so that only oral mucous membrane and hard palate remain. The graft is placed in gentamicin (Garamycin) solution for several minutes and is rinsed with balanced salt solution.

Suturing the Hard-Palate Graft to Lower Eyelid Retractors and Tarsus Muscle

The inferior edge of the graft is sutured to the lower eyelid retractors with a 5-0 chromic catgut suture run nasally to temporally (Fig. 25–1*K*). Each bite of the suture passes through the lower lid retractors and then the inferior edge of the hard-palate graft. The graft is placed so that the internal surface of the graft facing the eye is the mucosa-lined tissue.

The contact lens is removed, and the lower eyelid is placed in normal position. The surgeon judges the amount of excessive hard-palate graft that extends above the inferior tarsal border and trims this tissue off. Because it is usually better to have a slightly excessive hard-palate graft rather than a sparse one, the trimming of the excessive tissue should be done sparingly.

Next, the superior edge of the hard-palate graft is secured to the inferior tarsal border with another 5-0 chromic catgut suture (Fig. 25–1*L*). The suture is run continuously nasally to temporally and with the temporal and nasal knots buried deeply.

A suture tarsorrhaphy is formed nasally and temporally, with two 4-0 black silk, double-armed sutures. Each suture passes through the skin and orbicularis muscle of the lower eyelid and exits through the gray line. The sutures then enter the skin and orbicularis muscle above the eyebrow (Fig. 25–1*M*).

The contact lens is removed, and a 24- or 48-hour collagen shield is placed over the eye. The sutures are tied over cotton pledgets to keep the lower eyelid on an upward stretch. Gentamicin ointment is applied to the eyes and to the sutures.

POSTOPERATIVE CARE

Eye Care

To keep the graft flat against its orbicularis muscle bed, I usually prefer to apply a dressing of an eye pad, 4 ×

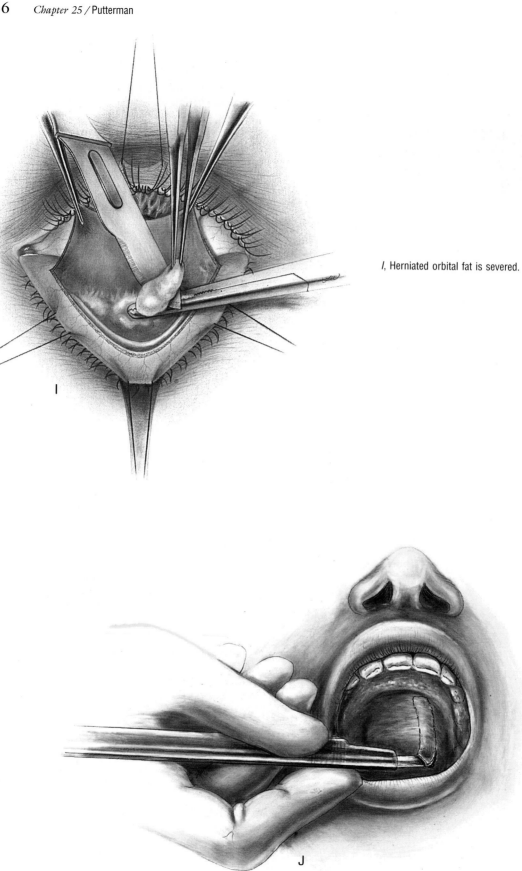

I, Herniated orbital fat is severed.

I

J

J, A hard-palate mucosal graft is harvested from the roof of the patient's mouth.

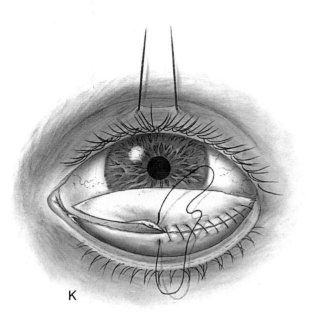

K, Severed borders of conjunctiva, Müller's muscle, and capsulopalpebral fascia are sutured to the hard-palate graft so that the mucosal surface faces the eye.

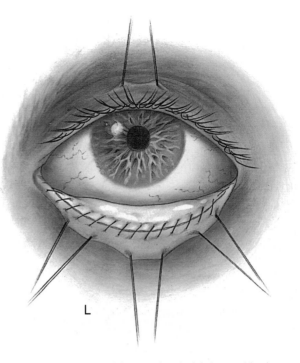

L, The hard-palate graft is sutured to the inferior tarsal border.

4 cotton pads, and tape (Microfoam, 3M Company, St. Paul, Minn.), to be reapplied for several days. It is important, however, to check under the dressings to make sure that a retrobulbar hemorrhage has not resulted from the fat removal. I do this frequently during the first few hours postoperatively and then instruct the patient's family how to do it periodically thereafter. The dressing is removed and reapplied the next day.

The patient is placed on a regimen of systemic antibiotics for 1 week and is instructed to apply gentamicin ophthalmic ointment to the eye and sutures twice a day for 2 weeks postoperatively.

Forty-eight hours after surgery, the dressing is completely removed and the patient is able to see through a separation of upper and lower eyelids, even with the tarsorrhaphy sutures in place. The tarsorrhaphy sutures are removed 1 week after surgery.

M, With 4-0 black silk sutures, the lower eyelid is pulled upward toward the eyebrow.

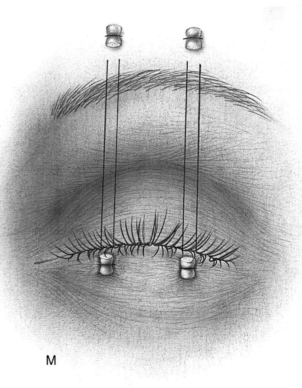

Mouth Care

The patient should remove the plastic plate from the roof of the mouth before eating. Patients should gargle twice a day with an antiseptic mouthwash, such as cetylpyridinium (Cēpacol). They also may use a numbing mouthwash, such as 2 per cent viscous lidocaine. Most patients use the roof plate for approximately 1 week postoperatively, and then they are usually comfortable.

Granulation of the roof of the mouth usually takes place 1 month after the procedure.

COMPLICATIONS

Complications include overcorrections and undercorrections, which can be diffuse or segmental. If slight retraction occurs, upward massage may be helpful. If moderate residual retraction results, further grafting may be necessary.

Other problems consist of loss of cilia, which is usually due to severing of the orbicularis muscle, and interference with the vascular supply to the eyelid.

Entropion and ectropion are other potential complications. If these occur, they are treated by appropriate correction procedures. At times, the ectropion can be eliminated simply by removal of excessive hard-palate grafting. Conjunctival granulomas occasionally occur, and these can be easily treated by a simple excision.

In my experience, I have encountered several cases of nasal entropion, which I treated by (1) splitting the eyelid into two lamellae; (2) excising the skin, orbicularis muscle, and offending eyelashes; and (3) letting the area granulate. I have treated several cases of granuloma with simple excision. In a couple of patients, the hard palate extended upward over the tarsal border and had to be trimmed off.

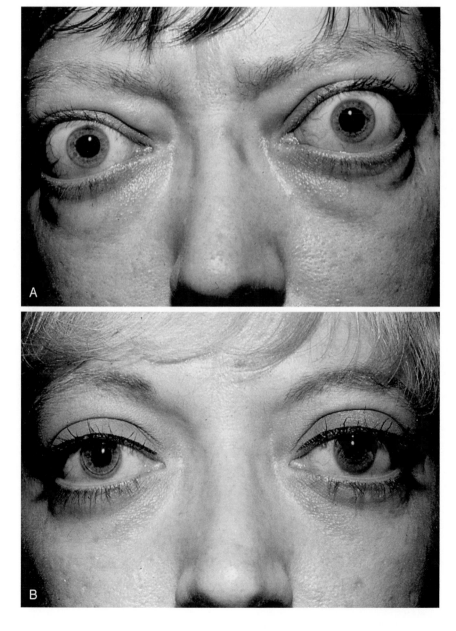

figure 25–2

A, Preoperative appearance of a patient with thyroid-related retraction of all four eyelids associated with lower eyelid herniated orbital fat. *B,* Same patient after lower lid elevation by recession of the retractors, placement of a graft between the retractors and the inferior tarsal border, and internal fat excision. The upper eyelids were lowered simultaneously by excision of Müller's muscle and recession of the levator aponeurosis through an internal approach (as described in Chapter 16), and lateral tarsorrhaphies were performed (as described in Chapter 26).

RESULTS

I have treated lower eyelid retraction in thyroid disease in more than 300 eyelids. Approximately 100 of these procedures have been completed with hard-palate grafts, and the others involved the use of sclera or ear cartilage (Fig. 25–2). Results were much better with hard-palate grafting, and complications were minimal. In no patient have I needed to add or remove the hard palate.

In most cases, this procedure has successfully relieved lower lid retraction, ocular irritation, and keratopathy.

References

1. Putterman AM: Basic oculoplastic surgery. In Peyman G, Sanders D, Goldberg MF (eds): Principles and Practices of Ophthalmology, vol 3, p 2248. Philadelphia, WB Saunders, 1980.
2. Mauriello JA Jr, Wasserman B, Allee S, et al: Molded acrylic mouthguard to control bleeding at the hard palate graft site after eyelid reconstruction. Am J Ophthalmol 1992; 113:342–344.
3. Shorr N, Enzer YR: Letter to the editor re Mauriello JA Jr, Wasserman B, Allee S, et al: Molded acrylic mouthguard to control bleeding at the hard palate graft site after eyelid reconstruction. Am J Ophthalmol 1992; 114:779–780.

Allen M. Putterman

Chapter 26

Lateral Tarsorrhaphy in the Treatment of Thyroid Ophthalmopathy

Lateral tarsorrhaphy is a new chapter in this textbook. I perform a lateral tarsorrhaphy in many patients whom I treat with upper or lower retraction surgery. This procedure enhances upper and lower eyelid retraction surgery and decreases the exophthalmic appearance from a lateral view. It also decreases ocular irritation and keratopathy.

ALLEN M. PUTTERMAN

A lateral tarsorrhaphy is useful in the treatment of many patients with thyroid ophthalmopathy. This technique can mask the protrusion of the eye, add protection to the cornea, and decrease ocular irritation.

I rarely perform the procedure by itself. Most often, it is an adjunct procedure to orbital decompressions, retraction, surgery of the upper and lower eyelids, and excision of herniated orbital fat.

SURGICAL TECHNIQUE

The patient is prepared and draped, as described in Chapter 10. Topical tetracaine is instilled over the eyes, and a scleral protective lens is applied over the eye and under the eyelids. Two per cent lidocaine (Xylocaine) with epinephrine is then injected subcutaneously over the temporal upper and lower eyelids and adjacent lateral canthus.

A No. 11 Bard-Parker blade is used to make an incision in the gray line of the eyelid margin over the temporal upper and lower eyelids (Fig. 26–1A). This incision is usually about 3 mm long but occasionally extends 4 or 5 mm. The extent of the incision is based on how much tarsorrhaphy is to be performed (Fig. 26–1B). I find that a small tarsorrhaphy produces more acceptable results than a large one does.

The edge of the posterior eyelid margins are excised with Westcott scissors over the length of the gray line incision (Fig. 26–1C). The skin, orbicularis oculi muscle, and eyelashes are excised over the anterior lamellae in the same area. Bleeding is controlled with a disposable cautery.

Two to three 6-0 polyglactin (Vicryl) sutures are passed through the internal lamellae of the upper eyelid, externally to internally, and then through the lower eyelid, internally to externally (Fig. 26–1D). I often make a full-thickness passage through these structures even though it means having an exposed suture under the closed flaps. If the patient has a thick tarsus, however, I make this bite two thirds of the way through the tarsus so it does not penetrate the internal aspect of the eyelid.

When these sutures have been placed, the surgeon moves the patient into a sitting position and judges the width of the eyelid as well as the patient's appearance. If too little or too much of the palpebral fissure is closed off, the surgeon extends the tarsorrhaphy or removes sutures, respectively. When the desired effect has been achieved, the surgeon places two or three 6-0 black silk interrupted sutures through the skin and orbicularis muscle of the upper and lower eyelids to unite the external lamellae (Fig. 26–1E).

Topical gentamicin (Garamycin) is applied over the sutures. The 6-0 black silk sutures are removed 1 week postoperatively.

COMPLICATIONS

Occasionally, the lateral tarsorrhaphy is too great, and in these cases it is necessary to open the lateral canthus. I do this by performing a lateral canthotomy to the level where I would like the new horizontal fissure to extend. Then I suture skin to conjunctiva over the severed upper

261

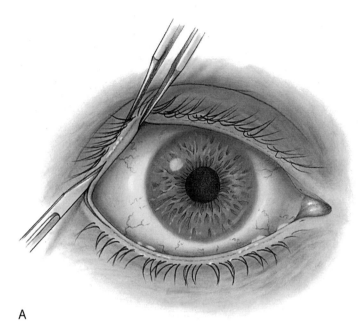

A

figure 26–1

A, A No. 11 Bard-Parker blade is used to divide the eyelid into anterior and posterior lamellae over the temporal 3–5 mm of the upper and lower eyelids.

B, The temporal 3–5 mm of upper and lower eyelids have been divided at the gray line to produce anterior and posterior lamellae.

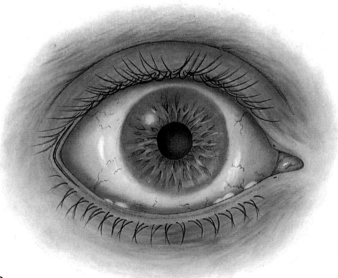

B

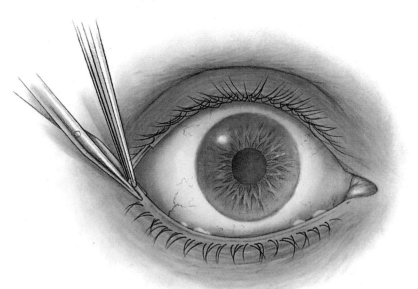

C, A sliver of eyelid margin is removed from the temporal upper and lower posterior lamellae.

C

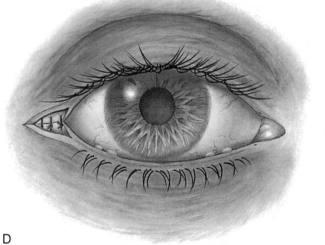

D

D, Several 6-0 interrupted polyglactin (Vicryl) sutures unite the posterior lamellae over the temporal 3–5 mm of the lateral upper and lower eyelids.

E, Several 6-0 black silk interrupted sutures unite the skin and orbicularis muscle of the anterior lamellae of the temporal upper and lower eyelids.

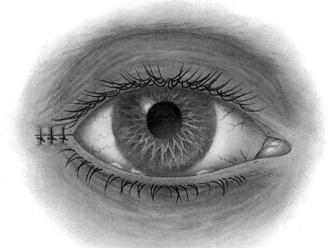

E

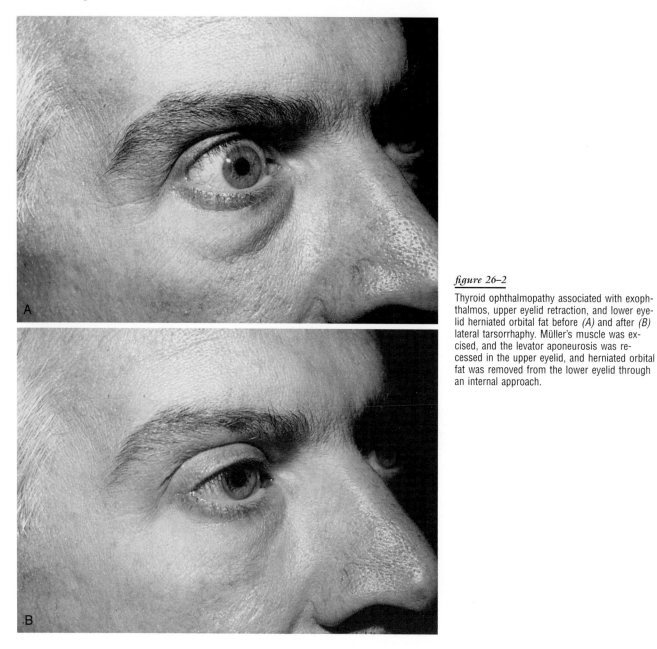

figure 26–2

Thyroid ophthalmopathy associated with exophthalmos, upper eyelid retraction, and lower eyelid herniated orbital fat before *(A)* and after *(B)* lateral tarsorrhaphy. Müller's muscle was excised, and the levator aponeurosis was recessed in the upper eyelid, and herniated orbital fat was removed from the lower eyelid through an internal approach.

and lower eyelid margins to prevent this area from re-uniting.

If the lateral tarsorrhaphy is not sufficient, the lateral upper and lower eyelids can be united to a greater extent according to the same technique described above.

RESULTS

I have performed the procedure in more than 300 patients with satisfactory results (Fig. 26–2).

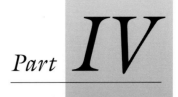

FOREHEAD, BROW, AND FACE LIFTS

M. Eugene Tardy
James Alex
David Hendrick

Chapter *27*

Rejuvenation of the Aging Brow and Forehead

Eyebrow ptosis is an important problem in cosmetic oculoplastic surgery. Frequently, a large upper eyelid fold is only partially caused by excessive upper eyelid skin and is significantly contributed to by ptosis of the brow. In these cases, elevation of the brow, in addition to excision of upper eyelid skin, is necessary to achieve the best cosmetic result. In Chapter 12, the authors described an internal brow lift, a procedure that elevates the central and temporal brow slightly. For patients needing a larger brow lift or lifting of the loose tissue above the nasal brow and the bridge of the nose, other techniques must be considered. Patients with deep wrinkles of the forehead and top of the nose also require other procedures.

In this chapter, M. Eugene Tardy, James Alex, and David Hendrick present multiple techniques to improve the appearance of the forehead, brow, and superior aspect of the nose. The techniques of direct brow, temporal, and coronal lifts are presented. The authors also discuss the pretrichal forehead lift, midforehead lift, midforehead browplasty, and treatment of glabellar creases. For each of these techniques, they present the indications; this information should be helpful in selecting suitable candidates.

Each of the various techniques has been beautifully illustrated to enable the cosmetic surgeon to perform these techniques with precision.

Endoscopically assisted forehead lifts are another alternative to raising the forehead and brows as well as eliminating frown lines. Because the endoscopic forehead lift is a relatively new technique and to differentiate it from the proven technique that Dr. Tardy and colleagues outline in this chapter, I have included this subject as a separate topic (see Chapter 28).

ALLEN M. PUTTERMAN

PATIENT SELECTION

Psychological Considerations

The orbit and its soft-tissue adnexa provide a challenging interface between the oculoplastic surgeon and the facial plastic surgeon. Although each specialist corrects deficiencies of anatomy from the perspective of his or her own subspecialty, improved understanding of the anatomic basis for orbital abnormalities has led to more uniform and unified surgical approaches by both subspecialties.

As highly motivated patients increasingly search for methods to forestall the inevitable evidences of aging in the orbital, forehead, and temporal regions, surgeons have responded with effective surgical remedies.[1-4] Lifting and repositioning operations designed to restore more normal anatomic relationships in the upper third of the face represent effective and safe adjuncts to traditional blepharoplasty.

Aesthetic surgery, by its very nature, differs considerably from surgical procedures employed to render sick patients well. Individuals seeking improvement in their appearance present as *well* patients seeking to look as well as they feel, and facial plastic surgeons accept a profound responsibility to achieve definitive improvement without making their patients *unwell*. The avoidance of even minor complications, then, ranks as the cardinal principle in all aesthetic surgery.

A further unique characteristic of aesthetic facial surgery relates to the inescapable fact that the surgeon's work—including incisions and scars—is on constant display for all to evaluate. Therefore, fastidiousness in incision siting and repair is paramount. Through thoughtful planning and scrupulously delicate surgical technique, scars (the inevitable sequelae of surgery) may be effectively camouflaged within the hair-bearing scalp or at the interface of hair to the non-hair-bearing scalp.

Careful patient selection to ensure effective, satisfactory outcomes, a significant part of all forms of aesthetic surgery, is especially important in rejuvenation of the orbital region. Patients who actually need forehead, brow, and temple lifting regularly request eyelid surgery. Educating patients about the most effective procedures often requires superior communication skills and gentle guidance because few patients are aware that ptosis of the forehead and brow is responsible for their age-

related orbital changes. Clearly, more of the surgeon's time must be expended to realize the laudable goals of effective patient understanding and truly informed consent. Surgeons unwilling to invest this added time should perhaps direct their talents to other fields of endeavor.

Patient selection, particularly from the viewpoint of *motivations* and *expectations*, assumes major importance in the magnitude and effectiveness of the surgical outcome. In aesthetic surgery, pure technical excellence does not always result in a happy, satisfied patient. Useful guidelines to patient selection (and rejection) exist, but each patient must be carefully and sensitively screened.

Anatomic Considerations

The aesthetic facial unit of the eyelid and orbital region, flawed by gradual aging, asymmetry, or familial abnormality, cannot always be satisfactorily rejuvenated by traditional blepharoplasty methods alone.[5-7] The ptotic eyebrow and temple commonly compound the problem of redundant upper eyelid skin by crowding the eye and producing an abnormal appearance of fatigue and premature aging (Fig. 27–1). If brow ptosis is sufficiently severe, visual deficits may even develop in the temporal quadrant. If upper blepharoplasty alone is employed in attempts at correction, the eyebrow is potentially drawn near the lid margin, obliterating adequate delineation of the supratarsal anatomy by sacrificing excessive upper eyelid skin.[8, 9] A preferred outcome would preserve sufficient upper eyelid skin to achieve a pleasant sweeping delineation of the upper eyelid cleft, incorpo-

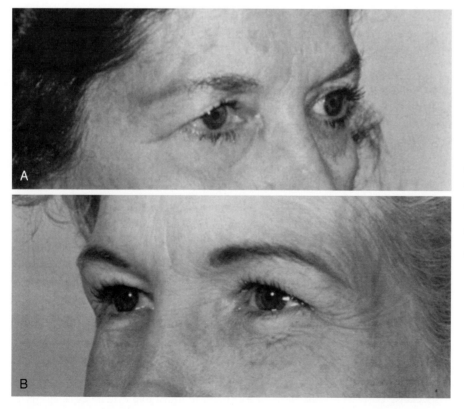

figure 27–1

A, Progressive age-related ptosis of the eyebrow and temporal region results in encroachment on the eyelid, characterized by loss of delineation of the normal supratarsal cleft. *B*, This tired and saddened appearance may be accompanied by a temporal visual deficit.

rating one of the brow elevation procedures to enhance the eyelid appearance.

Although different regions of the face age at variable rates and are influenced primarily by genetic factors, the upper third of the face ages in its own unique fashion (Fig. 27–2).[10] As skin elasticity progressively declines, the forehead, temple, and glabellar skin descend. Ptotic (low-positioned) brows ensue, crowding the orbital region and increasing the extent of skin redundancy in the upper eyelid area (Fig. 27–3). Fine lines, the result of the combination of gravity and repeated contraction of the orbicularis oculi muscle, appear at the lateral canthus and temple (Fig. 27–4). Progressively deep horizontal creases appear in the forehead, the consequence of repetitive frontalis muscle contraction and hypertonicity (Fig. 27–5). (The absence of these creases in the paralyzed forehead validates this observation.) Synergistic actions of the corrugator and procerus muscles produce vertical, oblique, and horizontal creases in the glabella and nasal root (Fig. 27–6).

Blepharoplasty alone is ineffective in improving and recontouring the lateral orbital rhytids (crow's feet or "laugh lines"), which contribute to the aging appearance and which displease patients.[11] Effective improvement of oblique vertical and transverse glabellar frown lines requires direct surgical interruption of the involved animation muscles. Some form of adjunctive lifting procedure, therefore, is required to augment the improvement achieved by blepharoplasty. Most useful among these are the following:

- Forehead (coronal and pretrichal) lift
- Midforehead lift
- Temporal (temple) lift
- Direct brow lift (browplasty)[12]

Indications for and limitations of each approach are explored in this discussion. The accurate selection of the most effective techniques is critical and is based on the unique anatomic factors in each individual (Table 27–1). Among these, mobility of the forehead and scalp dramatically influences the choice of procedure and ultimate result.

The recent introduction of minimally invasive, small-incision, endoscopically aided lifting procedures in the forehead region provides options for the cosmetic surgeon (see Chapter 28). These procedures, not yet stan-

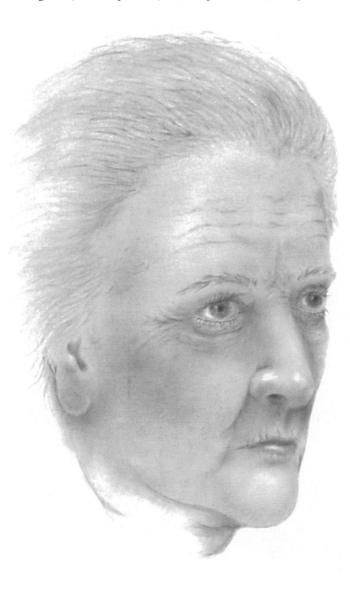

figure 27–2

Characteristics of the aging brow, temple, eyelids, and face. Although environmental influences may worsen or hasten aging changes, each person's genetic disposition plays the predominant role in the aging process.

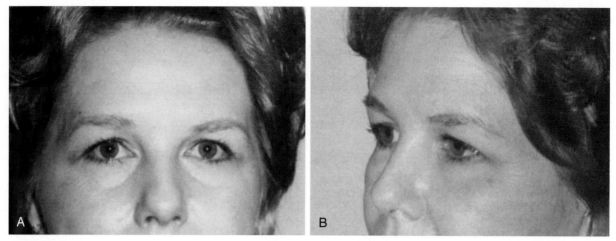

figure 27–3

A and *B*, Typical appearance of the ptotic forehead and brow. The eyebrows have descended to or below the level of the bony supraorbital ridges, with early rhytids ("crow's feet") forming at the root of the nose.

dardized in their approach, scope, or long-term outcome, are designed to *complement* rather than *replace* the more traditional approaches to forehead and brow lifting. Certain endoscopic procedures require extensive central and posterior scalp flap elevation, extending the magnitude of the procedure and the potential for complications. Time and careful observation of long-term outcomes will determine the degree of value that endoscopically assisted lifting procedures provide in facial rejuvenation. We predict that traditional forehead and brow procedures will continue to play a major role in patients seeking an improved appearance of the upper third of the face.

With rare exceptions, the indicated brow elevation procedure should be carried out *before upper blepharoplasty* so that the surgeon can judge the precise amount of upper eyelid skin to be excised. This prevents an overaggressive elevation of the brow–upper eyelid complex with the potential for causing difficulty in normal closure of the upper eyelids. In some patients, brow elevation procedures may eliminate the need for upper blepharoplasty altogether.

Forehead lifting procedures may be effectively combined with methods to rejuvenate the middle and lower thirds of the face (facelift and cervical lift). Because the various regions of the face may age at different rates, forehead or brow lifting is also commonly accomplished as an isolated procedure or as a preliminary to blepharoplasty.

Two factors bear heavily on the surgeon's choice of sequence and combination of operations:

- Relative position of the brows
- Patient's gender

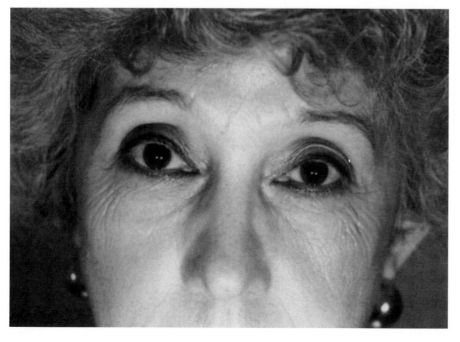

figure 27–4

Fine rhytids peripheral to the lateral canthus, the consequence of permanent skin etching from repeated contracture of the orbicularis oculi muscle, generally may be only partially improved by rejuvenation and lifting procedures around the orbit.

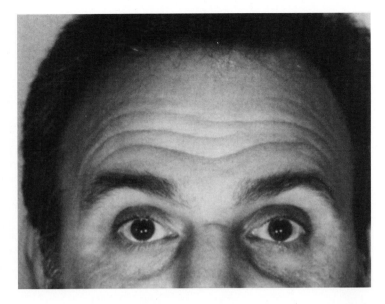

figure 27–5

Deep horizontal creases form in individuals with active, expressive foreheads, the consequence of repeated vertical contraction or hypertonicity of the paired frontalis muscles.

table 27–1

Patient Evaluation: Anatomic Factors

Forehead height relative to facial proportions
Hairline: frontal and temporal
Abundance of frontal and brow hair
Skin quality, texture, sebaceous quality, and thickness
Skin elasticity and mobility
Scalp (galeal) mobility
Degree of depth of forehead wrinkling
Eyebrow position and mobility
Eyebrow anatomy and symmetry
Degree of dermatochalasis
Lateral canthal hooding
Temporal rhytidosis

figure 27–6

Synergistic actions of the corrugator, frontalis, and procerus muscles produce progressively deep oblique and vertical creases in the glabellar area. Transverse rhytids may form at the nasal root. Forehead and brow ptosis accentuates the aging process produced by this combined muscle action.

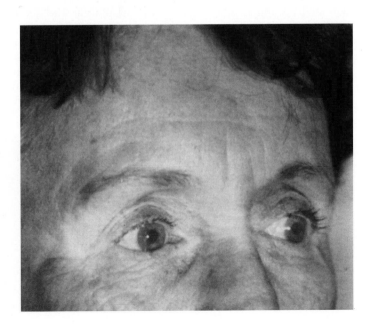

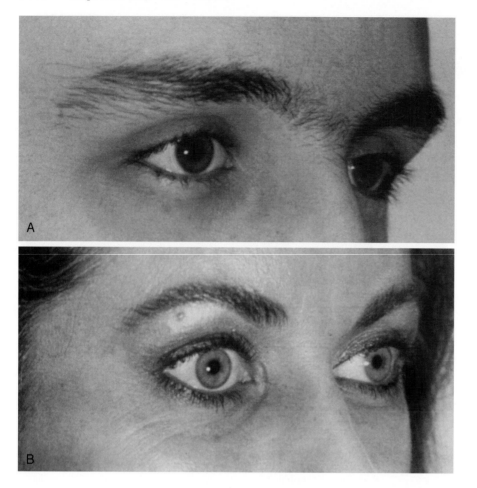

figure 27–7

Normal brow position in the male *(A)* differs from that in the female *(B)*, in that males ordinarily demonstrate a relatively transverse and flat brow position, which is less laterally arched than the female brow. The classic and desirable female brow arches higher laterally than the male brow and tends to thin as it courses temporally. (Females generally possess a thinner hair content.) Although ideal brow positions and shapes can be identified, many attractive variations exist.

The male brow classically is heavier in hair content, occupies a more inferior (caudal) position, and arches laterally less than the female brow (Fig. 27–7*A*). This typical horizontal brow configuration, although occasionally objectionable in women, is not usually displeasing in men. In contrast, the preferred female brow (many variations obviously exist) arches higher laterally than medially and assumes its highest point at about the junction of the middle and outer thirds (Fig. 27–7*B*). The female brow typically thins as it courses laterally, diminishing the ease of potential scar camouflage in the hair-skin junction.

Critical evaluation before selection of the technique includes assessment of the eyebrow position, attitude, and shape, completed with the patient sitting and in facial repose (Fig. 27–8). Through manual elevation of the brow with the patient gazing straight ahead, a tentative judgment can be made of the favorable effect of brow elevation on the aesthetic unit of the eye and orbit (Fig. 27–9). Individuals with ptotic brows often involuntarily attempt to elevate the brow, bringing about excessive forehead animation. This facial posture is ordinarily an unconscious habit, giving rise to a "surprised" facial expression as the drooping brow is temporarily elevated. Preoperative estimates of the benefits of surgical brow elevation are much more accurate if all animation is consciously eliminated and the brow position is judged with the patient in complete facial repose.

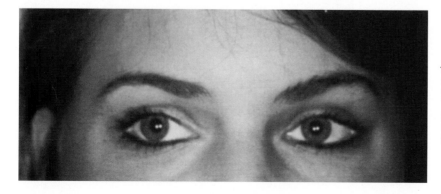

figure 27–8

An ideal female brow position, in which the brow rests well above the superior orbital bony margin. The brow arches gracefully upward and temporally, with the highest extent of the upward arch beginning between the lateral limbus and the lateral canthus.

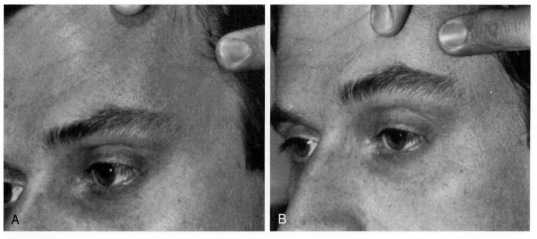

figure 27–9

Preoperative manual elevation of the eyebrow-temporal unit *(A)* and the eyebrow *(B)* offers an important diagnostic assessment of the impact of surgical correction on rejuvenation of the orbital appearance. Precise estimates can be made of the degree and angulation of surgical elevation desirable. In addition, the approximate postoperative improvement may be shown to the patient with the aid of a three-way mirror.

If the patient closes his or her eyes and then opens them slowly after allowing the facial muscles to relax, the surgeon can determine the true brow position in repose. The individual anatomic situation then dictates the choice of brow elevation procedure that would most favorably complement the planned blepharoplasty operation.

SELECTION OF APPROPRIATE PROCEDURE

The indications and contraindications for each forehead and brow-lifting procedure described are presented in Table 27–2.

Coronal Forehead Lift

For total forehead and brow elevation with reasonable longevity, consideration should be given to the forehead lift approach through a coronal incision posterior to the frontal and temporal hairline. All aspects of the aging forehead, including brow and forehead creases, are effectively treated with this approach, which thus allows a more comprehensive operation.[13]

The advantages of this procedure are:

1. Elevation of the entire brow, particularly when medial brow ptosis exists.
2. Complete camouflage in the scalp hair.
3. Direct attenuation of the action of the frontalis, corrugator, and procerus muscles.
4. Reduction of the transverse vertical creases.
5. If indicated, lifting of the drooping nasal skin.

Relative disadvantages include:

1. The potential for slight elevation of the frontal hairline.
2. Slightly less ability to fine-tune the ultimate brow posture and position from an incision sited a considerable distance away from the upper orbit.
3. A more complex and time-consuming operation.

Although the coronal forehead lift has been performed sparingly in the United States for many years, recently surgeons have come to appreciate the lasting quality and relative ease and safety of this approach. The current enthusiasm undoubtedly stems from the advantage of directly excising transverse portions of the frontalis muscle to release the overlying wrinkled forehead skin. Various surgeons accomplish the latter effect with muscle cross-hatching, incisions, and/or resection of transverse muscle segments.

Although it is a more extensive procedure, the forehead lift is, in reality, not complicated as long as the surgeon respects normal anatomy. General or local anesthesia may be used, and along with browplasty and temporal lift, the procedure can also be performed on an outpatient basis in well-motivated, healthy patients.

Surgical Technique

If a local anesthetic agent is chosen, infiltrations to block the supraorbital and supratrochlear nerves along the level of the eyebrows, augmented by infiltration along the intended line of incision, are sufficient to create excellent local anesthesia. (It is imperative to appreciate that the infiltration near the frontal branch of the facial nerve may result in a temporary partial or complete frontal paralysis.) A freshly mixed solution of 1 per cent lidocaine with 1:100,000 epinephrine is sufficient to provide excellent local anesthesia and aid in hemostasis. Approximately 10 ml suffices to render the forehead anesthetic; if required, more can be infiltrated later in the procedure.

The incision site is marked in a coronal fashion within the hair, far enough behind the frontal hairline that an excision of 1–2.5 cm of scalp anterior to the incision will place the resultant scar 2.5–4 cm behind the hairline (Fig. 27–10*A*). The lateral wings of the incision may extend to or beyond the tragus of each ear, carried in sinuous fashion from the temple into the junction of the auricle and the face (Fig. 27–10*B*).

An alternate scheme brings the incision to the hairline

table 27–2

Forehead and Brow-Lifting Procedures

Procedure	Indications and Advantages	Contraindications and Disadvantages
Coronal forehead lift	Ideal and immediate scar camouflage Treats all aspects of aging forehead and brow	Limited use in males Elevates hairline Vertically lengthens upper third of face Elongated scar Possible prolonged hypesthesia of scalp Less fine-tuning of brow position
Pretrichal forehead lift	High hairline No vertical forehead lengthening Preserves hairline Treats all aspects of aging forehead and brows Immediate scar camouflage (with hair)	Possible visible (exposed) scar Possible prolonged hypesthesia of scalp
Midforehead lift	Prominent horizontal forehead creases Preserves hairline Improved fine-tuning of brow position Corrects brow asymmetry	Possible visible (exposed) scar Avoid in oily, thick skin
Midforehead brow lift	Prominent horizontal forehead creases Improved fine-tuning of brow position Corrects brow asymmetry	Possible visible (exposed) scar Treats brows only Avoid in oily, thick skin
Direct brow lift	Accurate brow elevation Preserves forehead/scalp sensation Patients with abundant brow hair preferred Immediate scar camouflage (with hair) Corrects brow asymmetry	Possible visible (exposed) scar Treats brows only
Temporal lift	Ideal and immediate scar camouflage Improves brow position and temple laxity	Not useful for midforehead glabellar creases No effect on medial aspects of brow

junction in the midline, thus preserving the widow's peak in patients who so desire (Fig. 27–10C). Scar camouflage with these incisions is excellent as long as strong galeal and dermal-to-dermal closure is carried out fastidiously. Beveling the coronal incision along the axis of the residual hair follicles protects them.

The incision is made in short segments to allow control of bleeding by pressure, fine bipolar cautery, and, at times, Raney clips. Use of the Shaw hemostatic scalpel facilitates control of minor bleeding; for large vessels in the temporal area, ligation may be necessary for complete safety.

As the subgaleal supraperiosteal plane is entered, the operation may proceed rapidly and bloodlessly with largely blunt dissection (Fig. 27–10D), which is performed in this manner down to the level of the supraorbital ridges. The periosteum is left intact to this point in the procedure. The facial nerve frontal branch crosses the temporal region along the undersurface of the temporoparietal fascia, eventually penetrating the frontalis muscle along its deep surface. As long as surgical dissection remains deep to the subgaleal fascia (leaving the fascia on the elevated coronal flap), the frontal branch is protected.

With blunt dissection, the extent of the corrugator muscles is delineated and isolated from the bilateral supraorbital neurovascular bundles, which are scrupulously protected (Fig. 27–10E). The corrugator muscles are separated from their bony origin and cross-clamped, and 1–1.5 cm of muscle is excised. Cautery of the cut muscle ends ensures hemostasis.

If desired at this point, the procerus muscle may be partially removed and the dorsal nasal skin elevated as an additional lifting benefit (Fig. 27–10F). The previously

Text continued on page 280

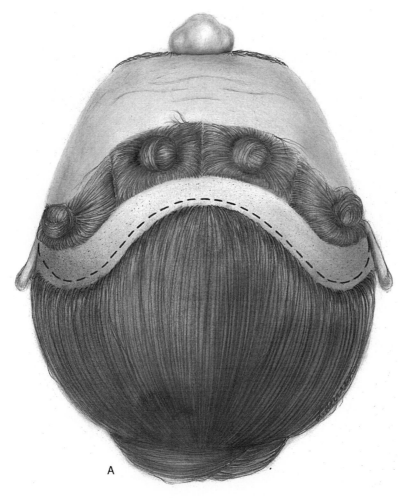

A

figure 27–10

A, The coronal forehead lift incision is sited 2.5–4 cm behind the frontal hairline, generally paralleling the shape of the hairline.

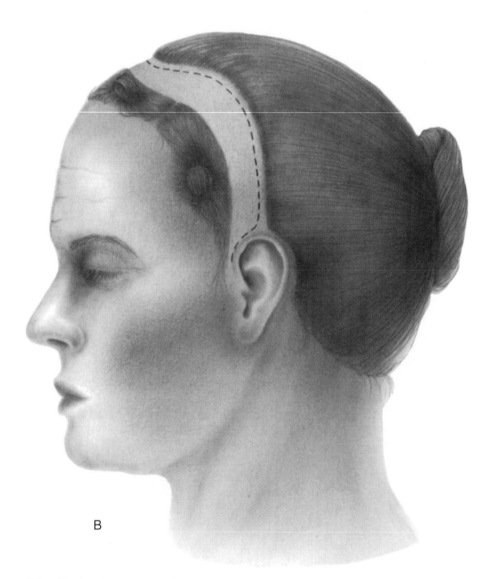

B

B, To achieve maximum exposure, the surgeon may carry the lateral excursions of the incisions to or beyond the tragus in the preauricular crease.

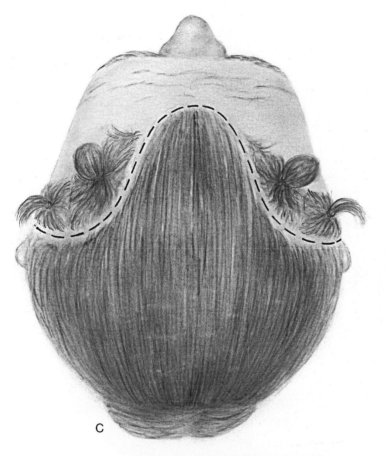

C, To avoid elevation of the widow's peak centrally, the surgeon may design an alternative coronal incision to sweep into the pretrichal extent of the midline hair pattern.

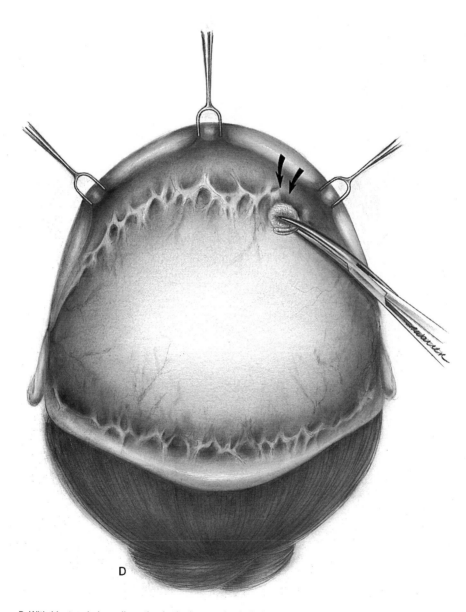

D, With blunt and sharp dissection in the loose subgaleal plane above the periosteum, the forehead-scalp flap is elevated and reflected. Bleeding in this plane is minimal and is effectively controlled by the Shaw hemostatic scalpel.

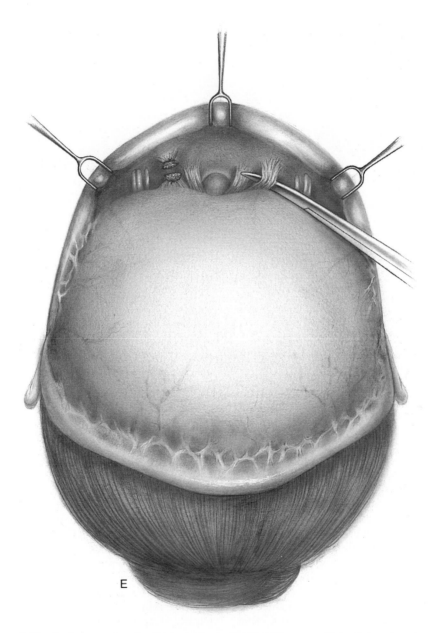

E

E, After the tissues surrounding the neurovascular bundles of the supraorbital complex are spread, blunt dissection with a fine hemostat aids in identifying, isolating, and preserving these important elements while exposing the corrugator muscle bundles for ligation and partial excision.

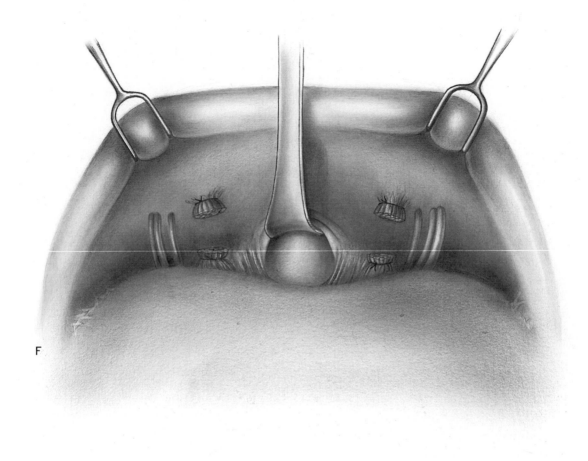

F, Elevation of the dorsal nasal tissues is easily accomplished to lift ptotic nasal tissues or to attenuate the action of the procerus muscle by division and ligation.

marked transverse skin creases on the forehead surface are then visually oriented to the undersurface of the forehead flap. Transverse narrow (0.5-cm) strips of galea, frontalis muscle, and subcutaneous tissue are excised by sharp dissection with the Shaw scalpel or the Bovie cutting cautery, preserving muscle intact laterally at the region of the supraorbital neurovascular bundles (Fig. 27–10*G*). This important resection releases the elastic tension effect of the frontalis muscle on the wrinkled ptotic forehead and is the principal factor in allowing a prolonged reduction of forehead creases. Total elimination of forehead creases should not be expected, however, because animation is preserved.

In most patients, further improvement is gained by incising the periosteum at the supraorbital rim, thus releasing the periosteum and orbital skin for increased upward elevation (Fig. 27–10*H*). After absolute and meticulous hemostasis is achieved, the forehead flap is advanced cephalically and redundant skin is excised segmentally in the hairline (Fig. 27–10*I*); this results in brow and forehead elevation and an immediate improvement in appearance. Before scalp skin is excised, the scalp posterior to the coronal incision should be pushed forward to determine its mobility and elasticity, a factor influencing the amount of skin excised from the forehead flap. Incision closure is relatively rapid, with multiple 3-0 polydioxanone (PDS) buried galeal and dermal

sutures to eliminate all tension, supplemented by surgical staples in the hair-bearing scalp (Fig. 27–10*J*). Drains are rarely necessary.

The coronal forehead lift can be expected to bring about a relatively long-lasting elevation of the entire forehead and brow (Fig. 27–11). Transverse forehead creases and wrinkles are considerably improved but should not be expected to disappear entirely, and normal animation is preserved. Congenitally low-placed brows assume a more normal cephalic position after a forehead lift, as do brows rendered ptotic by the aging process. Brow elevation thus exerts a salutary effect on redundant upper eyelid skin, allowing a more conservative and accurate skin resection during upper lid blepharoplasty. Clearly, deep vertical rhytids are best treated by muscle excision through the forehead lift.

Pretrichal Forehead Lift

An alternative approach to forehead and brow lifting, the pretrichal forehead lift is accomplished by siting the coronal incision at the junction of the hairline and cephalic forehead. Although the resultant scar is theoretically not as well camouflaged as that resulting from the coronal forehead lift, scars located at the junction of two major facial landmarks in the hairline-skin interface

Text continued on page 284

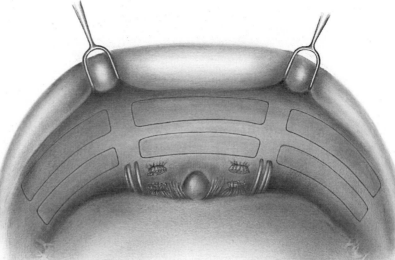

G, Fusiform excisions of the frontalis muscles, sited to conform with the areas of deepest wrinkling on the forehead, are carried out with the Shaw scalpel to reduce muscle bleeding. Generally, in order to preserve sensation, the surgeon does not extend the muscle excisions laterally beyond the level of the pupils and supraorbital nerves.

H, Freeing the forehead flap from the supraorbital regions by elevating the periosteum from the bony orbital rims provides superior elevation of the ultimate brow position.

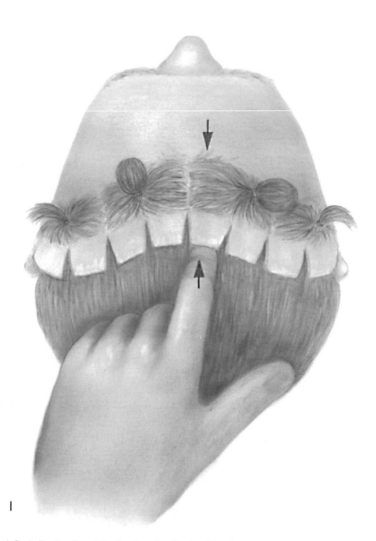

I, Cephalic elevation of the freed, mobile forehead flap is carried out, and the surgeon estimates the amount of redundant skin by manually pushing the cephalic margin of the coronal incision inferiorly, toward the flap edge. The excessive tissue is then excised in segments, and bleeding from the flap edge is controlled progressively with bipolar cautery. The excision must at all times parallel the direction of the hair follicles. Closure follows with multiple subcutaneous buried sutures of 3-0 polydioxanone (PDS) in the galea and dermis to eliminate all tension on the epithelial margins. Final closure of the incision is made with stainless steel skin staples.

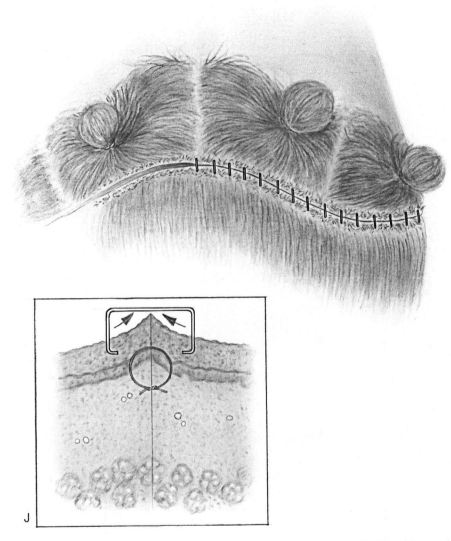

J, Following multiple dermal sutures to evert slim edges and provide stable flap opposition, stainless steel staples provide a rapid, effective scalp closure.

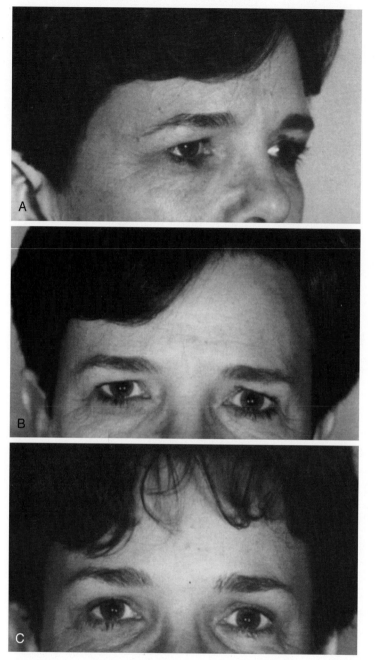

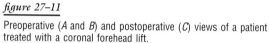

figure 27–11

Preoperative (*A* and *B*) and postoperative (*C*) views of a patient treated with a coronal forehead lift.

ordinarily heal in an inconspicuous manner if meticulously repaired, and the hair can be styled to completely hide the surgical scar. In patients with a more vertical proportion to the forehead, with a high hairline, this approach is useful because it avoids further elevation of the hairline with a consequent increase in forehead height.

Surgical Technique

The incision is made in a curvilinear fashion, following and parallel to the hairs of the frontal hairline. Occasionally, the incision be made irregular with Zs or steps to create an uneven scar, aiding in eventual scar camouflage (Fig. 27–12). Once the subgaleal plane is entered, the operation proceeds in essentially the same manner as in the coronal forehead lift procedure. Meticulous incision closure with dermis-to-dermis interrupted 4-0 polydioxanone sutures followed by a running locked epithelial suture of 6-0 polypropylene (Prolene) is necessary for ideal scar healing. On occasion, reverse beveling of the hairline incision, which separates some of the hairline hair follicles at varying levels, is useful because a portion of the frontal hairline hairs will grow back through the incision, thus improving scar camouflage (Figs. 27–13 to 27–15).

Midforehead Lift

Specific anatomic criteria must be met before the midforehead lift technique is contemplated; only certain

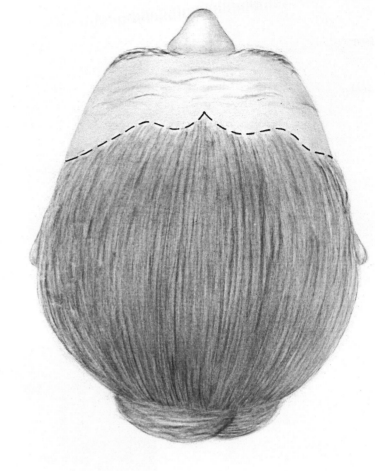

figure 27–12

The surgeon initiates the forehead lift through a pretrichal incision to avoid postoperative elevation of the frontal hairline, thus preserving pleasing forehead-facial proportions.

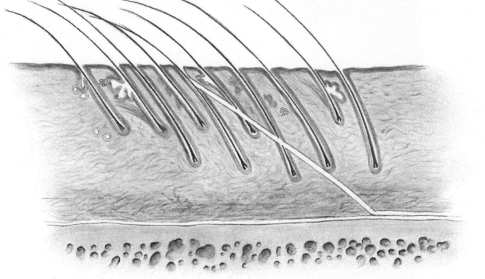

figure 27–13

Reverse beveling of the incision to partially transect several hairline hair follicles allows some eventual hair growth through the resulting scar, thus improving camouflage of the incision.

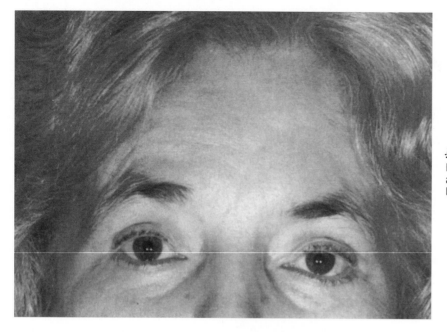

figure 27–14

Favorable healing camouflage of a pretrichal scar as a consequence of reverse beveling of the hair-line incision.

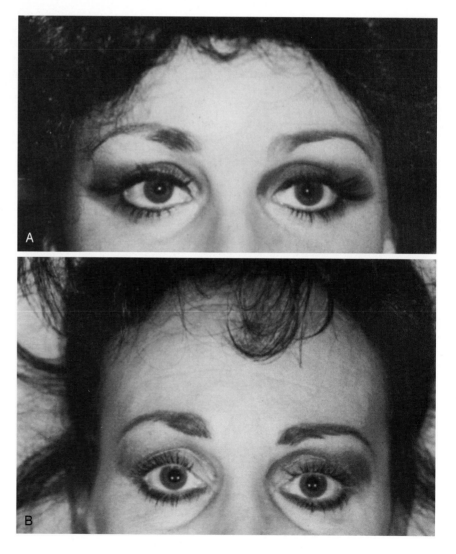

figure 27–15

Preoperative *(A)* and postoperative *(B)* views of a patient treated with a pretrichal forehead lift.

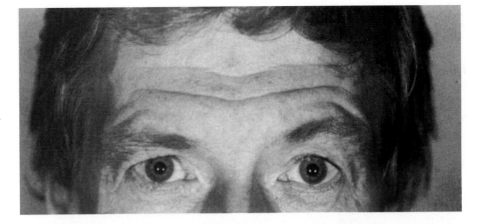

figure 27-16

Typical appearance of deep horizontal forehead rhytids.

patients are good candidates for this approach. A typical patient must possess prominent transverse forehead creases in which the incision and ultimate scar may be hidden (Fig. 27–16). Thinner nonsebaceous skin is preferred over thick, oily, textured skin, for better ultimate scar camouflage. Patients with high or progressively receding hairlines may benefit from this approach because the height of the upper third of the face is slightly reduced after surgery, improving overall facial proportions. Because the incision lies closer to the ptotic brows, more exact repositioning of the desired elevation of brow posture may be possible.

The midforehead lift differs substantially from the coronal and pretrichal forehead lifts, in that the plane of elevation of the flap is created subcutaneously rather than in a subgaleal plane.

Surgical Technique

A high, completely transverse forehead skin crease is selected for incision siting (Fig. 27–17A). The incision depth is limited to the *subcutaneous plane*, initially avoiding penetration of the galea. Creation of an irregular transverse skin incision during closure is useful in certain patients to optimize scar camouflage.

With blunt and sharp dissection using the Shaw he-

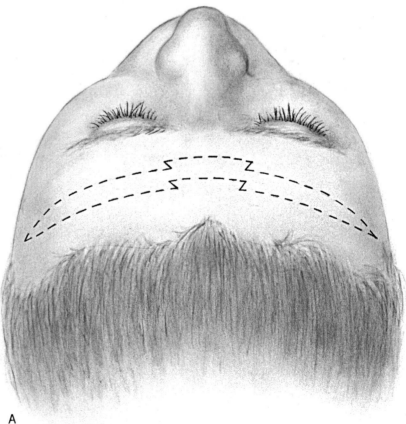

figure 27-17

A, Typical siting of incision within horizontal forehead crease. Making the incision irregular aids the ultimate camouflage of the scar.

A

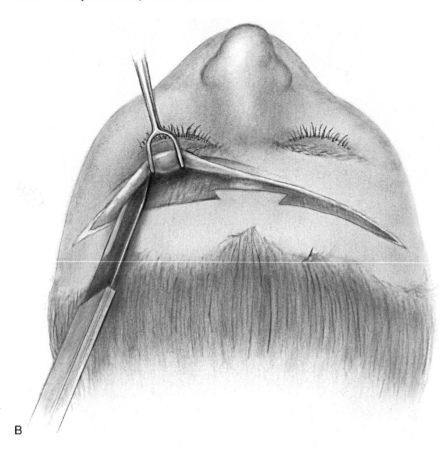

B, Inferior forehead flap elevated in the *subcutaneous tissue plane* with a Shaw hemostatic scapel.

B

mostatic scalpel, the surgeon elevates the inferior subcutaneous flap down to the level of the brow and root of nose (Fig. 27–17*B*). To isolate and resect or attenuate these muscles, the surgeon makes a transverse galeal incision 3 cm above the nasal root, entering the subgaleal plane (Fig. 27–17*C*). This incision must not extend beyond the supraorbital nerves if sensory innervation to the forehead is to be preserved. Meticulous hemostasis is paramount and is usually easily ensured with the hemostatic scalpel. This broad exposure maximizes visualization of the corrugator and procerus muscles (Fig. 27–17*D*), which are treated in the same fashion as in the coronal and pretrichal forehead lift procedures.

Excision of the overactive corrugator and procerus muscles at the glabella is now easily accomplished under direct vision in a manner similar to that described for the coronal forehead lift.

Cephalic subcutaneous elevation of the upper edge of the incision ensues for 1.5–2 cm to evert the skin edge for closure; selected incisions of the paired frontalis muscles are carried out to release overlying deep creases. Before skin closure, the transverse galeal incision is closed, after excision of any excess, with 4-0 polydioxanone sutures (Fig. 27–17*E*). With the inferior flap pulled upward, the amount of redundant skin created by the preferred degree of brow elevation may be accurately estimated and excised (Fig. 27–17*F*). The degree of medial and lateral skin excision may be tailored to create a desirable unequal elevation of asymmetric brows to achieve improved symmetry.

Exacting and meticulous dermal and epidermal suture closure is vital to the success of these techniques. Multiple buried, everting dermal sutures of 5-0 polydioxanone approximate the dermis and prevent even the slightest tension in the everted skin edges (Fig. 27–17*G* and 27–17*H*). Incision closure follows with a 6-0 running polypropylene suture (Fig. 27–17*I*), which is removed in 4–5 days and replaced with antitension skin strips. If the surgeon adheres to the anatomic criteria listed for this procedure in patient selection, a highly acceptable level of scar camouflage may be expected after ultimate healing.

Midforehead Browplasty

Men with ptotic brows and prominent midforehead or suprabrow skin creases are potential candidates for midforehead browplasty. In this procedure, the forehead incisions do not cross the midline and interconnect, further maximizing scar camouflage (Fig. 27–18). Siting incisions in creases at different levels on either side further enhances scar camouflage. Improved brow posture may be realized accurately and effectively with this more limited approach, but deep glabellar and horizontal forehead rhytids are better treated with the other forehead lifting procedures.

Surgical Technique

Forehead creases lying above the lateral aspects of the brows are selected for incision sites; often the second-

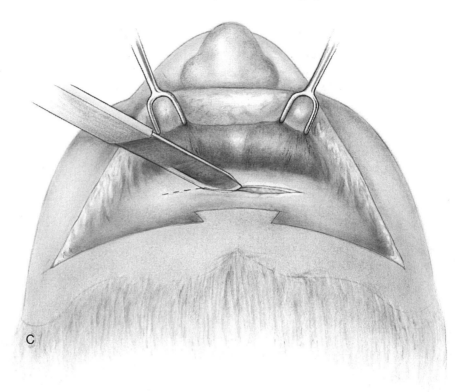

C, Transverse incision in midforehead galea to gain access to glabellar region.

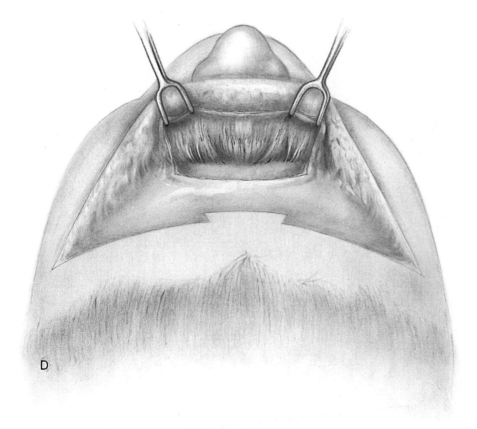

D, Exposure of the corrugator and procerus muscles via a horizontal incision in the galea. Attenuation of the activity of these muscles is accomplished in the same fashion as in the coronal forehead flap approach.

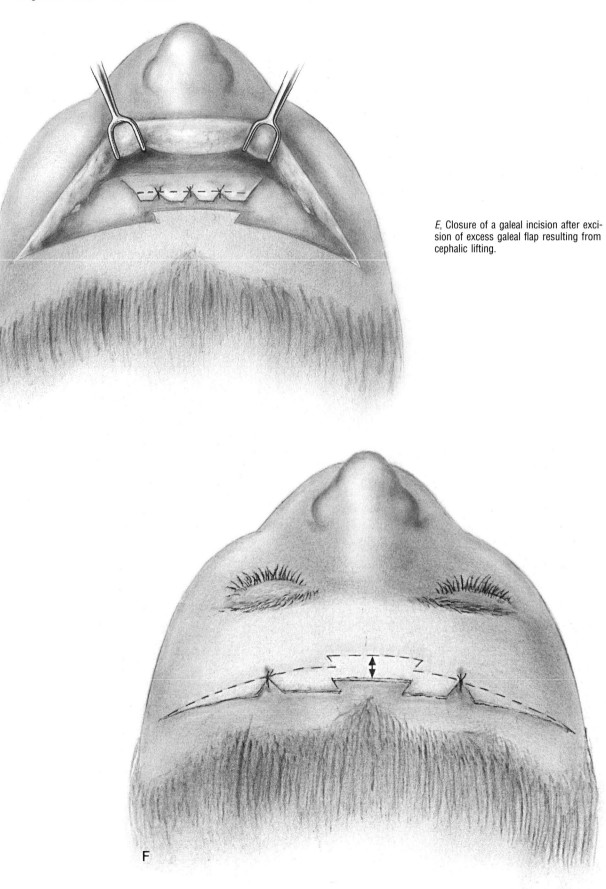

E, Closure of a galeal incision after excision of excess galeal flap resulting from cephalic lifting.

F, Meticulous closure of the skin incision with tension-relieving, buried 4-0 polydioxanone (PDS) sutures in the dermis, followed by closure of the skin with the use of eversion suture techniques and 6-0 polypropylene (Prolene) sutures.

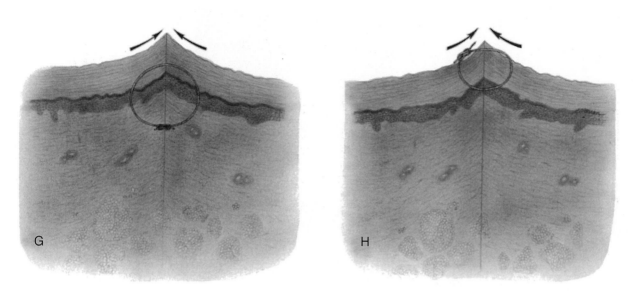

G, Interrupted, buried dermal sutures provide long-term strength of wound closure and facilitate significant hypereversion of the epithelial margins to eliminate the possibility of ultimate scar inversion and widening. *H*, Hypereversion may be facilitated by a series of 6-0 polypropylene sutures, placed without tension in mattress-suture fashion in the epithelial edge.

I, Running continuous intradermal closure of a midforehead lift incision.

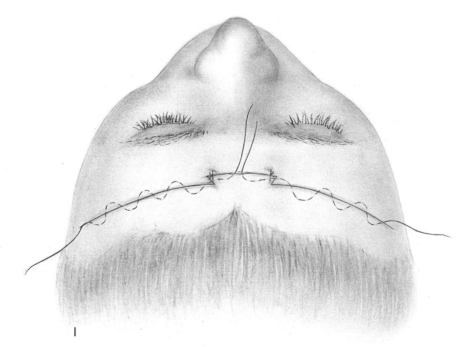

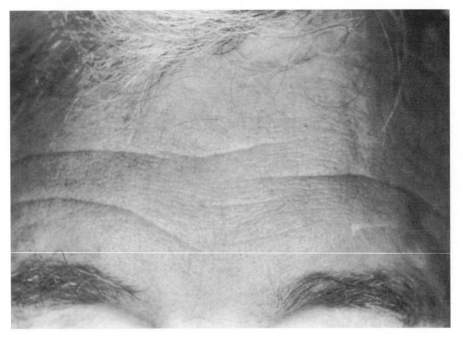

figure 27–18
Asymmetric suprabrow forehead creases, ideal for camouflage of incisions created for midforehead brow lift procedures.

encountered crease is chosen (Fig. 27–19*A*). If possible, incisions should be sited in creases at different levels above either brow because of the potential for superior scar camouflage.

The incision enters the *subcutaneous plane*, and the inferior flap is dissected to the level of the brow or just below, remaining superficial to muscle (Fig. 27–19*B*). If hypertrophic orbicularis muscle exists, selective transverse myectomy is performed. In selected patients, the muscle and dermis of the brow are suspended to periosteum superolaterally with three or four 3-0 nylon (Tevdek) sutures (Fig. 20–19*C*), but this additional maneuver is not always found to be necessary to effect lasting brow elevation. As the brow is retracted to the desired new cephalic position, excessive skin of the inferior flap becomes apparent and is excised (Fig. 27–19*D*).

Meticulous dermis-to-dermis opposition with multi-ple buried interrupted 5-0 polydioxanone sutures closes the wound firmly, followed by skin closure with everting, running 6-0 polypropylene sutures (Fig. 27–19*E*). Early removal of the sutures at 4–5 days prevents development of suture marks.

This procedure is thus quite limited in the treatment of forehead creases by myotomy but is highly effective in fine-tuning the ultimate brow position and shape in preparation for blepharoplasty. In addition, a significant improvement in lateral canthal hooding and temple ptosis results with proper incision placement because the incision generally courses more laterally than in the direct brow lift. At all times, the surgeon must respect the "danger zone" of the region of the frontal facial nerve branch in the temple by avoiding excessive dissection, cautery, and traumatic stretching and manipulation during flap retraction (Fig. 27–20).

Text continued on page 297

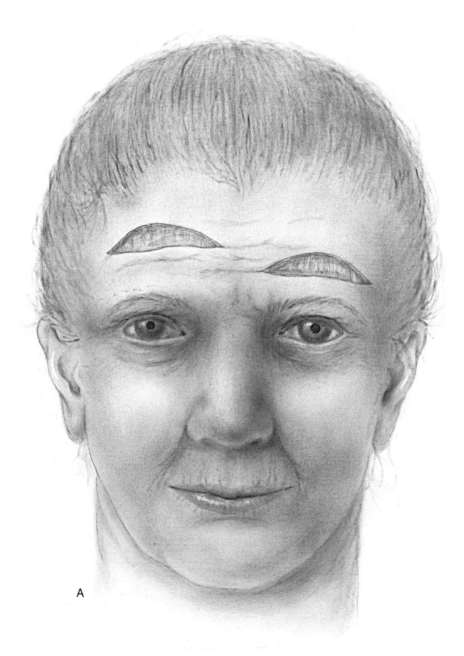

figure 27–19

A, Siting of incisions asymmetrically in midforehead brow creases.

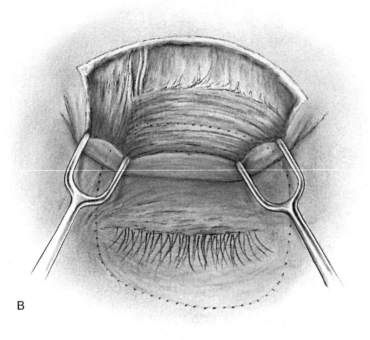

B, Exposure of orbicularis muscle and brow tissues through a midbrow lift approach.

B

C, Brow sutures elevated and suspended to the galea with the use of multiple 3-0 nylon (Tevdek) white sutures.

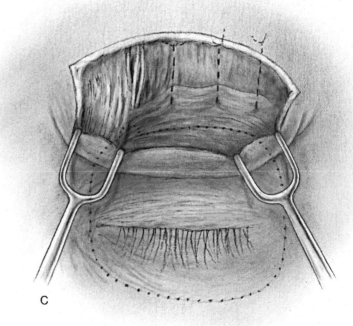

C

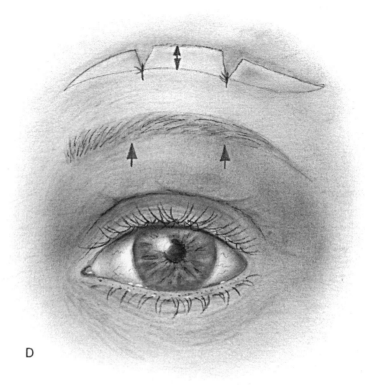

D, Elevation of brow position with resection of excess skin.

D

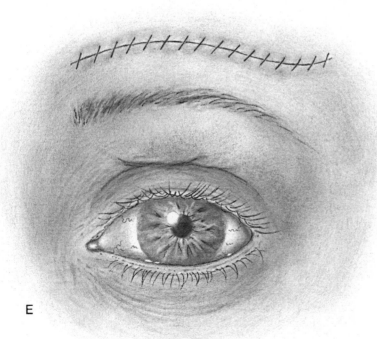

E, Meticulous tension-free incision closure with the brow elevated.

E

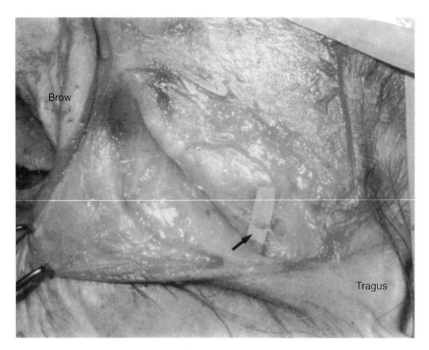

Brow

Tragus

figure 27–20

Dissection of the anatomic location of the frontal branch of the facial nerve.

figure 27–21

Typical example of brow and temple aesthetic ptosis *(A)*, amenable to temporal lift procedure *(B)*.

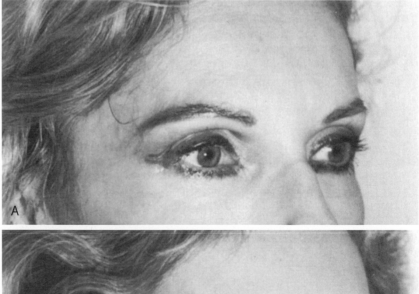

A

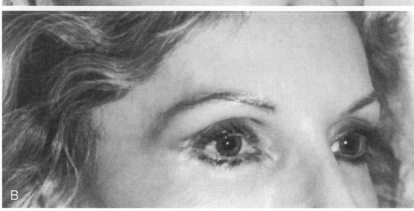

B

Temporal Lift

In selected patients, a lifting force can be applied to the eyelid–brow–lateral canthal aesthetic complex by carrying out an isolated temporal (temple) lift. The patient with early brow ptosis and lateral canthal ptosis and rhytids is a candidate for this approach (Fig. 27–21). We regularly employ this technique in concert with blepharoplasty and facelift in appropriate candidates.

Surgical Technique

The irregular incision is marked approximately 2.5–3.5 cm inside the temporal hairline and carried deep to the level of the hair follicles through the superficial tissues to the level just above the thick, shiny deep temporalis fascia (Fig. 27–22A). The precise geometrics of the irregular incision vary with and are guided by the patient's frontal lateral hairline. With more blunt than sharp dissection, the temporal flap is undermined essentially bloodlessly to just below the level of the static brow and redundant lateral canthal skin (Fig. 27–22B). Because the frontal branch of the facial nerve occupies a very superficial position here within the fascia, blunt dissection progresses under direct vision aided by good fiberoptic lighting. The frontal branch is probably more at risk from stretching or injury from cautery than from careful dissection. The skin is then advanced and rotated slightly (Fig. 27–22C), the excess is trimmed, and closure is completed in the hairline with staples after firm dermis-to-dermis opposition with multiple 4-0 polydioxanone dermal sutures (Fig. 27–22D).

This approach, which in reality is similar to the temporal extension of the traditional rhytidoplasty operation,

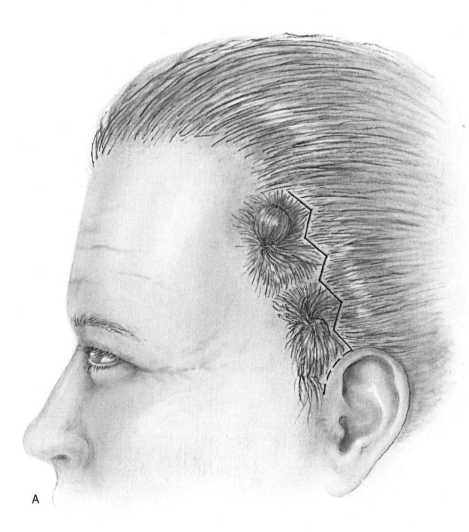

A

figure 27–22

A, The temporal lift incision is sited 2.5–3.5 cm cephalic to the temporal hairline and is made irregular to ensure maximum camouflage of the scar. Precise design of the incision varies from patient to patient according to surgical needs and differing anatomy and hair distribution. Patients should be made aware that a lifting procedure of this design may alter slightly the "double-tuft" anatomic distribution of the temporal hairline.

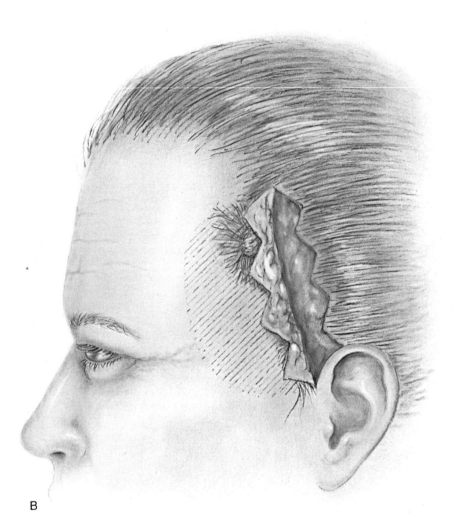

B

B, Blunt dissection in the loose areolar plane just superficial to the deep temporal fascia is carried infero-medially down to the supraorbital rim. At risk in this procedure is the frontal branch of the facial nerve; therefore, cautery and traumatic dissection should be avoided in this crucial area. In the proper plane, the or-bicularis muscle remains attached to the skin flap; if desired and indicated, its lateral margins may be plicated upward to the temporalis fascia.

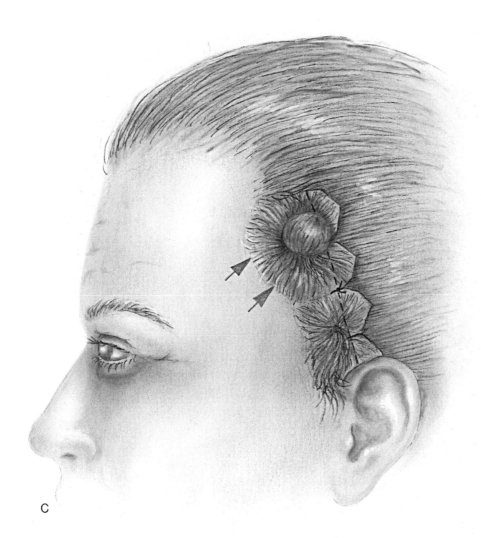

C, Posterocephalic advancement of the flap is carried out, and redundant tissue is excised. Aesthetic improvement of the orbitotemporal unit is immediately apparent. If concurrent upper blepharoplasty is contemplated, the degree and nature of skin removal may now be more accurately planned and executed.

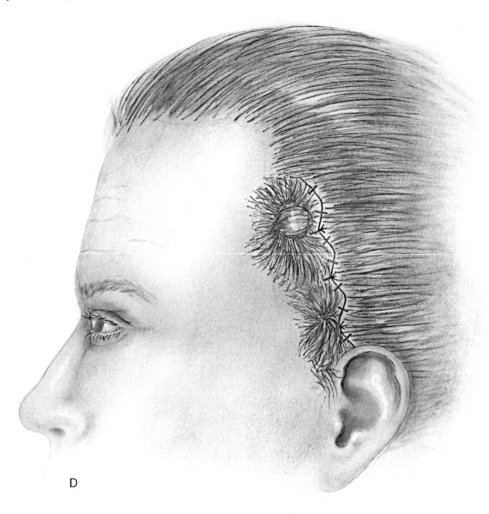

D, Wound closure is accomplished with multiple buried subdermal 4-0 polydioxanone (PDS) sutures to relieve all tension from the wound edges. Final rapid closure with stainless steel skin clips completes the procedure.

produces immediate and favorable elevation of the brows and temples (Fig. 27–23). One result, however, may be that the temporal hairline is slightly elevated. This may be objectionable in some patients with high hairlines or thinning hair and therefore must be discussed in detail with each patient preoperatively.

Direct Brow Lift

The choice of the most appropriate brow-lifting procedure rests on a combination of factors that should be weighed carefully before surgery. The direct brow lift (browplasty), the simplest and most direct approach, possesses significant advantages. The anticipated improvement can be rather accurately demonstrated to the patient preoperatively in a three-way mirror. If asymmet-

ries in brow position (often compounded by unequal frontalis muscle action during animation) exist, symmetric corrections are less difficult to achieve by accurate measurement with this direct approach. The direct brow lift, depending on the geometric pattern of the excision, may allow the selection of a favorable brow elevation in its nasal, middle, or temporal extent, sculpturing the brow position according to a preoperatively determined scheme (Fig. 27–24*A* to 24*C*). Surgical trauma is minimal, as are the recovery and healing processes. The improvement in appearance is immediately apparent.

A direct approach that interrupts the offensive action of the corrugator and procerus muscles is facilitated by medial dissection into the glabella. Fine-tuning the ultimate brow position is easily accomplished in browplasty; no vital motor nerves are at risk in the surgical

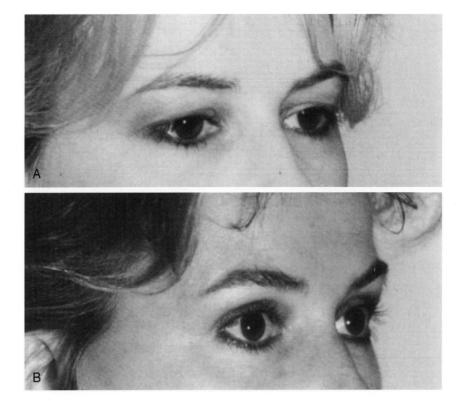

figure 27-23

Example of aesthetic improvement possible after an isolated temporal lift. A, Preoperative appearance. B, Postoperative appearance. Note the improved arch of the lateral eyebrows.

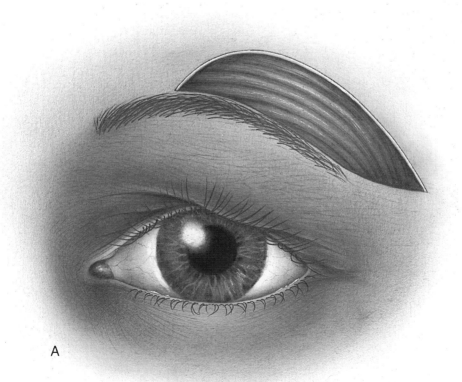

figure 27-24

A-C, The geometrics of the design of the suprabrow skin excision are determined by the final desired postoperative appearance as related to the anatomy of the brow. Many variations are possible, depending on the inclination and aged characteristics of the ptotic brow.

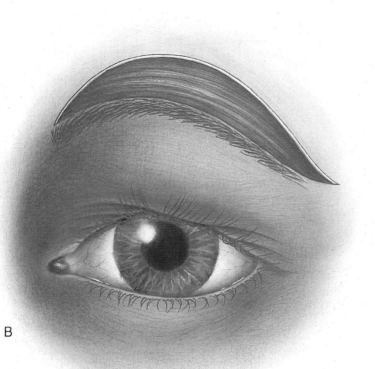

B, Continued

B

C, Continued

C

field, postoperative edema is ordinarily quite minimal, and the intended result is immediately apparent to patient and surgeon alike. If the incision is placed *just inside* the cephalicmost line of brow hairs and carefully repaired with eversion techniques, scar camouflage is generally satisfactory. A thin application of an eyebrow pencil can render the healing scar inconspicuous until nature provides normal scar maturation and obscurity. Combing the brow hair upward temporarily to cover the suprabrow incision aids in early incision camouflage. A drop of hair spray applied to the finger and brushed along the brow keeps brow hairs in a cephalic orientation. (Patients must, however, be willing to accept a lifelong scar at the brow-forehead interface.) Furthermore, subsequent brow lift operations may be carried out, if ever required, through the same incision.

The brow lift operation possesses significant limitations that will influence the surgeon's choice of procedure. Rhytids adjacent to the lateral canthus are improved to only a limited extent by direct browplasty approaches, and then only when the incisions are carried lateral to the hair-bearing brow. Undermining in this area is necessary for even limited improvement, thereby theoretically exposing the frontal temporal branch of the facial nerve at risk. Sensation in the suprabrow area quickly returns to normal.

Surgical Technique

Once the surgeon decides on the brow lift by developing a diagnostic distinction between isolated brow ptosis, temporal ptosis, and redundancy and ptosis of the entire upper face (forehead, temple, and brow), preoperative skin markings are positioned. The patient is evaluated while sitting upright and in facial repose. This position eliminates spurious brow elevation induced by voluntary or involuntary frontalis muscle action, a common circumstance. If manual elevation of the brow improves the upper orbital space and delineates the upper eyelid cleft pleasantly, browpexy is judged to be helpful.

Taking into account and compensating for the commonly encountered brow position asymmetries, the surgeon outlines fusiform patterns above the brow in the forehead skin, placing the site of the intended final scar just within the highest row of brow hairs (see Fig. 27–24). Making the incision irregular with small Zs or incision offsets to conform to the typical uneven distribution of brow hairs adds further finesse to scar camouflage.

Brow lift procedures are best carried out with the patient under local infiltration anesthesia, but incisional and excisional judgments must be finalized and marked before any infiltration distortion, however slight, occurs. Various options of geometric fusiform excisions are available, depending on the individual aging characteristics, the patient's sex, and the patient's preference for appearance. It can be helpful to create a pattern from x-ray film or other sterile suture packages to ensure bilaterally symmetric markings and excisions, although asymmetric brow positions may require asymmetric suprabrow excisions.

After injection, a delay of 10–15 minutes enhances maximum vasoconstriction. The surgeon then creates the initial lowest incision by beveling the scalpel blade obliquely to cut parallel to the shaft of the upper hair follicles, cutting just inside the top row of hairs (Fig. 27–25). Failure to bevel the scalpel blade can lead to hair loss, a visible scar lying slightly cephalic to the intended brow-forehead interface, or both. After the uppermost incision is completed, also beveled obliquely to facilitate a slightly everted skin closure, the circumcised fusiform segment of skin and subcutaneous tissue is excised with sharp knife dissection and the skin edges are undermined only enough to allow an eversion of the wound edges on closure.

If the lateral canthal rhytids are to be improved, the surgeon must superficially separate the skin from the underlying tissue to free the redundant skin from the effect of underlying muscle action. It is generally imprudent to carry any portion of the incision medial to the nasal extent of the brow. Meticulous hemostasis is ensured with a pinpoint bipolar cautery. Excision of orbicularis muscle is ordinarily unnecessary unless the muscle is hypertrophic and thus redundant. If the brow structures are deemed to be loose and excessively mobile, the brow muscle is suspended from the forehead periosteum with multiple 4-0 polypropylene sutures (Fig. 27–26).

The surgeon initiates meticulous closure by advancing both muscle and dermis, closing the dermis with buried everting sutures of 5-0 polydioxanone (see Fig. 27–17*G* and 17*H*). Accurate and fastidious closure of the dermis is a critical element in minimizing the eventual epithelial scar. The buried sutures should be uniformly positioned to effect a complete apposition of the epidermal skin edges, creating a distinct hypereversion to facilitate ultimate development of a mature, flat, thin scar that is camouflaged in the eyebrow-forehead junction. Even slight scar widening, particularly if associated with sufficient scar inversion to create a distinct shadow from incident light, will render the scar less than ideal. Further hypereversion of the closed skin edge with a running 7-0 nylon suture, removed after 4 days to avoid suture marks, ensures a favorable fine nondepressed scar line. If desired, a running intradermal subcuticular monofilament nylon suture may be substituted and left in place for 14 days (Fig. 27–27).

The wounds are dressed with a thin application of neomycin-dexamethasone (NeoDecadron) ophthalmic ointment (Merck & Co., West Point, Pa.). Petroleum gauze and a lightly compressing circumferential dressing are applied for 36–48 hours to diminish edema (Fig. 27–28). Swelling and ecchymosis are minimal if tissue handling has been gentle and hemostasis fastidious.

The direct brow procedure accomplishes a calculated isolated cephalic reposition of the ptotic brow and improves delineation of the infrabrow cleft (Figs. 27–29 and 27–30). If combined with blepharoplasty, the brow lift should always precede the eyelid operation, to avoid creating a permanent lagophthalmos secondary to excessive removal of eyelid skin. Marking the extent of removal of upper eyelid skin always is delayed until dermal closure of brow lift incisions is complete. At this point, the surgeon can accurately assess the degree of redundant eyelid skin and mark it. Anesthetic infiltration of

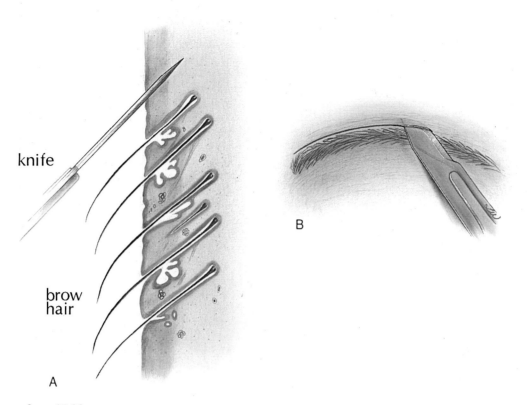

figure 27–25

A, Critical to the aesthetic outcome and scar camouflage in browplasty is the placement of the incision *just inside* the most cephalic row of hairs, with the blade angled and incising parallel to the hair follicle shafts. Because the brow line is often irregular in its hair distribution, the incision may also be sited in a curvilinear or irregular fashion. *B*, Brow lift incision with the blade beveled to parallel the hair follicles.

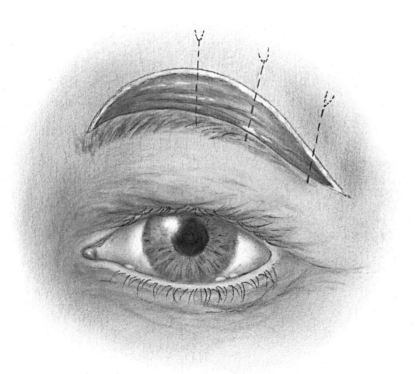

figure 27–26

Permanent suspension sutures (4-0 white braided nylon) from the brow tissues to the suprabrow galea.

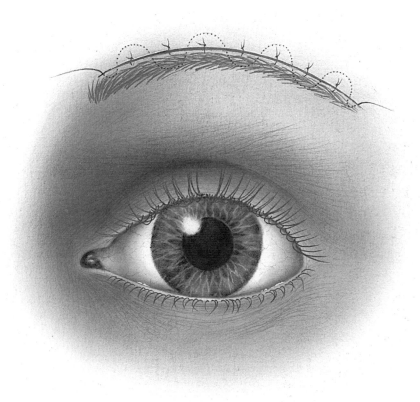

figure 27–27

A suitable alternative in epithelial closure is the running intradermal 6-0 monofilament nylon closure. This running suture may remain in place for as long as the surgeon desires (8 days or longer) without creating telltale suture marks and exerts no everting effort on the epithelial edges.

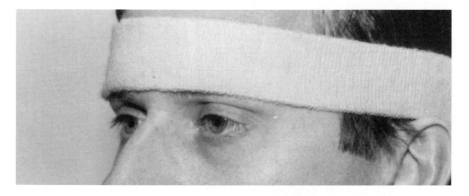

figure 27–28

In selected patients, a gently compressing colored elastic cotton headband serves well as a bandage, allowing early return to work and social activities during the healing process.

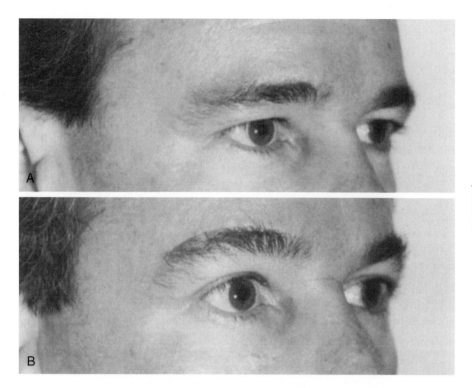

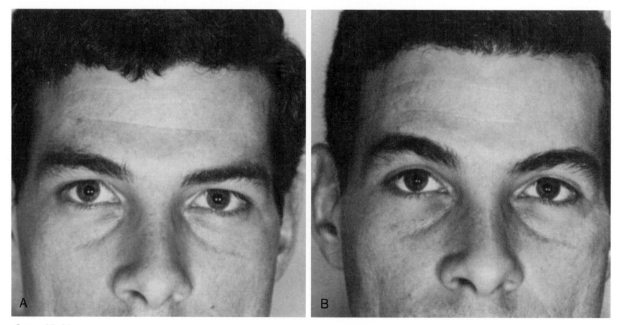

figure 27–29

Favorable improvement of brow position following a direct brow lift. *A*, Preoperative appearance. *B*, Postoperative appearance.

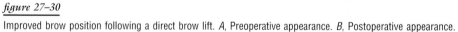

figure 27–30

Improved brow position following a direct brow lift. *A*, Preoperative appearance. *B*, Postoperative appearance.

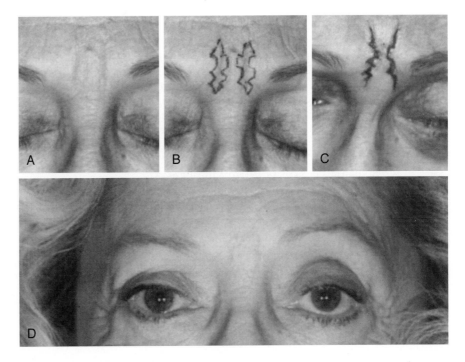

figure 27–31

A, Deep glabellar crease to be excised employing a geometric broken-line pattern to enhance eventual camouflage. *B*, Excision of a deep glabellar rhytid. *C*, Immediate geometric broken-line closure repair. *D*, Result obtained following a glabellar rhytid repair.

the eyelid then ensues, followed by final brow closure and then blepharoplasty.

Glabellar Creases

Glabellar creases may be modified through the brow lift approach by carrying the dissection into the midforehead subcutaneously to free the skin from the underlying muscles. Insertions of the corrugator muscles are delineated and elevated with a sharp periosteal elevator, and the muscle bellies are divided or partially resected to attenuate their crease-producing action. The synergistic action of the procerus muscle is similarly eliminated by isolating it with dissecting forceps and dividing or even avulsing its cephalic portion. Improvement in the glabellar rhytids may be expected, but total elimination of eventual glabellar creases is problematic at best.

Patients with excessively deep glabellar creases also require a direct surgical crease resection with scar camouflage technique (Fig. 27–31) in addition to the muscle attenuation techniques. A geometric broken line excision with closure facilitates camouflage, effectively and immediately effacing deep creases.

Light dermabrasion of the glabellar area 3–6 months later often complements the final effect; injectable collagen placed in the dermis temporarily effaces the superficial (but not deep) glabellar creases.[14] Either of these modalities may be carried out at the time of the glabellar muscle resection.

COMPLICATIONS AND SEQUELAE

A variety of complications are possible after forehead and brow-lifting procedures (Table 27–3).[15] Because the scalp and forehead are well vascularized and the technical procedures quite straightforward, complications are rare.

The most serious complication, requiring immediate drainage and wound exploration, is undoubtedly a postoperative expanding hematoma. Flap necrosis can occur if hemostasis is not immediately secured. No expanding hematoma has occurred in the several hundred patients we have operated on in the past 30 years.

Facial nerve injury is rare and, if experienced, is usually transient, the consequence of excess flap stretching (tension) or thermal cautery. Our lone case of nerve paresis, which developed immediately after a bilateral temporal lift, was judged to result from thermal injury

table 27–3

Possible Complications of Forehead and Brow-Lifting Procedures

Hematoma	Neuralgia
Flap necrosis	Incision pruritis
Infection	Widened or depressed scar
Alopecia	Scar depigmentation
Seventh nerve paresis	Brow asymmetry
Scalp hypesthesia	Elevated hairline
Scalp paresthesia	Abnormal soft-tissue contours

to the frontal branch of the facial nerve; function returned in 6 weeks.

All patients undergoing forehead lifting procedures experience hypesthesia of the scalp postoperatively, and they should be warned of this condition before surgery. Return of sensation is highly variable and may require from 6 weeks to 6 months to approach normal. We have never encountered a case of permanent forehead or scalp hypesthesia.

Revision of widened or depressed scars has been necessary in fewer than 5 per cent of patients in our series. Light dermabrasion may be useful several weeks after surgery to further camouflage scars.

References

1. Brennan GH: Aesthetic Facial Surgery. New York, Raven Press, 1991.
2. Tardy ME: Surgical Anatomy of the Nose. New York, Raven Press, 1990.
3. Tardy ME, Thomas R: Aesthetic Facial Surgery. St. Louis, Mosby-Year Book, 1995.
4. Becker FF, Johnson CM, Smith O: Surgical treatment of the upper third of the aging face. In Papel I, Nachlas N (eds): Facial Plastic and Reconstructive Surgery, pp 147–157. St. Louis, Mosby-Year Book, 1992.
5. Brennan GH: The forehead lift. Otolaryngol Clin North Am 1980; 13:209.
6. Kaye BL: The forehead lift. Plast Reconstr Surg 1977; 60:161–170.
7. Webster RC, Fanous N, Smith RC: Blepharoplasty: When to combine it with brow, temple, or coronal lift. J Otolaryngol 1979; 8:339–343.
8. Gleason MC: Brow lifting through a temporal scalp approach. Plast Reconstr Surg 1973; 52:141–144.
9. Castanares S: Forehead wrinkles, glabellar frown and ptosis of the eyebrows. Plast Reconstr Surg 1964; 34:406.
10. Pitanguy I: Indications and treatment of frontal and glabellar wrinkles in an analysis of 3,404 consecutive cases of rhytidectomy. Plast Reconstr Surg 1981; 67:157–166.
11. Spira M: Blepharoplasty. Clin Plast Surg 1978; 5:121–137.
12. Rafaty FM: Elimination of glabellar frown lines. Arch Otolaryngol 1981; 107:428–430.
13. Tardy ME, Parras G, Schwartz M: Aesthetic surgery of the face. Dermatol Clin North Am 1991; 9:169–187.
14. Stegman SJ, Tromovitch TA: Implantation of collagen for depressed scars. Dermatol Surg Oncol 1980; 6:450–453.
15. Baker TJ, Gordon HL, Stuzin JM: Surgical Rejuvenation of the Face. St. Louis, Mosby-Year Book, 1996.

Gregory S. Keller
Robert Hutcherson

Endoscopy-Assisted Small-Incision Forehead and Brow Lift

Endoscopy-assisted small-incision forehead and brow lifts are gaining popularity. The alternative technique of a coronal brow lift is unappealing to many patients because they view it as invasive. Most patients like the idea that their skin and hair are not being removed through the small-incision technique and that the procedure is being done with an endoscope, which they know from other surgical procedures in the body is usually less invasive.

It has been my experience that the endoscopy-assisted forehead and brow lift can achieve mild lifting of the forehead and brow, which in most patients is enough. It also is a good technique for patients who have asymmetric brow positions, which then lead to asymmetric upper lid skin folds. In these cases, the technique not only achieves more brow symmetry but also leads to more symmetric upper eyelid creases and folds, which are difficult to achieve without dealing with elevation of the forehead and brow.

Gregory Keller has had extensive experience with this technique and has performed it probably longer than most other surgeons. He and Robert Hutcherson graphically describe this procedure.

For the most part, I have been performing small-incision, endoscopy-assisted forehead lifts through a scalp approach and an upper blepharoplasty approach. My addendum to this chapter elaborates on my technique and contrasts it to that of the authors.

I believe that patients should be apprised that they may suffer hair loss around the incision sites with this procedure. In most cases, the hair grows back and patients find this acceptable.

ALLEN M. PUTTERMAN

Coronal and pretrichal forehead and brow-lifting techniques have provided surgeons with effective methods of brow elevation and removal of forehead wrinkles; however, these techniques carry a significant morbidity that is unappealing to many patients (see Chapter 27). Much of this morbidity has been linked to the size of the incision. Significant scarring, hair loss, numbness of the posterior scalp, and frontotemporal recession (even in pretrichal patients) are sequelae that cause many patients to reject forehead procedures that are otherwise bountiful in their rejuvenative capabilities.

Alternate treatments of brow ptosis have included direct browplasty, midforehead lifting techniques, and transblepharoplasty brow suspensions (see Chapters 12 and 27). Although useful in certain instances, these techniques often leave unacceptable scars or, in the case of transblepharoplasty brow suspension, are useful only for certain patients.

Endoscopic forehead and brow-lifting techniques, originally conceived of as laser-assisted procedures, were first introduced in 1991.[1-4] Since then, these procedures have been progressively refined and nonlaser techniques have been introduced.[5-27]

The primary advantage of these procedures is that they use smaller incisions in the frontal area that are minimally invasive compared with the larger incisions used in other techniques. The use of an endoscope or telescope enables the surgeon to work at a distance from the incisions.

INSTRUMENTATION

The Optical Chain

The endoscopic system (Fig. 28–1) is an "optical chain" consisting of the following:

1. A light source and the fiberoptic light delivery system, which is used to illuminate the object being imaged.
2. An endoscope, which carries a fiberoptic light delivery system and contains lenses to view the imaged object.
3. A camera with a device to couple it to the endoscope, which is used to transmit an electronic signal of the imaged object.
4. A central processing unit (CPU) to decode the signal received from the camera and send it to the monitor.
5. A monitor or viewing station to visualize the image.

Recent advances in endoscopes have allowed a digitalization of the image, so that it can be visualized more sharply.

It is important that all the components of the optical chain be engineered so that they produce an image that is always uniformly illuminated (without white "hot spots"), sharp, and in focus. The integration of these components by the engineers is what separates excellent systems from those that are barely usable. Because a detailed explanation of the optical chain is beyond the scope of this chapter, the reader is referred elsewhere for a clear and concise summary of this topic.[28]

History

The field of endoscopic surgery was begun by Nitzi, who in 1879 (1 year after Thomas Edison harnessed electricity) developed the first lighted cystoscope, a large primitive device. At the turn of the century, an otolaryngologist, Chevalier Jackson, developed distally lighted telescopes with small incandescent bulbs that could be miniaturized sufficiently for bronchoesophagology.

Although H. H. Hopkins, a British physicist, developed the Hopkins rod telescope in 1950, it did not find its way into general use until the 1970s. This device, which is in common use today, uses a system of glass rods, separated by air lenses. A fiberoptic light delivery system is integrated into the telescope so that the object can be illuminated and visualized through the same instrument.

The increased illumination, improved field of vision, and better contrast achieved with the Hopkins rod endoscope allowed the size of the telescope to be decreased so that access to smaller areas became possible. In addition, the lens system of the Hopkins rod telescope allows the surgeon to view magnified images of objects, making it an illuminated "telemicroscope."

Modern Instruments

Whereas smaller-diameter telescopes are possible, the 4-mm 30° endoscope is the one most commonly used for

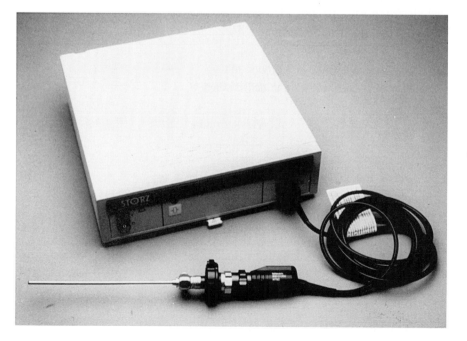

figure 28–1

A portion of the optical chain: Hopkins rod lens telescope, coupler, camera, and central processing unit. (Courtesy of Karl Storz International.)

facial plastic surgery applications today, particularly for the endoscopic brow lift. The 4-mm caliber is small enough to fit through small incisions and to be easily maneuvered around the optical cavity that the surgeon creates in the frontal and temporal regions, leaving room for instrumentation. The 4-mm size is also large enough to carry enough light to illuminate and visualize the relatively dark cavities, provided that sufficient engineering of the optical chain has been incorporated into the system.

Because there is no naturally occurring cavity in the forehead, the surgeon must create a cavity between the fascial layers of both the forehead and temple. A 30° telescope is used with a retractor sheath or system so that the surgeon can hold the overlying scalp out of the way, while visualizing the dissection field straight ahead.

Many surgeons, including one of us (G. S. K), have devised special instruments for the endoscopic brow lift, and the instrumentation has recently evolved. For the blind undermining over the frontal areas, the shape of the head of the instrument is the most important. This instrument must be turned downward at almost right angles, so that the periosteum can be dissected off the frontal bone. The shaft of the instrument should be straight or slightly curved.

For dissection over the temporal area, a straight or slightly curved dissector is preferable for dissecting the layers of temporal fascia apart (Fig. 28–2). Use of a straight endoscopic sheath with a flare to produce a wide, unrestricted field of view is helpful.

For dissection over the orbital rim, many surgeons have devised orbital rim dissectors. These usually have slightly curved shafts with heads that angle downward.

Recently, orbital dissection sheaths that allow the surgeon to dissect the periosteum over and in the area of the orbital rim have been devised. These sheaths allow the surgeon to visualize and dissect through one port and, because of their angulation, are especially helpful in patients with high foreheads.

To release the muscles of facial expression, we use long endoscopic scissors or a carbon dioxide laser with a thin, flexible waveguide (Fig. 28–3). The wide-angle sheath is used for visualization. Other surgeons use insulated endoscopic grasping forceps to coagulate and tear the muscles apart.

For coagulation of bleeding vessels, we use an insulated endoscopic suction bipolar cautery and pull the bleeding vessel away from the overlying skin. When the surgeon aims downward, or in protected areas, an insulated suction cautery can be useful and expedient. Other surgeons use endoscopic grasping forceps to pull the bleeding vessel away from the skin surface and to cauterize it (see Fig. 28–3).

PATIENT EVALUATION

With normal aging, relaxation of the forehead and descent of the brow cause a hooding of eyelid skin over the eye. The lateral brow, in particular, falls downward, producing lateral hooding that can extend past the lateral canthus and even past the lateral bony orbital rim. When hooding extends past the lateral canthus, brow descent should be assumed to exist. Brow lifting, particularly of the lateral brow (or brow "tail"), then becomes necessary to achieve an aesthetically pleasing eye.

The glabella and forehead also show signs of aging. Downward descent of the midbrow and medial brow occurs when the muscles that pull the brow downward and inward (corrugator, procerus, depressor supercilii, and orbicularis oculi) overcome their antagonists, which elevate the brow (occipitalis-galea-frontalis sling) (see Chapter 7).

Patients with brows that have descended frequently elevate them artificially as they open their eyes, producing horizontal lines across the forehead. These "brow elevators"[29] will lose their horizontal lines when their brows are surgically elevated. The brow position on

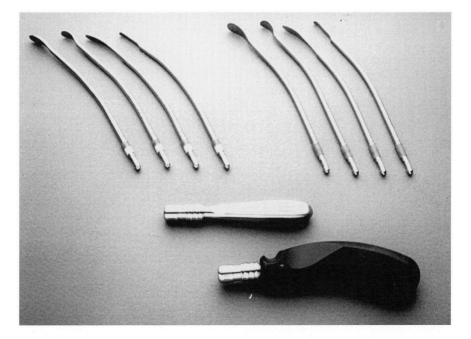

figure 28–2

Dissectors used for endoscopic facial plastic surgery. (Courtesy of Karl Storz International.)

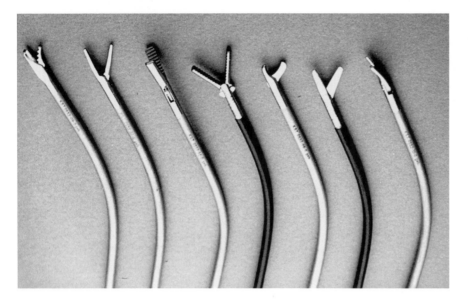

figure 28–3

Scissors, graspers, and bipolar coagulators used for endoscopic facial plastic surgery. (Courtesy of Karl Storz International.)

preoperative and postoperative photographs, however, will often appear the same (except that the forehead lines are gone) if the surgeon has not taken photographs with the patient's eyes closed, when the patient cannot elevate the brow.

"Frowners and squinters,"[29] by contrast, may have prominent vertical glabellar lines that are present from a relatively early age. These patients require special attention to release and deactivate the corrugator, depressor supercilii, and procerus muscles.

The frame height[30] and brow glide[31] indices are often used for the assessment of patients. The frame height is defined as the distance from the midpupil to the top of the brow. Brow ptosis is considered to exist if the frame height is less than 2.5 cm.

The brow glide test takes three successive measurements of brow excursion. While lifting the brow, the examiner takes measurements of maximal excursion of the medial, central, and lateral portions of the brow from the neutral position. Because the test is difficult to reproduce, measurements are taken three times and averaged.

The average brow glide is between 1 and 2 cm. Greater amounts of brow glide are seen in older Caucasians. Lesser amounts are observed in young Asians and African-Americans.[31]

SURGICAL TECHNIQUE

A spectrum of anesthesia types can be used, depending on the patient. A local anesthetic with supraorbital and supratrochlear nerve blocks may be used for the calm, accepting, and well-prepared patient. For most patients, however, either monitored anesthesia or general anesthesia, administered by an anesthesiologist and augmented by a local and nerve block injection, is preferable.

The local anesthesia consists of supraorbital and supratrochlear nerve blocks bilaterally and a "ring" block. Fifteen milliliters of lidocaine (Xylocaine) with epineph-

rine (1 per cent) and 15 ml of bupivacaine (Marcaine) (0.25 per cent) are mixed together and used for the blocks. Following this, the entire area is infiltrated with a tumescent anesthesia such as Klein's solution[32] (1000 ml normal saline, 12 ml sodium bicarbonate, and 1 ml of a 1:1000 solution of adrenaline) using a hydrodissection pump (Klein pump, Wells Johnson, Tucson, Ariz.).

After anesthesia, all endoscopic brow procedures use the following stages or components, albeit in different manners: (1) use of small incisions, (2) construction of an optical cavity, (3) release of periosteum and muscles, and (4) elevation and fixation of the brow.[33]

Use of Small Incisions

The use of small incisions that parallel the course of the supraorbital and supratrochlear nerves avoids the large incisions seen with pretrichal and coronal forehead lifting techniques. These incisions are quite difficult to find, do not change the hairline or hairline pattern, and preserve the sensation to the scalp (Fig. 28–4).

Four incisions over the frontal bone are constructed in vertical fashion in between the hairs. They are placed 1 cm behind the hairline and are 1 cm long.

The two medial frontal incisions are placed in the vertical plane of each medial brow. The two lateral frontal incisions are placed at the juncture of thick frontal hair and temporal thinning hair close to the temporal line. The temporal line is the juncture point at which the temporalis muscle and fascia meet the frontal bone. It is a palpable ridge where the soft temporalis muscle meets the hard bone. After an incision with a knife through the scalp skin that extends past the hair bulbs, a small self-retaining retractor is placed in the incision and the incision is carried down to the bone with a laser or a Colorado needle (see Chapters 35 and 36).

Two diagonal temporal incisions are then placed in the line where the surgeon would construct a facelift. The facelift incision is made in a line parallel to the anterior hairline, beginning at a point just posterior to the helical crus (root of the helix). The top of the two diagonal temporal incisions is over the superior portion of the temporal muscle. The midpoint of these incisions is located at the horizontal plane of the bony superior orbital rim. These temporal incisions are often extended to 2 cm in length if the hair is reasonably thick.

If a facelift is not performed, two diagonal temporal incisions are placed parallel to the anterior hairline and 2–3 cm behind it. One can find the midpoint of the 2-cm incision by drawing a line that begins at the nasal ala and extends through the lateral canthus until it intersects the prospective incision.

The incisions are beveled at an angle to preserve the hair bulbs and are carried downward to the temporoparietal fascia. The temperoparietal fascia is a bluish white layer that moves with the skin when the skin is pulled backward.

The temporoparietal fascia is then incised until the gleaming silver-white deep temporal fascia is seen. The deep temporal fascia does not move when the skin is grasped and pulled.

Creation of the Optical Cavity

In the forehead, there are no naturally occurring cavities for the placement of an endoscope, as there are in other parts of the body (e.g., the nose for sinoscopy or the bladder for cystoscopy). Consequently, an optical cavity must be constructed within the fascial layers of the forehead and temple (see Fig. 28–4). Creation of the optical cavity proceeds in three stages:

- Blind dissection over the frontal and parietal bones
- Temporal dissection
- Joining of the frontal and temporal dissections

Blind Dissection Over Frontal and Parietal Bones

For most procedures, the optical cavity over the frontal bone is created blindly in the subperiosteal plane until the plane of the brow is encountered, whereupon the dissection becomes supraperiosteal. A short elevator, with its tip angled downward at 80°, is placed into the right lateral incision, and the subperiosteal plane is gently uncovered with scraping and prying movements. By subperiosteal dissection through each of the four frontal incisions, the elevation is carried backward to the occiput, inferiorly and laterally over the parietal bone, and downward toward the brow. The surgeon should avoid blind dissection of a small area (2 cm above the central brow) in order to avoid the shearing off of a supraorbital nerve that emerges from a foramen above the bony rim in about 20 per cent of the cases.

In the central area, over the glabella, a restriction of the elevator's movement will be felt at approximately

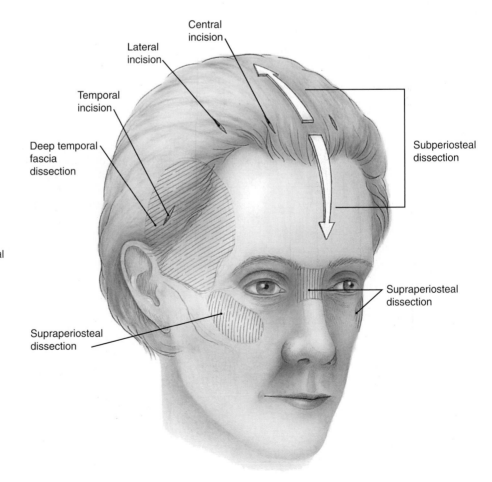

figure 28–4

Typical endoscopic incisions and optical cavity dissection planes.

the level of the brow. This point is at the origin of the corrugator muscles. The elevation is brought superficially at this point and extended supraperiosteally over the nose. The elevator is insinuated between the origins of the corrugator muscles with twisting motions, until a pop is felt into the supraperiosteal plane over the glabella and nose.

Temporal Dissection

Attention is then turned to the creation of the optical cavity over the temporalis muscle, the zygomatic process of the frontal bone, the frontal process of the zygomatic bone, and the malar eminence (see Chapter 7). The posterior edge of the temporal incision edge is grasped and pulled upward. The elevator is then used to lift the areolar tissue (innominate fascia) from the deep temporal fascia posteriorly, until bone is felt. A subperiosteal sweeping dissection over the temporoparietal and frontal areas is used to connect the temporal incision with the lateral frontal incision.

The anterior edge of the temporal incision is then grasped and pulled upward. The areolar tissue (innominate fascia) is separated from the deep temporal fascia to a point corresponding to the anterior edge of the hairline.

The endoscope and elevator are placed in the temporal incision (Fig. 28–5A), and the innominate fascia is then elevated and separated from the deep temporal fascia in a diagonal direction toward the malar eminence. Above the dissection, through a fascial layer, is the temporoparietal fat pad, which is yellow. As the dissection extends inferiorly to the level of the brow, a yellowish tinge may be seen in the deep temporal fascia. This represents the superficial fat pad, which sits between the superficial and deep layers of the deep temporal fascia.

At the level of the frontozygomatic suture, and about 1 cm lateral to it, a prominent vein can be seen. This vein, the "sentinel vein," is a branch of the zygomaticotemporal vein (Fig. 28–5B). As this vein proceeds superiorly, a branch can be seen about 1 cm lateral to the tail of the brow. This vein is a reliable marker for the facial nerve, which is just lateral to the vein.[34] As the surgeon dissects medially and inferiorly to the vein over the frontal process of the zygoma and the malar eminence in a supraperiosteal plane, another branch of the zygomaticotemporal vein, accompanied by a sensory nerve, is encountered immediately lateral to the malar eminence. Normally, identification of this second vein marks the inferiormost margin of the dissection. Occasionally, the dissection must be more extensive in order to free up the temple. In this case, the surgeon should proceed medial to the vein over the malar bone so that the zygomaticus muscle can be identified.

If the surgeon must free up the temple extensively, he or she should proceed laterally along the zygomatic arch so that another branch of the zygomaticotemporal vein can be identified. By gently pushing upward with the elevator along the vein, the surgeon can identify a nerve that does not accompany the vein but proceeds in a diagonal direction over the zygomatic arch. This nerve represents the frontal branch of the facial nerve.

With the elevator and endoscope turned laterally, the plane over the deep temporalis fascia is developed to the frontal bone. The areolar tissue (innominate fascia) is pushed upward until the frontal bone can be palpated beneath the elevator.

Joining the Frontal and Temporal Optical Cavities

The fusion of the galea and the temporoparietal fascia is termed the *conjoint fascia*. The conjoint fascia over the bone is pushed upward, and the elevator is inserted onto

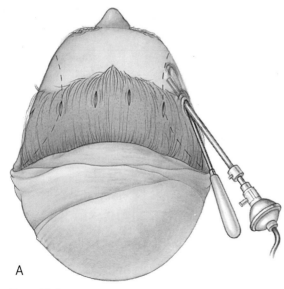

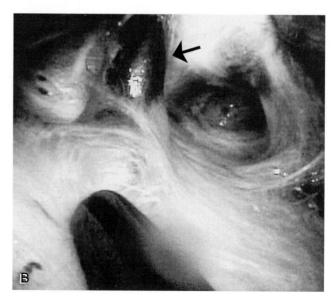

figure 28–5

A, Dissector and endoscope through temporal incision.

B, Dissection over superficial layer of the deep temporalis fascia. The sentinel vein *(arrow)* is seen just lateral to the frontozygomatic suture.

the bone at a point approximately 7 cm above the brow. If the surgeon initially elevates the periosteum 7 cm above the brow, the facial nerve is avoided while the periosteal plane is found.

The periosteum is then sharply elevated from the frontal bone at the temporal line, connecting the frontal and temporal cavities. The periosteal dissection proceeds inferiorly along the temporal line until a resistance to further dissection is felt at about the level of the brow. This thickening of the periosteum is termed the conjoint tendon and often contains a communicating vein, which is cauterized with the bipolar cautery. Approximately 1 cm lateral to this vein, a branch of the frontal nerve may be reliably identified in or immediately beneath the temporoparietal fat pad.[34]

The conjoint tendon is then incised sharply over the bone with the elevator or scissors. This maneuver connects the supraperiosteal dissection over the zygomatic process of the frontal bone with the subperiosteal dissection over the remainder of the frontal bone. An adequate release of the conjoint tendon is an essential part of the release of the tail of the brow.

Release of the Periosteum and Depressor Muscles

The release of the periosteum, galea, and depressor muscles (corrugator, procerus, orbicularis oculi, and depressor supercilii) is one of the most important aspects of the endoscopic brow procedure. Releasing the attachments of the brow allows the frontalis-galeal-occipitalis sling to exert a backward force on the brow and to smooth out the scalp posterior to the fixation points (Fig. 28–6).

The lack of a thorough release of the periosteum and depressor muscles is probably the most common reason that endoscopic forehead and brow procedures fail. The tail of the brow, in particular, can be elevated only when a complete release is performed.

The release of the periosteum and depressor muscles can be divided into three sections:

1. Periosteal release with exposure of the supraorbital nerve.
2. Release of the central musculature medial to the supraorbital nerve.
3. Release of the orbicularis oculi muscle lateral to the supraorbital nerve.

Careful attention to each of these steps is essential.

Periosteal Release With Exposure of the Supraorbital Nerve

The first part of this procedure, the release of the conjoint tendon, is completed with the joining of the frontal and temporal optical cavities, as described earlier. After this step, either a two-handed or a one-handed technique may be used.

In the one-handed technique, a dissecting sheath is placed into the lateral frontal incision. In the two-handed technique, the visualization sheath and telescope are placed in the central frontal incision and the dissecting instruments are placed in the lateral frontal incision.

The periosteum is then dissected to the orbital rim. As the rim is seen in the midpupillary area, supraorbital nerves that emerge from a foramen are visualized (Fig. 28–7). These may all emerge from a large foramen, or only a smaller, lateral branch may emerge from a foramen and the larger medial branch may sprout from a notch below the orbital rim. All supraorbital branches are preserved, whether or not they emerge from a foramen or a notch.

The periosteal dissection is continued over the lateral orbital rim. The dissector is then used to pry the arcus

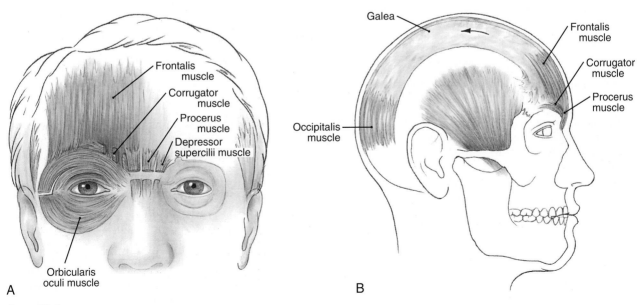

A

B

figure 28–6

A and B, When the brow depressors are released, the frontalis-galeal-occipitalis sling exerts upward traction on the brow.

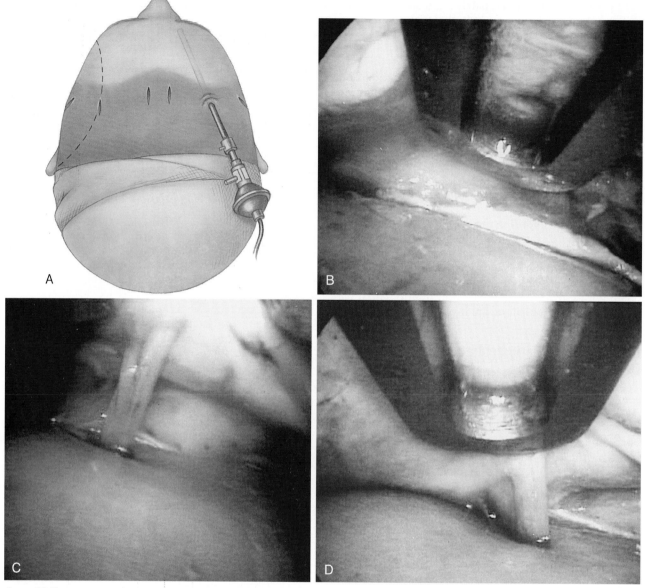

figure 28-7

A, Dissection over the frontal bone, with the dissecting sheath through the lateral incision.

B, Endoscopic photograph of dissection over the frontal bone.

C and D, The supraorbital nerve, emerging from a foramen above the orbital rim, is identified.

marginalis upward and to expose roof fat. As the surgeon continues in this plane medially, the supraorbital nerves that emerge from a notch below the rim are identified.

Medial to the supraorbital nerve, the periosteum is swept from the corrugator muscle with the elevator. The corrugator is identified as it attaches to the frontal bone between the brows. In this area, the subperiosteal dissection has transitioned to a supraperiosteal one and extends over the nose. Thus, the procerus muscle is already free of periosteum.

Two sets of veins can be identified at this point. The medialmost veins are branches of the facial and lateral nasal veins. The more lateral veins are branches of the supraorbital and supratrochlear veins (see Chapter 7).

By cauterizing these veins at this point in the procedure, the surgeon can prevent a great deal of troublesome bleeding. These veins can be cauterized with bipolar cautery because there is a significant amount of muscle mass between the veins and the skin.

Release of Central Musculature Medial to the Supraorbital Nerve

The muscles are incised. In order to avoid depressions where the muscle was taken, we do not remove muscle with forceps. The muscle incisions may be performed with either endoscopic scissors or a laser. If a laser with an endoscopic hand piece is available, use of the laser results in less patient bruising and ecchymosis.

The procerus muscle is incised horizontally (see Fig. 28–6). Most commonly, this incision is placed low, at a point corresponding to the nasion. This technique prevents a retraction of the corrugator into the nasion, producing a blunting of the nasal frontal angle.

If there is a nasal hump or a too-deep nasofrontal angle, the horizontal procerus incision may be placed high. This maneuver allows the corrugator muscle to retract into the nasion, blunting the nasal frontal angle or filling in the nasion above the nasal hump, thereby diminishing it.

The corrugator muscle is then incised, and the supratrochlear nerves are identified. These nerves are behind the corrugator muscle and in front of the depressor muscle (Fig. 28–8).

The supratrochlear nerves are distributed in many different ways. Two methods of distribution are the most common. If the surgeon sees a prominent stalk emerging and then branching, he or she may assume that the supratrochlear nerve emerges from its own foramen or notch (see Fig. 28-8). If multiple branches of the supratrochlear nerve are seen, the surgeon can assume that the nerve emerges from the same notch as the supraorbital nerve and rapidly gives off branches in all directions. In either case, it is desirable to preserve all branches of the nerve.

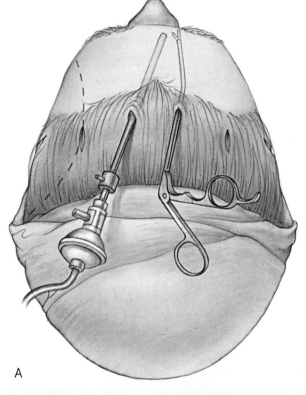

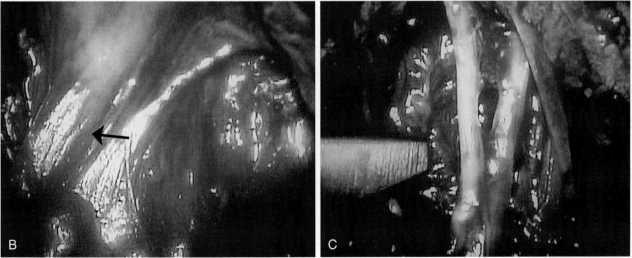

figure 28–8

A, Muscle release dissection. The endoscope is shown through the left central incision with an instrument through the right central incision.

B, Corrugator muscle *(arrow).*

C, Dissection of corrugator muscle demonstrating the supratrochlear nerve.

The corrugator muscle travels in front of the supra-trochlear nerves. Muscle that is behind the supratroch-lear nerve is the depressor supercilii. Muscle that is between the supratrochlear nerve and the supraorbital nerve is the corrugator.

Incision and release of both of these muscles is com-pleted medial to the supraorbital nerve and below the orbital rim (see Fig. 28–6). If the incision of these muscles is incomplete, stumps of muscle contraction may appear. If muscle resection and removal occurs, depressions may be seen as the swelling diminishes.

If there are prominent vertical glabellar rhytids and hypertrophic musculature, the musculature surrounding the rhytids must be cross-hatched to weaken it. Superior dissection of the nerve is first accomplished vertically through the muscle. Horizontal incision of the muscles can then be completed, with direct visualization of the nerves enabling the surgeon to avoid the nerves.

Release of Orbicularis Muscle Lateral to the Supraorbital Nerve

If at this point in the procedure the forehead is retracted upward from the lateral hairline, the tail of the brow will be tethered to some degree. If the orbicularis muscle is incised, the tail of the brow will retract freely.

Lateral to the supraorbital nerve, a horizontal incision below the bony rim is made in the orbicularis (see Fig. 28-6). This incision is carried vertically medial to the rim along its curve. A horizontal incision is made at the lower lateral portion of the rim, onto the malar emi-nence. At the junction of the malar eminence and the zygomatic arch, some adhesions may exist, which need to be lysed.

This incision creates a release of the lateral orbicularis, which can then retract upward. This release frees the tail of the brow for upward fixation.

Elevation and Fixation of the Brow

After release of the depressor muscles and periosteum, the brows are free for fixation. Although there are many methods of fixation, the most common is the method of screw fixation described (originally described by Isse[9]). A screw is placed into the outer table of the frontal bone at the lateral frontal incision. The screw is placed a predetermined distance (usually 5–15 mm) from the anterior margin of the incision. The distance from the anterior incision is equal to the amount of brow eleva-tion desired multiplied by a factor of 1.2. The incision is then pulled backward with a skin hook, and a staple bridging the incision is placed in back of the screw to hold the upward fixation (Fig. 28–9). Except in unusual circumstances, screws are not placed in the central inci-sions. They are usually unnecessary if the muscle release is adequate. The brow should elevate by the temporalis muscle pull. If screws are placed in the central incisions, they sometimes can lead to a sad look, with the central brow becoming higher than the lateral tail.

The placement of the screw, in the lateral frontal incision at the junction of the frontal bone and temporal line, provides the maximum upward pull at the level of the tail of the brow. The tail of the brow requires the most support, because it is the portion of the brow that is not pulled upward by the frontalis muscle.

An additional fixation is provided at the temple inci-sion. The anterior margin of the incision is pulled back-ward, and the temporoparietal fascia is sutured to the deep temporal fascia with a 4-0 polypropylene (Prolene) suture at the point of fixation. This maneuver fixates the temporal and lateral brow position.

For patients with an unstable tail of the brow (older patients with a great deal of brow glide) or patients who would like to change the shape of their sagging lateral brow, a suspension suture can be used to stabilize the tail of the brow. The suspension suture is placed from the orbicularis oculi muscle under the tail of the brow to the deep temporal fascia. To avoid a pucker at the brow level, the surgeon should not pull this suspension suture tight. The suture is not used to elevate the brow; it is used only to stabilize a brow tail that has a high probability of descent.

Achieving a satisfactory result is most difficult in pa-tients with unstable brow tails. These patients should be appropriately counseled before the operation about possible outcomes.

ALTERNATE SMALL-INCISION TECHNIQUES

Even though the endoscope provides excellent visualiza-tion and surgical precision, numerous authors, including ourselves, have used small-incision techniques without the laser. Two of the most common of these small-incision techniques are (1) the retrograde blepharoplasty technique and (2) the central horizontal incision tech-nique.

In the retrograde blepharoplasty technique, an upper blepharoplasty is first performed (see Chapter 10). Dis-section medially under the orbicularis leads to the corru-gator muscle, whose origin is medial to the brow and whose insertion is in the skin, anterior to the supraor-bital nerve and posterior to the supratrochlear nerve.

By marking the origin of the supraorbital nerve (by palpating the notch), the surgeon can take down the corrugator muscle. Care must be taken to preserve the various branches of the nerve. Medial dissection can then reveal the supratrochlear nerve branches.

The incision or removal of the medial muscle bundles is relatively more difficult. Blind dissection and incision can lead to troublesome bleeding from the veins in this area.

Further dissection under the orbicularis muscle later-ally leads to the bony rim. The lateral orbicularis can also be released.

If brow elevation is desired, small vertical incisions can be placed and blind dissection over the frontalis, occipital, and parietal bones can be performed in the manner described above.

A larger temporal incision can then be made, and under direct vision or magnification the temporalis dis-section can proceed, with the surgeon connecting the temporalis and frontalis optical cavities as described ear-lier.

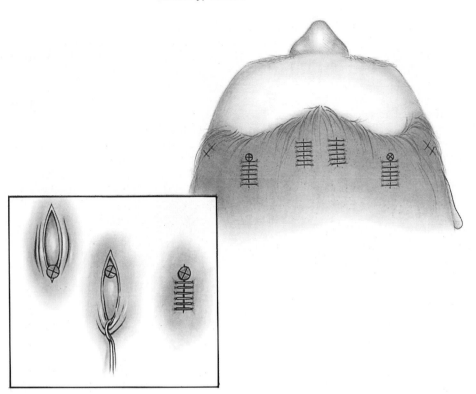

figure 28-9

Upward fixation of the brow is maintained by pulling the incision backward and using a screw to stabilize the upward movement.

Alternately, a larger horizontal incision can be made in the midfrontal area, behind the hairline. With the use of lighted retractors and magnification (loupes), the corrugator, procerus, and occipitalis muscles can be identified and modified.

Although these techniques are useful, they do not provide the direct visual control that the endoscopic techniques afford for muscle dissection. Portions of the medial musculature are invisible through this approach. Connections of the blepharoplasty to the frontal and temporal optical cavities are also associated with increased ecchymosis and adhesions. To combat the possibility of adhesions and removal of muscle, fat and fascia grafts must be used as fillers.

POSTOPERATIVE CARE

After the operation, a drain is commonly placed and a bulky pressure dressing is worn for 24 hours. The patient sleeps sitting up in a semi-Fowler's position for 72 hours and wears a headband for pressure. Strenuous activity is restricted for 3 weeks. Postoperative pain is usually minimal, and mild analgesics usually suffice.

COMPLICATIONS

Side effects and complications can occur. These complications seem to occur less often than with larger-incision forehead lifting procedures.

Seroma, ecchymosis, numbness, paresis, stitch abscess, relapse of brow ptosis, neuropraxia of the temporal branch of the facial nerve, skin burns from cautery, transient alopecia, hematoma, hypertrophic scars, irregularities, pruritus, and asymmetric brows have all been reported as side effects and/or complications. The authors[35-38] reported them as temporary and relatively minor compared with those caused by the larger-incision procedures (e.g., alopecia might consist of a 1–2 cm patch rather than involving a great deal of the frontal scalp). It was of great significance that no permanent injury of the facial nerve was reported.

It has been our experience, as well as that of other surgeons,[35] that complications are fewer and less severe than those after larger-incision procedures. This is logical, in that the endoscopic lift avoids large incisions, with the resulting supraorbital nerve interruptions, hair-bearing scalp resections, and flap tension of the standard operations.

RESULTS

Endoscopic brow-lifting procedures have supplanted open coronal and pretrichal techniques in our practices. We believe that endoscopic techniques allow us to tailor brow shape, forehead size, and brow elevation. The ability to precisely alter the muscles of facial expression to eliminate glabellar and brow wrinkles is unsurpassed when these muscles can be viewed under the 10× magnification provided by the endoscope (Fig. 28–10).

In a survey of plastic surgeons, most believed that their ability to achieve results comparable to those with coronal forehead lifting improved as they achieved familiarity with endoscopic techniques.[35] Two thirds of surgeons surveyed believed that they could achieve better control of the brow with an open technique but that

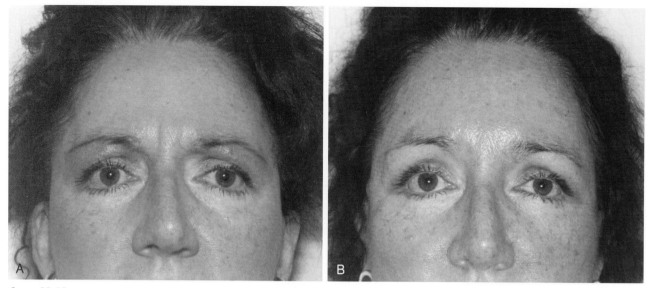

figure 28–10

Patient before *(A)* and after *(B)* endoscopic forehead and brow-lifting procedures.

the morbidity associated with this procedure was unacceptable. The conclusion of two thirds of the surgeons surveyed was that patients tolerated the endoscopic procedures better than open coronal or pretrichal procedures. For this reason, two thirds of the surveyed surgeons shifted to endoscopic techniques after only 1 year of experience with them.

PUTTERMAN UPPER BLEPHAROPLASTY APPROACH TO ENDOSCOPIC FOREHEAD AND BROW LIFT

In this chapter, Drs. Keller and Hutcherson have indicated their preference for lifting the forehead and brows solely through incisions in the scalp. In their subsection, "Alternative Small-Incision Techniques," the authors mentioned the possibility of accomplishing much of this procedure through an upper blepharoplasty incision. Since the upper blepharoplasty approach has become my standard technique except in rare instances, I decided to describe it here.

Surgical Technique

I make four central incisions as described by the authors. In addition, I make two temporal incisions; they are made vertically rather than horizontally, as described by the authors (Fig. 28–11*A*). The positions of these temporal incisions are made in alignment with the nasal alar base and corresponding lateral canthus extending into the hairline.

My dissection of the subgaleal and subperiosteal space through these incisions is similar to that of the authors. I perform the dissection, usually without the endoscope, to a position 3 cm above the brows.

I then proceed with an upper blepharoplasty with

excision of skin and orbicularis muscle but without invasion of the orbital septum, according to the technique I describe in the addendum to Chapter 12, "Internal Brow Lift." I then dissect under orbicularis muscle and over orbital septum to the level of the superior orbital rim.

I expose the superior orbital rim periosteum by retracting the skin and orbicularis muscle upward with a large Desmarres retractor. A No. 15 Bard-Parker blade is used to make an incision over the superior orbital rim periosteum temporal to the supraorbital notch (Fig. 28–11*B*). This incision is also extended over the superior lateral orbital rim. The sharp edge of a Tenzel periosteal elevator is used to dissect periosteum from the superior orbital rim, and the blunt end of the retractor is used to dissect periosteum from frontal bone until this periosteal dissection meets the previous downward dissection that had been accomplished through the scalp incisions (Fig. 28–11*C*). I take care to avoid the area of the supraorbital nerve and notch while dissecting periosteum nasally by staying at least 1 cm above the areas of the superior orbital notch in case the nerve is exiting above the superior orbital rim.

I use a small Desmarres retractor to retract the skin-orbicularis flap superiorly and nasally while cotton-tipped applicators isolate the corrugator muscles (see Chapter 43). The corrugator muscle is severed through the upper blepharoplasty approach.

At this point, the endoscope is inserted through the scalp incisions to allow for further dissection of periosteum around the supraorbital nerve and the areas above the nose. Any periosteum that has not been detached from the inferior aspect of the subperiosteal dissection is released, as described by Drs. Keller and Hutcherson.

I move the forehead and brow back and stabilize them with the two screws that the authors describe, but I also place two screws over the left and right central incisions. I pull the incision sites backward with a skin

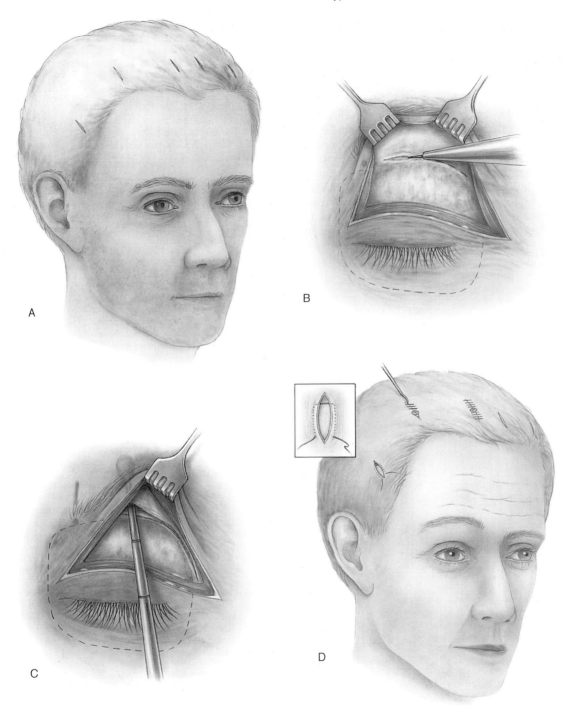

figure 28–11

A, Six 1.5-cm incisions are made beginning 1–1.5 cm posterior to the hairline. The central two incisions are 1.5 cm from the midline. The temporal incisions are made directly above the lateral canthus and are oblique, being more temporal posteriorly than anteriorly. The temporal brow incisions are made in alignment with the nasal alar base and the corresponding lateral canthus.

B, After excision of the eyelid skin and orbicularis oculi muscle and dissection of the suborbicularis superiorly, the periosteum is severed over the superior orbital rim.

C, Periosteum is reflected over the superior orbital rim and then superiorly over the frontal bone to meet the previous dissection from the scalp incisions.

D, A skin hook is used to retract the central four incisions backward to allow placement of a screw at the posterior aspect of the incision site. Several staples are placed behind the screw to connect the incisions while the skin hook holds the posterior incision backward under slight tension. Additional staples are placed behind the screw. The forehead and brow elevation is monitored by having the patient sit up on the operating table. The temporal brow is elevated by passing a 3-0 black silk suture through the anterior edges of skin and hair and posterior deep temporal fascia *(inset).*

hook in order to place a screw at the posterior aspect of the incision site. I place staples in back of this screw, while pulling the wound backward, to further elevate the lid (Fig. 28–11*D*).[39] The patient is seated up during these procedures so that the brow elevation can be titrated according to a technique I previously describe. I elevate the temporal incision with a 3-0 black silk suture placed through posterior temporalis fascia and then through the anterior skin edges.

After elevation of the forehead and brows and incision of the corrugator and procerus muscles, the upper eyelid crease is reconstructed. The orbital septum is opened, orbital fat is excised, and the upper eyelid crease and skin closure are performed according to the steps outlined in my modification of the internal brow lift (see Chapter 12).

Complications

Small areas of hair loss occurred around the four central incisions in approximately 50 per cent of patients. This resolved without surgery, with topical application of minoxidil (Rogaine). Additionally, a few patients noted numbness above the nose in the area of the supratrochlear nerves.

Results

My modification of the small-incision forehead and brow lift has been performed in more than 30 patients with good results.

References

1. Keller GS: U.S. Patent No. 5,370,642: Endoscopic facial plastic surgery, 1994.
2. Keller GS: Small incision frontal rhytidectomy with the KTP laser. Presented at the American Academy of Cosmetic Surgery World Congress, October 13, 1991, Scottsdale, Ariz.
3. Keller GS: Use of the KTP laser in cosmetic surgery. Am J Cosmetic Surg 1992; 9:177–180.
4. Keller GS: Endolaser excision of glabellar frown lines and forehead rhytids. Presented at the American Academy of Facial Plastic and Reconstructive Surgery meeting, February 1, 1992, Los Angeles.
5. Core GB, Vasconez LO, Askren C, et al.: Coronal face-lift with endoscopic techniques. Plast Surg Forum 1992; 15:227–228.
6. Liang M, Narayanan K: Endoscopic ablation of the frontalis and corrugator muscles—a clinical study. Plast Surg Forum 1992; 15:58–60.
7. Keller GS, Razum N.: Small incision laser lift for forehead creases and glabellar furrows. Arch Otolaryngol Head Neck Surg 1993; 119:632–635.
8. Keller GS: KTP laser rhytidectomy. Facial Plast Surg Clin North Am 1993; 1(2):153–162.
9. Isse NG: Endoscopic facial rejuvenation: Endoforehead, the functional lift. Aesthetic Plast Surg 1994; 18:21–29.
10. Daniel RK, Ramirez OM: Endoscopic-assisted aesthetic surgery. Aesthetic Surg 1994;14:14.
11. Ramirez OM: Endoscopic options in facial rejuvenation: An overview. Aesthetic Plast Surg 1994; 18:141–147.
12. Ramirez OM: Endoscopic full face lift. Aesthetic Plast Surg 1994; 18:363–371.
13. Fodor PB: Endoscopic plastic surgery: A new milestone in plastic surgery (editorial). Aesthetic Plast Surg 1994; 18:31–32.
14. Toledo LS: Video-endoscopic facelift. Aesthetic Plast Surg 1994; 18:149–152.
15. Chajchir A: Endoscopic subperiosteal forehead lift. Aesthetic Plast Surg 1994; 18:269–274.
16. Vasconez LO, Core GB, Gamboa-Bobadilla M, et al.: Endoscopic techniques in coronal brow lifting. Plast Reconstr Surg 1994; 94:788–793.
17. Keller GS, Cray J: Laser-assisted surgery of the aging face. Facial Plast Surg Clin North Am 1995; 3(3):319–341.
18. Nahai F, Eaves F, Bostwick J: Forehead lift and glabellar frown lines. In Bostwick J, Eaves F, Nahai F (eds): Endoscopic Plastic Surgery, pp 166–230. St. Louis, Quality Medical Publishing, 1995.
19. Core GB, Vasconez LO, Graham HD III: Development and current status of endoscopic browlifting. Clin Plast Surg 1995; 22:619–631.
20. Graham HD, Core G: Endoscopic forehead lifting using fixation sutures. In Friedman M (ed): Operative Techniques in Otolaryngology-Head and Neck Surgery, vol 6, No. 4, pp 245–252. Philadelphia, WB Saunders Co, 1995.
21. Matarasso A, Matarasso SL: Endoscopic surgical correction of glabellar creases. Dermatol Surg 1995; 211:695–700.
22. Ramirez OM: Endoscopically assisted biplanar forehead lift. Plast Reconstr Surg 1995; 96:323–333.
23. Song IC, Pozner JN, Sadeh AE, et al.: Endoscopic-assisted recontouring of the facial skeleton: The forehead. Ann Plast Surg 1995; 34:323–325.
24. Fuente del Campo A: Subperiosteal facelift: Open and endoscopic approach. Aesth Plast Surg 1995; 19:149–160.
25. Hamas RS: Reducing the subconscious frown by endoscopic resection of the corrugator muscles. Aesthetic Plast Surg 1995; 19:21–25.
26. Aiache A: Endoface-lift: Subcutaneous approach. In Ramirez O, Daniel R (eds): Endoscopic Plastic Surgery. New York, Springer-Verlag, 1996.
27. Abramo AC: Forehead rhytidoplasty: Endoscopic approach. Plast Reconstr Surg 1995; 95:1170–1177.
28. Keller GS (ed): Endoscopic Facial Plastic Surgery, pp 34–40. St. Louis, Mosby-Year Book, 1997.
29. Ellis DA, Masai H: The effect of facial animation on the aging upper half of the face. Arch Otolaryngol Head Neck Surg 1989; 1155:710–713.
30. McKinney P, Mossie RD, Zukowski ML: Criteria for the forehead lift. Aesthetic Plast Surg 1991; 15:141–147.
31. Sasaki G: Brow ptosis. In Sasaki G (ed): Endoscopic, Aesthetic, and Reconstructive Surgery, pp 19–28. Philadelphia, Lippincott-Raven, 1996.
32. Klein JA: Tumescent technique for regional anesthesia. J Dermatol Surg Oncol 1990; 16:248–263.
33. Keller G, Hutcherson R: Endoscope forehead and brow lift. In Keller G (ed): Endoscopic Facial Plastic Surgery, pp 46–70. St. Louis, Mosby-Year Book, 1997.
34. Nahai F: Interdisciplinary approaches to facial rejuvenation. Harvard University course, Vail, Colo, March 1996.
35. Sasaki G: Questionnaire analysis for endoscopic forehead lift procedures. In Sasaki G (ed): Endoscopic, Aesthetic, and Reconstructive Surgery, pp 72–89. Philadelphia, Lippincott-Raven, 1996.
36. Fodor P, Isse N (eds): Endoscopically Assisted Aesthetic Plastic Surgery, pp 57–61. St. Louis, Mosby-Year Book, 1996.
37. Bostwick J, Eaves F, Nahai F (eds): Endoscopic Plastic Surgery, pp 78–79, 228–229. St. Louis, Quality Medical Publishing, 1995.
38. Ramirez O, Daniel R (eds): Endoscopic Plastic Surgery, pp 65–67. New York, Springer-Verlag, 1996.
39. Putterman AM: Intraoperatively controlled-incision forehead and brow lift. Plast Reconstr Surg 1997; 100:262–266.

Jonathan A. Hoenig
Henry I. Baylis
David M. Morrow

Chapter **29**

Simplified Face and Neck Lift

Face lifting may not seem to be an understandable extension of this text, unlike the other new areas of treatment, including laser resurfacing, subperiosteal cheek lifts, and forehead and brow lifts, which perhaps have a greater impact on the eyelids. More and more patients, however, want to have a facelift along with a cosmetic blepharoplasty. Although face lifting is new territory for ophthalmologists, most oculoplastic surgeons who are building a cosmetic practice must consider performing facelifts. Therefore, I believe this book would be incomplete without including information about face lifting.

Multiple face-lifting techniques exist, including deep plane facelifts. I felt it was important to keep this chapter simple and introductory. Consequently, it describes an approach to performing facelifts that should not be too difficult for most oculoplastic surgeons to master and one that can be performed with minimal chances of complications.

Jonathan Hoenig, Henry Baylis, and David Morrow have created an outstanding chapter on simplified face and neck lifting. They give an overview of facial anatomy, as specifically related to this surgery, and describe facial aging changes, patient evaluation, and patient selection. The main thrust of the description of the procedure includes incision planning, neck dissection, liposuction, platysmaplasty, skin undermining, tightening of the superficial musculoaponeurotic system (SMAS), and skin resection. The authors also concisely describe possible complications and how to handle them.

I believe that this chapter will help oculoplastic surgeons expand their armamentarium of techniques.

ALLEN M. PUTTERMAN

Oculoplastic surgeons are increasingly expanding their horizons and venturing outside the traditional periorbital domain. Many routinely perform aesthetic midfacial lifts, total facial skin resurfacing, and even face lifting. As patients have become increasingly educated in the varied ways to forestall and reverse the aging process, more are requesting face-lifting and neck-lifting procedures. There are numerous procedures that rejuvenate the aging face. Obviously, it is beyond the scope of this chapter to attempt to describe them all. The goal of this chapter is to describe a safe and relatively simple technique to correct the structural defects that occur in the aging face. The technique described is by no means

exclusive, and we do not mean to imply that this is the best face-lifting technique. However, it is a starting point and hopefully the first of many techniques that you will employ in your armamentarium of rhytidectomy procedures.

FACIAL ANATOMY

An understanding of the anatomy of the face and neck is critically important for any surgeon performing cosmetic surgery in this region. We advise surgeons who are novices in performing facelifts to learn the anatomy by studying facial anatomy texts in combination with fresh-cadaver dissections.[1] The following is a brief review of the pertinent surgical anatomy of the face.

The facial soft tissue is arranged in concentric layers: skin, subcutaneous fat, SMAS, mimetic muscles, deep facial fascia, and a plane containing the facial nerve and parotid duct. The skin and subcutaneous layer vary in thickness throughout the face. The skin is thinnest in the eyelids and thickest in the cheek. The subcutis is composed of various amounts of adipose tissue, lobulated by thin fibrous septa called the retinacula cutis.[2] These septa connect the dermis to the underlying fasciae and muscles. The interlacing septa are often perpendicular or oblique to the skin surface. In the lip region, the dermis is directly in contact with the orbicularis oris muscle and subcutaneous fat is minimal or absent.[3,4]

The SMAS is a tissue plane composed of fibrous and muscle tissue, and it forms a continuous sheath throughout the head and neck (Fig. 29–1). The SMAS was originally described by Mitz and Peyronie,[5] and the understanding of this important structure has revolutionized facelift surgery.

The SMAS envelops the superficial facial mimetic muscles (platysma, orbicularis oculi, levator labii superioris alaeque nasi, zygomaticus major, zygomaticus minor, and risorius) and is present along the superficial and deep surfaces of the muscles. In the cheek, the SMAS blends with the more continuous muscle fibers of the orbicularis oculi of the lower eyelid. The subcutaneous fascial-fatty layer overlying the SMAS is abundant in the cheek and thins within the lower eyelid to terminate superficial to the periorbital portion of the orbicularis oculi muscle.[6–8] In the infraorbital region, the subcutaneous fat abruptly assumes a greater thickness (Fig. 29–2). This bulky, subcutaneous fat is triangular and has its base at the nasolabial fold. It is called the malar fat pad and lies superficial to the SMAS.[9] Medial to the fold, the mimetic muscles insert directly into the skin and support this area against the effects of aging. Lateral to the fold, there are no cutaneous muscle attachments, and this skin, with its thick subcutaneous fat, is not supported by the mimetic muscles. When a person smiles, the nasolabial crease is pulled laterally by the contraction of the mimetic muscles, allowing the overlying cheek fat to bulge medially, thus increasing the prominence of the nasolabial fold.

The levator labii superioris alaeque nasi muscle defines the medial nasolabial fold. This muscle arises from the frontal process of the maxilla and inserts into the alar cartilage and medial upper lip. The levator labii superioris muscle arises several millimeters inferior to the inferior orbital rim and overlies the infraorbital nerve. It inserts into the upper lip and on contraction accentuates the midnasolabial fold. The zygomaticus muscle complex is composed of the zygomaticus major and minor and originates from the zygoma. Contraction of these muscles deepens the lateral nasolabial fold (see Fig. 29–1).[4]

A deep fascial layer also exists in the face.[7,10] It begins in the neck as a layer superficial to the strap muscles. Overlying the parotid gland, the fascia is quite thick and is known as the parotid-masseteric fascia. In the cheek region, it overlies the masseter muscle and extends into the malar region, lying deep to the elevator muscles of

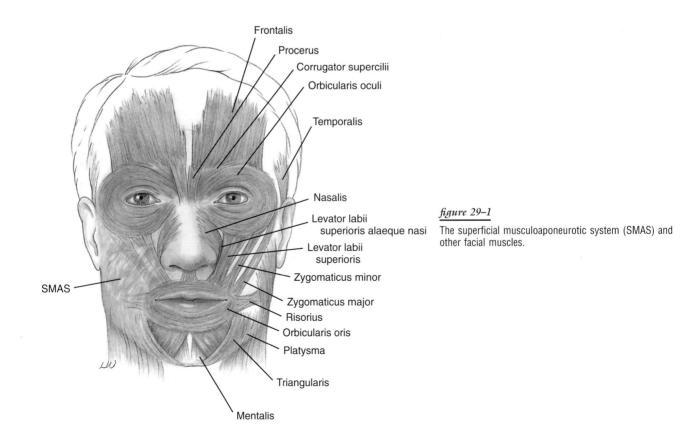

figure 29–1

The superficial musculoaponeurotic system (SMAS) and other facial muscles.

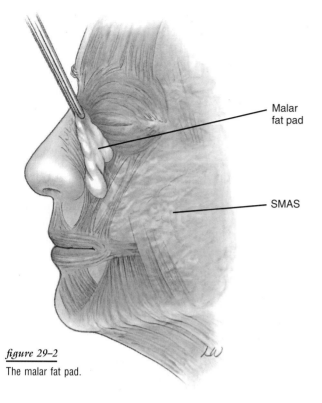

figure 29–2
The malar fat pad.

are situated deeper in the face and deep to the facial nerve. They therefore receive their innervation from their superficial surface.[7]

The mandibular nerve exits the parotid and courses inferiorly. The course of the mandibular nerve is described in Chapter 7.

The great auricular nerve (a sensory nerve), which is the largest branch of the cervical plexus, is vulnerable to injury during a facelift. Injury to the nerve can result in hypesthesia in the region of the ear. The nerve crosses the midbelly of the sternocleidomastoid muscle about 6.5 cm below the external auditory canal. The nerve is superficial and runs just deep to the skin in the sternocleidomastoid muscle's superficial fascia (see Fig. 29–3).

FACIAL AGING CHANGES

As our lives proceed, we are all subject to structural deformity of the face. Some of the characteristic changes that occur are due to our genetic makeup, whereas some are due to our lifestyle. Smoking and exposure to ultraviolet light are certainly two factors that contribute to the aging process. As we age, there is a progressive loss of skin thickness, elasticity, and adherence to the underlying subcutaneous tissues. This sagging is accentuated by the progressive atrophy of fat, muscle, and bone. This process first becomes noticeable in the third decade of life.

Predictable morphologic changes occur as we age. Among the first changes that occur are descent of the eyebrows, resulting in fullness of the upper eyelids, lateral orbital rhytids (crow's feet), and a trapezoidal configuration of the glabellar region. At the same time, as a result of years of contraction of the mimetic muscles, the attachments of the malar fat pad to the underlying SMAS begins to deteriorate. This results in an increasingly prominent nasolabial fold (Fig. 29–5*A*).[12]

In the upper cheek and eyelid region, the inferior orbicularis muscle becomes increasing ptotic and lengthens.[13] Normally, the orbicularis oculi muscle is firmly attached to the tarsal plate of the lower eyelid and to the lateral palpebral raphe. The inferior border of the orbicularis, however, has attachments only to the suborbicularis oculi fat (SOOF) and SMAS.[14] With age, the SOOF and SMAS attachments to the zygomaticus muscles deteriorate and the orbicularis oculi fibers become stretched. The orbicularis muscle migrates inferolaterally and becomes crescent-shaped, resulting in malar festoons and malar bags.[6] The SOOF and SMAS migrate inferomedially, resulting in deepening of the nasolabial fold[15] and an indentation in the infraorbital region. The superior edge of the descended SOOF is noticeable 5–10 mm inferior to the rim, particularly in the central and lateral regions (Fig. 29–5*B*). These structural changes result in a multicontoured configuration of the midfacial area.

In the lower cheek region, droopiness causes prominence of tissue in the midmandibular region, resulting in jowl formation. Normally, ligaments and fascial attachments anchor the subcutaneous tissues to the underlying deep structures. These attachments extend from

the lip (Fig. 29–3). The premasseteric fascia is an important landmark because the buccal branches of the facial nerve and the parotid duct lie on its surface.

The facial nerve exits the stylomastoid foramen and is encompassed by the parotid gland.[11] The main trunk is consistently located within the gland, whereas there is significant variation in the location of the distal branches. The frontal branch exits from the superior portion of the parotid gland at a point approximately halfway between the lateral canthus and the tragus. As it reaches the caudal portion of the zygomatic arch, it lies superficial to the periosteum. It then travels in the superficial temporal fascia and pierces the frontalis muscle about a finger breadth above the eyebrow. The frontal branch innervates the frontalis, corrugator, and procerus muscles and the cephalic portion of the orbital orbicularis oculi muscles. The zygomatic branches exit the parotid gland, cross the cephalic buccal space, run parallel to the parotid duct, and transverse the facial artery and vein. The branches then innervate the undersurface of the orbicularis and mimetic muscles. There are numerous anastomoses between the zygomatic and buccal branches (Fig. 29–4).

Medially, the buccal nerve leaves the parotid gland and traverses along the surface of the masseter muscle. In this location, it lies deep to the deep fascial layer. As the nerve proceeds medially, it penetrates the parotid-masseteric fascia, enters the buccal fat compartment, and lies superficial to the fat pad to innervate the overlying mimetic muscles. The zygomaticus and levator labii muscles lie superficial to the plane of the facial nerve and receive their innervation from their deep surfaces. The buccinator, levator anguli oris, and mentalis muscles

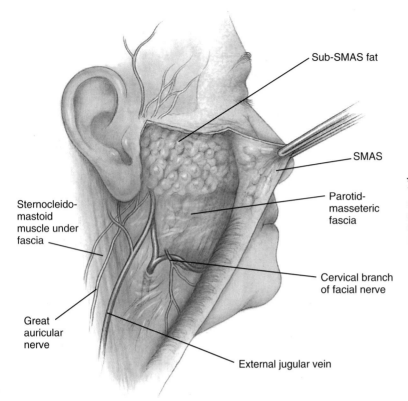

figure 29–3

The deep fascial layer. The sub-SMAS dissection plane, sub-SMAS fat, and parotid-masseteric fascia are demonstrated. The great auricular nerve, which runs within the sternocleidomastoid fascia, is most vulnerable to injury during face-lifting procedures.

figure 29–4

Branches of the facial nerve. The frontal and marginal mandibular branches are terminal branches, without anastomoses to other facial nerve branches. Damage to these nerves during face lifting can result in permanent paresis of the muscles supplied by these branches.

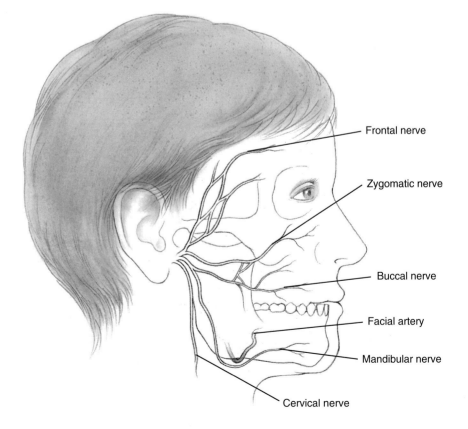

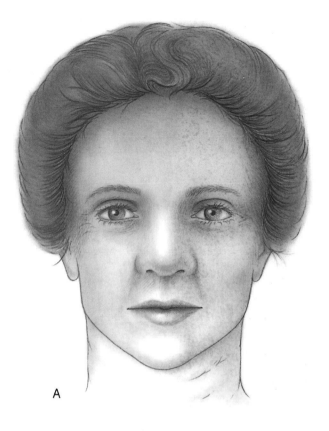

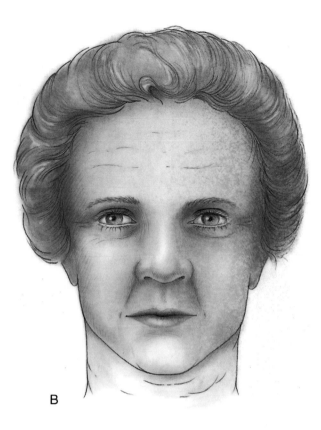

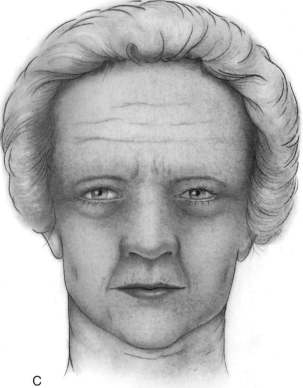

figure 29–5

Facial aging changes. *A,* Descent of the forehead and midface, resulting in eyebrow ptosis and deepening of the nasolabial fold. *B,* More pronounced lower and midfacial descent, resulting in a hollow appearance under the eyes, deeper nasolabial folds, and jowls. *C,* Significant descent of all the facial structures.

the zygoma to the mandible along a vertical line. Jowls occur as a result of loss of adherence between the superficial and deep fasciae along the line of attachment at the anterior aspect of the masseter muscle (Fig. 29–5C).

In the neck, there is a progressive loss of skin and muscle tone and an increase in the amount of fat stored. These changes result in a loss of the normal sharp cervicomental angle and a double chin. The platysma muscle, which extends from the shoulder to the cheek, may lack decussation and may develop multiple vertical folds, known as neck cords or bands.

PATIENT EVALUATION AND SELECTION[16, 17]

The goal of any aesthetic surgical procedure is to provide a result that pleases the patient. A careful assessment of the patient's motivations and expectations is paramount for a satisfactory result. A detailed consultation is required, one that evaluates the facial and neck structural abnormalities and includes a discussion of proposed options to address these abnormalities. Both the surgeon and the patient should understand the possibilities and limitations of facelift procedures. Facelift surgery is intended to reposition the deeper facial structures and improve the geniomandibular region, thereby removing the jowls. It can also rejuvenate the neck by restoring a sharper cervicomental angle and eliminating platysmal bands. Problems that are not treated by face lifting include perioral rhytids, skin atrophy and mottling, skeletal involution, and loss of facial fat. These problems are best treated by other techniques used in conjunction with the facelift. For example, we routinely perform skin peeling or resurfacing after the patient has undergone a facelift. Thus, the facelift recontours the structural problems of the face and the skin peeling or resurfacing improves the quality, texture, and color of the skin.

There is no magic age at which one should have a facelift. Although the first signs of aging appear in the mid to late 20s, most patients do not appear to be bothered by these structural changes until their late 30s or early 40s. Facelifts performed in patients in their 40s provide a moderate improvement in appearance, allowing the patient to maintain this youthful look for 10–15 years. Facelifts performed in patients in their 50s and 60s cause a more dramatic result, making it less likely to hide the fact that cosmetic surgery has been performed.

The preoperative evaluation includes assessment of facial asymmetries; skin laxity; solar damage; position of the eyebrows, eyelids, cheeks, and chin; and degree of jowls. The neck should be evaluated for submental fat, cervicomental angle, and platysma cords.

Patients may be classified into several categories according to the severity of the deformities. Some patients have minimal jowls and platysmal cords but may have significant cervical lipomatosis and an obtuse cervicomental angle. These patients will benefit from cervical liposuction and a conservative skin flap with or without SMAS plication. Other patients have more advanced laxity and jowl formation with or without submental lipomatosis. These patients will benefit from cervical liposuction, if indicated; SMAS plication; and skin excision. Finally, some patients have moderate to severe tissue laxity with prominent jowls and platsymal bands and varying amounts of cervical lipomatosis. These patients will require submental liposuction, platsymaplasty, SMAS plication, and excision of redundant skin.

A thorough medical history should be taken, including use of medications, tobacco, alcohol, and illicit drugs. The novice facelift surgeon should not operate on diabetic patients or patients who smoke on a regular basis. These patients are at risk for extensive flap necrosis resulting from underlying vascular insufficiency. Patients older than 60 years of age or those with a history of a chronic medical illness may require consultation with an internist. Patients with uncontrolled hypertension, upper respiratory tract infections, gastrointestinal problems (e.g., nausea, vomiting, hiccups, constipation), or heavy alcohol ingestion are at risk for postoperative hematoma. These medical abnormalities should be rectified before surgery. Patients should also be questioned about any prior facial surgery. Scars from previous thyroidectomy, parotidectomy, and mastoidectomy may traverse the cervicofacial flaps and increase the risk of skin necrosis.

Routine preanesthetic tests often include a complete blood cell count, prothrombin time and partial thromboplastin time, chemistry panel, hepatitis screen, human immunodeficiency virus (HIV) tests, urinalysis, and electrocardiogram.

Preoperative photographs are taken to document the structural facial changes that have occurred. Photographs are an extremely important tool in the management of patients undergoing cosmetic surgery. The patients quickly forget their preoperative condition and tend to focus on mild postoperative scarring and asymmetry. After surgery, we routinely give preoperative and postoperative instant (Polaroid) photographs, allowing the patient to compare the difference.

The details of the surgery are explained, including the anticipated scars and possible change in hairline position. We often have the patients speak with or meet other patients who have had similar surgery to discuss the postoperative course and view the resultant scars. It is beneficial to perform aesthetic surgery in one or more members of the office staff, since they are readily available and help guide the patient through the surgical and postoperative course.

SURGICAL TECHNIQUE
Preoperative Planning

Through observation and palpation of the tissues, the surgeon can assess the degree of submental lipomatosis. The fullest areas are marked with cross-hatching so that they can be appropriately addressed at the time of surgery. The amount of skin laxity and redundancy of the cheek and neck is assessed. Platysmal bands are marked.

Anesthesia

Usually, local anesthesia with intravenous sedation is administered. The preauricular region is bilaterally infiltrated with 1 per cent lidocaine with epinephrine (1:100,000). A total of 10 ml is used. Four stab incisions are then made with a No. 11 Bard-Parker blade on one side of the face. The contralateral side is infiltrated in a similar manner 30 minutes later. The first incision is vertical, in the superior preauricular region just anterior to the helical margin (Fig. 29–6). The second incision is made horizontally in the posterior auricular region at the mid-ear level. The third incision is made horizontally in the occipital region at the same vertical level as the posterior auricular incision. Finally, a horizontal incision is placed in the submental region just posterior to the normal crease. These incisions extend to the subcutaneous level only.

A Stevens scissors is then used to open a small subcutaneous pocket around the incision sites. A spatulated dissecting cannula is used to infiltrate a tumescent solution (1 liter of normal saline, 50 ml of 1 per cent lidocaine, 20 ml of 8.4 per cent sodium bicarbonate, and 2 ampules of 1:1000 epinephrine) into the subcutaneous space in the entire neck, cheek, posterior auricular, and occipital regions (see Fig. 29–6). The skin in the posterior auricular region overlying the mastoid bone is quite thin. The surgeon must be careful not to buttonhole the skin while injecting in this region. A period of 20 minutes is allowed to pass to provide for adequate vasoconstriction.

Incision Planning

The placement of the incision depends on many factors, including the degree of skin laxity, hair pattern, hair

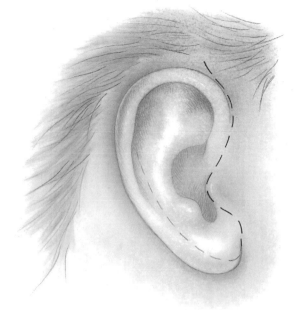

figure 29–7

The preauricular aspect of the incision follows the curvature of the ear and is hidden behind the tragus.

distribution, estimated hair recession, and previous surgery. A pen is used to mark the incisions.

The superior portion of the *preauricular incision* should parallel the curve of the posterior helical margin (Fig. 29–7). The incision extends into the superior tragal depression and is carried along the tragal rim. There

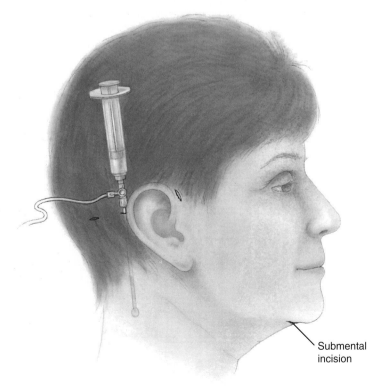

figure 29–6

One side of the face is infiltrated with the tumescent solution. A dissecting cannula is inserted through three stab incisions in the periauricular region. The entire neck is infiltrated through a submental stab incision.

Submental incision

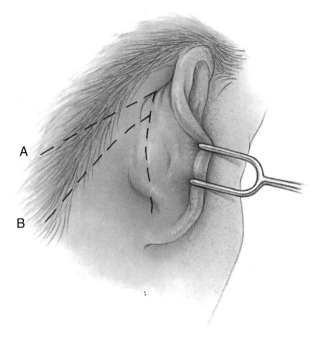

figure 29–8

The location of the occipital incision depends on the amount of skin redundancy in the neck. If the patient has little skin redundancy, the incision extends posteriorly into the occipital scalp *(A)*. If moderate to significant neck skin redundancy exists, the incision is placed along the hairline several millimeters superior to the fine hair on the nape of the neck *(B)*. The incision is beveled allowing the hair follicles to grow through the scar line.

should be a sharp angle between the superior preauricular incision and the posterior tragal incision. At the inferior aspect of the tragus, the incision acutely turns, continuing just anterior to the ear lobe. The ear lobe is totally disinserted from the cheek.

The *posterior auricular incision* should fall into the conchal sulcus and extend to the mid-ear level. If the patient has redundancy of the skin in the posterior auricular region, the incision should be placed directly on the posterior conchal surface, to the extent necessary to excise this skin redundancy (Fig. 29–8).

The location of the *occipital incision* depends on the amount of skin redundancy in the neck. If the patient has little skin redundancy, the incision extends posteriorly into the occipital scalp. If moderate to significant

neck skin redundancy exists, the incision should be placed along the hairline several millimeters superior to the fine hair on the nape of the neck. The incision is beveled, allowing the hair follicles to grow through the scar line.

The *submental incision* for a midline corset platysmaplasty is usually 2.5–4 cm in length and situated posterior to the submental crease. The surgeon determines the location of the incision by placing gentle superior traction on the cheeks. The incision should be well hidden in the submental region after the cheeks are elevated. Placement of the incision too anteriorly results in a noticeable scar. The incision site usually falls at a point halfway between the anterior chin and hyoid bone (Fig. 29–9).

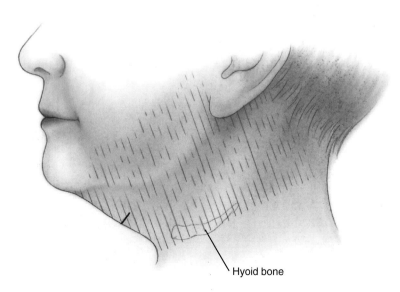

Hyoid bone

figure 29–9

The submental incision site usually falls at a point halfway between the anterior chin and hyoid bone.

Neck Dissection, Liposuction, and Platysmaplasty

Ear plugs are placed in both ears to prevent blood from pooling in the ear canals. The neck is addressed first. A 5-mm liposuction cannula is inserted into the submental stab incision. The submental tissues are grasped between the fingertips, and the excess fat is suctioned. The surgeon must stay superficial with the liposuction cannula to avoid damage to the underlying platysma muscle. At the same time, one must maintain the dermal fat layer or scarring and adhesions between the skin and platysma muscle may develop. The liposuction cannula should not be directed above the mandible. The end point of the liposuction occurs when the tissues of the neck are thinned and have a uniform thickness. One can judge the end point by pinching the skin between the fingertips. There should be an obvious improvement in the cervicomental angle at this point. If laxity of the platysma muscle and prominent platysmal bands are present, a platysmaplasty is indicated.[15]

If an anterior platysmaplasty is performed, a No. 15 Bard-Parker blade is used to lengthen the submental incision to approximately 2.5 cm. The liposuction will have already dissected most of the skin off the underlying platysma muscle. A lighted angled retractor is placed through the incision. Using a long facelift scissors, the surgeon cuts the remaining adhesions between the skin and the platysma muscle. Any bleeding points on the muscle are cauterized with the bipolar cautery. Attention is focused on the central submental region. The edges of the platysma muscle are identified, and the degree of muscle redundancy is determined. If significant redundancy exists, a strip of midline platysma muscle is excised. Subplatysmal fat, which lies between the muscle and the deep cervical fascia, may be sculpted as needed. Often small arteries lie in this fat layer, and will need to be cauterized. The surgeon must take care not to remove too much fat, for this will lead to a hollowness, known as a cobra deformity.

The platysma is then divided horizontally for 1–2 cm on either side of the midline, at the level of the hyoid bone. This allows the formation of a sharp cervicomental angle (Fig. 29–10). The medial edges of the platysma are grasped and pulled toward the midline. The edges of the platysma muscle are sutured together with buried

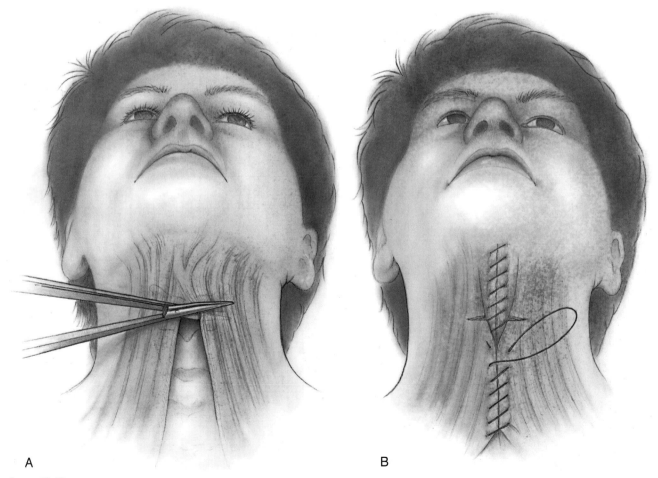

A   B

figure 29–10

Platysmaplasty. *A,* A vertical strip of platysma muscle is excised as needed. A horizontal relaxing incision through the platysma muscle is performed at the level of the hyoid bone. *B,* The edges of the platysma are sutured together with a buried running 2-0 polyglactin (Vicryl) suture. If significant laxity exists, the muscle can be imbricated by another row of sutures.

3-0 polyglactin (Vicryl) sutures on a cutting, semicircular needle. These sutures should proceed from the mandible to the level of the thyroid cartilage. Because the surgeon must work in a confined space, we find it helpful to suture with a long endoscopic needle holder. If platysmal redundancy still exists, the muscle can be imbricated inward and sutured with a 3-0 polyglactin running stitch.

Skin Undermining

Attention is then turned to the preauricular region. A No. 15 blade is used to make an incision along the previously demarcated lines. A facelift scissors, with the tips pointing down, is used to dissect in the subcutaneous plane. Once the proper plane is developed, the scissors can be used in a pushing rather than a cutting fashion. As the dissection proceeds toward the midcheek and along the mandible, sharp dissection is avoided because there is a potential to damage superficial branches of the facial nerve. Rather, the scissors are held with the blades in a vertical direction and a gentle spreading motion is used.

Attention is then turned to the posterior auricular and occipital regions. A No. 15 blade is used to make the incision along the previously demarcated lines. A No. 10 blade can be used along the hairline, and the incision is beveled inferiorly at a 45-degree angle. The dissection proceeds in the subcutaneous plane. The skin is very thin and bound down in this region, and the surgeon must be careful not to buttonhole the skin. Conversely, it is important to stay superficial so as not to damage the sternocleidomastoid muscle. Approximately 6.5 cm inferior to the external auditory meatus, the greater auricular nerve crosses the sternocleidomastoid muscle. The skin continues to be very thin at this point. If the dissection plane is too deep, the nerve can be easily cut. It is best to dissect by spreading vertically in this region. Once this point has been passed, the scissors can be used to push the skin off of the underlying tissues. The subcutaneous plane should now connect to the previously dissected region of the neck. At this point, the skin has been completely undermined in the cheek and neck regions.

SMAS Tightening

The surgical assistant places an Army-Navy retractor to retract the skin flap of the cheek. The surgeon views

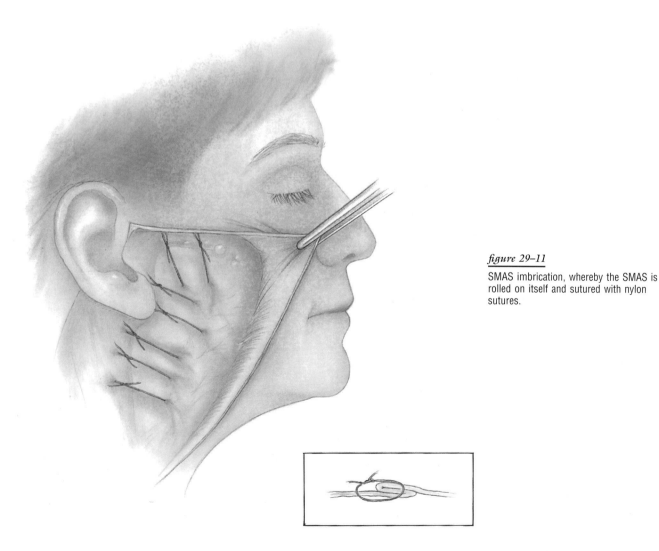

figure 29–11

SMAS imbrication, whereby the SMAS is rolled on itself and sutured with nylon sutures.

the SMAS, which is covered by subcutaneous fat. The surgeon can grasp this layer and note the degree of laxity and mobility. The SMAS can be tightened by either imbrication or plication. Imbrication involves grasping the SMAS anteriorly, stretching it posteriorly, and rolling it on itself. The rolled SMAS is then secured to its new position with sutures. SMAS plication involves dissection of the SMAS off the parotid-masseteric fascia and creation of a flap. The SMAS is pulled superoposteriorly, and the excess is excised. The edges of the cut SMAS are then sutured in place. Since the branches of the facial nerve lie just deep to the parotid-masseteric fascia, there is greater risk to them with the use of the SMAS flap. Thus, the novice facelift surgeon should begin with SMAS imbrication.

For the first imbrication suture, the surgeon grasps the tissue at the level of the angle of the mandible and pulls the tissue superoposteriorly toward the inferior tragus (Fig. 29–11). Either 2-0 or 3-0 nylon or polydioxanone (PDS) buried sutures are used to imbricate the tissue. A second suture is used to imbricate the anterior midcheek tissue posteriorly to the pretragal region. Numerous sutures are then used to imbricate the tissues from the lateral neck superoposteriorly to the mastoid region. The knots are rotated and buried. With proper imbrication, the SMAS becomes very taut.

Alternatively, the surgeon can develop a SMAS flap by incising through the SMAS to the underlying fascia. The fascia can be identified as a white fibrous sheet several millimeters deep to the top layer of the SMAS. The flap is created with a horizontal incision 1 cm inferior to the zygomatic arch and a vertical incision 1 cm anterior to the tragus (Fig. 29–12). The vertical incision extends down to the angle of the mandible. The SMAS is undermined approximately 2–3 cm. Once again, a vertical spreading technique is used (Fig. 29–13). Allis clamps are then used to pull the SMAS superoposteriorly. The surgeon should inspect the cervical and mandibular regions and determine the angle of pull that creates a defined neck and jawline. The excess SMAS is then excised, and the SMAS is sutured with 3-0 buried nylon or PDS sutures to the pretragal and mastoid regions (Fig. 29–14). It is imperative that the underlying fascia *not* be incorporated into the suture; this may damage the underlying nerves.

Skin Resection

Whether SMAS imbrication or plication has been performed, the SMAS should feel taut and the skin flap will lie in an advanced position without tension. The skin flap in the posterior auricular region is then pulled superiorly and clamped with a towel clip. The patient's face is turned, and the contralateral side of the face is addressed in a similar manner.

When the surgeon has completed SMAS plication or imbrication on both sides of the face, he or she proceeds

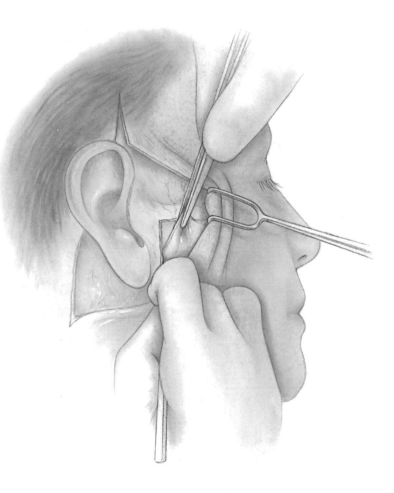

figure 29–12

SMAS plication. A horizontal incision through the SMAS is made several millimeters inferior to the inferior border of the arch. A vertical incision in the SMAS is made several millimeters anterior to the ear.

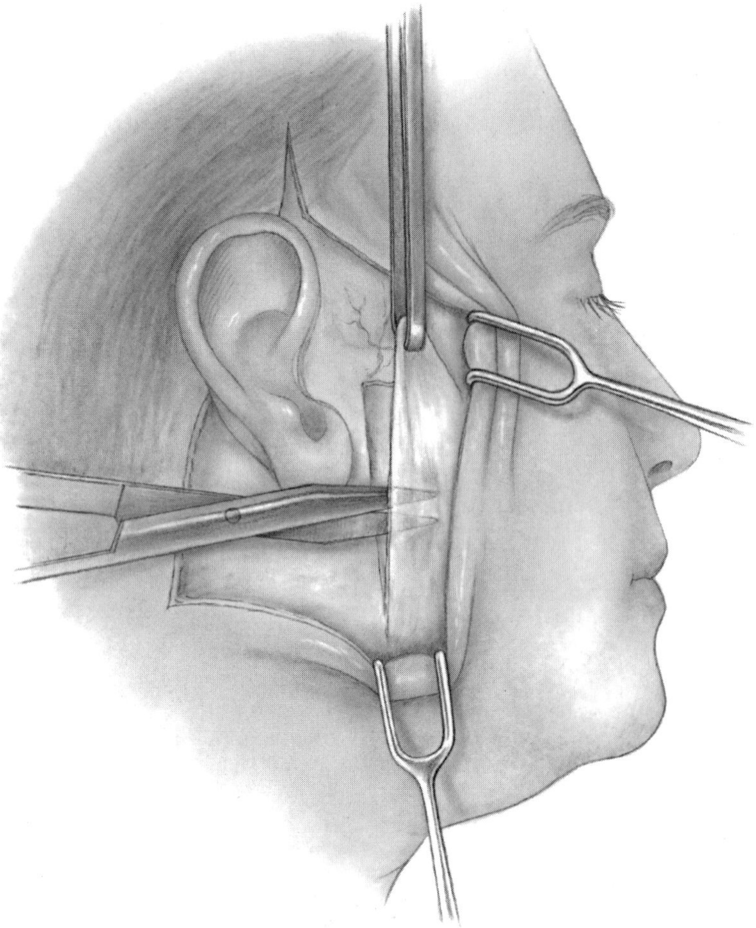

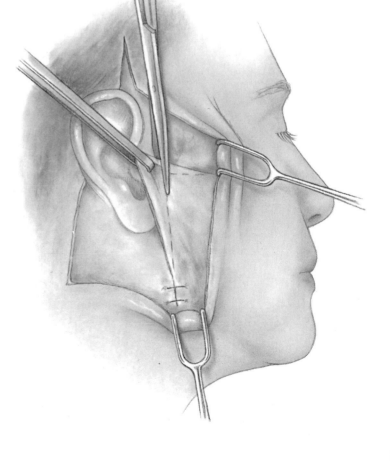

figure 29–13

The SMAS is undermined for approximately 2–3 cm. The sub-SMAS dissection should be performed with a vertical spreading motion once the plane is created.

figure 29–14

The SMAS is pulled superolaterally, and the excess SMAS is trimmed.

with advancement and closure of the skin flaps. This is the most critical portion of the procedure because improperly tailored skin flaps result in scarring and thus an unhappy patient. The skin flap is grasped along the angle of the jaw and gently pulled toward the inferior aspect of the tragus. A Brown-Adson forceps is used to grasp the point where the tissue meets the tragus. A No. 11 blade is then used to make an oblique incision through the skin flap. A 4-0 nylon suture is used to tack the cut edge of the skin flap to the inferior tragus (Fig. 29–15).

Attention is turned to the superior helix, where the skin flap is pulled superoposteriorly and stapled in place. The excess skin is excised with a No. 15 blade. A fold of excess tissue is sometimes created superior to the helix, resulting in a "dog-ear" deformity. The surgeon can manage this dog ear by excising a triangle of the temporal hair-bearing tissue and advancing this tissue inferiorly toward the ear (Fig. 29–16). The base of the triangle should lie in the coronal plane. The superior helix wound is then closed in two layers with 4-0 PDS buried subcuticular and 4-0 nylon skin sutures.

Attention is turned toward the preauricular tissue. The skin flap is grasped with a forceps and pulled posteriorly (Fig. 29–17). Then the skin flap is thinned so that all of the subcutaneous fat is removed. The excess skin is meticulously trimmed and sutured in place with 4-0 nylon sutures.

The posterior auricular region is then addressed. The skin flap is pulled superiorly and stapled in the mastoid region. The dog ears and excess tissues are excised and closed with staples. If the incision extended along the hairline, the incision is closed in two layers. The posterior auricular incision is also closed in two layers. The deep closure incorporates the tissue in the posterior auricular sulcus, thereby creating a sharp angle between the skin overlying the mastoid and the posterior auricular skin. It is imperative that no tension exist on the skin flaps (Fig. 29–18).

Finally, attention is turned to the ear lobes. The lobes should fall in the same anterior position as the superior helix. If the lobes are excessively long, the surgeon can shorten them by taking out a wedge of tissue, as described by Ellenbogen.[18] A No. 11 blade is then used to make an incision in the prelobular skin. The lobe is sutured to the face with 4-0 nylon sutures.

The face and hair are then washed, and a pressure dressing is applied to prevent formation of a hematoma. The dressing can be removed in 24 hours. Some surgeons prefer to insert a Jackson-Pratt drain to drain the neck region. We occasionally use a drain.

POSTOPERATIVE CARE

Patients are usually discharged on the day of surgery and are given written instruction sheets. The patient is started on a regimen of ciprofloxacin to minimize the risk of chondritis. Pain medications are prescribed, although severe postoperative pain is rare. Severe pain in the immediate postoperative period may represent hematoma formation and must be evaluated immedi-

ately. An expanding hematoma of the neck can potentially compromise respiratory function. Patients are instructed to apply ice to the face as much as possible in the first 24 hours after surgery.

The patients are examined the first postoperative day, and the dressing and drain (if used) are removed. The patients are followed up frequently so that the postoperative course can be monitored. The preauricular and posterior auricular sutures are removed in 5–7 days. Staples and sutures in the temporal and occipital region are removed in 10–14 days.

COMPLICATIONS

All surgical procedures can have complications. The complications that occur in aesthetic surgical patients may be especially difficult to manage because these patients originally were healthy individuals seeking to improve their looks. An astute and understanding surgeon is the key to managing complications in these patients.[19]

Hematoma

Hematoma is the most common complication, occurring in about 4 per cent of cases. Patients using aspirin or nonsteroidal anti-inflammatory medications are at risk. Hypertension, coughing, or vomiting in the immediate postoperative period are also risk factors. Acute expanding hematomas occurring immediately after surgery are usually localized to the lateral neck or posterior auricular regions. A staple or suture can be removed and the hematoma suctioned or expressed. Manual pressure to the affected area is applied for 5–10 minutes. If the patient's blood pressure is elevated, it should be controlled as well; this usually alleviates the problem. If the hematoma recurs, the wounds must be opened and the bleeding vessels must be identified and cauterized. If a hematoma is generalized and extends both in the preauricular and postauricular regions, the wounds should be opened and the bleeding points controlled. If this is not done, the skin flaps will develop ischemia and will be at risk for flap necrosis.

At times, the surgeon may notice a hematoma several days after the surgery. These hematomas can be aspirated with a needle. If these hematomas are not evacuated, the patient is at risk for scarring, infection, skin necrosis, and wrinkling of the skin.

Skin Necrosis

The incidence of skin necrosis following facelift procedures is approximately 2 per cent. Patients who have diabetes, smoke, or use steroids over a long term are at risk. The most common site of necrosis is over the mastoid region, since this portion of the skin flap is closed under the greatest tension. When the skin flap is compromised, it shows signs of blanching, erythema, cyanosis, and superficial blistering. It is imperative that this region be kept moist because desiccation of the

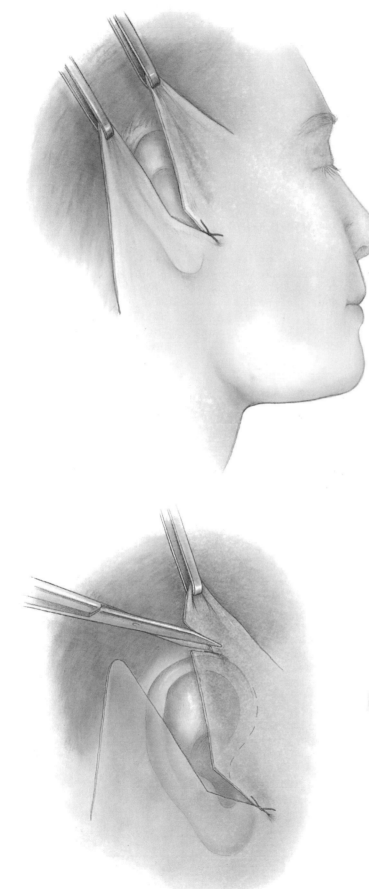

figure 29–15

The first cardinal suture is placed at the inferior aspect of the tragus.

figure 29–16

The second cardinal suture is placed superior to the ear.

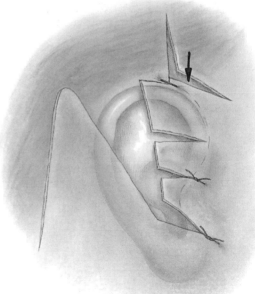

figure 29–17

The excess skin is excised as needed and the hair-bearing scalp tissue is rotated inferiorly. The third cardinal suture is at the superior aspect of the tragus.

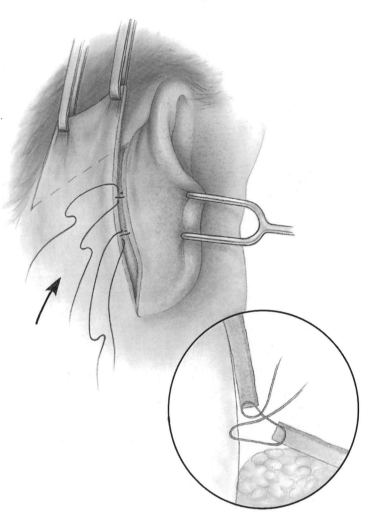

figure 29–18

The posterior auricular skin is pulled superiorly and slightly anterior.

ischemic areas deepens the zone of necrosis. We have found it useful to apply 2 per cent nitroglycerin paste to these areas, which dilates the vasculature and increases blood flow. If necrosis occurs, débridement of the eschar should be performed and the tissue should be cleaned with hydrogen peroxide and lubricated with an antibiotic ointment. The tissue usually heals remarkably well with proper wound care.

Nerve Injury[20]

All patients undergoing facelift surgery will have some degree of hypesthesia, especially in the lower third of the ear and preauricular regions. The sensation usually returns in several weeks. Damage to the greater auricular nerve can result in periauricular numbness and pain. If the nerve is lacerated during surgery, the surgeon should immediately repair the nerve to prevent the development of a painful neuroma.

The various branches of the motor facial nerve are at risk during facelift surgery. The buccal branch is the one most often injured in facelift surgery. Fortunately, true long-lasting paralysis is rare. Usually, blunt trauma during the dissection or edema of the nerve results in temporary paresis. The frontal and mandibular branches

have few anastomoses with other branches of the facial nerve, and injury to these nerves can cause paralysis.

Infection

Infections of the face are rare but may occur in areas of hematomas secondary to the proliferation of *Staphylococcus aureus*. There is also a risk of infection of the ear cartilage because sutures are often passed through this structure. We prescribe a regimen of prophylactic broad-spectrum antibiotics for all patients; we give intravenous antibiotics during surgery followed by oral antibiotics for 5–10 days.

Cutaneous Changes

Hyperpigmentation may occur in areas of hematomas as a result of deposition of hemosiderin. Telangiectasias sometimes appear on the cheek and preauricular regions, especially in patients with thin skin. The patients can easily cover up these abnormal vessels with makeup. The pulsed dye laser is also effective in removing telangiectasias.

Scarring can occur and is most noticeable in the pre-

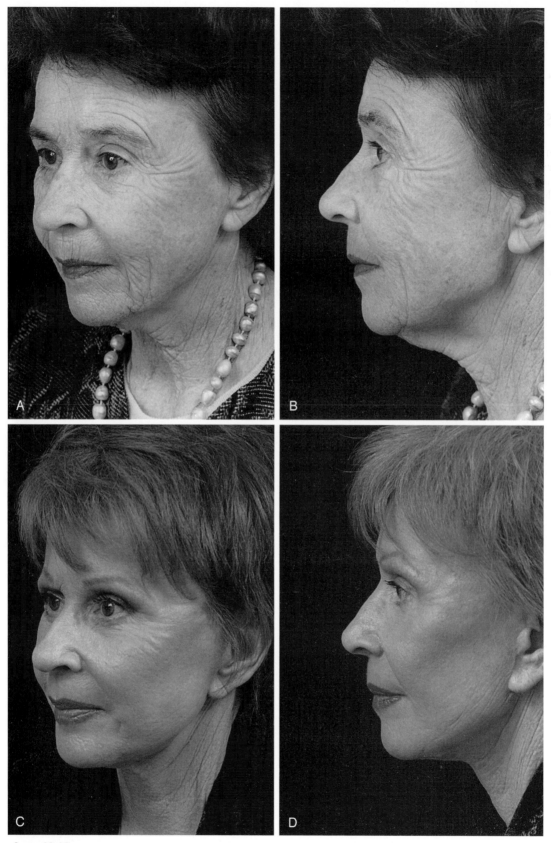

figure 29–19

A and *B*, Preoperative front and side views of a 70-year-old woman with solar damage, moderate jowls, and significant laxity of the neck. *C* and *D*, Same patient 6 weeks after endoscopic forehead, cheek, and neck lift and facial peel. The patient subsequently underwent a light chemical peel of the neck.

auricular region. Meticulous two-layer closure should minimize the incidence of scarring. The scars can be managed by laser treatment, dermabrasion, or skin resurfacing. We have found it particularly useful to use silicone gel to reduce hypertrophic scars.

RESULTS

Face lifting, especially combined with other cosmetic procedures, such as skin resurfacing, can create dramatic improvements in appearance (Fig. 29–19). We have performed close to 1000 face-lifting procedures over the past 15 years, with excellent results and high patient satisfaction.

References

1. Larrabee W, Makielski KH: Surgical Anatomy of the Face. New York, Raven Press, 1993.
2. Wassef M: Superficial fascial and muscular layers in the face and neck: A histological study. Aesthetic Plast Surg 1987; 11:171–176.
3. Barton FE Jr: The SMAS and the nasolabial fold. Plast Reconstr Surg 1992; 89:1054–1057.
4. Pensler JM, Ward JW, Parry SW: The superficial musculoaponeurotic system in the upper lip: An anatomic study in cadavers. Plast Reconstr Surg 1985; 75:488–492.
5. Mitz V, Peyronie M: The superficial musculoaponeurotic system (SMAS) in the parotid and cheek area. Plast Reconst Surg 1976; 58:80–88.
6. Ruess W, Owsley JQ: The anatomy of the skin and fascial layers of the face in aesthetic surgery. Clin Plast Surg 1987; 14:677–682.
7. Stuzin JM, Baker TJ, Gordon HL: The relationship of the superficial and deep facial fascias: Relevance to rhytidectomy and aging. Plast Reconstr Surg 1992; 89:441–449.
8. Gosain AK, Yousif NJ, Madiedo G, et al: Surgical anatomy of the SMAS: A reinvestigation. Plast Reconstr Surg 1994; 92:1254–1263.
9. Fuleihan NS: The nasolabial fold and the SMAS. Plast Reconstr Surg 1994; 94:1091–1093.
10. Maillard JF, Cornette de St Cyr B, Scheflan M: The subperiosteal bicoronal approach to total facelifting: The DMAS—deep musculoaponeurotic system. Aesthetic Plast Surg 1991; 15:285–291.
11. Rudolph R: Depth of the facial nerve in face lift dissections. Plast Reconstr Surg 1990; 85:537–544.
12. Yousif NJ, Gosain A, Matloub HS, et al: The nasolabial fold: An anatomic and histologic reappraisal. Plast Reconstr Surg 1994; 93:60–69.
13. Furnas DW: Festoons, mounds and bags of the eyelids and cheek. Clin Plast Surg 1993; 20:367–385.
14. Hamra ST: Repositioning the orbicularis oculi muscle in the composite rhytidectomy. Plast Reconstr Surg 1992; 90:14–22.
15. Feldman JJ: Corset platysmaplasty. Clin Plast Surg 1992; 19:369–382.
16. Hamra ST: Composite Rhytidectomy. St. Louis, Quality Medical Publishing, 1993.
17. Owsley JQ: Aesthetic Facial Surgery. Philadelphia, WB Saunders, 1994.
18. Ellenbogen R: Avoiding visual tipoffs to face lift surgery. Clin Plast Surg 1992; 19:447–454.
19. Courtiss E: Aesthetic Surgery Trouble: How to Avoid It and How to Treat It. St. Louis, CV Mosby, 1978.
20. Seckel B: Facial Danger Zones: Avoiding Nerve Injury in Facial Plastic Surgery. St. Louis, Quality Medical Publishing, 1994.

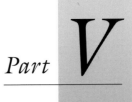

Part V

ADJUNCTIVE PROCEDURES AND TECHNIQUES

Norman Shorr
David M. Morrow
Jonathan A. Hoenig

Chemical Peel: Eyelid, Periorbital, and Facial Skin Rejuvenation in Conjunction with or Independent of Cosmetic Blepharoplasty

Norman Shorr has popularized eyelid and facial skin peeling with and without a blepharoplasty and has had good results. In this chapter, Drs. Shorr, Morrow, and Hoenig explain the various chemicals that can be used for an eyelid and facial chemical peel, explain how to identify candidates for the procedure, and detail how to apply the chemicals.

The authors also discuss how to care for the patient postoperatively and how to handle possible complications. Sometimes a change in skin color and exposure keratopathy seem to result.

When I see patients with wrinkly lower lid skin associated with herniated orbital fat, I commonly treat them with laser skin resurfacing, a transconjunctival blepharoplasty, and plication of the lateral lower orbicularis oculi muscle to the periosteum. I have had minimal experience with chemical peeling.

I believe that the procedure described in this chapter will add to the surgeon's armamentarium for treating cosmetic oculoplastic surgery patients.

ALLEN M. PUTTERMAN

The skilled surgeon and the skilled seamstress can each change the dimensions and the draping of the skin or cloth with which he or she works, but neither can change the type of skin or material. The most skilled seamstress cannot turn a cotton shirt into a silk blouse. Traditional surgery cannot change the quality, texture, or elasticity of the skin. This reality is a major limitation to surgery alone.

Fortunately, skin rejuvenation procedures do improve the quality, texture, and elasticity of the skin.[1] *Chemical peeling*, or *chemexfoliation*, is the process in which the skin is wounded or burned with a chemical agent. The zone of cellular destruction and depth of the wound are dependent on several variables, including the peeling agent and its concentration and skin thickness and permeability.[1] The immediate reaction of the skin is a second-degree, chemically induced burn and inflammation that may extend variably into the epidermis and dermis. The inflammatory response peaks at 48 hours, but skin rejuvenation and collagen remodeling may last for weeks or months. Regeneration of the surface epithelium begins almost immediately and should be complete by 5–14 days.

Several methods may be used to remove the layers of

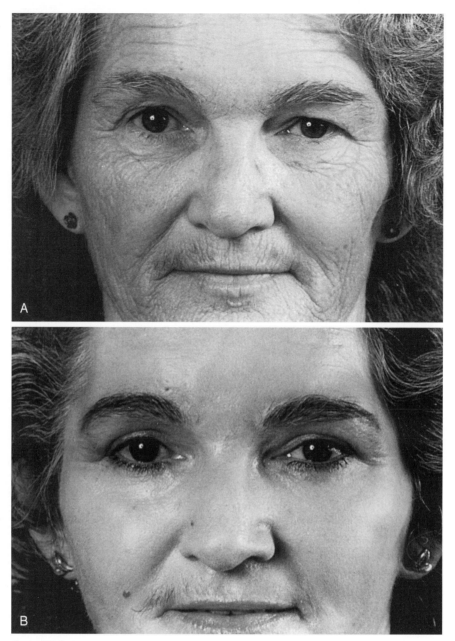

figure 30–1

A 65-year-old woman before *(A)* and after *(B)* a chemical peel (untaped) of the eyelids and face with Baker's phenol mixture. She has never had surgery. Note the resolution of dermatochalasis (excess skin) and the improvement of skin texture.

the skin. The most superficial layer, the stratum corneum, may be removed with *exfoliants*, mild alpha-hydroxy acids, or abrasive agents. This process gives the skin a healthy glow by removing the outer thickened dead keratin layer and may soften fine rhytids (crow's feet). Removal of skin layers can also be accomplished with a mechanical method, such as *dermabrasion*, pulsed lasers, or even fine sandpaper. Each method is effective in rejuvenating the skin but is operator-dependent for greater or less control of wound depth. We perform all of these techniques, individualizing the procedure to the patient's needs and desires. This chapter emphasizes

chemexfoliation as the time-tested and still popular method of skin rejuvenation.

No matter which technique is used, if the wounding depth is significant, there will be some permanent changes to the skin. The papillary dermal collagen changes from a wavy pattern to straight and parallel beneath the epidermal layer. The dermis shows fibroblastic proliferation and replacement of much of the old deformed elastic fibers with new elastic fibers.[2] Again, depending on the degree of wounding and chemicals used, there may be fewer melanocytes both in the basal layer and in the dermis. This accounts for the lightening

table 30–1

Grades of Depth of Chemical Peels

Chemical Agent	Indication	Anticipated Depth†	Anatomic Depth
TCA			
25%	Superficial wrinkling	Superficial depth	Upper papillary dermis
25%	Mild-moderate wrinkling	Superficial to medium depth	Papillary dermis
Phenol			
89%	Moderate wrinkling	Medium depth	Upper reticular dermis
Baker's*	Deep wrinkling	Deep depth	Midreticular dermis

*Baker's phenol is also known as Baker-Gordon formula. See Table 30–3.
†Clinically anticipated degree of wounding depth.
Abbreviation: TCA, trichloroacetic acid.

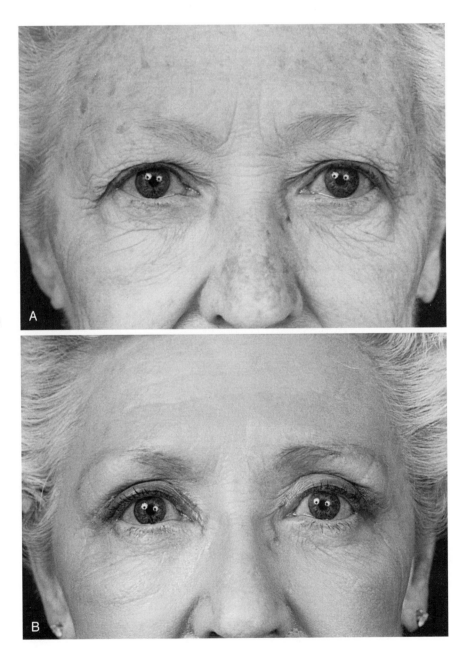

figure 30–2

A 75-year-old woman before *(A)* and after *(B)* an upper blepharoplasty, a lower transconjunctival blepharoplasty, and a simultaneous eyelid and periocular chemical peel. An improvement in skin texture is evident.

in color after peeling. This lightening is a spectral change and may be permanent, depending again on the degree and agent of wounding. With fewer melanocytes, the ability to tan is diminished accordingly. In terms of texture, the skin itself becomes smoother and more light-reflective (shinier), which is generally a healthy replacement for the previously sun-damaged skin (Fig. 30–1). The potential increased sun sensitivity due to decreased melanocytes makes it very important for patients to protect themselves against the sun's rays.

In general, the deeper the wound, the deeper the zone of replacement of old, damaged, and disorganized skin structural elements with new, healthy, and well-organized elements.[3] By the same token, the deeper the wound, the greater the potential for scarring and pigment changes.

Chemical peels may be divided into three types, graded by the depth of the wound (Table 30–1):

- *Superficial-depth* wounding, to the stratum granulosum, papillary dermis
- *Medium-depth* wounding, to the upper reticular dermis
- *Deep-depth* wounding, to the midreticular dermis

INDICATIONS AND PATIENT SELECTION

The primary aim of lower blepharoplasty is the removal of fat to address the undesirable convexity (bulging) of the lower eyelid. Approximately 70 per cent of patients who want to undergo lower blepharoplasty have such a small component of excess skin that the risk of the transcutaneous approach outweighs the advantage of removing a few millimeters of vertical skin, particularly when the skin problem is mostly a result of actinic damage. We have been performing only transconjunctival blepharoplasty in these patients for the past 20 years.

One of the authors (D.M.M.) developed and refined the technique of simultaneous transconjunctival blepharoplasty and chemical skin peeling.[4] We all now routinely use this combination procedure (Fig. 30–2). The 70 per cent of patients in whom skin removal has too great a potential risk may potentially benefit from simultaneous transconjunctival blepharoplasty and chemical peel rejuvenation of the skin of the lower eyelids; in fact, many of the 30 per cent in whom the risk of blepharoplasty is acceptable can also significantly benefit from simultaneous blepharoplasty and chemical peeling without the risk of an infralash incision.

Chemical peeling is indicated in any patient whose skin may benefit from greater elasticity, increased smoothness, removal of fine wrinkles, softening or obliteration of deep creases, lessening of pigmentary irregularities, or the replacement of a sallow, aged appearance of sun-damaged skin with a healthy and youthful glow. Thus, virtually all patients requesting blepharoplasty or any other facial cosmetic procedures may be candidates for a chemical peel.

EVALUATING THE SKIN[5]

Hypopigmentation (loss of skin color) after a chemical peel is a concern. Certainly, the issue of skin color change must be thoroughly discussed with the patient preoperatively. Permanent hypopigmentation presents little or no problem for light-skinned patients, according to Fitzpatrick's classifications I–III (Table 30–2).[6] If hypopigmentation occurs, it can be adequately camouflaged in patients with lighter skin because the color contrast is less drastic than in patients with darker skin (Fitzpatrick's classifications IV–VI). The deeper the wounding, the more hypopigmentation. In addition, as a chemical, phenol is melanotoxic. In patients with skin classifications IV–VI, hypopigmentation cannot be readily camouflaged.

CONTRAINDICATIONS

Although there are few absolute contraindications to chemical peeling, three groups of patients must be considered cautiously as candidates:

1. Patients with olive or darkly pigmented skin. The peel may permanently remove too much pigment or may result in a blotchy or hyperpigmented appearance.
2. Patients whose skin is fair but has been frequently sun-exposed for many years. These patients now have

table 30–2

Reaction to Sun by Skin Pigment Type

Classification (Fitzpatrick)*	Pigment Type	Reaction to Sun
I	Medium pigment	Always burns, never tans
II	Blue eyes, red hair	Usually burns, rarely tans
III	Average pigment	Sometimes burns, average tans
IV	More pigment	Rarely burns, usually tans
V	Much pigment	Minimum burns, mostly tans
VI	Most pigment	Never burns, always tans

*From Fitzpatrick TB: The validity and practicality of sun-reactive skin types I through VI. Arch Dermatol 1988; 124:869. Copyright 1988, American Medical Association.

permanently pigmented skin, and chemical peeling may result in an obvious demarcation between the treated area and the untreated area even if careful feathering is performed.

3. Fair-skinned, freckled individuals. These patients risk an odd appearance if they lose all of their facial freckles in one area but retain freckles in adjacent areas.

CHEMEXFOLIATION AND WOUNDING AGENTS

Chemical peeling is a commonly performed procedure. The depth (and thus the effectiveness) varies with the chemical agent used, its concentration, and the conditions under which it is applied. The wide spectrum of agents and formulas for peeling includes retinoic acid (Retin-A), solid carbon dioxide, sulfur solutions, resorcinol, salicylic acid, alpha-hydroxy acids, trichloroacetic acid (TCA), and phenol and phenol formulas. Table 30–1 lists the most common peeling agents, concentrations, and formulations and the depth to which they can wound.

The surgeon must determine the depth to which he or she wishes to wound the skin, since it is wound depth that determines the potential for the final result. Unfortunately, depth is not simplistically determined by chemical formulas and concentrations, as implied in Table 30–1. Other major factors that help determine wound depth are:

- Skin type (Fitzpatrick's skin classifications I–VI)
- Skin condition and thickness
- Pretreatment with retinoic acid, alpha-hydroxy acids, alpha-keto acids, low-dose *cis*-retinoic acid, epidermabrasive exfoliants, and defatting preparations

These agents alter the permeability of the skin to the wounding agent. Furthermore, the larger the amount of agent applied, the longer and harder the agent is rubbed onto the skin, and the longer the duration of contact between agent and skin, the deeper the wounding caused by the same agent. Finally, applying tape over the agent (*occlusion*) drives the chemical deeper into the skin.

Each of the several chemical wounding agents (see Table 30–1) may be used in various strengths. The most common agents, in increasing order of strength, are TCA (15, 20, 25, 35 per cent) and phenol (89 per cent). Most wounding agents can be driven deeper into the skin and thus cause a deeper burn by (1) occlusion (taping or ointments), (2) wetter applications, (3) multiple applications, or (4) vigorous scrubbing of the agent into the skin. As a result of the increased risk of scarring due to uneven penetration, we do not use taping as a method of penetration enhancement. Thus, we do not discuss taping in this chapter.

The 15 and 20 per cent dilutions of TCA are used as "freshening peels"; in a single application, they have a minimal potential for complications and provide minimal long-term improvement. We suggest to participants

in our teaching courses that they begin their experience in chemical peeling with these 15–20 per cent TCA freshening peels independent of or in conjunction with lower transconjunctival blepharoplasty. Compared with blepharoplasty alone, patient healing time is increased only slightly. Usually, the skin is fully reepithelialized so that the patient can comfortably return to socializing and, if desired, wearing makeup within 7–10 days.

After achieving a great deal of experience, we find that our most commonly used agent is TCA 35 per cent for combined simultaneous transconjunctival blepharoplasty and chemical peeling. In our experience, this concentration produces satisfactory results with one application in most patients if patient selection, application of the chemical, and aftercare are appropriately carried out. Minimal risks of scarring, textural change, eyelid contracture, and undesirable pigmentary changes still occur. On occasion, and for selected patients, we use phenol 89 per cent or Baker's phenol mixture combined with transconjunctival blepharoplasty. These agents, however, are not for the novice, and they carry a much greater risk of complications.

For eyelid skin peeling, other than in conjunction with blepharoplasty, we routinely use the phenol preparations. Phenol wounds more deeply than TCA and, as such, is very effective in treating deeper rhytids and creases in the eyelids.

It is thought, although still not proven, that phenol's ability to wound increases with the dilution; that is, the more dilute the phenol preparation, the greater the penetration. Phenol preparations, such as *Baker-Gordon formula* (Table 30–3), dilute the phenol and contain additional ingredients. Studies have shown that the most toxic phenol preparation is a phenol-and-water combination of 2:1. Thus, any dilution of full-strength phenol preparation, as occurs when tears run onto the eyelid, may increase the depth of penetration.

In choosing the chemical agent, the surgeon must keep in mind differences in wounding agents, the preparation of the skin, and the anatomic variations in the skin of each area of the face. For example, one may apply Baker-Gordon formula laterally, to the crow's feet and in the deep rhytids of the glabella and perioral region; 35 per cent TCA to the forehead and infrabrow area; 25 per cent TCA inferiorly to the upper blepharoplasty incision line, on the medial canthus, and over the bridge of the nose at the radix; and continue with 25 or 35 per cent TCA from the lower eyelid lash line inferiorly over the remainder of the face. The solutions should be applied in a feathered fashion to provide a natural look without a demarcation line. It is imperative that the solutions *not* be applied inferior to the jawline because this may result in scarring.

To determine the appropriate depth of wounding in any one area, the surgeon must evaluate at least the following skin factors:

- Amount of redundancy
- Thickness
- Quality
- Degree of oil production
- Laxity of the lower eyelid margin

table 30–3

Baker-Gordon Chemical Peel Formula

3 ml 89% liquid phenol (USP)	8 drops liquid soap (Septisol)
2 ml tap water	3 drops croton oil

- Prior upper or lower blepharoplasty or skin peel
- Actinic damage, rhytids
- Pigment and skin color

This customized approach is used for all peeling procedures whether the full face or only specific anatomic regions are peeled. After these factors are considered, the appropriate chemical agent is selected.

The chemical solutions themselves must be reliably mixed and fresh. TCA solutions are mixed from crystals every 180 days and stored in amber bottles. The mixed solution may be purchased from a pharmacy. A 35 per cent TCA concentration is obtained by mixing 35 g of TCA (USP) crystals with 100 ml of distilled water. The solution should be stirred before use in case some of the crystals may have come out of solution. Evaporation increases the concentration of TCA; therefore, bottles must be securely closed.

Baker-Gordon formulas are mixed fresh daily. Full-strength phenol (89 per cent) remains stable on a long-term basis in the manufacturer's amber glass bottle. Acetone may be purchased from the pharmacy and is used straight out of the bottle on a gauze pad (2 × 2 or 4 × 4 in) for cleansing the skin.

PRETREATMENT WITH RETINOIC ACID AND BLEACHING AGENTS

Topical retinoic acid is the acid form of vitamin A. Studies of daily use of retinoic acid for 6 months have shown that it is an effective treatment for wrinkling and actinic and pigmentary changes.[7] Pretreatment with retinoic acid for 2 weeks before chemical peeling usually results in a more even uptake and penetration of the chemicals and a quicker reepithelialization. In addition, this pretreatment may allow for deeper wounding with a given chemical concentration and application technique.

Retinoic acid is available in varying concentrations. The most potent and irritating forms, in descending order, are: 0.025 and 0.01 per cent gel and 0.1, 0.05, and 0.025 per cent cream. The preparation should be applied daily in gradually increasing potencies over weeks or months. Retinoic acid commonly causes a retinoid dermatitis, which is a pharmacologic irritation and not an allergy. The potency and frequency of application should be adjusted to minimize excessive irritation, but the patient must recognize that some degree of irritation must occur for benefit to be attained.[8]

Beginning again 2 weeks after peeling (after significant inflammation is resolved), regular use of retinoic acid may be continued indefinitely. The use of retinoic acid (just like the chemical peel itself) causes an acceleration in healing and a reduction of blotches, pigmentary changes, and fine wrinkling, with a smoothing of the surface and an improvement in color from the sallow complexion of actinically damaged and intrinsically aged skin to a healthy, rosy glow. All of these results should enhance all types of cosmetic surgery of the face.

Because chemexfoliation induces inflammation, there is always a risk of postinflammatory *hyperpigmentation* (darkening) of the skin. All patients are at risk, although the darker the skin, the greater the risk. Hydroquinone, kojic acid, and azelaic acid are agents that inhibit tyrosinase and decrease the skin's ability to produce melanin. These bleaching agents come in various strengths and combinations. We prefer to use 4 per cent hydroquinone or a combination of 2 per cent hydroquinone and kojic acid (Pigment Gel, Physicians Choice, Scottsdale, Ariz.). These bleaching agents should be started along with the retinoic acid 2 weeks before the peel, restarted approximately 2 weeks after the peel, and continued for several months.

SKIN CLEANSING

The presence of skin oils or grease on the skin inhibits an even and predictable penetration of the wounding agent. The patient's face and eyelids should be clean, dry, and free of oil before the procedure is begun. The patient is therefore asked to wash the face with soap and water the night before and the morning of surgery and to not apply makeup or moisturizers on the face or eyelids on the day of surgery. Cleansing with soap may be adequate but also may leave soap residue. For these reasons, the already clean face is degreased by the physician with acetone as the first step in the procedure. Even the acetone degreasing must be standardized because more rubbing will disrupt the epidermal barrier and allow for greater penetration. The skin should be stretched during this procedure to ensure degreasing at the depth of the rhytids.

TIMING RELATIVE TO SURGERY

Chemical peeling causes a contraction of the skin in both horizontal and vertical meridians while improving the texture and quality of the skin. Upper and lower eyelid chemical peeling may be performed without surgery or before, in conjunction with, or subsequent to eyelid surgery. Chemical peeling may also be used as an adjunct to endoscopic eyebrow and forehead elevation procedures. As long as the blood supply to the skin has not been disrupted, there is no contraindication to performing a chemical peel at the same time of surgery. For example, we commonly perform an endoscopic eyebrow lift and simultaneously peel the skin of the forehead. In contrast, at the time of a facelift, we peel the perioral skin but not the skin of the cheeks, since the cheek skin has been undermined and its vascular supply theoretically may be compromised.

When chemical peeling is performed simultaneously with upper eyelid surgery (immediately on completion of the surgical procedure, while the patient is still in the operating room), the upper eyelid skin incision and the skin between the upper eyelid incision and the upper eyelid margin are not treated. Alternatively, at the surgeon's discretion, the pretarsal skin may be treated very lightly.

ANESTHESIA AND PATIENT MONITORING

The patient is kept comfortable throughout the procedure and during the postoperative course. Some authors have stated that specific regional skin anesthesia is not necessary for 35 per cent TCA and lighter peels. We have found that many patients do, in fact, have pain with these concentrations and, thus, we use regional block anesthesia for all chemical peels of 35 per cent TCA and the phenol preparations. For greater patient comfort, regional block anesthesia may be administered along with intravenous sedation.

In all cases of simultaneous blepharoplasty and chemical peeling, adequate infiltrative anesthesia exists such that a regional block using 0.5 ml of 2 per cent lidocaine (Xylocaine) with epinephrine and 0.5 ml of hyaluronidase (Wydase) may be infiltrated around the supratrochlear, supraorbital, zygomaticofacial, and infraorbital nerves (see Fig. 31–4). For chemical peels performed independent of surgery, the same regional blocks are given provided that the wounding agent is 35 per cent TCA. The pain resulting from the use of 35 per cent TCA in eyelid and facial peels seems to last no longer than a few minutes as long as iced compresses are used. Because phenols may burn for several hours after application, 0.5 per cent bupivacaine (Marcaine) with 1:200,000 epinephrine is used. Marcaine provides postoperative anesthesia for 4–6 hours and may be repeated if desired.

Cardiac monitoring is standard procedure for full-face phenol peels. Phenol, which is absorbed systemically, is cardiotoxic and may cause arrhythmias. The amount of phenol in the blood stream at any one time is controlled by application of the phenol to segments of the face at 15-minute intervals. If arrhythmias develop, the applications are stopped until the cardiac rate has been regular for 15 minutes. Subsequent phenol applications are placed on smaller surface areas, timed further apart. Lidocaine can be injected intravenously in doses of 5–10 mg for control of arrhythmia.

We have never seen or heard of an arrhythmia resulting from a localized application of phenol to the eyelids. Therefore, we do not use cardiac monitoring for regional applications of phenols. TCA is not absorbed and produces no systemic symptoms other than transient pain.

During full-face peels independent of surgery, many patients desire intravenous sedation. For those who choose not to have intravenous medication, we routinely administer a cocktail of clonidine, which controls acute rises in blood pressure, meperidine (Demerol) and hydroxyzine (Vistaril) for pain control, and flurazepam (Dalmane), which has a sedative and hypnotic effect. The patient is then given regional blocks as described earlier.

CHEMICAL PEEL TECHNIQUE

The same techniques of application are used for all chemical peeling agents. As stated earlier, various wounding agents may be used in different areas and in different manners for each area of the face. When eyelid chemical peeling is performed simultaneously with surgery, the method of application differs from that used for an eyelid chemical peel performed independent of surgery because the agent must avoid the suture lines. The independent procedure is described fully first, and the modifications to be used when a chemical peel is performed in conjunction with blepharoplasty are then detailed.

In all peeling procedures, the skin surface must be adequately prepared. As instructed, the patient has already washed the face before surgery. The surgeon vigorously scrubs the patient's skin with an acetone-moistened gauze pad.

Application of 35 Per Cent TCA

TCA is applied to the skin by means of one or two nonsterile, cotton-tipped applicators with wooden sticks. The use of wooden stick applicators allows the physician to rub the acid vigorously into the skin without breaking the applicator. The applicator is dipped into the TCA. The cotton tip of the applicator is pressed against the side of the container until excess liquid is removed, so that TCA does not drip onto the skin. TCA is applied in the desired manner, with one or more applications according to the depth of wounding desired (Fig. 30–3).

Ideally, the chemical is applied with the patient lying supine. The chemical may be applied to corresponding segments of the eyelids sequentially (i.e., to the right lower eyelid, then to the left lower eyelid) while the amount of chemical and anticipated depth of wounding in the first segment are still fresh in the surgeon's mind.

Some surgeons prefer the eyelids to be closed during application as additional protection for the cornea; others prefer the eyelids to be open in order to avoid the "wick" phenomenon of pulling the chemical agent along rhytid creases (especially in the canthi) into the eye by capillary attraction. Some surgeons advocate using no bland ointment in the eye for fear that it will get onto the skin and cause uneven wounding; others prefer using ointment to protect the cornea and avoid tearing, which will dilute the chemical agent. We place a drop of topical tetracaine and a small amount of bland ophthalmic ointment in each eye.

On the upper eyelid, we prefer to apply the chemical

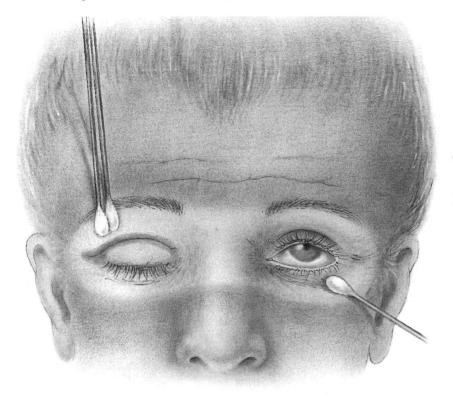

figure 30–3

Application of a chemical wounding agent. *Left (patient's right eyelid),* Immediately on completion of standard upper and lower transconjunctival blepharoplasty. The wounding agent is applied to within several millimeters of the incision lines. *Right (patient's left eyelid),* Independent of blepharoplasty procedure. The chemical is applied to the lower eyelid with the eyelids open and the patient looking up.

while the patient's eyelids are closed. We recommend beginning with the crow's feet superior to the lateral canthal angle and proceeding across the upper eyelid laterally to medially along the inferior border of the eyebrow, then inferiorly down to the eyelash margin, the inner canthus, and the radix of the nose. This is in contrast to the method of McCollough and Hillman,[8] who perform the peel no closer than 2–3 mm from the eyelash margin. The chemical is carried into the eyebrow. There is no damage to the eyebrow cilia from chemical peeling in the eyebrow. (By the same token, the chemical peeling on the forehead is carried into the scalp in a full-face peel.)

On the lower eyelid complex, we apply chemicals with the patient's eyelids open and the patient looking superiorly. The application proceeds from the lateral malar area and orbital rim, across the crow's feet, moving superiorly and medially to the eyelash margin; again, this is in contrast to the method of McCollough and Hillman. The chemical is applied more lightly to the extremely thin skin on the inner canthus and the thin skin over the tarsal plates. The thicker skin of the crow's feet, infrabrow areas, and upper and lower eyelids can tolerate a stronger solution applied with one or two cotton-tipped applicators. Wherever the solution is applied, the edges should be feathered to avoid a sharp line of demarcation and objectionable color contrast.

For peeling an entire face, the TCA solution is applied with two or three cotton-tipped applicators. It is best to apply the solution in a methodical manner to each anatomic region so that areas are not skipped. For example, the solution is first applied to the right cheek, then the left cheek, then the right jowl, then the left jowl. For areas with deeper rhytids, the surgeon can apply the

solution more vigorously, thereby achieving a deeper peel.

Once applied, the chemical produces a white blanching or frosting of the skin. This frosting becomes more prominent over 5–10 minutes, signifying a deeper chemical burn. The extent and speed of frosting are determined by the concentration and amount of TCA applied and by how briskly the applicators are rubbed into the skin. In another 5–10 minutes, the frosting begins to fade and a deep erythema is manifested. The surgeon must look through the frosting to see the erythema. With experience, the surgeon can judge the depth of wounding by the relative timing of onset and density of the frosting and the erythema. Generally, the "whitening" of the skin signifies epidermal protein coagulation and is the end point of the application. Deep frosting may last 20–30 minutes before it begins to fade.

Modifications

Just as different depths of wounding are appropriate for different skin thicknesses and different degrees of actinic change, the experienced surgeon can also use differential depth wounding to tailor the results of the procedure. For example, if an increased superior lateral lift or tightening of skin is desired in the lateral canthus, the surgeon may apply larger amounts of chemical agent in the lateral canthus to cause further vertical shortening of skin and, therefore, a relative "lift" in this area.

Technique for Chemical Peeling Combined with Blepharoplasty

Chemical wounding, performed immediately after the completion of blepharoplasty, is performed in the same way and following the same general scheme just described. If the procedure was an isolated lower transconjunctival blepharoplasty, the upper eyelid and, in fact, all skin surfaces may be treated exactly as if the peel were being performed entirely independent of the surgical procedure.

If the surgical procedure was an upper blepharoplasty and a lower transconjunctival blepharoplasty, the chemicals are applied as described previously, with the following exception. A feathering begins 1 or 2 mm superior to the suture line in the upper eyelid and the chemical application becomes denser up to approximately 3–5 mm superior to the suture line, where the wounding depth is the same as it would be without surgery. A very light "feathering depth" application may be placed on the pretarsal skin, beginning several millimeters inferior to the suture line and continuing to within 1 mm of the lash line. The medial canthus and lower eyelid are peeled exactly as if there had been no surgery.

In the lateral canthus, the surgeon again takes care to stay several millimeters away from the suture line and to feather the edge of the chemical peel adjacent to the suture line to avoid a demarcation line. When a lateral canthal procedure has been performed, the chemical agent is kept away from the suture line as described.

After the chemical peel is completed, nonsterile gauze pads soaked in iced water are applied immediately to the eyelids and peeled areas. Acid applied to the skin surface burns to completion very rapidly. If there is any question as to whether the chemical peeling agent remains on the skin, the skin is immediately dried with the gauze before the cool compresses are applied.

The gauze pads are changed frequently so that they can be kept cool. To minimize the discomfort and burning sensation after a chemical peel, many surgeons instruct patients to use continuous cool compresses for the first day after application of 35 per cent TCA or for 2 days after applications of phenol.

Once the patient is comfortable in the recovery room, a thin coat of petroleum jelly or polymyxin B-bacitracin ointment (Polysporin) is applied to the peeled skin. Patients are instructed to continue cool compresses at home (primarily to offset postoperative swelling) until bedtime and to sleep with their head elevated on two pillows.

The theory and techniques for peeling the remainder of the face in conjunction with facial cosmetic surgery are similar to those for the eyelid. When peeling the forehead region, we routinely use TCA 35 per cent or other agents, depending on the desired depth of penetration. In the glabellar region, a Baker's phenol solution can be applied specifically to any deep rhytids. The perioral rhytids are often difficult to eradicate, and a phenol or Baker-Gordon phenol peel is often required. Peeling of the perioral region can be performed in conjunction with a facelift.

MANAGEMENT AFTER A CHEMICAL PEEL

Management is similar after all chemical peeling procedures, varying only with regard to the total area peeled and the depth of wounding in that area. A partial thickness of the peeled skin dies on the first postoperative day. This dark or ashen-gray skin begins to spontaneously peel off on the first to third postoperative day. Beginning on the first day after a chemical peel, the patient should institute a regimen of facial cleansing twice a day, followed by application of a thin film of ointment.

This regimen begins with the cleansing afforded by either cool or warm, wet compresses, followed by the application of 3 per cent hydrogen peroxide to the skin peel area with cotton-tipped applicators. After sloughing of skin has started, the patient can encourage this process by brisk but light scrubs with the nonsterile cotton-tipped applicators dipped in 3 per cent hydrogen peroxide to remove all debris and dead skin that comes off easily. Skin should never be peeled off manually. With the use of cotton-tipped applicators, a coating of petroleum jelly or polymyxin B-bacitracin ointment is then applied to keep the skin smooth, supple, and lubricated.

If a patient does not take off enough dead skin after a large area of skin is peeled with TCA 35 per cent or a deeper peeling agent, the area may become hot and inflamed. A cellulitis along with a fever may even develop. This does not happen after peels with concentrations below 35 per cent TCA. The surgeon should remind the patient that showers and scrubs always must be followed by coating the area with petroleum jelly to prevent skin desiccation and to promote reepithelialization. Mechanical debridement with scissors and forceps should never be performed because it may damage tissue and cause scarring.

After both blepharoplasty and chemical peels, we generally advise the use of cool-water compresses on the first 2 postoperative days and warm-water compresses to increase circulation and carry away edema beginning on the third postoperative day. The patient, of course, may add cool-water compresses for comfort as needed. Although codeine or hydrocodone (Vicodin) is often prescribed for postblepharoplasty pain, no pain medicine is generally required after TCA skin peels.

This regimen of cleansing and using compresses is continued until the skin is fully reepithelialized, which occurs in 7–10 days. When the upper and lower eyelids have been peeled without surgery, the upper eyelids generally heal 1–2 days more slowly compared with the lower eyelids. This may be because the upper eyelid folds in on itself at the crease, an action that continually reopens the skin and delays reepithelialization in this area.

Once eyelids are fully reepithelialized, the patient may again apply makeup. During the first 2 weeks after the peel, the patient is instructed not to wipe the eyelids when drying with a towel because this may damage new skin. The patient should perform all drying in the peeled area by patting. Sunscreen should not be applied until 4 weeks after peeling, because there is a significantly increased likelihood of contact allergy before then. For the first postoperative month, the patient is instructed to stay out of the sun and to wear a hat when outside.

Sunlight can burn the skin and cause hyperpigmentation.

REPEATED CHEMICAL PEELS

Chemical peeling may be repeated one or more times to achieve the desired result. Whereas some clinicians encourage deep-depth wounding on the first peel, theorizing that the first peel has the least risk of scarring and complications, others advise the use of repeated medium-depth peels to lessen the shock of pigment changes and to reduce the risk of complications. We discuss the options with the patient and decide on the depth of peeling and considerations for subsequent peeling on the basis of all factors, including how soon afterward the patient must resume appearing in public. We frequently perform a simultaneous upper blepharoplasty, a lower transconjunctival blepharoplasty, and a chemical peel with 35 per cent TCA. This may be followed as early as 14 days later by a second peel using TCA 35 per cent or 89 per cent phenol if it is deemed appropriate. If further improvement is desired, a third peeling procedure may be performed after completion of healing of the second peel, usually at 4 days or longer.

The same basic parameters are assessed for each repeated chemical peel as though it were the first time. These parameters are as follows:

- Amount of redundant skin
- Degree of lower eyelid margin laxity
- Existence of lagophthalmos
- Possibility of precipitating corneal exposure
- Degree of actinic damage
- Skin color

Chemicals may be applied to scar lines from previous blepharoplasties. Peeling over the scar does not cause hypertrophy of the scar and tends to lighten its color.

Repeated applications with milder chemical solutions also are appropriate for individuals whose skin is dark (Fitzpatrick's classifications IV–VI) and who want to reduce the risk of hypopigmentation as well as for those who want a brief and easy recovery after each application.

COMPLICATIONS

Complications include ocular damage, prolonged erythema, unexpected hypopigmentation, splotchy hyperpigmentation, scarring (including textural changes), cicatricial ectropion, eyelid retraction, and lagophthalmos.

Ocular Damage

Chemical solutions may burn the cornea or conjunctiva. This may occur either when an applicator accidentally strikes the cornea or conjunctiva or when the welling up of tears along the eyelid margins and canthal areas exerts a wick effect, channeling the chemical to the eye. If the chemical solution strikes the cornea or conjunctiva, it instantly produces a whitish gray burn on the exposed area.

Appropriate treatment consists of immediate irrigation with sterile saline or artificial tears. Pain is managed with one application of topical 1 per cent tetracaine. An antibiotic ointment or antibiotic-steroid ointment is applied. Routine management of a corneal or conjunctival surface burn includes reevaluation at the end of the procedure with regard to the extent of epithelial damage and existing pain. Patching or a corneal bandage contact lens, in addition to antibiotic coverage and continuing ophthalmologic care, may be appropriate.

One of us (D.M.M.) has seen three minor corneal epithelial burns with 35 per cent TCA, all of which healed uneventfully within 2 weeks. This dilution of TCA causes a superficial burn, with instant epithelial coagulation of protein. None of us has experience with burns to the eye caused by 50 per cent TCA or phenol.

Prolonged Erythema

Deeper wounding causes more pronounced and longer-lasting erythema. In general, erythema resulting from the use of 35 per cent TCA lasts 2–4 weeks; from 89 per cent phenol, about 3 months; and from Baker-Gordon formula, 5–8 months. Until erythema resolves, it can usually be camouflaged successfully with makeup.

Unexpected Hypopigmentation

A 35 per cent TCA concentration usually causes minimal permanent hypopigmentation. When phenols are used, there is some permanent hypopigmentation in every case. Thus, it is mandatory that the surgeon carefully evaluate skin color and feather the edges of the treatment areas in order to avoid a sharp line of demarcation, which would draw attention to objectionable color contrast.

Splotchy Hyperpigmentation

Hyperpigmentation is thought to result from exposure to ultraviolet A (UV-A) light in pigment-prone individuals, those who are pregnant, or those who are taking birth control pills, exogenous estrogens, or photosensitizing drugs. It is easier to avoid this complication than to manage it. As mentioned earlier, the skin of each patient is primed with bleaching agents before and after the peel. Every patient should also wear wraparound ultraviolet-filtering protective sunglasses, which shield the upper and lower eyelids and lateral canthi, including the crow's feet areas, from light for 4–6 weeks. The patient must wear a wide-brimmed hat for 6 weeks after surgery and must begin using a UV-A sunscreen with a sun protection factor (SPF) of 15 as soon after healing as possible. In patients who are especially susceptible to hyperpigmentation, the physician may advise the use of sunscreen as early as 2 weeks after a chemical peel and may insist that the sunscreen be applied every hour while the patient is outdoors.

If splotchy hyperpigmentation occurs, it usually can be successfully treated with a combination of 0.05 per cent retinoic acid cream at bedtime and 4 per cent hydroquinone cream in the morning for a few weeks. If this regimen is not successful, the skin may be repeeled to remove the splotchy hyperpigmentation. Strict avoidance of sunlight on the repeeled skin should prevent any recurrence.

Scarring and Other Textural Changes

Scarring and textural changes can occur with wounding depths of TCA 35 per cent or higher. These changes may present as (1) flat, shiny (*atrophic*) areas, (2) as web-type contracture at the inner or outer canthus, or (3) as elevated, thickened (*hypertrophic*) areas of skin.

We know of no effective therapy for atrophic scarring.

Elevated, thickened types of scarring respond favorably to biweekly injections of approximately 0.1 ml of triamcinolone at a concentration of 10 mg/ml. Topical silicone gels are also effective, as are potent topical steroids.

For minor, slight elevations of scarring, twice-daily applications of 1 per cent hydrocortisone ointment also are helpful.

Cicatricial Ectropion, Lid Retraction, and Lagophthalmos

One benefit of chemical eyelid peeling is a vertical shortening of the skin. If more vertical shortening than is desirable occurs, it manifests as lagophthalmos with corneal exposure, lower eyelid retraction, or early lower eyelid margin ectropion or frank ectropion.[9] Exposure symptoms are far more common in patients with an underlying case of dry eyes. Management of these patients includes artificial tear supplementation, bland ointment at night, bandage soft contact lenses, and punctal occlusion.

The lower eyelid is managed with weekly or biweekly injections of triamcinolone (Kenalog). A total of 0.2–0.3 ml (10 mg/ml) is injected into the skin in a horizontal line just inferior to the lower eyelash margin. Further help can be achieved by support of the lower eyelid with sterile gauze strips (Steri-strips) or tape, as is standard for management of postblepharoplasty eyelid retraction or ectropion. These methods, combined with time, can be expected to resolve the majority of such problems related to chemical peeling.

Infections

Bacterial infections, usually secondary to *Staphylococcus aureus*, can occur. We routinely have patients take oral antibiotics for a week following a full facial peel of TCA 35 per cent or deeper. The most feared infection is that due to the herpes simplex virus. Because most people have been exposed to the virus, all patients are at risk for infection. Herpes infection usually occurs 10 days after a peel. The patient may have fever, pain, erythema, and sometimes vesicles, which are seen as punched-out ulcerations.

All patients undergoing one of the more major full-face peels are started on a regimen of oral antiviral agents on the day of the peel, which is continued for 2 weeks. Patients who are undergoing just periorbital peels usually do not require prophylactic antiviral agents.

RESULTS

We have performed more than 10,000 chemical peels over the past 20 years. In general, the procedure has been extremely safe and effective. In our combined experience, we have not had any complications when 25 per cent TCA or less was used. The complications that have occurred were in 35 per cent TCA and phenol peels. There were two cases of herpetic infections after full-face phenol peels that resulted in significant scarring. Both of these patients were receiving prophylactic acyclovir and had breakthrough infections.

Within the past few years, several new antiviral agents have appeared on the market. We recommend that if a herpetic infection develops even if a patient has received acyclovir, a second antiviral agent should be added to the medical regimen.

Mild hypertrophic scarring developed in approximately 1 per cent of our patients who underwent perioral phenol peels. We have been able to reduce these scars with a combination of silicone gels, pulsed dye laser treatments, and intralesional steroid injections. Many patients experienced mild textural skin changes, even after a 35 per cent TCA peel. In general, these changes were mild but problematic to the patient because makeup does not adhere well to these areas to provide camouflage. We recommend that if textural changes are noticed early in the postoperative period, the patient should start using a mild topical steroid.

Two of us (N.S. and J.A.H.) have performed lateral canthal resuspension with a suborbicularis oculi fat (SOOF) and cheek lift,[10–13] which gave satisfactory final results in seven patients referred with lower eyelid retraction after chemical peeling. The use of a hard-palate graft, which is successful for lower eyelid retraction following transcutaneous blepharoplasty,[14] is usually not necessary after a chemical peel because the midlamella has not been manipulated and therefore is not scarred.

CONCLUSION

Chemical peeling alone or in conjunction with surgery can vastly improve the quality of the skin. The procedure is safe and effective but a knowledge of skin cosmetic pathology, wounding and its management, and proper patient selection is required. The potential for improvement by adding chemical peeling to blepharoplasty is significant, and the risk of significant complications in properly selected patients is relatively small. With these considerations in mind, we routinely perform upper blepharoplasty and lower transconjunctival blepharoplasty combined with simultaneous chemical peelings.

REFERENCES

1. Morrow DM: Chemical peeling of the eyelids and periorbital area. J Dermatol Surg Oncol 1992; 18:102–110.
2. Brody HJ: The art of chemical peeling. J Dermatol Surg Oncol 1989; 15:918–921.
3. Stegman SJ, Tromovitch TA: Cosmetic Dermatologic Surgery, pp 27–46. Chicago, Year Book Medical Publishers, 1984.
4. Morrow DM: Simultaneous CO_2 transconjunctival lower lid blepharoplasty and chemical skin peeling. Presented at the Third International Congress of Aesthetic Surgery, Paris, May 20–22, 1989.
5. Hoenig JA, Morrow D: Patient evaluation. In Carniol PJ (ed): Laser Skin Rejuvenation. Philadelphia, JB Lippincott, 1997.
6. Fitzpatrick TB: The validity and practicality of sun-reactive skin types I through VI. Arch Dermatol 1988; 124:869–871.
7. Kligman AM, Grove GL, Hirose R, Leyden JJ: Topical tretinoin for photoaged skin. Am Acad Dermatol 1986; 15:836–859.
8. McCollough EG, Hillman RA: Chemical face peel. Otolaryngol Clin North Am 1980; 13:353–365.
9. Wojno T, Tenzel R: Lower eyelid ectropion following chemical face peeling. Ophthalmic Surg 1984; 13:596–597.
10. Shorr N, Fallor MK: Repair of post blepharoplasty "round eye" and lower eyelid retraction, combined cheek lift and lateral canthal resuspension. In Ward PH, Berman WE (eds): Plastic and Reconstructive Surgery of the Head and Neck, vol 1. Aesthetic Surgery, pp 279–290. St Louis, CV Mosby, 1984.
11. Shorr N, Fallor MK: "Madame Butterfly" procedure: Combined with cheek and lateral canthal suspension procedure for post blepharoplasty "round eye" and lower eyelid retraction. Ophthalmic Plast Reconstr Surg 1985; 1:229–235.
12. Shorr N, Goldberg RA: Lower eyelid reconstruction following blepharoplasty. J Cosmetic Surg 1989; 6:77–82.
13. Hoenig JA, Shorr NS, Shorr J: The suborbicularis oculi fat in aesthetic and reconstructive surgery. Int Ophthalmol Clin 1997; 37:3.
14. Shorr N: Management of post-blepharoplasty lower eyelid retraction with palate mucosal graft. Presented at the American Society of Ophthalmic Plastic and Reconstructive Surgeons, 21st Annual Scientific Symposium, October 1990.

Arthur L. Millman

Chapter *31*

Eyelid and Facial Laser Skin Resurfacing

Carbon dioxide (CO_2) laser resurfacing of the eyelids and face has gained tremendous popularity during the last few years. There is no doubt that this is a useful instrument in smoothing the skin of the face and reducing facial wrinkles.

Debate continues as to whether using this expensive equipment has any significant advantage over using the traditional chemical peels, which are certainly much less costly (see Chapter 30). There is also a question whether laser resurfacing produces more redness of the skin and for a longer time compared with chemical peeling. However, laser resurfacing is appealing to patients, and cosmetic surgeons therefore are encouraged to learn how to use this technology.

In this chapter, Arthur Millman describes the various instruments that can be used to achieve CO_2 laser resurfacing. He also demonstrates how to use this equipment and suggests certain power settings and number of passes to achieve the desired effect.

I continue to use CO_2 laser resurfacing and have had most of my experience with the Luxar equipment. I have found it most useful in smoothing out lower eyelid wrinkles and lateral canthal crow's feet (rhytids). When this technique is added to removal of herniated orbital fat through an internal blepharoplasty approach (see Chapter 20) along with lateral canthal plication (see Chapter 22), I seem to find my best lower eyelid cosmetic results. Although Dr. Millman advocates doing 2½ passes in the lower eyelid, I have found that one pass suffices in most of my patients and has the advantage of reducing the duration of postoperative redness from months to weeks.

Dr. Millman also alerts us to the possible complications of laser resurfacing, which include prolonged skin redness, photosensitivity to the sun, scarring, infections, and abnormal skin pigmentation.

ALLEN M. PUTTERMAN

Aesthetic laser surgery has come to the forefront of oculoplastic and facial surgery technique. This technologic advance has occurred over many years and is most recently attributable to significant changes in technology with the application of the CO_2 laser. This laser, which has been used in medicine for almost a decade, has been associated with recent advances, including the superpulsed CO_2 laser mode, higher-power versions, radiofrequency excited sealed vacuum laser tubes, and hollow-fiber delivery modality. Last, the introduction of an advanced computer chip program and computer pattern generator modalities have allowed for three-dimensional control of the delivery of CO_2 laser energy to wide areas of the eyelid and facial anatomy.

These advances have made aesthetic surgery more viable and the results more predictable and desirable.[1, 2] However, an element of informed skepticism and surgical conservatism should always be used in the application of a new technology. Longitudinal studies are ongoing in this contemporary technique.

LASER SURGICAL SETUP

Oculoplastic surgery with the CO_2 laser calls for a number of special instruments and precautions in the setup of the surgical field for laser efficacy and safety. These include the use of protective eyewear for all persons in the operating room.

Contact lenses or eye shields are necessary for the patient and preferably should be made of metallic surgical steel (Bemsco Surgical Supply, West Seattle). The internal surface of the steel contact lenses should be smooth, and the external surface should be sandblasted for antireflective properties. Topical tetracaine and ophthalmic ointment are usually applied on the inner surface of the shield for patient comfort.

All surgical personnel should wear wavelength-appropriate eyewear, such as eye goggles, surgical loupes, or eyeglasses. Sandblasting the surface of all metallic instruments used in the surgical procedure is recommended. In particular, this antireflective status prevents the inadvertent reflection of the CO_2 laser beam in unwanted areas or tissue.

The surgical field should include the use of wet towels and dressings soaked in sterile water or saline to surround the face or surgical area. Some surgeons use aluminum foil, although I find it cumbersome and do not recommend it.

A smoke or laser plume evacuator is mandatory. Improper laser plume evacuation results in chronic pharyngitis for the surgeon, and biologic and viral particles have been shown to be recovered and transmissible in the laser plume. Standard operating room suction will not suffice.

If general anesthesia is used, anesthetic agents should be nonflammable and the endotracheal tubes should be wavelength-appropriate, usually with a metallic or antireflective coating. A large basin of water should be on or near the surgical field for lavage should a fire start, and an Underwriters Laboratories–approved fire extinguisher should be present in the surgical suite.

CARBON DIOXIDE SURGICAL LASER

A number of CO_2 lasers are available for plastic surgery. This modality is rapidly changing in regard to the technology and equipment available. I have extensive experience with the Coherent Ultrapulse, Luxar Novapulse, and Sharplans Silk Touch and Feather Touch systems.

Although new instruments and companies continually are entering the market, instrumentation is basically divided into two groups. The first group (e.g., Luxar and Coherent) are those that provide a *superpulsed laser*. Used for incisional and resurfacing surgery, this laser can deliver CO_2 energy in very short ($< 1/500$ μsec) bursts, so as to maximize tissue ablation and minimize thermal damage or heat capacitance within the tissue to be treated. In my experience, the ability to use the superpulsed laser for some incisional and all resurfacing surgery is ideal.

The second group (e.g., Sharplans Silk Touch and Feather Touch) consists of *continuous-wave* lasers that deliver energy in a continuous mode. These lasers are frequently presented to the tissue by means of a mechanical mirror-reflecting system, which rapidly moves the laser energy spot in a spiral pattern to perform resurfacing or which remains a stationary spot for incisional surgery.

Each laser uses different settings and terminology (Table 31–1).

LASER PHYSICS PRINCIPLES

The surgeon should understand basic laser physics principles, which guide laser settings in the practice of laser surgery.[1, 2]

For incisional surgery, a small spot size delivers a more precise cutting incision width and delivers more power per unit area, or *fluence*; however, it has a decreased thermal or hemostatic effect. In general, a spot size of 0.2–0.4 mm is ideal for cutting at 7–8 watts of power in a standard continuous-wave mode. The surgeon can accurately modify the amount of energy delivery by focusing and defocusing the laser spot through positioning of the laser hand piece. Laser energy is delivered at a maximum energy level at the exact focal point of the given laser.

The working distance (*focal point*) of each unit is determined by the manufacturer and the given model. This focal point is usually delineated by a footplate attached to the hand piece, which reminds the surgeon of the working distance. The focal point measures 2.5–3.75 cm (1–1.5 inches) in the Coherent and Sharplans models. The exception is the Luxar Novapulse unit, which works on a hollow-fiber delivery system (instead of the mirror-reflected beam in articulated arms for the Sharplans and Coherent models) and in a near-contact mode. Its focal point is simply adjacent by 2–3 mm to the tip of the laser hand piece. The surgeon can thus deliver maximum energy and maximum vaporization or cutting, with minimal thermal or peripheral damage to the surgical tissue, by working at the laser's exact focal point (Fig. 31–1*A*).

table 31-1

Suggested Laser Settings for Cosmetic Skin Resurfacing

Laser Unit	Program		Power	
	Eyelid	*Facial*	*Eyelid*	*Facial*
Luxar Novapulse (3-mm Novaspot scanner)*	E 5–8	E 7–10	5–7 W	6–8 W
Computer pattern generator				
Surescan				
Parallelogram	7.6 × 7.0 mm	12.4 × 7.0 mm	6–8 W	7–10 W
Rectangle	8.0 × 6.3 mm	12.0 × 9.8 mm	6–8 W	7–10 W
Coherent Ultrapulse				
3-mm spot or computer pattern generator:				
(shape) (size) (density)	(3) (3) (3–5)	(3) (6–9) (4–8)	250–350 mJ	350–500 mJ
Sharplans				
Continuous-wave (Silk Touch)	4 mm spiral	6–9 mm spiral	10–14 W	16–18 W

*Program E indicates how fast and large an area will be treated; power, how deep tissue ablation is intended.
Abbreviations: mJ, millijoules; W, watt; mm, millimeter.

Conversely, the surgeon can defocus by withdrawing or increasing the distance of the hand piece to the tissue, thus creating a decrease in power delivered, which decreases the laser's cutting ability but maximizes its thermal or coagulative ability (Fig. 31–1*B*). This is useful for hemostasis and for contouring or ablating tissue. The superpulsed cutting mode increases the depth of the incision by approximately 10–20 per cent and, most importantly, decreases the charring or thermal component by 20–30 per cent.

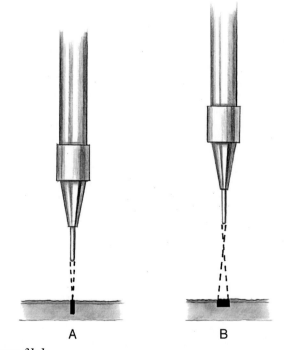

figure 31–1

A, Carbon dioxide (CO₂) laser showing 0.4-mm cutting hand piece focused at the exact focal point of CO₂ beam. Note its thin, deeper incision profile. *B,* The CO₂ laser has been defocused by increasing its distance from the tissue. Note the shallower and wider burn with increased coagulation.

Histopathologic evaluation of continuous-wave versus superpulsed cutting modes has demonstrated that the zone of necrosis or the area of peripheral damage surrounding the actual incision is reduced by almost 30 per cent in the superpulsed mode (compared with the continuous-wave mode), giving a cleaner incision with significant reduction of postoperative inflammation, scarring, and contracture of tissue. Histopathologic samples show an average peripheral zone of necrosis of 130 μm at 7 watts of continuous-wave energy in contrast to 100 μm in the superpulsed mode at the same 7-watt power level.[4]

For resurfacing and tissue ablation, the reader should be familiar with two concepts:

1. *Laser fluence* is defined as the energy per unit area density of the CO_2 laser, that is, the amount of laser energy expressed in millijoules (mJ), or the amount of work, expressed as a numerator, over a denominator expressing the amount of surface area. The unit of millijoules per millimeter squared (mJ/mm²) is used as a convention (J/mm² is rarely used).

2. The *tissue ablation threshold* is the minimum amount of energy required to ablate eyelid and facial skin with a minimal amount of thermal energy. It has been established that 50 mJ/mm² is an accepted minimum threshold for facial skin resurfacing laser ablation.

Because power settings for laser resurfacing refer to a two-dimensional area, the power required for an increased spot size varies exponentially in proportion to the area to be treated. Therefore, the power setting is exponentially proportional to the spot size to achieve ablation threshold.

Different spot sizes are used for different laser instruments. It is most useful to convert the individual terminology into laser fluence levels or the necessary amount of work per unit surface area, as described in millijoules per millimeter squared, to accomplish tissue ablation. For example, a 0.8-mm spot requires 25 mJ/mm² to accomplish ablation threshold. A 3-mm spot requires

353 mJ/mm^2 and a 6-mm spot requires 1413 mJ/mm^2 to achieve ablation threshold. It is obvious that the amount of energy required goes up dramatically with increases in spot size.

COSMETIC SKIN RESURFACING

Eyelids

Cosmetic skin resurfacing (CSR) is the latest advance in cosmetic laser surgical techniques.[1,2] Use of various CO_2 laser systems for careful and discrete resurfacing removal of epithelial and anterior papillary and reticular dermal layers allows for contracture of the skin and collagen matrix. The technique also provides contouring or skin sculpting of the lower eyelid to complete cosmetic blepharoplasty (see Chapter 35). The CSR technique can also be used in the upper eyelid as a touch-up for patients with previous blepharoplasty when a small amount of redundant skin remains and a small amount of tissue contracture will be suitable for a cosmetic effect (Fig. 31–2; see Color Figure). In suitable candidates, there is no need for lower lid skin excision, therefore dramatically diminishing the possible side effects of ectropion and eyelid retraction.

It is important to both select and prepare patients properly for CSR. I do this meticulously to achieve optimal results.

Patient Selection

Patient selection is by far the most important part in the engineering of a successful CSR of the eyelids. Familiarity with dermatologic technique and with the dermatologic and laser literature is paramount to successful skin resurfacing.

A careful history should be obtained as to skin tanning, hair and skin pigment, ethnic history, previous acne or acne treatment, and isotretinoin (Accutane) therapy. Isotretinoin is an absolute contraindication to laser skin resurfacing if it has been used within a 1- to 2-year period. This drug eliminates the adnexal glandular architecture to provide the substrate for reepithelialization and will interfere with proper wound healing. Additionally, the surgeon should identify patients who have sensitive skin, problems using cosmetic products, and hypersensitivities to topical agents and cosmetics.

Careful attention should be made to the patient's geographic origins and ethnicity, childhood hair color, complexion, and tanning history. A familiarity with the Fitzpatrick classification of skin type is required (see Chapter 30, Table 30–2). Fair-complexioned patients, types I and II, are ideal for skin resurfacing. Asian, Hispanic, and Mediterranean patients (types III and IV) are at increased risk for hyperpigmentation after laser resurfacing, and CSR is contraindicated for African-Americans (types V and VI). (Skin preparation and treatment are described in Chapter 30.) Finally, patients whose pigmentation puts them at higher risk for complications after CSR, types III and IV, should be considered for preoperative treatment with melanocyte-suppressing and melanin-suppressing agents (see next). The ideal is to select patients whose skin is clear, healthy, and minimally pigmented.

Preparation for Surgery

Patient preparation begins with proper informed consent and a discussion to ensure that the patient's expectations, are realistic. It is a good idea to show the patient preoperative and postoperative photographs, including pictures of skin erythema and sequential steps in healing. This allows the patient to make an informed decision whether to proceed with skin resurfacing. Additionally, during consultation and on the day of surgery, I use a felt-tipped marker to identify wrinkles in areas to be treated (Fig. 31–3).

Skin preparation can be approached by several methods and should be individualized to the patient's skin care history and skin quality. Any relative risks to hyperpigmentation can be reduced with skin-bleaching agents that suppress melanocytes and melanin. A common preoperative regimen that can be instituted 4–6 weeks before CSR includes the daily use at bedtime of retinoic acid (Retin-A or Renova) cream in either a 0.05 or 0.025 per cent strength. This allows for rejuvenation of the epithelial layer of the skin surface and thinning of the epithelial layer for ideal CSR. In addition, if pigmentation is suspected or a deep tanning history is obtained (Fitzpatrick classification types III and IV), hydroquinone with or without kojic acid can be prescribed. I recommend the use of pigment cream, available from Physicians Choice (Scottsdale, Ariz.), which contains 2 per cent hydroquinone and sunblock sun protection factor (SPF) of 25. An alpha-hydroxy acid can also be used to accomplish a light exfoliation in the preoperative period, optimizing CSR. This can be used daily for 4–6 weeks for melanocyte and melanin granule inhibition and then again after reepithelialization of the skin resurfacing wound (see Postoperative Care later).

Additional preoperative pharmacologic preparation includes antibiotic prophylaxis and anti-inflammatory and antiviral medications, which are all started 1 day preoperatively. Prophylaxis against herpes simplex virus outbreak is mandatory before CSR. It is thought that without prophylaxis approximately 10 per cent of patients undergoing CSR will suffer from herpetic complications. Either a cephalosporin, 250 mg orally four times a day, or tetracycline or erythromycin in penicillin-allergic patients, may be combined with acyclovir (Zovirax), 400 mg orally three times a day, beginning a full 24 hours preoperatively and continuing for 5 days after resurfacing. It is important for patients using these medications to avoid sun-related pigmentation damage by applying a proper sunblock (ultraviolet A and B SPF 15–30). Lastly, systemic steroids can be used before and after CSR. The easiest to use is oral methylprednisolone (Medrol Dosepak), which can be started 1 day before surgery and used as directed as a self-tapering diminishing dosage regimen over a 5-day period.

It is advised to train a member of the office staff, preferably a surgical nurse skilled in dermatologic and postoperative skin care, to prepare the patient for CSR

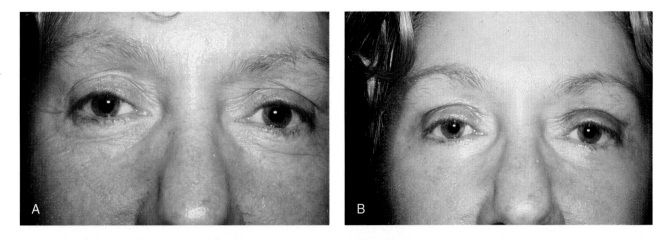

figure 31–2 *A,* Preoperative view of a patient 5 years after conventional four-eyelid blepharoplasty, with recurrence of upper eyelid dermatochalasis (excess skin) and loss of skin fold and lower lid wrinkling. *B,* Postoperative view after CO_2 laser skin resurfacing at 350 mJ and two cosmetic skin resurfacing (CSR) passes to the upper eyelid above the eyelid crease and to lower eyelids and lateral canthus. Note the absence of dermatochalasis and the reformation of the eyelid crease in the upper eyelid as well as the absence of lower eyelid wrinkles. (No incisional surgery or skin incision was performed.)

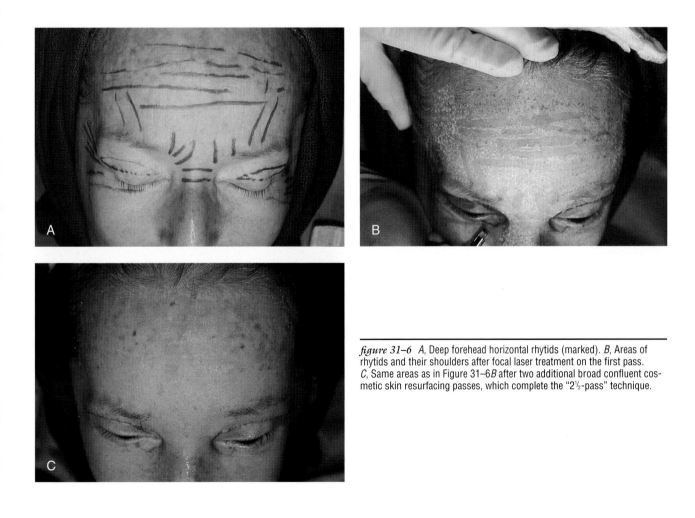

figure 31–6 *A,* Deep forehead horizontal rhytids (marked). *B,* Areas of rhytids and their shoulders after focal laser treatment on the first pass. *C,* Same areas as in Figure 31–6*B* after two additional broad confluent cosmetic skin resurfacing passes, which complete the "2½-pass" technique.

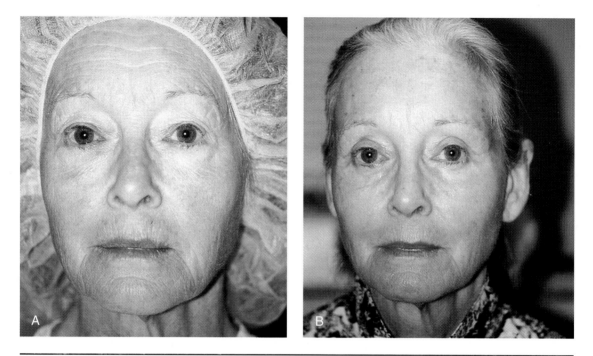

figure 31–8 A woman before (*A*) and after (*B*) full-face cosmetic skin resurfacing in two passes at 350 mJ and focal treatment at 350 mJ (2½-pass technique) and four-lid blepharoplasty using the CO_2 laser technique. Note the significant improvement in facial dyschromias and rhytids, specifically forehead, eyelid, and perioral.

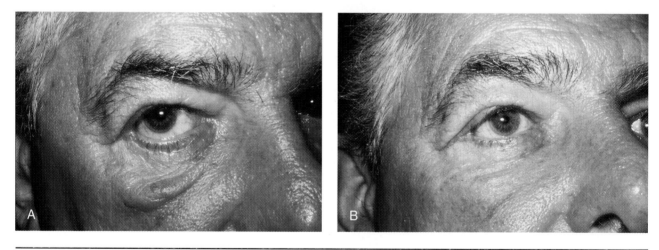

figure 31–9 A man with a malar festoon (cheek bag) before (*A*) and after (*B*) three passes of 300-mJ cosmetic skin resurfacing. He previously had undergone two blepharoplasties.

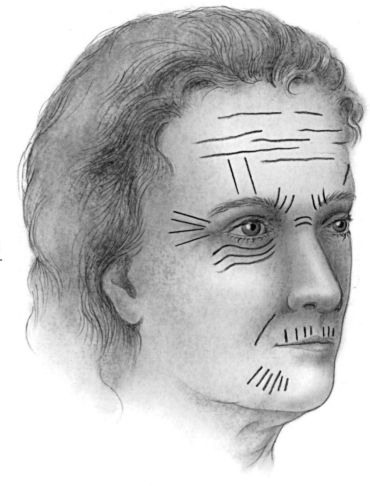

figure 31–3

Marks applied with a felt-tipped marker indicate areas of concern needing focal treatment. The "shoulders" of the highlighted wrinkles will be pretreated in the "2½ pass" technique. (See Eyelid and Periorbital Cosmetic Skin Resurfacing Incisions in text.)

preoperatively and help in the perioperative and postoperative period. The patient should obtain all prescriptions, dressings, and sunblock preparations before surgery.

Surgical Technique

Marking. With the patient in a fully alert status, the cosmetic surgical areas should be marked with a felt-tipped marker. The areas to be marked include excess skin for upper eyelid blepharoplasty, the lateral canthus, and areas of periorbital static and kinetic wrinkling. Generally, I ask the patient to view what I mark in a hand-held mirror so we reach agreement on areas to be treated (see Fig. 31–3). In addition, extremely deep wrinkles should be marked in their "deepest valley," and the "shoulders" (the high points of the wrinkle) should be marked to accentuate and allow for laser sculpting of these areas with additional laser passes. The proper markings should be done before sedation and before instillation of local anesthesia, which distorts the area of static and kinetic wrinkling.

The surgeon at this point should pay careful attention to the proposed plan of resurfacing, including the area to be treated, depth of resurfacing, and probable power settings and number of laser passes to be used. The surgeon should refer to a preoperative facial diagram

and make careful preoperative notes and markings, including any benign tumors to be removed or other ancillary surgery to be performed simultaneously and planned areas of treatment.

If facial or perioral areas are to be treated, these need to be marked at this time (see Perioral and Facial Cosmetic Skin Resurfacing).

Anesthesia. There are two components to proper anesthesia of the laser surgical patient. The first is preoperative sedation with an anxiolytic, such as diazepam (Valium); typically, 5–10 mg is suitable. An analgesic medication can be used additionally, either oral hydrocodone and acetaminophen (Vicodin extra strength) or oxycodone and acetaminophen (Percocet), or intramuscular meperidine (Demerol), 75 mg, and hydroxyzine (Vistaril), 25 mg, for narcotic analgesia. Intravenous sedative anesthesia monitored by an anesthesiologist is recommended. A propofol (Diprivan) infusion pump is ideal.

Eyelid resurfacing can be conducted with proper local or regional nerve block anesthesia (Fig. 31–4). The surgeon must have an intricate familiarity with trigeminal nerve distribution in the ophthalmic maxillary, mandibular, and precervical and postcervical areas. All peripheral nerve branches, especially mental, submental, nasociliary, nasopalatine, supraorbital, supratrochlear,

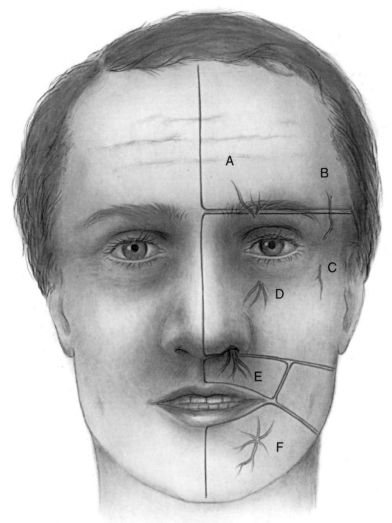

figure 31–4

Trigeminal regional nerve blocks for facial sensory blockade in facial cosmetic skin resurfacing. A, supraorbital nerve; B, zygomaticofrontal nerve; C, zygomaticotemporal nerve; D, infraorbital nerve; E, nasopalatine nerve; F, mandibular nerve.

and frontal nerve branches, are used.[3] Proper use of regional nerve blockade allows for a minimum amount of lidocaine to be instilled, with maximum sensory blockade, and allows the surgeon to minimize the use of direct infiltration. There are three important benefits. First, local-regional blockade lessens epinephrine vasoconstriction, which masks the depth of laser penetration and blanches tissue, making it more difficult to "read" the color or depth of dermal penetration. Second, it avoids direct infiltration, which balloons the tissue-masking skin rhytids and proposed areas of wrinkle removal and treatment. Third, the volume of lidocaine necessary can be kept to a minimum, which avoids toxicity with full facial blockade.

Regional nerve blockade (most necessary for large areas of full facial CSR and when combined with incisional blepharoplasty) is generally done after the initialization of intravenous sedation. Intravenous sedation should be performed by a board-certified anesthesiologist or under direct supervision of a well-trained and experienced nurse anesthetist. Ideally, intravenous sedation is delivered with a combination of sedative, analgesic, and amnestic medications. The use of medications,

such as propofol medazepam, and fentanyl in proper combination provides ideal patient comfort and cooperation. (See Chapter 8 for additional discussion of anesthesia in oculoplastic surgery.)

Patient sedation optimizes the surgeon's ability to perform laser surgery. It is even more critical than in conventional surgery that the patient be made comfortable so that a movement is minimized. Even small degrees of patient movement or muscle animation result in high degrees of inaccuracy in laser delivery, in both an incisional and a resurfacing mode.

Eyelid and Periorbital Cosmetic Skin Resurfacing Incisions. CSR of the eyelids and periorbita should always be performed with the use of proper laser safety (see Laser Surgical Setup). The resurfacing surgeon can think of the eyelid area as broken down into anatomic regions corresponding to pretarsal, preseptal, and orbital areas correlating with the orbicularis anatomy. Each of the skin surfaces associated with these regions varies in thickness, with the pretarsal being the thinnest and the thickness increasing to the orbital region and the cheek.

Power settings vary with the different instruments

(see Table 31–1). Generally, power settings correspond to the amount of work or millijoules used, which correspond to the amount of tissue to be removed or depth of penetration.

Program settings generally refer to a two-dimensional surface area, either a 0.8- or 3-mm spot matrix. Program settings are in a geometric pattern, usually squares, parallelograms, or rectangles (in the case of superpulsed instruments such as the Coherent and Luxar systems) or as 4-mm, 6-mm, and larger circles done as a spiral of continuous-wave laser applications (in the Sharplans Silk Touch and Feather Touch systems). Table 31–1 demonstrates typical programs suggested for the eyelid and facial areas separately.

Techniques for resurfacing vary greatly among different surgeons, and new techniques are developing at a rapid rate. It is rare to use more than two passes of CSR in the eyelid area, and the beginning surgeon would be well advised to begin with slower repetition, small geographic area programs, and lower-power laser settings. Additionally, some surgeons advocate very light treatment, including only single passes in the eyelid area, which accomplish epithelial ablation with minimal or no dermal penetration. In the periorbital and orbital regions and adnexal areas (cheek, lateral canthus, and temples), deeper penetration can be used. The surgeon should avoid the medial one third or peripunctal area of the upper and lower eyelids to prevent punctal ectropion.

Advanced techniques include pretreatment by laser resurfacing and tissue ablation of specific wrinkles, scars, or acne pits and the treatment of the shoulders (the high-sided ridges) of deep static wrinkles. Ideally, the shoulders of these wrinkles are treated first (Fig. 31–5A and B), and ablated debris is removed after CSR by wiping with saline-moistened gauze. Uniform confluent passes of laser CSR over the entire area to be resurfaced are then done in layers (Fig. 31–5C to E). One to two additional confluent passes of CSR can be used in addition to the focal treatment of shoulders already described.

After each pass of laser resurfacing, the ablated tissue should be wiped away meticulously with a moistened gauze pad. The skin should be kept taut for a consistent and accurate application of the laser energy so that a reproducible consistent pattern can be used from patient to patient and to avoid overlapping or skipping of each burn. The surgeon must not fail to remove ablated debris and should avoid an overlap of any burn pattern because either will allow for significant uncontrolled application of energy. Ablated debris or overlap acts as a heat sink and delivers a much higher degree of thermal energy and, therefore, more tissue damage than desired.

In review, previously identified areas of deep rhytids (crow's feet) and/or their shoulders, creases, or scars are treated focally, and two broad confluent passes of CSR are then accomplished over the entire area to be treated. As an example, compare the marker-highlighted areas in Figure 31–6A (showing where deep forehead horizontal rhytids are present; see Color Figure) with Figure 31–6B (showing a smooth area that received focal treatment with 350 mJ along the areas of the horizontal rhytids and their shoulders). Subsequently, an additional two broad confluent CSR passes at 350–450 mJ are performed (Fig. 31–6C), for a total of three passes in the focal areas and two broad confluent passes over the entire treatment area. I call this the *2½ pass* technique.

In the eyelid and periorbital area, the 2½ pass technique is especially useful in the lateral canthus and lateral cheek area for rhytids and areas of facial mimesis (Fig. 31–7). Focal treatment to the rhytids and then broad confluent passes at 250–350 mJ in the lateral canthus and lower eyelid, comprising the 2½ pass technique, are very effective for aesthetic lower eyelid results, especially in combination with transconjunctival removal of fat pads for blepharoplasty. Judgment as to depth and penetration is aided by tissue color differentiation.

Generally, a first pass allows for complete removal of epithelium and a pink erythematous appearance of the skin. Each pass, ideally, removes 60–80 μm of tissue (see Fig. 31–5A to E).[4] A second pass allows for entry into the papillary dermis and an orange-like tinge to the skin that begins to border on yellow-orange. High-power second passes or medium-power third passes

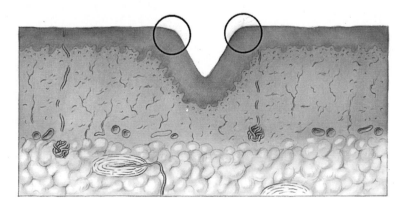

figure 31–5

The "2½ pass" technique. *A*, Rhytid with "shoulders" marked in circles.

A

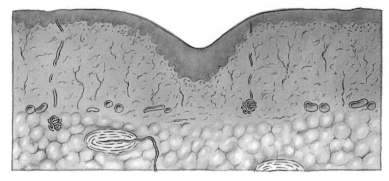

B

B, The first pass or half pass of laser cosmetic skin resurfacing (CSR) is made over the shoulders only.

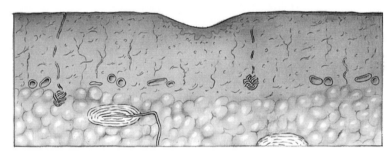

C

Second-pass CSR penetration into papillary dermis

C, The second pass confluently removes all epithelium.

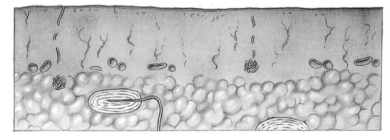

D

D, The third pass removes and contracts the upper papillary dermis.

E, Skin layers are vaporized in the "2½ pass" technique. Shown are three distinct maneuvers: I, the epithelium is focally removed from the shoulders of the wrinkle; II, a confluent pass is made over the entire area entering the papillary dermis of the shoulder or high point of the wrinkle, simultaneously completing epithelial removal confluently elsewhere; and III, maximum ablation (~150–180 μm in depth) is achieved at the shoulder or high point of the wrinkle, entering deep into the papillary dermis after a total of three passes (two passes over the confluent surrounding skin area).

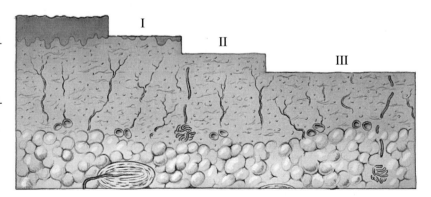

E

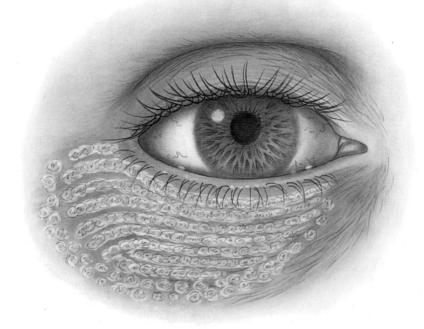

figure 31–7

Lower eyelid cosmetic skin resurfacing pattern with 3-mm spot matrix at 300 mJ.

allow for entrance into the reticular layer of the dermis and begin to bring out a chamois-yellow and white appearance. This should be a definite end point to skin resurfacing. A white or grayish appearance to the resurfaced area indicates deep reticular layer penetration and can allow coagulative necrosis. Coagulative necrosis, which stimulates the need for healing by secondary intention and granulation tissue, of course, leads to subsequent hypertrophic scarring.

The beginning surgeon is advised to be very conservative in initial treatments and, again, to use lower power settings and slower program settings with small geographic areas to be treated. Fewer passes or a single pass would be well advised.

At the completion of CSR, the surgeon can treat regional areas and fine-tune and accomplish *feathering* (blending an area of CSR with an area not to be treated). For example, if a blepharoplasty is to be done alone with lower eyelid resurfacing, this area may be blended with the surrounding cheek and temples so as not to create a regional demarcation of untreated area. This is generally best done at decreasing power levels in a layered technique (i.e., in decreasing amounts of penetration and ablation) to allow for a transition zone between the areas to be resurfaced and the untreated area. Typical power settings are presented in Table 31–1; in general, 250–350 mJ is a good power level for the eyelid area.

The 3-mm spot is the most useful and controllable in eyelid and periorbital resurfacing and is available in all three of the laser systems described in this chapter (see Fig. 31–6, Color Figure). Large geographic patterns using a computer pattern generator in the Coherent or Luxar system can be used; however, I find that using larger than 6-mm patterns can be difficult to lay down systematically and perfectly evenly and confluently in the eyelid area.

Feathering (blending) is generally done by both decreasing the power level to 200 mJ and decreasing the density of the 3-mm spots to be delivered so that there are gap areas in between. Feathering also can be performed using lower densities in the computer pattern generator of numbers 2 and 3 in the Coherent laser and −1 and −2 in the Luxar system. In the Sharplans system, a gradual reduction in wattage accomplishes the same result, particularly going from a 6-mm pattern in the main areas to be treated down to 4-mm spots in the peripheral area and reducing from 14 watts in the main area to be treated to 9 or 10 watts in the peripheral feathering area (see Table 31–1).

Perioral and Facial Areas

Patient selection, preparation for surgery, marking, and anesthesia are similar to those described for eyelid resurfacing. The surgeon must be careful when marking in the perioral, cheek, forehead, and glabellar areas in order to ascertain areas to be treated and the proposed thickness of skin and depth of resurfacing to be accomplished (see Fig. 31–3). Carefully delivered regional trigeminal nerve blocks are used, as for eyelid CSR (see Fig. 31–4).

Resurfacing the perioral, cheek, and forehead areas allows for a higher depth of penetration and, therefore, a higher power setting and use of deeper ablation programs (Fig. 31–8; see Color Figure). It is also easier for the surgeon to use larger geometric patterns, including the larger computer pattern generator program patterns available. The large square and parallelogram patterns measuring almost 1.5 cm are easily used in the forehead and broad cheek areas and can be linked as a tiling pattern quite easily. The density usually can be quite high; however, overlap of burns should be consistently avoided. Typical power levels include 350–500 mJ (see Table 31–1) for the forehead and cheek area and in the upper eyelid and perioral area.

Resurfacing of the facial area needs to be done carefully if the patient has a previous history of chemical peels, specifically a phenol peel or multiple trichloroacetic acid peels. This, of course, also applies to patients who have had previous CSR and are being retreated. These patients have thinner epithelial and dermal areas after laser resurfacing and achieve a deeper penetration more quickly with less power and fewer laser surgical passes.

An additional note of caution in the perioral area is to protect the teeth enamel by covering the teeth in the surgical field with moist gauze pads. The laser will "resurface" the enamel of normal teeth and the porcelain layer of capped teeth.

The area of the vermilion border in the perioral area, in addition to perioral "lipstick" lines, may be treated. The surgeon should visualize the resurfacing pattern measuring 3–5 mm across the vermilion border and use slightly lower energy settings to prevent slow epithelial regeneration in this area and morbidity while the patient is eating. Again, the shoulders of deep rhytids and wrinkles should be treated and marked preoperatively and then followed by uniform patterns of CSR. The outer corner of the lip or oral angle should be treated lightly or omitted to avoid delayed wound healing due to constant wetting of this area with salivation and eating.

The lower lip and chin can be included in the perioral treatment area. This is also a frequent area for acne scarring, as are the malar eminence and cheek in patients with acneiform history. The surgeon can best treat these areas by marking the center of the acne crater and avoiding laser treatment to those areas. The surgeon then uses the laser to shape or plane the circular area surrounding the depth of the acne crater or the ring surrounding the acne pit. This allows for contraction of this tissue and laser "planing," which creates a more uniform surface. These areas are generally treated at higher-power settings, such as 450–500 mJ (see Table 31–1).

BROW

The brow area most commonly treated is the *glabella*, or the area between the eyebrows extending onto the nasal bridge. The horizontal furrows of the nasal bridge and vertical creases of the glabella are due to the corrugator and procerus protractor muscles of the forehead.

The patient's expectations must be realistic because complete ablation usually is not possible with CSR alone. Entire forehead resurfacing can be used and, because the brow area generally has thicker skin, second and third passes are frequently used at higher power levels (e.g., 350–500 mJ). The combination of endoscopic brow lifting with CSR of the forehead area is remarkably effective in treating forehead and glabellar creasing (see Chapter 28). However, patients should be instructed that CSR most successfully treats areas of static wrinkling, whereas areas of facial mimesis and kinetic wrinkling or areas that wrinkle on movement and facial animation are treated least successfully.

MIDFACE, NOSE, AND CHEEK

The cheek area, which has a very thick dermis, can be treated with high-power settings, again in the range of 350–500 mJ (Fig. 31–9; see Color Figure). This area is also easily treated with large computer pattern generator geometric areas of 8, 10, and 12 mm. High-density programs can also be used where essentially confluent passes can be made (see Table 31–1).

POSTOPERATIVE CARE

After CSR is completed, the surgeon irrigates the treated surface area with copious saline. The surface should then be towel-dried gently. The use of a hair dryer gun on a cool setting can be used to further dry the treated area. A dry occlusive dressing, such as Flexzan, is then applied (Fig. 31–10). I prefer the use of a dry dressing technique. The advantage of a Flexzan dressing is that it has an adhesive component; used dry, it allows absorption of the serous transudate in the healing skin resurfacing wound. The Flexzan dressing also can be left in place for 2–5 days and acts as a scaffolding for more rapid epithelialization and diminished postoperative edema. Its drawback, however, is that it is opaque and does not allow for viewing of the skin surface during this healing period.

Alternatives include wet dressing techniques, which can be as simple as using petroleum jelly (Vaseline) or vegetable oil (Crisco); some surgeons prefer the use of bacitracin antibiotic ointment. It should be noted that a percentage of patients who have or will develop hypersensitivities to topical antibiotics in the early postoperative period experience deepithelialization (see Complications). Wet dressings also include Vigilon or plastic wrap (Saran Wrap), which are clear and thus allow the wound to be visualized at all times. These dressings are changed daily, with repeated application of lubricants, ointments, or antibiotics, and need to be fixated with Micropore paper tape. In either case, it is important to use ice masks, which diminishes postoperative edema.

Epithelialization generally occurs at 10–14 days, and at that point makeup can be applied. Initially, there is a markedly erythematous phase, which is best concealed with a green concealer. I recommend Gentle Cover Green Concealer and a flesh-tone cover-up that includes an SPF-15 sunscreen, called Le Velvet film make-up. Dermablend postoperative concealer is a commonly available alternative. For more information on the use of makeup postoperatively, see Chapter 39. For maximum suppression of postoperative and inflammatory pigmentation, a daily regimen of pigment cream (Physicians Choice) can be restarted at 3–4 weeks postoperatively.

COMPLICATIONS

Common postoperative difficulties after CSR are mainly related to skin care. Exaggerated hypersensitivity, even

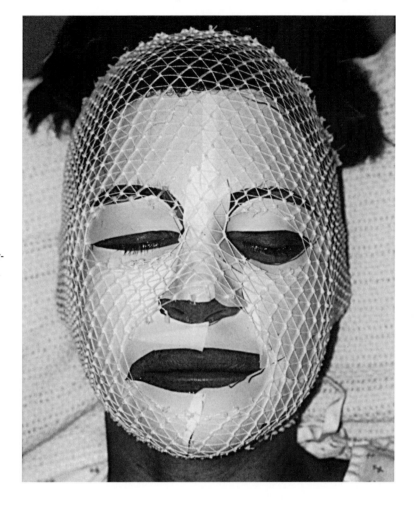

figure 31–10

Patient with a full-face dry occlusive dressing (Flexan) covered by a facial net.

to previous products the patient regularly used, is common. Topical medications and moisturizers should therefore be simple and plain. Allergies to the soy in Crisco oil and to SPF-sunblock lotions and soaps are frequently seen and can result in skin ulceration and delayed healing. Herpes simplex infection can mimic this effect and needs to be ruled out or treated. With acyclovir prophylaxis, I have not had one case of herpetic infection. Similarly, no bacterial infections have yet occurred with the oral antibiotic and methylprednisolone regimen (Medrol Dosepak).

Erythema is expected and usually can be covered with makeup at 2 weeks. The erythema gradually resolves over 6–12 weeks, depending on depth of treatment. I have not seen persistent erythema with the methods and settings described in this chapter.

I have encountered temporary eyelid retraction and a few cases of temporary ectropion (everted eyelid). These complications were always in patients who had undergone previous skin excision blepharoplasty, and all cases resolved without treatment.

RESULTS

I have treated more than 180 patients with CSR. Overall, patients find the improvement in skin texture, complexion, and rejuvenation gratifying after CSR. Often,

patients describe the procedure as painless. Patients typically can resume normal lifestyles after avoiding social activity for 7–10 days.

CSR, in combination with conventional eyelid and facial plastic surgical techniques, allows for optimal results, although CSR can be used alone for more moderate results. Indeed, this technique represents an exciting addition to the armamentarium of the ophthalmic plastic and facial plastic surgeon.

ERBIUM LASER

Laser surgery continues to evolve rapidly. Already, new lasers and techniques for laser skin resurfacing are being considered in addition to the previously established techniques designated in this chapter.

One of the most promising new developments is an erbium:YAG laser system whose absorption spectrum is 2.94 μm, in contrast to the 10.6-μm absorption output characterizing the CO_2 laser. At the 2.94-μm level, there is a tenfold increase or improvement in energy absorption of intracellular water (H_2O). This tremendous increase in energy absorption spectrum of the erbium:YAG laser allows for increased tissue ablation with decreased thermal conductivity and zone of thermal damage. In clinical practice and after a 1-year trial of the erbium:YAG laser, the depth of tissue ablation with multiple, repetitive "impacts," or applications, of this laser can be made equivalent to those of the CO_2 laser, and the amount of tissue damage, postoperative inflammation, and erythema is dramatically reduced. With the erbium:YAG laser, patients are free of erythema in 7–14 days; with the CO_2 laser, 6–12 weeks is the norm. Consequently, patients with Fitzpatrick's skin classification types III and IV (including Hispanics and Asians) can be treated with dramatic reduction of short-term and long-term pigmentary conditions.

Disadvantages of the erbium:YAG laser include a lack of coagulation resulting from the lack of thermal content, so that it cannot be used for incisional surgery or cutting. Also, when deep resurfacing is performed, there is breakthrough punctate bleeding by the capillaries of the papillary dermis. Finally, there is no contracture effect because there is neither thermal damage nor a zone of necrosis.

The Energy Systems Corporation and I are exploring the possibility of combining the erbium:YAG and CO_2 lasers into one medium and application. In this experimental modality, the epithelium is removed with the erbium:YAG laser at 1–1.5 joules and 10 impacts per second (15 watts), and initial penetration to the papillary dermis is accomplished. At that point, the CO_2 pulsed laser, at 300–400 mJ with the computer pattern generator, within the thermal relaxation of the dermis, is used to further deepen the removal of tissue and create contracture in the dermis, where long-term cosmetic improvement of skin and ablation of rhytids are accomplished. In this way, postoperative morbidity, erythema, inflammation, and risks of pigmentation are noticeably reduced, and the positive effects of wrinkle removal and tissue contracture are maintained at a level slightly less than with the CO_2 laser alone but with morbidity significantly reduced.

There will no doubt be continued evolution of both equipment and application of the erbium:YAG laser. Aesthetic surgeons will be well served, as will their patients, by keeping current with and participating in the development of this technology. My personal eyelid and facial surgical technique has greatly changed from what it was 6 years ago, with the routine inclusion of at least a laser surgical component, if not comprehensive laser surgical technique. I am sure that other oculoplastic surgeons have increased their experience with lasers as well. Consequently, our patients are now able to obtain a more predictable, refined result, with significantly lessened postoperative morbidity and increased satisfaction.

References

1. Waldorf HA, Kauvar AN, Geronemus RG: Skin resurfacing of fine to deep rhytides using a char-free carbon dioxide laser in 47 patients. Dermatol Surg 1995; 21:940–946.
2. Keller GS, Cray J: Laser-assisted surgery of the aging face. Facial Plast Surg Clin North Am 1995; 3:319–341.
3. Tu N: Dermabrasion, chemical peel and laser procedures. In Tu N (ed): Anesthesia and Facial Plastic Surgery. New York, Thieme, 1994.
4. Millman A: Comparison of histopathology of superpulse laser in carbon dioxide cosmetic skin resurfacing. Presented at the American Society of Plastic and Reconstructive Surgeons–American Academy of Ophthalmology Meeting, November 1996, Chicago.

Steven Fagien

Chapter 32

Facial Soft-Tissue Augmentation with Autologous Injectable Collagen

Soft-tissue facial insufficiencies manifest themselves as grooves and depressions in the face. Surgical tightening of the facial and eyelid tissues and administration of botulinum toxin (Botox) help minimize these problems. However, some patients will have a good result by soft-tissue augmentation alone.

Augmentation with injectable materials is certainly an important part of cosmetic facial surgery and is a new topic to this edition. In the past, soft-tissue augmentation was performed by the injection of nonautologous injectable collagen, mostly with xenogeneic bovine collagen (Zyderm and Zyplast). In this chapter, Steven Fagien brings us up to date on how to test patients for nonautologous collagen, determine candidates for the procedure, and inject this material. He also elaborates on other augmentation materials, such as silicone fluid, polytetrafluoroethylene (polytef, Teflon) paste (Plastipore), hydroxyapatite, and expanded polytef (Gore-tex).

The main thrust of this chapter is on autologous injectable collagen (Autologen). Dr. Fagien has had considerable experience with this new material. Autologous injectable collagen has advantages over other injectable materials because it is produced from the patient's own skin, therefore eliminating the allergenic problems that can occur with nonautologous materials. Also, this material possibly has a longer lasting effect than the nonautologous injectable materials, specifically Zyderm and Zyplast.

Autologen is still new in its use by cosmetic surgeons, and only time will tell its lasting effect. At this time, however, Autologen seems to be a promising new injectable material for soft-tissue augmentation.

ALLEN M. PUTTERMAN

Over the past few decades, specialists who offer remedies for facial rejuvenation have balanced the efficacy of surgical and nonsurgical options. The surgical approach is evolving. Particular attention has been directed to the gross anatomy of aging (e.g., submuscular aponeurotic system, canthal ligaments, platysma, suborbicularis oculi fat [SOOF], malar fat, brow position) with solutions that attempt to reverse the effects of aging in these areas.[1, 2] Surgical solutions are typically directed at restoring the anatomic position and otherwise excising redundant soft tissue in three dimensions. Many surgical options have proved less effective in enhancing the qualitative aspect of soft tissue (wrinkling, dermal contour defects, and dermal and subcutaneous volume losses that occur with aging)—the fourth dimension. Educated surgeons (and patients) are demanding treatment solutions to the aged face that not only are "nonsurgical" in appearance but also yield longer-lasting beneficial effects. This concern is clearly evident in the surgical arena by comparing the superficial musculoaponeurotic system (SMAS) or composite approach to face lifting versus a mere "skin lift."[1–4] This segregation has enlightened many of us to the realization that not every case of facial rejuvenation is a surgical problem.

Nonsurgical approaches to the aging face have also covered the spectrum of obvious triumphs and unfortunate failures. Skin resurfacing with topically applied agents such as trichloroacetic acid (TCA)[5] and phenol,[6] chemodenervation (Botox),[7] and laser exfoliation[8] still has a stronghold in the war against wrinkles (see Chapters 30, 31, and 33). Skin resurfacing by any method, including dermabrasion, is mostly useful for fine and medium wrinkles, with less attention paid to the "deeper" components of facial aging.

Understanding the anatomy of the aging face on a microscopic level allows us to realize where some of the aforementioned options for facial rejuvenation fall short. Aging affects not only the gravitational influence on a macroscopic level (e.g., ptosis of the brow, SMAS, canthal tendons) but also the qualitative and quantitative integrity of the soft tissue, including dermal collagen and subdermal fat.[9]

ALLOPLASTIC AGENTS FOR SOFT-TISSUE AUGMENTATION

Many dermal fillers have been tried during the 20th century in an attempt to augment facial soft tissue.[10] Mineral oil, paraffin, and similar oils and waxes were used for various purposes during the early part of the 20th century.[11] Complications, such as local chronic edema, lymphadenopathy, granulomata, scarring, and ulcerations, were common.

In the past 20 years, other alloplastic injectable and surgically implanted materials have been used with varied success in an attempt to create an "off-the-shelf" substance to be used for soft-tissue augmentation.[12–17] Such materials include:

- Silicone fluid
- Polymethylmethacrylate microspheres (Artecoll)
- Cross-linked polydimethylsiloxane (Bioplastique)
- Teflon paste (Plastipore)
- Porous/mesh-form polyethylene (Marlex)
- Hydroxyapatite
- Multiple variations of expanded polytetrafluoroethylene (ePTFE; Gore-tex)

The advantages of these substances, although touted for efficacy as a result of their inert behavior, mostly reflect availability and cost. Concerns regarding the use of these products include chronic inflammation, infection, extrusion, and migration of the substance, which often necessitates removal. In addition, these alloplastic

agents are technically difficult to administer and have yielded lesser aesthetic effects. Injectable alloplastic agents have typically been designed for intradermal injection. Surgically implantable agents are administered subcutaneously either with the use of a trocar or in a surgical plane (i.e., skin-muscle-subcutaneous flap) at the time of a facial plastic surgical procedure, for instance, a facelift.

HETEROLOGOUS AGENTS FOR SOFT-TISSUE AUGMENTATION

Xenogeneic fillers have also been used to correct facial wrinkles, furrows, and other dermal defects. Such materials include:

- Reconstituted bovine collagen (Zyderm and Zyplast)[18, 19]
- Other biologic injectable heterologous products (Fibrel)[20]
- Surgically implantable homologous tissue (Alloderm)[21]

Of all of the nonautologous injectable agents commercially available, Zyderm and Zyplast (Collagen Corporation, Palo Alto, Calif.) have enjoyed considerable popularity because of their availability and immediate aesthetic effects. Zyderm I is a 3.5 per cent suspension of bovine dermal collagen fiber fragments. Zyplast is a glutaraldehyde cross-linked variety initially formulated to be more resistant to *in vivo* enzymatic degradation. Zyderm I was designed for the correction of superficial facial wrinkles and to be injected into the papillary dermis. Zyplast, on the other hand, was designed for placement into the middle to deep (reticular) dermis.[18]

Patients with a history of autoimmune disease typically have been excluded from treatment with bovine collagens. Some examples include:

- Rheumatoid arthritis
- Systemic lupus erythematosus
- A history of anaphylactoid reactions or hypersensitivity to lidocaine
- A history or established positive skin test to the Zyderm/Zyplast implant)

Skin testing is mandatory and is easily performed by injection of a 0.1-ml test dose of Zyderm I into the dermis of the skin on the volar forearm of the patient. A positive skin test is defined as an indurated erythematous papule that lasts for more than 6 hours or appears 24 hours or more after testing. Reportedly, at least 3 per cent of those tested have a positive result. In an additional 2 per cent of patients, an allergic reaction develops at the treatment site despite an initial negative skin test; therefore, most physicians who use bovine collagen advocate double skin testing.[18]

The technique of injecting bovine collagen is similar to that for injecting autologous collagen and is detailed later in this chapter. Zyderm I is typically administered with a slight overcorrection and associated blanch (whiteness). The injection of Zyplast is commonly followed by massage to smooth out any beading that might occur with a more superficial placement of the implant. In thicker skin, a layering technique may be employed whereby a more superficially placed Zyderm I is injected over a more deeply placed Zyplast. Despite the excellent aesthetic effects that can be achieved with bovine collagen, in most patients these beneficial effects last only several months.

Replacing or augmenting an individual's dermal collagen with processed animal or skin-banked/cadaveric human collagen for the correction of wrinkles also heralds concerns of immunogenicity and transfer of a communicable disease.[22-34] Our increased knowledge of collagen biochemistry and our clinical experience indicate that the efficacy of the xenogeneic collagen implants has fallen short of our expectations. Although the overall safety of the xenogeneic collagen implant has been relatively well established, clinicians and the consumer have become wary of its use because of its lack of efficacy. The knowledge gained, however, has cleared the way for the creation of the ideal autologous implant.

AUTOLOGOUS AGENTS FOR SOFT-TISSUE AUGMENTATION (AUTOLOGEN)

Autologous injectable collagen (Autologen, Collagenesis, Inc., Beverly, Mass.) is the ideal implant for facial soft-tissue augmentation because it is efficacious, biocompatible, easy to administer, and exceeds all safety requirements. It is not apparent (except for its augmentative effect), it remains immobile (no migration), it induces no short-term or long-term inflammatory effects, and it poses no risk of communicable or immune-mediated diseases. Autologous tissue grafting[35-45] has been universally successful in such reconstructive surgical procedures as:

- Dermis-fat grafting
- Skin grafting
- Ear, nasal, and hard palate cartilage grafts
- Muscle transplants
- Fascial grafts
- Bone grafts
- Hair transplants
- Mucous membrane grafting
- Corneal autografts
- Coronary artery bypass grafting
- Pericardial patches

A commercial process for preparing intact collagen fibers from the dermal tissue has been made available.[11, 46-49] This process is being used to prepare a sterile, injectable dispersion of collagen fibers (Autologen), for correcting cutaneous wrinkles and smoothing dermal contour defects. Autologen fulfills the criteria for the next generation of injectable filler materials that is safe and longer-lasting than other currently available agents.

Autologous harvesting of skin typically occurs during planned cosmetic or reconstructive plastic surgery. Injectable autologous collagen can be produced from skin removed during any plastic surgical procedure. Normally discarded skin, in these instances, can now be transformed into injectable autologous collagen or stored indefinitely if autologous collagen injection is not contemplated for the near future. Advanced technology is now being developed for producing autologous collagen in growth factor–enriched media to produce larger volumes of Autologen from small samples of skin, such as from a simple punch biopsy.

Dispersion

Autologen is composed of intact autologous collagen fibers dispersed into an injectable form derived from the patient's own dermis via a proprietary patented process.[47, 48] The collagen fibers are suspended in a neutral pH phosphate buffer. Autologen generally is offered in two forms: (1) Autologen (standard, 4 per cent) and (2) Autologen XL (cross-linked, 6 per cent). Autologen contains intact dermal collagen fibers with natural cross-links inherently formed during collagen fibril formation in the body. These characteristics contribute to the durability and efficacy. Autologen XL is more tightly cross-linked than native autologous collagen and has shown enhanced efficacy, which is especially useful for deep dermal and subcutaneous augmentation.

To date, Autologen has been produced from excessive skin removed during blepharoplasty, facelift, brow lift, abdominoplasty, breast reduction, scar revision, brachioplasty, scalp reduction, and transcutaneous general surgical procedures in which additional skin is removed from the incision site before closure. It also has been produced from inconspicuous donor sites, such as the suprapubic region, for patients not undergoing planned cosmetic surgical procedures.

Harvesting

After skin is excised during a plastic surgical procedure, it is promptly wrapped with saline-moistened gauze and placed in a sterile container supplied by the manufacturer. Collagenesis also supplies Styrofoam Express mailers, requisition and consent forms, sealable pouches, and dry ice packs for refrigeration and mailing. The excised skin may be refrigerated for several days before mailing. It is preferable to freeze Autologen while it is in the supplied sterile container if mailing is delayed for any reason. The specimens can be safely frozen at standard freezer temperatures for up to 2 weeks.

Containers should be carefully labeled with the requested vital information as soon as the skin is harvested. Specimens are sent to Collagenesis Laboratories (Beverly, Mass.) via Express Mail in the provided self-addressed mailer kit.

Preparation and Yield

Once the container is received at Collagenesis Laboratories, skin specimens are dissected to remove epidermis and subcutaneous tissues, leaving only the dermal skin layer. The dermis is minced and mechanically pulverized in sterile buffer into a dispersion of intact collagen fibers via a patented proprietary process. The dispersed collagen fibers are extensively washed in sterile phosphate buffer and concentrated by centrifugation. A range of collagen concentrations can be prepared by controlling the configuration speed. The final concentrate is then placed into sterile, 1-ml Luer-Lok syringes and hand-labeled with the donor-recipient's identification codes.

All procedures are performed aseptically, and each processed issue lot is tested for sterility. Quality control is meticulously executed. Each specimen is thoroughly processed from start to finish in a single sterile Class 100 laminar flow hood by a highly trained technician, with careful labeling identification throughout each step of the procedure. Total procurement and analysis generally require 3–4 weeks, including processing, testing for sterility, receipt of certificate of sterility, and delivery to the physician in carefully labeled and sealed 1-ml syringes. If Autologen is not immediately requested, a highly sophisticated storage system is available using bar-coded, inventoried, low-temperature freezers. Inventoried skin specimens can be stored for at least 5 years.

The yield of Autologen having an average solid content of 40 mg/ml (4 per cent) is approximately 1 ml per square inch of donor skin (excluding blepharoplasty and eyelid skin, which yield approximately half of this amount because of the relative thicknesses of the corresponding dermis).

Autologen has been used for many facial cosmetic and reconstructive treatments. Among these are:

- Glabellar frown lines
- Nasolabial folds
- Perioral rhytids ("smoker's" or "lipstick lines")
- Periocular rhytids
- Oral commissures
- Depressed scars
- Augmentation of the lip, including the vermilion ridge

Small to medium wrinkles, furrows, and rhytids are best treated with the use of Autologen (standard, 4 per cent), which can be delivered through a 30-gauge needle; defects requiring significant volume for augmentation are best treated with Autologen XL (cross-linked, 6 per cent), which requires a slightly larger-bore (27-gauge) needle for administration. The implant effect is mostly related to the autologous collagen deposition in the dermis. Only a small residue of the autologous collagen implant remains after the phosphate-buffered saline has resorbed.

Several injections into the same dermal defect are required over a finite period to fill a defect completely. The "booster theory" (Fig. 32–1) has been clinically proven when multiple injections of Autologen are given at intervals of 2–4 weeks that eventually fill a defect for a prolonged period. For the correction of larger defects, Autologen XL (cross-linked, 6 per cent) may be used. Typically, fewer injections are required (often only one) to fill a particular defect; however, for moderate to deep furrows, three to four injections are required for long-term correction.

Method of Injection

Autologen can be injected without local infiltrative or regional anesthesia. The injection may be painful (especially Autologen XL), and this ultimately may affect the patient's experience and result. Use of local or regional anesthesia is suggested when applicable. EMLA cream (2.5 per cent lidocaine and 2.5 per cent prilocaine) and other topical anesthetic agents may be useful in some instances but afford only superficial anesthesia. These agents, however, can be used in conjunction with other anesthetic methods. Table 32–1 suggests the preferred method of anesthesia for certain facial regions (Fig. 32–2).

After the designated area has received the appropriate local anesthesia (with a wait of at least 10 minutes), the region is wiped clean with an alcohol pad. Autologen should be removed from the refrigerator (*not frozen*) at least 30 minutes before use. A 27- or 30-gauge needle is then firmly affixed to the Luer-Lok end of the Autologen syringe. A small test amount should be injected into the needle, and Autologen should be seen exiting the lumen of the needle. This ensures normal syringe and needle function and allows the physician to evaluate the resistance to injection and ease of application. Loupe magnification and good lighting are essential. Administration commonly is performed with the patient sitting or slightly reclining in an examining chair.

Autologen is injected into the mid-dermis, not into

table 32–1

Prefered Anesthesia Methods for Facial Regions

Area*	Target Lesion/Defect	Regional/Local Anesthetic Agent
A	Glabellar frown lines (and horizontal furrows at root of nose/overlying procerus muscle)	Infratrochlear nerve block or frontolacrimal nerve block
B	Horizontal forehead furrow	Frontolacrimal nerve block
C	Lateral canthal rhytids	Transconjunctival/local
D	Nasolobial folds	Infraorbital nerve block (transcutaneous or transbuccal)
E	Lip augmentation (including vermilion ridge)	Transbuccal/local
F	Marionette lines	Transbuccal (lower gingival sulcus)
G	Perioral rhytids (vertical)	Transbuccal

*Areas correspond to letters on facial wrinkles in Figure 32–2.

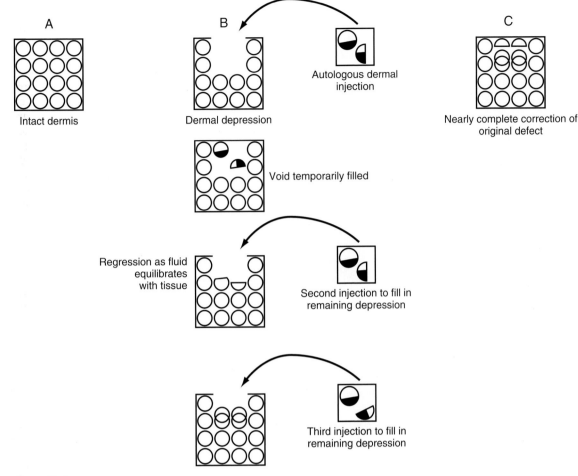

figure 32–1

A, Intact dermis, with no wrinkle or contour defect. *B*, Booster theory for a dermal depression (wrinkle). A dilute concentration of injectable autologous collagen (Autologen, standard, 4 per cent) is injected into the target region. With resorption of the fluid vehicle or buffer, a small residue remains and acts as the foundation for subsequent layered injections to achieve a desired effect. After each additional injection, more filling of the dermal defect occurs. *C*, A nearly complete correction of the original defect results.

the immediate subepidermal or superficial dermis or into the subcutaneous space. The physician can facilitate this process by stretching the patient's skin and straddling the dermal defect between the physician's thumb and index finger while using the other hand for injecting. Multiple small-volume injections are given from the periphery of a particular defect at an angle of approximately 30 degrees. The defect should be overcorrected by approximately 20 per cent (Fig. 32–3). A blanch associated with a slight elevation of the dermal defect usually indicates appropriate dermal placement of the implant (Fig. 32–4).

Repeated injection of the area, if necessary, should be scheduled 2–4 weeks after the first procedure. For most defects, three or four injections of Autologen are needed to achieve resolution of facial wrinkles, furrows, and other skin defects (Fig. 32–5).

ADVERSE REACTIONS AND COMPLICATIONS

At times, mild erythema and edema may be noted at the treatment site for 24–48 hours; prolonged erythema or edema has not been reported. No allergy-type or other adverse reactions or complications have been documented with the use of Autologen.

POSTINJECTION CARE

Ice, topical antibiotics, and/or steroid ointments are optional and at times useful for the patient's enhanced comfort. Most patients require no postinjection care.

RESULTS

More than 800 patients and 100 physicians have had experience with Autologen. Clinical results have been subjective and documented by serial photography.[50] Most physicians note superior results with Autologen compared with reconstituted bovine collagen, degraded porcine collagen, and fat. One small retrospective analysis of a group of more than 25 patients of one physician with a 1-year follow-up period showed 50–75 per cent correction of a facial wrinkle after a single injection for

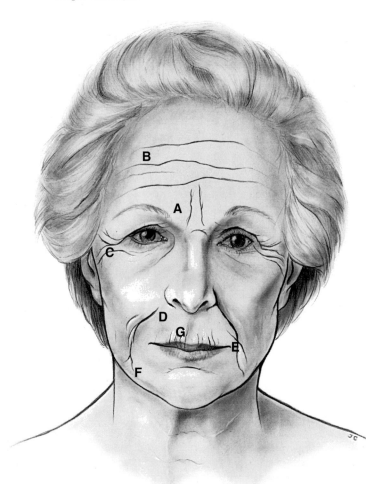

figure 32–2

Acquired facial wrinkles and dermal contour defects. See Table 32–1 for corresponding areas and facial wrinkles amenable to local anesthesia to reduce pain during injections.

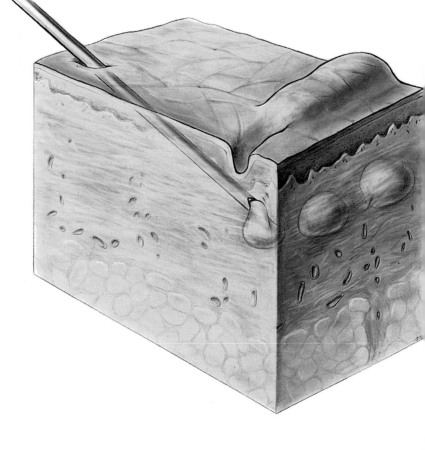

figure 32–3

Multiple boli of Autologen are administered into the approximate mid-dermis along a facial wrinkle or dermal contour defect. The needle is directed tangential to the skin at an angle of approximately 30 degrees.

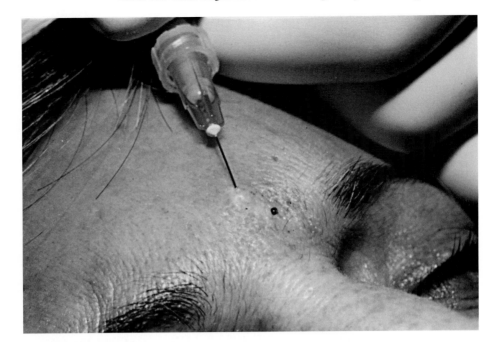

figure 32–4

Typical blanch (white) appearance at end point of an Autologen injection, shown here in the glabellar region.

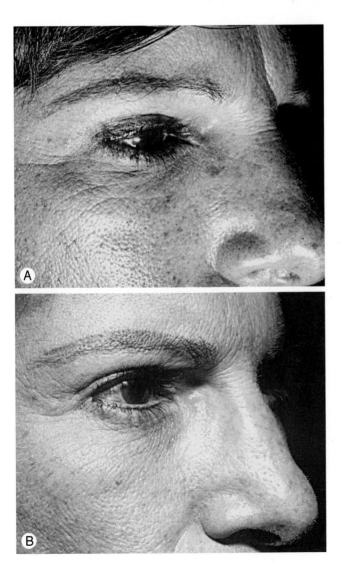

figure 32–5

Before *(A)* and 4 years after *(B)* treatment with Autologen in a patient with a deep glabellar frown line (vertical forehead furrow).

up to 3 months and 50 per cent correction up to 6 months.[47] Two injections provided 75 per cent correction for up to 6 months. Three or more injections to a site provided greater than 75 per cent correction beyond 12 months. This observation is consistent with many other experienced Autologen users. Several early investigators and clinicians with experience using Autologen (including myself) have achieved full correction with three to four injections to a particular site, with the effect lasting more than 2 years.[50]

I have had personal experience with Autologen in more than 30 patients and have treated glabellar forehead furrows, horizontal furrows of the nasal bridge, nasolabial folds, "marionette" lines, perioral rhytids, and distensible facial scars. Results have been excellent, especially in patients who have had at least three treatments in the target region or lesion.

CONCLUSION

Autologen appears to be the ideal material for facial soft-tissue augmentation. The experience of investigators who have used more than 2000 injections of autologous collagen suggests that it is both safe and effective for the treatment of facial wrinkles and dermal contour defects. Skin sources are typically obtained from patients who are undergoing elective plastic surgical procedures in which skin is removed and transformed into injectable autologous collagen to be used for future use. Clinical trials to establish efficacy and to compare Autologen with other injectable fillers in a controlled fashion are under way at three centers (Stanford University Medical Center, University of Miami School of Medicine, and New York University Medical School). Formal histopathologic evaluation is being performed at the New York Eye and Ear Infirmary. Also, research and development efforts are ongoing to establish the feasibility of producing autologous collagen from skin biopsy specimens.

Treatment of the aging face requires a multidisciplinary approach. Facial rejuvenation can be facilitated by surgery, chemical and laser resurfacing, skin care and topical exfoliants, chemical denervation, and soft-tissue augmentation. The use of Autologen should be added to the cosmetic surgeon's armamentarium.

References

1. Stuzin JM, Baker TJ, Gordon HL: The relationship of the superficial and deep facial fascias: Relevance to rhytidectomy and aging. Plast Reconstr Surg 1992; 89:441.
2. Hamra ST: Composite Rhytidectomy. St. Louis, Quality Medical Publishing, 1993.
3. McCord CD: Eyelid Surgery: Principles and Techniques. Philadelphia, Lippincott-Raven Publishers, 1995.
4. Baker TJ, Gordon HL, Stuzin JM: Facial soft tissue anatomy and rhytidectomy. In Baker TJ, Gordon HL, Stuzin JM (eds): Surgical Rejuvenation of the Face, pp 143–383. St. Louis, Mosby-Year Book, 1996.
5. Resnick SS: Chemical peeling with trichloracetic acid. J Dermatol Surg Oncol 1989; 10:549.
6. Baker TJ: Chemical face peeling and rhytidectomy: A combined approach for facial rejuvenation. Plast Reconstr Surg 1962; 29:199.
7. Carruthers JDA, Carruthers JA: Treatment of glabellar frown lines wth botulinum-A exotoxin. J Dermatol Surg Oncol 1992; 18:17–21.
8. Weinstein C, Alster TS: Skin resurfacing with high energy, pulsed carbon dioxide lasers. In Alster TS, Apfelberg DB (eds): Cosmetic Laser Surgery, pp 9–27. New York, John Wiley & Sons, 1996.
9. Kohn RR, Schnider SL: Collagen Changes in Aging Skin. In Balin AK, Kligman AM (eds): Aging and the Skin, pp. 121–139. New York, Raven Press, 1989.
10. Boyce RG, Toriumi DM: Considerations in the use of biologic grafts and alloplastic implants in facial plastic and reconstructive surgery. J Long Term Effects Med Implants 1992; 2:199–220.
11. DeVore DP, Hughes E, Scott JB: Effectiveness of injectable filler materials for soothing wrinkle lines and depressed scars. Med Prog Technol 1994; 20:243–250.
12. Lemperle G, Hazan-Gauthier N, Lemperle M: PMMA microspheres (Artecoll) for skin soft-tissue augmentation. II: Clinical investigations. Presented at the 12th International Congress of International Society of Aesthetic Plastic Surgery, Paris, September 1993.
13. Ersek RA, Beisang AA: Bioplastique: A new textured copolymer microparticle promises permanence in soft-tissue augmentation. Plast Reconstr Surg 1991; 87:693–702.
14. Landman MD, Strahan RW, Ward PH: Chin augmentation with Polytef paste injection. Arch Otolaryngol 1972; 95:72–75.
15. Maas CS, Gnepp DR, Bumpous J: Expanded polytetrafluoroethylene (Gore-tex soft tissue patch) in facial augmentation. Arch Otolaryngol Head Neck Surg 1993; 119:1008–1014.
16. Waldman RS: Gore-tex for augmentation of the nasal dorsum: Preliminary report. Ann Plast Surg 1991; 26:520–523.
17. Stucker FJ, Hirokawa RH, Bryarly RC: Technical aspects of facial contouring using polyamide mesh. Otolaryngol Clin North Am 1982; 15:123–131.
18. Hanke CW, Coleman WP: Collagen filler substances. In Coleman WP, Hanke CW, Alt TH (eds): Cosmetic Surgery of the Skin: Principles and Techniques. Philadelphia, BC Decker, 1991.
19. Knapp TR, Kaplan EN, Daniels JR: Injectable collagen for soft tissue augmentation. Plast Reconstr Surg 1977; 60:398–405.
20. Ruiz-Esparza J, Bailin M, Bailin PL: Treatment of depressed cutaneous scars with gelatin matrix implant: A multi-center study. J Am Acad Dermatol 1987; 16:1155–1162.
21. Jones R, Schwartz BM, Silverstein P: Use of a nonimmunogenic acellular dermal allograft for soft tissue augmentation: A preliminary report. Aesthetic Surg Q 1996; 16:196–201.
22. Cooperman L, Michaeli D: The immunogenicity of injectable collagen: I. A 1-year prospective study. J Am Acad Dermatol 1984; 10:638–646.
23. Clarke DP, Hanke CW, Swanson NA: Dermal implants: Safety of products injected for soft tissue augmentation. Dermatol Surg 1989; 21:992–998.
24. Charriere G, Bejot M, Schnitzler L: Reactions to a bovine collagen implant. J Am Acad Dermatol 1989; 21:1203–1208.
25. McCoy JP, Schade WJ, Siegle RJ: Characterization of the humoral immune response to bovine collagen implants. Arch Dermatol 1985; 121:990–994.
26. Trentham DE: Adverse reactions to bovine collagen implants (editorial). Arch Dermatol 1986; 122:643–644.
27. DeLustro F, Smith ST, Sundsmo J: Reaction to injectable collagen: Results in animal models and clinical use. Plast Reconstr Surg 1987; 79:581–594.
28. Vanderveen EE, McCoy JP, Schade W: The Association of HLA and immune responses to bovine collagen implants. Arch Dermatol 1986; 122:650–654.
29. Barr RJ, Stegman SJ: Delayed skin test reaction to injectable collagen implant (Zyderm). J Am Acad Dermatol 1984; 10:652–658.
30. Cooperman L, Michaeli D: The immunogenicity of injectable collagen: II. A retrospective review of 72 tested and treated patients. J Am Acad Dermatol 1984; 10:647–651.
31. Murayama Y, Satoh S, Oka T: Reduction of the antigenicity and immunogenicity of xenografts by a new cross-linking reagent. Trans Am Soc Artif Intern Organs 1988; 34:546–549.
32. Siegle RJ, McCoy JP, Schade W: Intradermal implantation of

bovine collagen: Humoral immune responses associated with clinical reactions. Arch Dermatol 1984; 120:183–187.

33. Frank DH, Vakassian L, Fisher JC: Human antibody response following multiple injections of bovine collagen. Plast Reconstr Surg 1991; 86:1080–1088.

34. Trautinger F, Kokoschka EM, Menzel EJ: Antibody formation against human collagen and C1q response to a bovine collagen implant. Arch Dermatol Res 1991; 283:395–399.

35. Levine MR, Fagien S: Dermis fat grafts. In Stewart WB (ed): Surgery of the Eyelid, Orbit, and Lacrimal System, vol 3, pp 104–110. San Francisco, American Academy of Ophthalmology, 1993.

36. Baylis HI, Rosen N, Neuhaus RW: Obtaining auricular cartilage for reconstructive surgery. Am J Ophthalmol 1982; 93:709–712.

37. Cohen, MS, Shorr N: Eyelid reconstruction with hard palate mucosal grafts. Ophthalmic Plast Reconstr Surg 1992; 8:183–195.

38. Hankelius L, Olsen L: Free autogenous muscle transplantation in children: Long term results. Eur J Pediatr Surg 1991; 1:353–357.

39. Wiggs EO: Extrusion of enucleated implants: Treatment with secondary implants and autogenous temporalis fascia or fascia lata patch grafts. Ophthalmic Surg 1991; 23:472–476.

40. Tessier P: Autogenous bone grafts taken from the calvarium for facial and cranial applications. Clin Plast Surg 1982; 9:531.

41. Rassman WR, Carson S: Micrografting in extensive quantities: The ideal hair restoration procedure. Dermatol Surg 1995; 21:306–311.

42. McCord CD, Chen WP: Tarsal polishing and mucous membrane grafting for cicatricial entropion, trichiasis, and epidermalization. Ophthalmic Surg 1983; 14:1021–1025.

43. Hodkin MJ, Insler MS: Transplantation of corneal tissue from a blind eye to a high-risk fellow eye by bilateral penetrating keratoplasty (letter to the editor). Am J Ophthalmol 1994; 117:808–809.

44. Favaloro RG: Current status of coronary artery bypass graft surgery. Semin Thorac Cardiovasc Surg 1994; 6:67–71.

45. Del Campo C, Love J, Bowes F: Prosthetic replacement of the superior vena cava with a custom made pericardial graft: An experimental study. J Cardiovasc Surg 1992; 35:305–309.

46. Fagien S: Autologous collagen injections to treat deep glabellar furrows. J Plast Reconstr Surg 1994; 93:642.

47. DeVore DP, Kelman CD, Fagien S, Casson P: Autologen: Autologous injectable dermal collagen. In Bosniak S (ed): Principles and Practice of Ophthalmic Plastic and Reconstructive Surgery, pp 670–675. Philadelphia, WB Saunders, 1995.

48. Kelman CD, DeVore DP: Human collagen processing and autoimplant use. U.S. patent No. 4,969,912; November 13, 1990.

49. Kelman CD, DeVore DP: Human collagen processing and autoimplant use. U.S. patent No. 5,332,802; July 26, 1994.

50. Fagien S: Autologen: Autologous injectable collagen for facial soft tissue augmentation. Presented at the annual meeting of the British Association of Aesthetic Plastic Surgeons, Royal College of Surgeons, London, December 3, 1996.

Steven Fagien

Chapter 33

Treatment of Hyperkinetic Facial Lines with Botulinum Toxin

An adjunct to eyelid and facial cosmetic plastic surgery is the injection of botulinum toxin into hyperactive facial and eyelid muscles. This technique helps to smooth deep furrows. It commonly produces a softer, smoother skin surface and a more rested, youthful appearance. Because botulinum toxin injection offers patients the ability to improve their appearance without being subjected to major surgery, it is an appealing procedure for many patients.

I have used botulinum toxin injections in the treatment of blepharospasm and hemifacial spasm for approximately 15 years. Additionally, I found the drug to be effective in decreasing hyperactive corrugator and procerus muscles when I first used it for this purpose about 8 years ago. In 1990, I reported on the ability of botulinum toxin to create facial and eyelid symmetry in a patient with aberrant regeneration of the facial nerve.

Steven Fagien demonstrates the use of botulinum toxin injections for treatment of lateral canthal rhytids ("crow's feet"), asymmetric eyebrows, forehead wrinkles, prominent nasolabial folds, and perioral rhytids ("lipstick lines") as well as for eyebrow contouring. He also emphasizes that botulinum injection into hyperkinetic muscles can be used along with carbon dioxide laser resurfacing to create a result that is superior to that obtained with either modality alone.

ALLEN M. PUTTERMAN

An improved understanding of the pathophysiology of facial lines, wrinkles, and furrows has broadened the treatment options for a variety of facial cosmetic blemishes. For years, the nonsurgical approach involved the use of various topical formulations created to alleviate skin aging to yield a more youthful appearance. Despite years of effort by the consumer with such products, the skin succumbs to time, gravity, and personal habits. Individuals seeking a renewed appearance typically consult a cosmetic surgeon. Careful patient and treatment selection is necessary to maximize aesthetic outcome.

The logical approach to facial rejuvenation is facilitated when one differentiates quantitative from qualitative changes in facial soft tissue. *Quantitative* changes (excess) typically require a surgical approach: the excision of excessive soft tissue (skin, muscle, and fat). Conversely, *qualitative* changes require the following:

1. Fortification of the soft tissue (resurfacing with exfoliation or soft-tissue augmentation).
2. Reduction of causative factors, including hyperkinetic (muscular) components (chemodenervation).
3. Long-term maintenance (e.g., skin care, sun protection, changes in diet and habits).

In this chapter, I discuss the use of chemodenervation

to weaken hyperkinetic facial muscles and enhance facial appearance.

HISTORY

The interest in chemodenervation, and specifically the use of botulinum toxin as a therapeutic agent for muscle weakening, dates back to the 1920s. Almost 30 years later, Dr. Alan Scott collaborated with Dr. Edward J. Schantz[1] in the preparation of a batch of crystalline toxin to determine its effectiveness as a drug for producing transient weakness of extraocular muscles and permanent changes in ocular alignment.[2] This batch remains the source of botulinum toxin type A for the present-day commercially available product Botox (Allergan, Inc., Irvine, Calif.).

The toxins of *Clostridium botulinum* are classified into eight immunologically distinguishable exotoxins. The type A toxin is most easily produced in culture and was the first one obtained in a highly purified, stable, and crystalline form.

The principal effect of muscle paralysis is caused by the inhibition of the release of acetylcholine at the neuromuscular junction. The paralytic effect of the toxin is dose-related, with the peak of the effect occurring 5–7 days after injection. Denervated muscle histopathology shows muscle atrophy and mild degree of demyelinative changes at the nerve terminal.[3] Single-fiber electromyographic (EMG) studies indicate abnormal neuromuscular transmission in muscles distant from the site of injection despite the absence of clinical weakness indicating the potential for spread of the toxin, which can be significant at higher doses.[4] These effects, supported by some good experimental data, provide a rationale for treatment protocols for a variety of disorders.

Botox has been approved by the Food and Drug Administration (FDA) for the treatment of strabismus and blepharospasm associated with dystonia, including benign essential blepharospasm or seventh cranial nerve disorders, in patients 12 years of age and above.[5] Although Botox is not FDA-approved for the following uses, many physicians have experience with a multitude of other clinical applications of botulinum toxin, including the treatment of bruxism, stuttering, painful rigidity, lumbosacral pain and back spasms, radiculopathy with secondary muscle spasm, spasticity, spastic bladder, achalasia, tremor, and involuntary tics.[6] Additional ophthalmologic applications of the toxins evolved to include the treatment of lower eyelid entropion, aberrant regeneration of the facial nerve (after Bell's palsy), acquired nystagmus, and corneal pathology and amblyopia therapy aided by the effects of occlusion.[3]

Many experienced clinicians who were keen on facial aesthetics and received favorable comments from their patients regarding their chemodenervation treatment, mostly of the eyelid and facial spastic disorders, began to notice the beneficial effects of the skin appearance in contrast to the contralateral side in those with unilateral abnormalities (Fig. 33–1). Some physicians noted the improvement of the appearance of glabellar frown lines in patients treated for benign essential blepharospasm

(Fig. 33–2).[7] This discovery, in conjunction with a better understanding of the anatomic basis of several facial frown lines,[8] forced the question of the possible benefit of chemodenervation for certain facial wrinkles.

The treatment of glabellar frown lines with Botox enjoyed early attention as a result of the experience of those versed in the treatment of benign essential blepharospasm, which typically involved injection of toxin into the medial eyebrows (Fig. 33–3). Other targeted facial hyperkinetic lines that gained early popularity included the treatment of lateral canthal rhytids and horizontal forehead furrows. More recently, the applications have extended to congenital and traumatic[9] facial asymmetry, postsurgical eyebrow asymmetry (including dyskinesis) and facial paralysis, and orbicularis oculi muscle hypertrophy of the lower eyelids and as an adjunct to endoscopic forehead lifts and injectable agents for soft-tissue augmentation (Table 33–1).[10]

ANATOMY AND PHYSIOLOGY OF FACIAL WRINKLES

The pertinent anatomy of facial expression has been well described in Chapter 7 and elsewhere (Fig. 33–4).[11] An understanding of the anatomic relationships and functional features of these muscles to the surrounding soft tissue provides the necessary groundwork for the treatment rationale of chemodenervation for various aesthetic imperfections.

The palpebral component of the orbicularis oculi muscle surrounds the pretarsal and proximal septal aspects and is the sphincter muscle of the eyelids responsible for blinking and gentle eyelid closure. Its direct antagonist is the levator palpebrae muscle. Forceful contraction of the orbital component of the orbicularis oculi muscle induces concentric folds emanating from the lateral canthus. Some of the fibers of the orbital component function as depressors of the eyebrow. These fibers constitute the depressor supercilii.[11] Its antagonist in this function is the frontalis muscle. The corrugator supercilii muscle serves to draw the eyebrow inferiorly and medially, producing the vertical glabellar frown lines.

The procerus muscle, in part, draws the medial eyebrows inferiorly and produces the transverse wrinkles over the bridge of the nose. The zygomaticus major muscle draws the angle of the mouth superiorly, laterally, and posteriorly with actions of laughing, smiling, and chewing. The zygomaticus minor muscle, in conjunction with the various levator muscles of the lip, forms the nasolabial fold (see Fig. 33–4). Forceful contraction of the zygomaticus muscles in animation (smiling) produces synergistic effects in the periorbital region. It does so by accentuating the contraction of the orbital orbicularis muscle and enhancing the radially oriented folds at the lateral canthus, by contracting the lower eyelid orbicularis muscles, and by recruiting lower eyelid soft-tissue redundancy (by elevating the cheek) that is not evident in the nonanimated state.

An understanding of the basic anatomy of facial expression is essential not only for the appropriate ap-

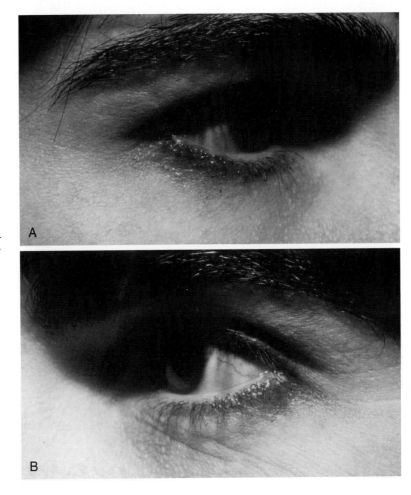

figure 33–1

In a patient treated for several years for aberrant regeneration of the right facial nerve after a Bell's palsy, hyperkinetic periocular (lower eyelid and lateral canthal) lines are absent on the treated, right side *(A)* and evident on the untreated, left side *(B)*.

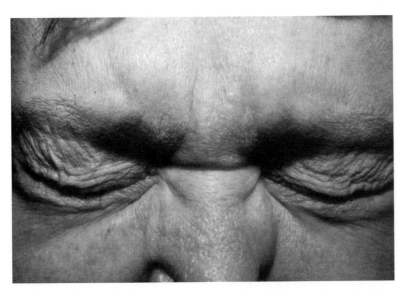

figure 33–2

Typical significant glabellar frown lines in a patient with benign essential blepharospasm.

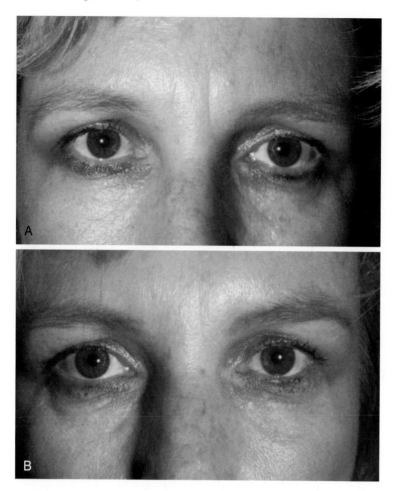

figure 33-3

A, Glabellar furrows before treatment with botulinum toxin A (Botox). *B*, After injection of Botox to the corrugator muscles in the described locations. The patient also demonstrated the beneficial effects of injections to the lateral sub-brow (orbital-orbicularis) region to achieve subtle lateral brow elevation for the enhancement of brow contour and for treatment of mild lateral eyebrow ptosis.

proach to the treatment of hyperkinetic facial lines and furrows but also as a way to avoid complications (see later in this chapter).

PREPARATION AND DILUTION

Botulinum toxin A is a labile but highly potent toxin. Each vial of Botox supplied by Allergan contains 100 units of toxin in a crystalline complex. The toxin should be stored immediately on receipt in the office freezer at $-5°C$ or lower in this crystalline form. For maximal potency, the toxin should be reconstituted just before actual injection.

Dilution should be followed carefully with the diluent of nonpreserved saline, as instructed for specific concentrations in the package insert[5]; however, most clinical uses of Botox are well suited for a dilution of 2.5 units/ 0.1 ml. This concentration is easily obtained by mixing 4 ml of nonpreserved saline to the vial. Some authors

---

table 33-1

Cosmetic Applications of Botulinum Toxin A

For treatment of:

Horizontal forehead furrows	Orbicularis oculi muscle hypertrophy of
Glabellar frown lines	the lower eyelids
Horizontal furrows at the nasal bridge	Aberrant regeneration of the facial
Eyebrow asymmetry	(seventh cranial) nerve
Eyebrow contour	Facial asymmetry and paralysis
Eyebrow ptosis	Facial dyskinesis
Lateral canthal rhytids (crow's feet)	Perioral rhytids ("smoker's"/"lipstick
Dynamic lower eyelid rhytids	lines")

For adjunctive treatment in:

Endoscopic forehead lifting	
Laser exfoliation of lower eyelid and	Facial soft-tissue augmentation
lateral canthal rhytids	Canthal suspension procedures
	Lip augmentation

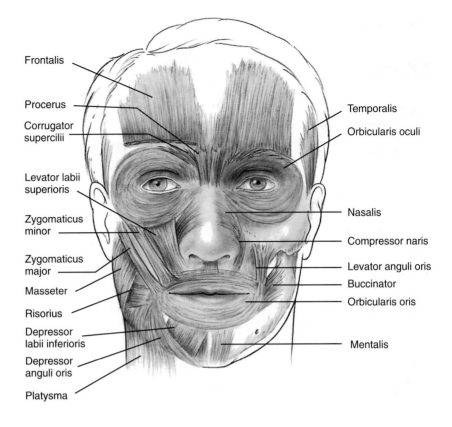

Frontalis

Procerus

Corrugator supercilii

Levator labii superioris

Zygomaticus minor

Zygomaticus major

Masseter

Risorius

Depressor labii inferioris

Depressor anguli oris

Platysma

Temporalis

Orbicularis oculi

Nasalis

Compressor naris

Levator anguli oris

Buccinator

Orbicularis oris

Mentalis

figure 33–4
Pertinent facial muscular anatomy.

have suggested the use of preserved saline in hopes of extending the shelf life and potency once the toxin has been reconstituted. However, there has been concern regarding the effect of the preservative on the denaturing of the delicate toxin. Some have even raised concern about the possible effects of the alcohol used to swab the vial stopper before needle insertion and withdrawal in addition to the possible effects of a high-velocity, turbulent dilution and agitation.

Once reconstituted, the toxin should be used as quickly as feasible. The package insert suggests that the product be used within 4 hours; however, many physicians have noted reasonable effects with the use of the product for up to 30 days.[12] In my experience, a significant decline in clinical potency occurs after 48 hours of reconstitution. Furthermore, the relative stability of the toxin is believed to be best maintained by refrigeration. To my knowledge, there have been no studies to substantiate or refute claims of the duration of potency of the toxin after reconstitution.

Early investigators have suggested 10–20 units or more of toxin per site to weaken the targeted muscles of facial expression.[7] However, one can achieve effects with far less toxin (2.5 units per site) and maintain longevity of effect. In my experience, a dose of 2.5 units per site is effective for an average of 4–6 months. These lower doses in smaller volumes serve to reduce unwanted effects and complications. Concentrations much less than 2.5 units/0.1 ml can induce a weakening effect on the targeted muscle but appear to do so for a much shorter duration. Diluted toxin should be drawn up into 1-ml tuberculin-type syringes through an 18-gauge needle to minimize physical trauma to the toxin.

METHOD OF INJECTION

As in all procedures, patients desire maximum benefit with minimal side effects. It may be advisable, therefore, that patients temporarily discontinue aspirin and other drugs that can lead to bleeding before receiving a Botox injection; this recommendation is similar to general instructions given prior to surgery. This precaution is not mandatory but may reduce or eliminate facial bruising that can last for several weeks.

The use of local anesthesia is generally contraindicated and unnecessary. Alcohol may be applied to the injection sites, but it should be allowed to dry fully before injection of toxin because of toxin lability.

After the toxin is drawn up by 18-gauge needles into 1-ml syringes, the needle is replaced by a short 30-gauge needle for injection. Most of the scant literature on the cosmetic applications of botulinum toxin A describes and illustrates sites for injection with reference points targeted at the actual wrinkle line rather than the causative associated muscular component.[7]

For physicians just starting to use this modality, it is often helpful to mark the skin while observing the affected hyperkinetic lines with frowning, smiling, and generalized facial expression. Currently, I do not employ the use of EMG guidance, as I find this cumbersome and mostly unnecessary; however, EMG guidance may be useful when the physician is getting started with chemodenervation for general orientation. Skin demarcations and sites of eventual injections of toxin should be made over the presumed belly or muscle mass of the regional muscle of facial expression (Fig. 33–5) and not typically at the site of the maximal dermal depression,

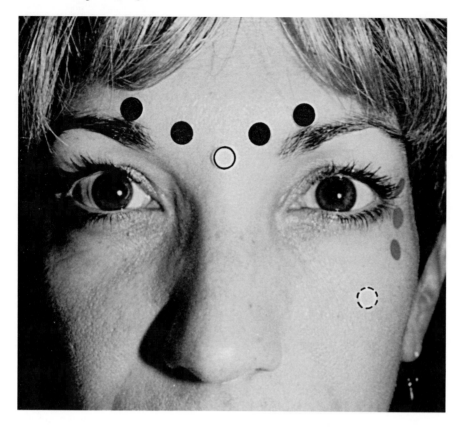

figure 33–5

Typically, four injection sites are satisfactory in eliminating focal muscle tone and voluntary contraction of the corrugator muscles. Black circles indicate approximate areas of treatment of the corrugator muscles for diminishing the glabellar forehead furrows. White circle with solid black lines (nasal bridge) indicates the approximate location of the midaspect of the procerus muscle that effects medial eyebrow depression and the creation of the horizontal furrows at the bridge of the nose. Gray circles indicate the approximate area of treatment for lateral canthal rhytids. White circle with dashed lines indicates the approximate region of the proximal aspect of the zygomaticus major muscle, which recruits significant lower eyelid and lateral canthal rhytids in hyperanimation.

which at times may be quite distant from the mass of the target muscle.

For the larger, deeper muscles, such as the corrugator supercilii, the physician will find it most useful and efficacious to inject toxin deep to the overlying muscles (frontalis and orbicularis) or directly into the belly of the targeted muscle. Typically, four injection sites (see Fig. 33–5) at a dose of 2.5–5 units per site are satisfactory for eliminating focal muscle tone and voluntary contraction of the corrugators. More superficial application tends to weaken the more superficial muscles predominantly, without achieving the desired effect. The physician can most easily facilitate this procedure by becoming familiar with the pertinent facial soft-tissue anatomy and observing the dermal and muscular effects of the frown line on command, inserting the needle (after immediate relaxation on command) deep to the level of the periosteum beneath the muscle, withdrawing slightly into the presumed muscle mass, and then injecting the toxin (typically 0.1 ml).

I treat the thinner orbicularis oculi muscle (and even the procerus) quite differently. I have not found it necessary, advantageous, or even advisable to attempt injection of toxin directly into the orbicularis oculi muscle. Unlike the other larger muscles of facial expression that may require direct contact of the toxin to the majority of the muscle mass, hence requiring injection directly into the muscle, the relatively thin orbicularis oculi muscle (and isolated procerus) appears to be satisfactorily affected when the toxin is injected into the subcutaneous space overlying the muscle. This not only reduces the chance of significant ecchymoses but also may maintain the potency that might be reduced by bleeding. Addi-

tionally, injection into the subcutaneous space may allow for more local and even diffusion over the targeted muscle and may provide an additional safety barrier to structures deep to the muscle. For lateral canthal rhytids, three injections are given; the physician should particularly avoid the pretarsal orbicularis muscle of the upper and lower eyelid by keeping the injections temporal to the lateral canthus and distant to the eyelid margin (see Fig. 33–5).

The procerus muscle can be injected at one or two sites just beneath the skin transverse wrinkle at the nasal bridge. Hyperkinetic horizontal forehead furrows[12, 13] appear to respond favorably to either subcutaneous or intramuscular injection of the toxin, presumably because the frontalis is the only active muscle in this region. Weakening, rather than complete frontalis denervation, may be preferable in some individuals to avoid brow ptosis. Results may be most effective when the physician injects a "uniform grid,"[13] whereby approximately nine sites are injected across the forehead (Fig. 33–6). Three sites over each side are positioned in a vertical line above the mideyebrow. Three additional sites are positioned vertically in the midforehead region.

Typically, 2.5 units (0.1 ml) is administered at each site. To minimize gross lateral brow ptosis, the physician should avoid injections over the lateral eyebrow.

POSTINJECTION CARE

Contrary to the reported suggestion that the patient "stay upright for several hours" after the injections,[13] I have not found it necessary to instruct patients to do

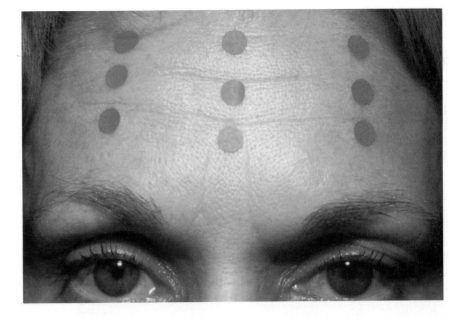

figure 33–6

The "grid pattern" is often used for treatment of horizontal forehead furrows.

so. Patients typically resume normal activity immediately after injection.

COMPLICATIONS

Reported adverse reactions to Botox for all approved applications include blepharoptosis, diplopia, globe perforations, retrobulbar hemorrhage, Adie's pupil, worsening of dry eye symptoms, lagophthalmos, photophobia, epiphora, ectropion, and exposure keratitis.[5] Complications that have arisen with the cosmetic applications of Botox have included most of the above-noted reactions and additional unwanted effects, including ecchymoses, eyebrow ptosis and asymmetry, and mouth droop. My experience of complications has been limited to transient ecchymoses and worsening (or induction) of dry eye symptoms that was significant in two patients (both treated for aberrant regeneration of the seventh nerve); temporary discontinuation of contact lens wear was necessary for several weeks.

RESULTS

Although the botulinum toxin is described as taking effect between 3 and 7 days, I have consistently noted an earlier onset of effect in cosmetic surgery patients compared with patients who undergo Botox treatment of eyelid and facial spastic disorders, such as benign essential blepharospasm and hemifacial spasm. Occasionally, for reasons not well understood, a recipient of Botox for treatment of hyperkinetic facial lines experiences the effects within several hours. Although the immediate treatment benefits reflect the toxin's ability to temporarily weaken or paralyze those muscles responsible for the muscular component of the hyperkinetic facial lines, it is theorized (but not yet proven) that repeated injections into the same muscles over time may produce a sort of "dis-use" atrophy[14] that would limit

the development of such hyperkinetic lines in younger individuals and possibly eliminate or reduce, over time, established facial lines and furrows.

Most effects of the various cosmetic applications of Botox last from 2–6 months, a duration similar to that obtained for treatment of functional and spastic disorders. Patients must be counseled and made aware of the typical transient effects of chemodenervation on their hyperfunctional lines and the likely need for repeated maintenance treatments.

OTHER USES OF TOXIN

Aberrant Regeneration of Facial Nerve

Botulinum toxin A is helpful for a variety of other facial cosmetic problems. I have found it useful in even subtle cases of aberrant regeneration of the seventh nerve (e.g., after recovery of a Bell's palsy), a condition that may not induce a significant visual impairment but may pose significant embarrassment to some patients (Fig. 33–7). Putterman[15] first reported on the use of botulinum toxin for this disorder. At times, very low doses are quite effective, such as 1 unit or less per site administered over the pretarsal orbicularis muscle in the same manner as in treatment of benign essential blepharospasm.

Eyebrow Asymmetry

Eyebrow asymmetry can be seen in a variety of scenarios, including facial nerve trauma after brow lifts, surgically induced facial paralysis, in those with long-standing (even postsurgically corrected) ipsilateral blepharoptosis, and asymmetric nonpathologic facial expression. As an alternative to brow lifting of the more ptotic eyebrow, one might consider eyebrow chemodenervation to enhance symmetry for patients who are unwilling to undergo surgery but who desire more symmetric features.

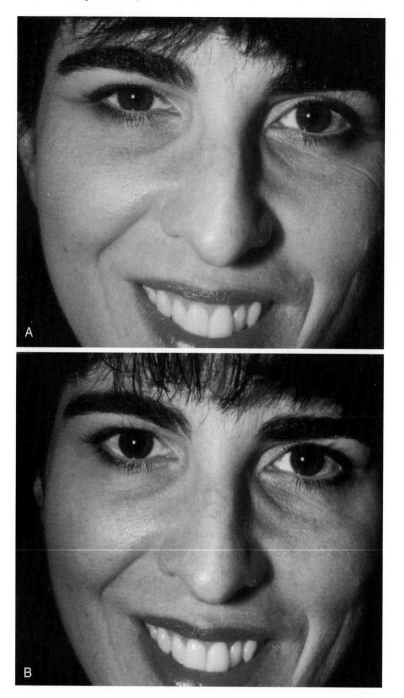

figure 33–7

A patient with aberrant regeneration of the facial (seventh cranial) nerve before *(A)* and after *(B)* treatment with botulinum toxin A (Botox; 1 unit/0.05 ml per site).

The sites and number of injections depend on where the effect is desired and usually. The injections are administered into or overlying the frontalis muscle approximately 1 cm above the eyebrow to avoid the brow depressors.

Dermal Depressions

Another very useful application of botulinum toxin A has been in patients with significant dermal depressions or subcutaneous defects (e.g., in the glabellar region) that are only partially or minimally aided with chemodenervation alone and require, in part, some soft-tissue augmentation[10] (see Chapter 32). Preceding the injectable soft-tissue augmentation material by at least 1 week, Botox (2.5 units/0.1 ml per site) is administered to bring about focal weakness or paralysis. The dermal filler or subcutaneous fat is then injected into the now paralyzed or muscularly weakened area.

The denervation serves two distinct purposes:

1. It eliminates or reduces the muscular component of frowning.
2. It may increase the longevity of the dermal filler or subcutaneous fat by reducing supposed muscular atrophy of the implant and may reduce the immediate microextrusion at the injection sites by repetitive muscular action.

One can see this enhancing effect by weakening the lip elevators before soft-tissue augmentation of the nasolabial folds and in lip augmentation by performing selective chemodenervation with low-dose, low-volume injections (<2 units/0.1 ml) confined to the vermilion ridge. The combination of chemodenervation and soft-tissue augmentation (particularly with autologous collagen) in these areas is highly synergistic (see Chapter 32).

Hypertrophy of the Orbicularis Oculi Muscle

Orbicularis oculi muscle hypertrophy of the lower eyelids may also be effectively treated with very low concentrations (1 unit/0.05 ml) of toxin into or overlying the visibly hypertrophic (thickened) muscle. Two or three injections are administered at the central lower eyelid and lateral canthus overlying the affected areas. Higher concentrations, however, may induce paralytic ectropion or significantly impair the nasolacrimal outflow by inhibiting the pumping action of the orbicularis oculi muscle, inducing epiphora.

Similar caution and consideration can be applied to tone down the effects of the zygomaticus muscles. The zygomaticus major muscle affects the elevation of the corner of the mouth with smiling and in doing this recruits the enhancement of rhytids, which can be quite exaggerated in some individuals. The zygomaticus minor muscle originates similarly to the zygomaticus major muscle and inserts more medially into the upper lip. Both these muscles, in part when acting, deepen the nasolabial fold. By treating the most proximal aspects (far from the mouth) near the areas of origin, with efforts made to inject toxin mostly at the level of the

edge of the inferior aspect of the orbicularis or subcutis, one can soften the additive effects on the lateral canthal rhytids and nasolabial folds. One or two injections (5 units) administered over the lateral malar eminence are usually satisfactory in obtaining the desired effect without incurring complications, particularly paralysis of the ipsilateral upper lip (Fig. 33–8).

Lateral Canthal Suspension Reinforcement

Reinforcement during lateral canthal suspension procedures, such as the lateral tarsal strip, can be aided by Botox injections (2.5 units/0.1 ml) around the lateral canthus in a method similar to that described for treatment of lateral canthal rhytids. This technique not only diminishes the regional rhytids but also reduces local orbicularis muscle function, which may compromise the position and security of the lateral canthus with repeated muscular contraction (Fig. 33–9).

Eyebrow Shape and Position

With botulinum toxin A, the physician can also induce creative changes in eyebrow shape and position. For instance, with injection of Botox into the medial eyebrow for glabellar frown lines, the adjacent medial frontalis muscle can also be affected. Treatment induces a mild relative medial brow ptosis and at times causes a more pleasing contour to the eyebrow, especially in "flat" brows, because there is an induced relative lateral brow elevation, particularly with animation. Many patients, in fact, have commented that some of their friends asked whether they had undergone a brow lift.

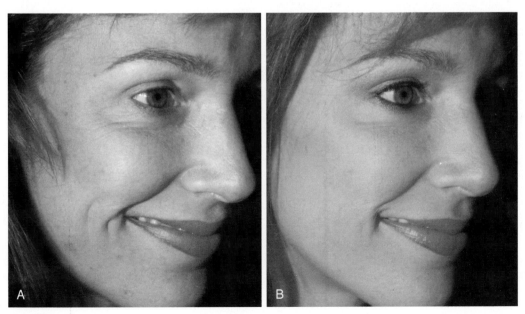

figure 33–8

A, In a patient who had undergone four-quadrant blepharoplasty and a modified cheek lift, significant recruitment of lower eyelid and lateral canthal rhytids during hyperdynamic facial animation (e.g., smiling) was still present. *B*, Defects are diminished after treatment of 5 units/0.1 ml of botulinum toxin A (Botox) at one site over the lateral malar eminence.

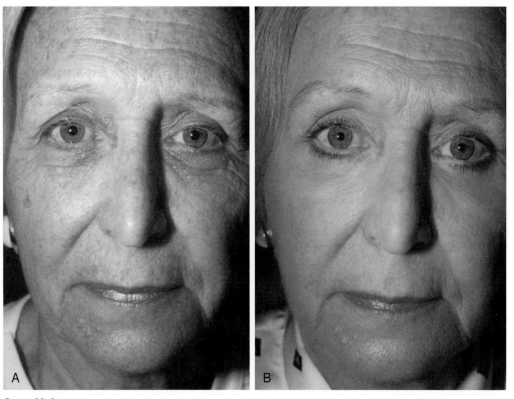

figure 33–9

A, Appearance of a patient before periorbital rejuvenation. Preoperative findings are eyebrow ptosis, upper and lower eyelid dermatochalasis, substantial lower eyelid laxity, and lateral canthal dystopia associated with dense lower eyelid rhytids. *B*, Four months after brow lift, upper and lower (transconjunctival) blepharoplasty, transpalpebral lateral retinacular suspension, and lower eyelid and lateral canthal carbon dioxide laser resurfacing. Botulinum toxin (Botox; 2.5 units/0.1 ml) was administered to the lateral sub-brow region, lateral canthus, and glabella (see Fig. 33–5) 1 week before surgery.

Similarly, it is useful to understand that the lateral, orbital aspect of the orbicularis oculi muscle above the lateral retinaculum serves as an antagonist muscle to the lateral (temporal eyebrow) frontalis muscle. One can achieve mild brow elevation by injecting toxin into this orbicularis muscle region, enhancing the effect of the antagonist frontalis muscle. I often employ this method when injecting Botox for treatment of rhytids with extension of the lateral canthal area injections (2.5 units/ 0.1 ml) into the lateral sub-brow region (see Fig. 33–3). Similarly, this approach is possibly most useful in enhancing the effects of endoscopic brow lifting by weakening the inferior vector force (antagonist) and promoting the maintenance of the elevated brow position (see Fig. 33–9).

Adjunct to Laser Resurfacing

Physicians experienced with carbon dioxide laser abrasion have noted that the first recurrent rhytids in lower eyelid and canthus after resurfacing occur as animation lines accentuated by facial expression (see Chapter 31). Pretreatment (or treatment immediately after "epidermalization") with Botox may maintain the smoothing effect of the resurfaced skin long enough to cause more permanent eradication of wrinkles (Fig. 33–10).

Lipstick Lines and Lip Augmentation

Botox has been useful in reducing fine perioral rhytids (lipstick lines).[16] Approximately 1–2 units (0.05 ml) of toxin is injected adjacent to the fine vertical rhytids overlying the orbicularis oris muscle close to the vermilion ridge. An added aesthetic effect, noted at times with this treatment, is the appearance of fuller (pseudoaugmented) lips, since the sphincter muscle is weakened, allowing the vermilion border to assume a more everted position (Fig. 33–11).

Tension Relief

Not uncommonly, patients receiving Botox (most often when the injections are in or around the eyebrows and forehead) report a generalized, almost euphoric feeling of improved sense of well-being; that is, they feel "less stressed." I assume that this may be related to the relief of muscular contraction (tension), similar to that in the classic muscular contraction or tension headaches. This finding has been ubiquitous and possibly suggests even more expanded uses for botulinum toxin A.

CONCLUSION

The use of botulinum toxin A for the treatment of hyperkinetic facial lines and furrows is another effective

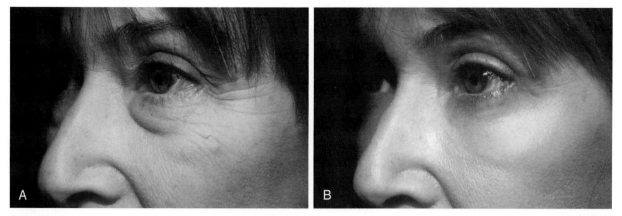

figure 33–10

A, Appearance of a patient before periorbital rejuvenation. Preoperative findings are dermatochalasis and herniated orbital fat of the upper and lower eyelids and severe lower eyelid and lateral canthal rhytids, which are largely hyperfunctional in origin. B, Four months after upper and lower (transconjunctival) blepharoplasty, transpalpebral lateral retinacular suspension, and lower eyelid and lateral canthal carbon dioxode laser resurfacing. Botulinum toxin (Botox; 2.5 units/0.1 ml) was administered to the lateral canthus (as in Fig. 33–5) 1 week before surgery.

figure 33–11

Perioral rhytids ("lipstick lines") before (A) and after (B) treatment with botulinum toxin A (Botox; 1–2 units/0.05 ml) to the orbicularis oris muscle along the vermilion border. Note the pseudoaugmentation, or fuller appearance, of the lips caused by the weakening of the sphincter action of this muscle.

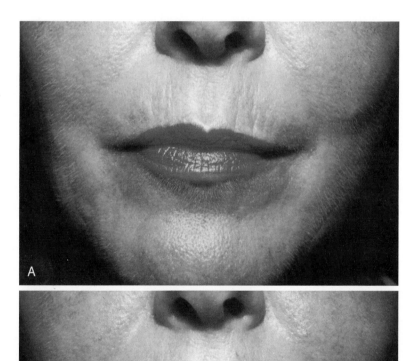

adjunct in the spectrum of treatment options for full facial rejuvenation. Unwanted side effects can be minimized and beneficial effects maximized with a thorough understanding of the facial soft-tissue anatomy, proper patient selection, and administration of the lowest effective doses with minimal volume of delivery. Botox injections do not always replace surgery, laser skin resurfacing, soft-tissue augmentation, or skin care; however, they can be useful alone or in conjunction with other treatment options to give selected patients the most effective and comprehensive solutions for a more youthful appearance.

References

1. Schantz EJ, Scott AB: Use of crystalline type A botulinum toxin in medical research. In Lewis GE (ed): Biomedical Aspects of Botulism, pp 143–149. New York, Academic Press, 1981.
2. Scott AB, Rosenbaum A, Collins CC: Pharmacologic weakening of extraocular muscles. Invest Ophthalmol 1973; 12:924–927.
3. Osako M, Keltner JL: Botulinum A toxin (Oculinum) in ophthalmology. Surv Ophthalmol 1991; 36:28–46.
4. Sanders DB, Massey W, Buckley EG: Botulinum toxin for blepharospasm: Single-fiber EMG studies. Neurology 1986; 36:545–547.
5. Botox (botulinum toxin type A) purified neurotoxin complex. Irvine, Calif, Allergan, Inc, package insert, September 1995.
6. Jankovic J: Botulinum toxin in movement disorder. Curr Opin Neurol 1974; 7:358–366.
7. Carruthers JDA, Carruthers JA: Treatment of glabellar frown lines with *C. botulinum*-A exotoxin. J Dermatol Surg Oncol 1992; 18:17–21.
8. Pierard GE, Lapiere CM: The microanatomical basis of facial frown lines. Arch Dermatol 1989; 125:1090–1092.
9. Clark RP, Berris CE: Botulinum toxin: A treatment for facial asymmetry caused by facial nerve paralysis. Plast Reconstr Surg 1989; 84: 353–355.
10. Fagien S: Facial soft tissue augmentation with autologous injectable collagen (Autologen). In Klein AW (ed): Tissue Augmentation in Clinical Practice: Procedures and Techniques, pp 87–124. New York, Marcel Dekker, 1998.
11. Clemente CD (ed): Gray's Anatomy, 30th American ed, pp 438–444. Philadelphia, Lea & Febiger, 1985.
12. Garcia A, Fulton JE: Cosmetic denervation of the muscles of facial expression with botulinum toxin: A dose-response study. Dermatol Surg 1996; 22:39–43.
13. Klein AW: Cosmetic therapy with botulinum toxin. Dermatol Surg 1996; 22:757–759.
14. Wojno T, Campbell P, Wright J: Orbicularis muscle pathology after botulinum toxin injection. Ophthalmic Plast Reconstr Surg 1986; 2:71–74.
15. Putterman AM: Botulinum toxin injections in the treatment of seventh nerve misdirection. Am J Ophthalmol 1990; 110:295–206.
16. Foster JA, Wulc AE, Barnhorst D: The use of botulinum toxin to ameliorate dynamic lines. Int J Aesthetic Restorative Surg 1996; 4:137–144.

Mark R. Levine

Chapter 34

Blepharopigmentation

Blepharopigmentation is a controversial method of applying eyeliner by tattooing pigment within and adjacent to the upper and lower eyelashes. It is used at times as an adjunct to cosmetic blepharoplasty procedures and at other times alone. Many cosmetic surgeons are strongly against the use of blepharopigmentation. However, I included this chapter because I believe that, when used in selected patients, blepharopigmentation does have a place in the cosmetic surgeon's armamentarium.

Mark Levine has had extensive experience in blepharopigmentation. He tells us how to evaluate and select a patient for this technique. He describes the various instruments that can be used. In addition to demonstrating the technique, he gives us pointers on how to apply the pigment for the various eyelid types and how to choose specific pigments for patients of different ethnic backgrounds and different skin and hair colors. He also explains how to deal with some of the complications and how to remove pigment.

I have found that women who do not see well enough to apply makeup, as well as those who are athletic, are good candidates for this procedure. I have also found that the main complaints following this technique are asymmetry and overpigmentation. I warn patients that it is almost impossible to apply this pigment so that there is absolute perfection in the simulated eyeliner and that they must accept slight areas of overpigmentation, underpigmentation, or asymmetry. I have also had the opportunity to deal with complications of blepharopigmentation performed by other surgeons, in which I have been able to excise the pigment with minimal loss of lashes.

ALLEN M. PUTTERMAN

Blepharopigmentation was described by Angres[1] in 1984. The procedure involves the introduction of ferrous oxide pigment into the dermis along the eyelash line to simulate the appearance of cosmetic eyeliner. Pigment is placed between and along the base of the lashes, so that the result does not look like a line but gives a halo effect, hence the term *eyelash enhancement*.[1, 2]

Histopathologically, the pigment is located in the dermis and sometimes in the superficial orbicularis oculi muscle, with many fine pigment granules engulfed by macrophages. No acute or chronic inflammatory cells are found.[3–7]

Candidates for eyelash enhancement[8] are women who:

- Cannot apply makeup because of physical infirmities or visual problems
- Have allergies to conventional eye makeup
- Have lost eyelashes secondary to trauma or alopecia universalis
- Are athletic
- Have oily skin and whose makeup smears and fades
- Prefer the convenience of permanent makeup

EYELASH ANATOMY

The configuration of every person's eyelids and lashes is different. The lashes on the upper eyelid are larger and thicker and consist of three rows laterally that taper to a single row nasally. The lashes on the lower eyelid are generally delicate and consist of one row. The ideal anatomic landmarks are the medial punctum and the lateral canthus. It should not be necessary to place pigment medial to the punctum or to "unite" the upper and lower lateral canthus with pigment. The most common surgical error in blepharopigmentation is failure to remain close to the lower eyelid margin.

PREOPERATIVE EVALUATION

It is important that the physician evaluate each patient with her makeup in place while considering her skin texture and hair color. The surgeon should find out the following:

- Has the patient always worn makeup this way?
- Does she apply makeup (especially eyeliner) lightly or heavily?
- Does the patient apply eyeliner along the entire upper and/or lower eyelid or just the lateral or medial area?
- Does the makeup extend laterally beyond the canthus or medially beyond the punctum?
- What are the patient's favorite colors, and why does she prefer light or dark colors?

EYE EXAMINATION

A complete eye examination should be performed to rule out trichiasis, benign or malignant eyelid lesions, blepharitis, and meibomianitis. These conditions should be recognized and treated before eyelash enhancement.

HISTORY

A medical history should document any allergies. Contact allergies to paints, crayons, or makeup, all of which contain iron (ferrous oxide), may suggest a potential sensitivity to the ferrous oxide in the eyeliner pigment. This type of allergy, however, seems to be uncommon. When a skin test is indicated, a scratch test or impregnation of pigment between the toes, behind the ear, or on the forearm may be performed. These tests are repeated 2 and 7 days later to verify a skin reaction. If no reaction occurs, blepharopigmentation may be performed.

EYELID TYPES

Optimal placement of the pigment varies slightly, depending on the patient's eye type. There are six types of eyes: (1) close-set, (2) deep-set, (3) small, (4) wide, (5) Asian, and (6) prominent. See Modifications of Pigment Placement later.

INFORMED CONSENT

The patient must sign a consent form that explains possible complications. Complications can include loss of eyelashes, fading of the pigment, allergic reactions, asymmetry, skin sloughing, and penetrating injuries of the globe.

TYPES OF INSTRUMENTS

A number of units are available for blepharopigmentation. Three of the more popular units are Accents* (Fig. 34–1), Permark† (Fig. 34–2), and Natural Eyes‡ (Fig.

---

*Dioptics, 15550 Rockfield Boulevard, Suite C, Irvine, CA 92718.
†Permark, a division of M.P.D., 450 Raritan Center Parkway, Edison, NJ 08837.
‡Alcon Surgical, Natural Eyes Department, P. O. Box 19587, Irvine, CA 92713.

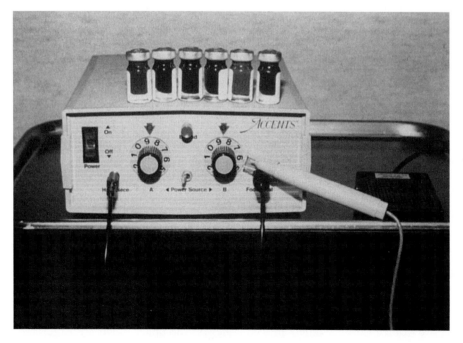

figure 34–1

Accents blepharopigmentation unit, consisting of hand piece (single-pronged needle), power supply, and pigment vials.

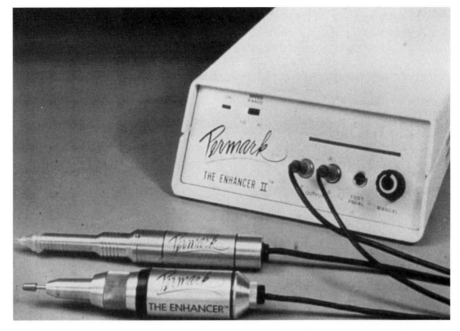

figure 34–2

Permark blepharopigmentation unit, consisting of power supply and two hand pieces: a single-pronged needle and a dermabrasion hand piece.

34–3). All three offer a choice of single-pronged or three-pronged (Fig. 34–4) needles. It is debatable as to which unit is more effective. I have used only the Accents unit. Its single-pronged needle has allowed for accurate results and good control. The three-pronged needle works best for eyebrows.

PIGMENT COLORS

There are three groups of pigment: black, brown, and gray. Brown pigment has dark, medium, and light shades. Black or brown-black pigment is most suited to African-Americans, Asians, and Hispanics. Black pigment is too harsh for Caucasians. Gray or light brown pigment is used for fair-skinned, blonde, and red-haired women.

SURGICAL TECHNIQUE

Sedation is seldom necessary. However, an anxious patient may benefit from taking 5–10 mg of oral diazepam 1 hour before surgery.

The patient, dressed in loose clothing, is placed on the operating table. Tetracaine (0.5 per cent) is instilled in both eyes. A 2.5-cm, 30-gauge needle is attached to a syringe containing a 10-ml preparation of 2 per cent lidocaine with epinephrine and hyaluronidase (Wydase). A frontal nerve block is given with 2 ml of the anesthetic

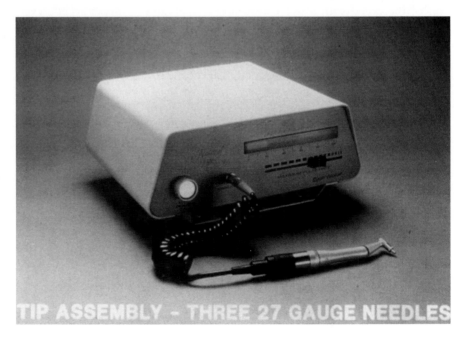

figure 34–3

Natural Eyes blepharopigmentation unit, consisting of power supply and hand piece.

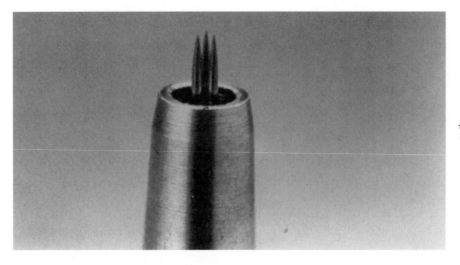

figure 34–4

Close-up view of triple-pronged needle from Natural Eyes blepharopigmentation unit.

agent in the center of the brow below the orbital rim. In addition, an infraorbital block is given by palpating for a depression 10 mm below the inferior rim and injecting 2 ml of the anesthetic agent.

Next, a cotton-tipped applicator soaked with 4 per cent topical lidocaine is placed in the inferior cul-de-sac, and 2 ml of anesthetic is injected along its length. The upper eyelid is everted over a Desmarres retractor, and topical 4 per cent lidocaine is applied. Then 1 ml of anesthetic is injected subconjunctivally above the tarsus. The upper and lower pretarsal eyelid skin is injected along its length behind the eyelashes.

The medical team prepares the patient for surgery, either by swabbing the eyelid skin with an alcohol pad or by a face preparation with povidone-iodine (Betadine) solution. The surgeon sits at the patient's right side, facing the patient, with two-power to six-power loupes. The surgeon applies an antibiotic ointment to the skin and eyelashes to prevent staining and to facilitate easy removal of excess pigment. An eyelid speculum may be used for keeping the eyelid fixed, or a simple manipulation of the eyelid with a wet cotton-tipped applicator may be all that is necessary to stabilize it.

The surgeon uses a pigmentation instrument with either a single-pronged or three-pronged needle. It is easiest to start on a lower eyelid. The surgeon identifies medial, central, and lateral landmarks by implanting tiny dots of pigment in these locations at the base of the lash (Fig. 34–5). Medially, the first dots should be 2–3 mm lateral to the punctum, and laterally they should be just short of the last lateral lash. The needle is frequently dipped in the stirred pigment (Fig. 34–6). The surgeon connects the first dots of pigment by adding dots that barely overlap (Fig. 34–7). An application of pigment that is slightly too heavy rather than too light is preferable. The same procedure is performed on the other lower eyelid.

The technique for the upper eyelids is slightly different. The pigment line is applied to the upper row of lashes in confluent dots. The surgeon may create an even line with a temporal flare by making two to three additional rows above the first, with the dots touching. Applying more rows laterally gives more flare. The central eyelid serves as a transition zone. The nasal third of the eyelid generally consists of one line of dots. For the upper eyelid, several dots are applied within the superior row of eyelashes laterally, centrally, and nasally, 1 mm lateral to the punctum (see Fig. 34–5). The areas be-

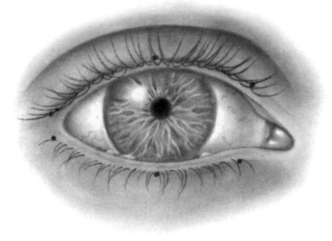

figure 35–5

Dots are applied to lower and upper eyelids to serve as guides for placement of pigment.

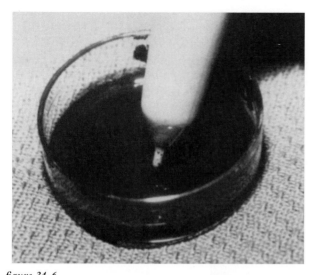

figure 34–6

The blepharopigmentation needle is dipped in the pigment.

tween the dots are then filled in (see Fig. 34–7). Then the other upper eyelid is pigmented.

At this point, a mirror is given to the patient for viewing, and further enhancement is performed if desired.

At the end of the procedure, the eyelids and eyelashes are cleaned of excess pigment and antibiotic ointment with a saline-soaked, cotton-tipped applicator. A new coating of antibiotic steroid ointment is applied.

POSTOPERATIVE CARE

Artificial tears are given for treatment of any exposure keratitis. Ice-cold compresses are applied for 4 hours to reduce edema and to increase comfort. Antibiotic steroid ointment is applied twice a day for 4 days.

MODIFICATIONS OF PIGMENT PLACEMENT

Optimal results are achieved when the procedure is begun 2 mm lateral to the punctum on the lower eyelid and when the pigment extends slightly toward the punctum superiorly on the upper eyelid (Fig. 34–8). For patients with a large nose or a wide and flat bridge, the optimal treatment is to place the pigment even further laterally to the punctum.

Close-Set Eyes. Close-set eyes can be made to appear more widely set if pigment is applied more intensely to the lateral aspect of the eye. It is best to leave 1–2 mm free in the lateral aspect of the lower eyelid so that the eyes look more open.

Deep-Set Eyes. An illusion of bringing the eyes forward can be created. The surgeon applies the pigment less intensely from the inner canthus to the middle upper eyelid and more intensely toward the outer canthus. In the lower eyelid, the application should be maintained lightly from the medial canthus to the outer canthus and then tapered medially toward the punctum.

Small Eyes. Pigment should be contoured in the base of the lashes in the lower eyelid. To make the eyes appear larger, the surgeon should apply pigment in the uppermost row of the three rows of lashes in the upper eyelid.

Wide-Set Eyes. To minimize wide-set eyes, the surgeon should apply pigment evenly from the medial canthus, stopping short of the lateral canthus.

Asian Eyes. The natural uplift should be emphasized. The surgeon starts pigment application 1–2 mm lateral to the punctum, a technique that makes the eyes appear more widely set and that emphasizes the almond shape.

figure 34–7

Blepharopigmentation of upper and lower eyelids connects the dots applied as guides.

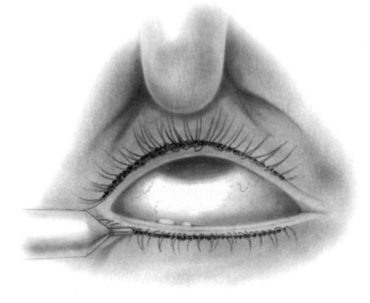

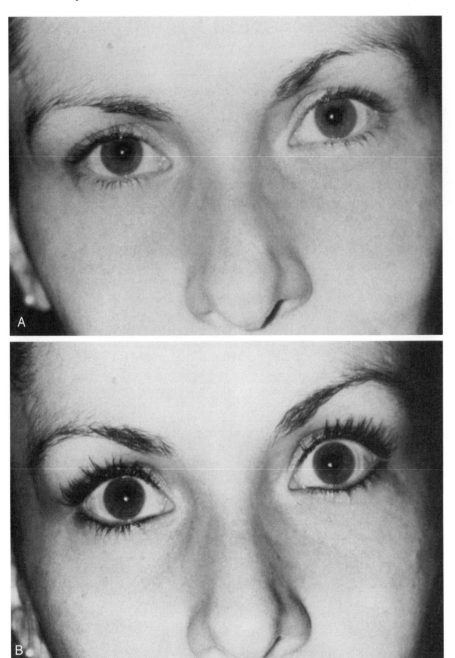

figure 34–8
Patient before *(A)* and after *(B)* blepharopigmentation.

Prominent Eyes. Eyes that appear pronounced can be softened if pigment is applied lightly around the perimeter of the eye.

COMBINING BLEPHAROPIGMENTATION WITH BLEPHAROPLASTY

If a patient undergoing a cosmetic blepharoplasty also desires blepharopigmentation, the blepharoplasty should be performed before the blepharopigmentation so that the line of pigmentation is not displaced by the surgery.

COMPLICATIONS

The most common complications of blepharopigmentation are caused by an improper technique. If the pig-ment is implanted too superficially, it will slough off as the epidermis desquamates or it may slowly fade over 1–2 years as macrophages engulf it.[9] If some of the pigment is improperly placed, it may be excised surgically with a small ellipse and gentle cautery to close the defect.[10] Large misplaced segments are linearly excised and sutured, then repigmented 4–6 weeks later.[11] The use of the argon blue-green laser to break up the pigment may be helpful. A laser setting of 50-μm spot size and 0.05-second exposure time, with a power of 0.3–0.8 mW, is used; approximately 100–150 burns are necessary for pigment dispersion.[12]

Postoperative loss of eyelashes has been reported in the literature. This problem is probably due to mechanical trauma to the eyelash bulbs from improper placement of the needle.[10] Pigment itself has not been shown to be responsible because it does not cause an inflammatory response.

There have been no reports of allergic reactions to pure iron oxide pigments. Eyelid swelling and puffiness have occurred after blepharopigmentation in patients who received magnetic resonance imaging of the head.[13] Swelling in these cases subsided in 48 hours, with no sequelae.

RESULTS

I have performed approximately 75 blepharopigmentations. I emphasize more pigment implantation rather than less because, in my experience, some fading occurs after 1 year, requiring a touch-up.

References

1. Angres GG: Blepharopigmentation and eyebrow enhancement techniques for maximum cosmetic results. Ann Ophthalmol 1985; 17:605–611.

2. Angres GG: Blepharo- and dermapigmentation techniques for facial cosmesis. Ear Nose Throat J 1987; 66:344–353.

3. Patipa M, Jakobiec FA, Krebs W: Light and electron microscopic findings with permanent eyeliner. Ophthalmology 1986; 93:1361–1365.

4. Hurwitz JJ, Brownstein S, Mishkin SK: Histopathological findings in blepharo-pigmentation (eyelid tattoo). Can J Ophthalmol 1988; 23:267–269.

5. Simons KB, Payne CM, Heyde RRS: Blepharopigmentation: Histopathologic observations and x-ray microanalysis. Ophthalmic Plast Reconstr Surg 1988; 4:57–62.

6. Wolfley DE, Flynn KJ, Cartwright J, Tschen JA: Eyelid pigment implantation early and late histopathology. Plast Reconstr Surg 1988; 82:770–773.

7. Tse DT, Folberg R, Moore K: Clinicopathologic correlate of a fresh eyelid pigment implantation. Arch Ophthalmol 1985; 103:1515–1517.

8. Patipa M: Eyelid tattooing. Dermatol Clin 1987; 5:335–348.

9. Wilkes TDI: The complications of dermal tattooing. Ophthalmic Plast Reconstr Surg 1986; 2:1–6.

10. Goldberg RA, Shorr N: Complications of blepharopigmentation. Ophthalmic Surg 1989; 20:420–423.

11. Putterman AM, Migliori ME: Elective excision of permanent eyeliner. Arch Ophthalmol 1988; 106:1034–1037.

12. Tanenbaum M, Karas S, McCord CD: Laser ablation of blepharopigmentation. Ophthalmic Plast Reconstr Surg 1988; 4:49–56.

13. Weiss RA, Saint-Louis L, Haik BG, McCord CD, Taveras JL: Mascara and eyelining tattoos: MRI artifacts. Ann Ophthalmol 1989; 21:129–131.

Arthur L. Millman

Chapter 35

Carbon Dioxide Laser Blepharoplasty

This revision includes a new chapter on carbon dioxide (CO_2) laser blepharoplasty in addition to the chapter on blepharoplasty with a neodymium:YAG laser, cautery, and Colorado needle (see Chapter 36).

Use of the CO_2 laser for laser resurfacing has been receiving an immense amount of publicity. This laser is also useful in cosmetic eyelid and facial surgery. Controversy continues as to whether the CO_2 laser is worth the time and expense compared with electrocautery, such as with a Colorado needle. Also, the decision whether to completely stop performing neodymium:YAG laser blepharoplasties has yet to be made.

There is no doubt that use of a CO_2 laser in blepharoplasty produces minimal bleeding and less discomfort in fat excision compared with the use of a hemostat clamp with secondary Bovie cautery. Whether less postoperative swelling and bruising also result remains to be determined.

Arthur Millman beautifully describes the technique for CO_2 laser blepharoplasty and all of the associated considerations, advantages, and disadvantages. He demonstrates a technique using the laser to develop the upper eyelid crease by forming a fusion between the orbicularis oculi muscle and the levator aponeurosis at the site of the crease.

One disadvantage of laser blepharoplasty, besides the time in setting up the laser and the expense, is that wound healing takes longer. Therefore, sutures must be left in place for a longer time than with conventional surgery.

I continue to refrain from using the CO_2 laser in performing blepharoplasty in most of my patients, and I prefer using a knife for my skin incision and a Colorado needle for making all other incisions and dissections. I clamp orbital fat with a hemostat and apply a Bovie cautery to the fat stump. By having the anesthesiologist administer a bolus of intravenous anesthesia at the time of fat removal, I minimize my patient's discomfort at this point in the procedure.

ALLEN M. PUTTERMAN

Advances in technology with the CO_2 laser have made its use in cosmetic surgery more viable and the results more predictable and desirable.[1,2] The tremendous improvement of intraoperative hemostasis shortens the duration of surgery. Additionally, the postoperative course has little morbidity, including minimal edema and ecchymosis. Minimized swelling and bruising allow patients an early return to normal functioning, usually 4–6 days compared with 10–12 days in conventional blepharoplasty.

LASER SURGICAL SETUP

Oculoplastic surgery with the CO_2 laser calls for a number of special instruments and precautions in the setup of the surgical field for laser efficacy and safety. These include the use of protective eyewear for all persons in the operating room.

Contact lenses or eye shields are necessary for the patient and preferably should be made of metallic surgical steel (Bemsco Surgical Supply, West Seattle.) The internal surface of the steel contact lenses should be smooth, and the external surface should be sandblasted for antireflective properties. Topical tetracaine and ophthalmic ointment are usually applied on the inner surface of the shield for patient comfort.

All surgical personnel should wear wavelength-appropriate eyewear, such as eye goggles, surgical loupes, or eyeglasses. It is recommended that the instrument manufacturer sandblast the surface of all metallic instruments used in the surgical procedure. In particular, Desmarres retractors and any broad metallic surface should be sandblasted. This antireflective status prevents the inadvertent reflection of the CO_2 laser beam in unwanted areas or tissue.

The surgical field should include the use of wet towels and dressings soaked in sterile water or saline to surround the face or surgical area. Some surgeons use aluminum foil, although I find it cumbersome and do not recommend it.

A smoke or laser plume evacuator is mandatory. Improper laser plume evacuation results in chronic pharyngitis for the surgeon, and it has been shown that biologic and viral particles have been recovered and transmissible in the laser plume. Standard operating room suction will not suffice.

If general anesthesia is used, anesthetic agents should be nonflammable and endotracheal tubes should be wavelength-appropriate, usually with a metallic or antireflective coating. A large basin of water should be on or near the surgical field for lavage should a fire start, and an Underwriters Laboratories–approved fire extinguisher should be present in the surgical suite.

CARBON DIOXIDE SURGICAL LASER

A number of CO_2 lasers are available for plastic surgery. This modality is rapidly changing in regard to the technology and equipment available. I have extensive experience with the Coherent Ultrapulse, Luxar Novapulse, and Sharplans Silk Touch and Feather Touch systems.

Although new instruments and companies continually are entering the market, instrumentation is basically divided into two groups. The first group (e.g., Luxar and Coherent) are those that provide a *superpulsed* laser. Used for incisional and resurfacing surgery, this laser can deliver CO_2 energy in very short ($<1/500$-μsec) bursts, so as to maximize tissue ablation and minimize thermal damage or heat capacitance within the tissue to be treated. In my experience, the ability to use the superpulsed laser for some incisional and all resurfacing surgery is ideal.

The second group (e.g., Sharplans Silk Touch and Feather Touch) consists of *continuous-wave* lasers that deliver energy in a continuous mode. These lasers are frequently presented to the tissue by means of a mechanical mirror-reflecting system, which rapidly moves the energy spot in a spiral pattern to perform resurfacing or which remains a stationary spot for incisional surgery.

Each laser uses different settings and terminology (see Chapter 31, Table 31–1).

LASER PHYSICS PRINCIPLES

The surgeon should understand basic laser physics principles, which guide laser settings in the practice of laser surgery.[1,2]

For incisional surgery, a small spot size delivers a more precise incision width and more power per unit area, or *fluence*; however, it has a decreased thermal or hemostatic effect. In general, a spot size of 0.2–0.4 mm is ideal for cutting at 7–8 watts of power in a standard continuous-wave mode. The surgeon can accurately modify the amount of energy delivery by focusing and defocusing the laser spot through positioning of the laser hand piece. A position further from the tissue defocuses the laser beam. Laser energy is delivered at a maximum level at the exact focal point of the given laser (Fig. 35–1).

The working distance (*focal point*) of each unit is determined by the manufacturer and the given model. This focal point is usually delineated by a footplate attached to the hand piece, which reminds the surgeon of the working distance. The focal point measures 2.5–3.75 cm (1–1.5 inches) in the Coherent and Sharplans models. The exception is the Luxar Novapulse unit, which works on a hollow-fiber delivery system (instead of the mirror-reflected beam in articulated arms) and in a near-contact mode. Its focal point is simply adjacent by 2–3 mm to the tip of the laser hand piece. The surgeon can thus deliver maximum energy and maximum vaporization or cutting, with minimal thermal or peripheral damage to the surgical tissue, by working at the laser's exact focal point.

Conversely, the surgeon can defocus by withdrawing or increasing the distance of the hand piece to the tissue, thus creating a decrease in power delivered, which decreases the laser's cutting ability but maximizes its thermal or coagulative ability (see Chapter 31, Fig. 31–1). This is useful for hemostasis and for contouring or

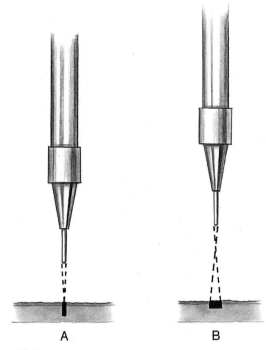

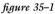

figure 35–1

A, Laser 0.4-mm cutting hand piece focused at the exact focal point of the carbon dioxide (CO_2) beam. Note the thin, deeper incision profile. *B,* Laser is defocused by increasing distance to tissue. Note the shallower and wider burn with increased coagulation.

ablating tissue. Cutting can also be done in a super-pulsed mode (available on the Luxar Novapulse and Coherent Ultrapulse) set at 25-μsec and 30-Hz (hertz) program settings with power levels of 7–8 watts.[4]

SURGICAL TECHNIQUE

Patient marking of excess upper eyelid skin to be removed should first be completed. Areas to be treated by cosmetic skin resurfacing (CSR) should be marked as described in Chapter 31.

The steps of laser blepharoplasty follow conventional blepharoplasty closely (see Chapters 9 and 10 for upper lid blepharoplasty and Chapter 20 for lower eyelid transconjunctival blepharoplasty). However, some important techniques are specific to the use of the CO_2 laser, as described next.

Upper Lid Laser Blepharoplasty

The laser is set on a continuous-wave setting of 0.2–0.4 mm spots at approximately 7–8 watts of power. The smaller spot size accomplishes a more precise and thin incision line but has a decreased coagulative or hemostatic effect. Conversely, the 0.4-mm spot has a slightly larger incision profile but increased hemostasis. I prefer the 0.4-mm spot because the level of hemostasis is substantially greater without significant compromise of incision quality.

A careful tempo is necessary, and the incision should

not be rushed. A rapid incision or fast movement of the hand piece allows for only superficial cutting. Conversely, an overly slow progression of incision allows for significant increase of depth of cutting and buildup of thermal capacitance, with possible charring and scarring of the surrounding tissues. Incisions should be made at exactly the working distance or focal point of the given laser. At a careful and deliberate tempo, the surgeon makes the incision along first the upper eyelid crease and then the superior aspect of the resection line (Fig. 35–2*A*).

The skin should be kept taut to allow accurate delivery of laser energy. In general, the assistant should allow for a taut upper eyelid (or the use of a David-Baker clamp for eyelid stabilization) and tension on all skin wounds to allow for separation of the incision line. Use of a 4-0 silk traction suture is recommended. This suture is placed pretarsally at the eyelid margin, and the eyelid is drawn downward.

Dissection is begun from the lateral aspect of the wound, where in a slightly "defocused" mode the hand piece is used to elevate the skin flap using a to-and-fro motion across the base of the elevating flap (Fig. 35–2*B*). Either a skin flap can be elevated, or a skin-muscle flap can be done as an en block method.

In general, hemostasis is automatic because the laser seals all blood vessels as it goes. The skin-muscle flap requires a deeper incision, and this is controlled by a slower tempo and deeper cut. Alternatively, two incisional passes can be used to each of the skin and then muscular planes so that each layer of skin and muscle is incised individually. Should breakthrough bleeding occur, the hand piece can be slightly withdrawn and defocused to allow for instant cauterization of all vessels. Again, a proper tempo is necessary to avoid charring and increased thermal ablation and contracture of tissue.

With the skin flap elevated, as the dissection is brought to the medial canthus, the surgeon should take care when severing the skin flap or skin-muscle flap to avoid an inadvertent burn to the medial canthus. The medial canthus is thus frequently protected with a saline-moistened gauze pad.

At this point, an incision is made through either the remaining orbicularis muscle or, in the case of the skin-muscle flap, the remaining orbital septum to prolapse both nasal and central orbital fat pads. A combination of direct cutting and defocused coagulation of the orbital fat pad can be used. The fat pad is usually grasped with a forceps and withdrawn (Fig. 35–2*C*). The surgeon then amputates the fat and by cutting directly with the laser at the exact focal length or working distance. The surgeon removes any remaining fat or contouring of the fat at the orbital rim by defocusing the hand piece and vaporizing the remaining fat directly. The lack of clamps and minimum manipulation of the fat pad allow for increased patient comfort as the surgeon uses gentle retropulsion of the globe and easy prolapse of the orbital fat pad for laser cutting and ablation. A Desmarres retractor with a sandblasted surface is used for retraction of the septum and to allow easy exposure of the fat pad (Fig. 35–2*C*).

The upper eyelid skin is closed, either directly with a

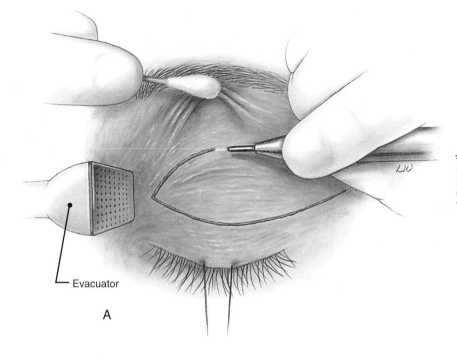

Evacuator

A

figure 35–2

Carbon dioxide (CO_2) laser upper eyelid blepharoplasty procedure. *A,* Redundant skin has elliptical incision using a 7-watt CO_2 laser with a 0.4-mm cutting tip profile.

6-0 nylon suture or with a more advanced technique that employs a supratarsal levator fixation for eyelid crease reconstruction (see Chapter 10). A modification of eyelid crease reconstruction uses the CO_2 laser in a defocused mode to accomplish "laser fusion" of the leading edge of the levator aponeurosis, the pretarsal orbicularis muscle, and the pretarsal skin surface. (All fat and septum have now been removed.) Figure 35–2*D,* which demonstrates this "fusion contracture" of the eyelid crease, shows the leading edge and how it is brought in direct apposition to the pretarsal skin edge, with ablation of pretarsal orbicularis muscle and con-

tracture bringing all the tissues into direct apposition so that suture closure can be accomplished directly.

The surgeon then closes the wound by using a 6-0 nylon suture from a nasotemporal direction, with every other bite capturing both proximal and distal skin edges with the levator aponeurosis in between. This suture is removed 6–7 days after surgery and leaves an excellent, formed crease. This crease is similar to that accomplished in conventional surgery (see Chapter 10) but without the use of the cutaneous and subcutaneous polyglactin (Vicryl) and polyester fiber (Mersilene) suturing used in conventional surgery.

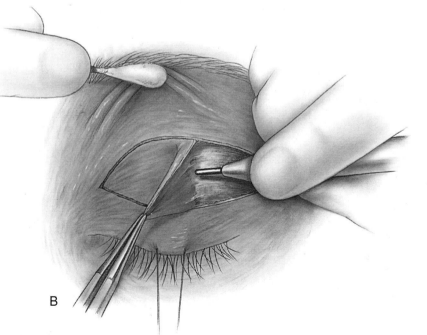

B, A skin or skin-muscle flap is raised with immediate hemostasis with a CO_2 laser in the cutting mode.

B

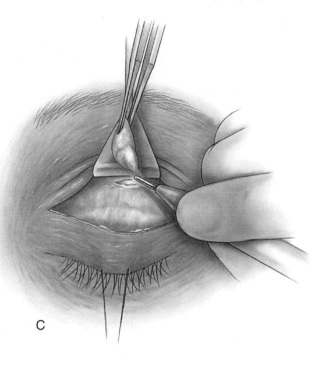

C, The CO_2 laser directly cuts and seals herniated orbital fat pads.

C

Lower Lid Transconjunctival Laser Blepharoplasty

Basic anatomy and technique for lower lid transconjunctival CO_2 laser blepharoplasty follow those of conventional transconjunctival blepharoplasty (see Chapter 20). Some laser techniques, however, allow for greater ease in performing the procedure and a decrease in morbidity and recuperative time. Gentle retropulsion on the contact lens allows for prolapse of the inferior fornix and a temporal to nasal direction incision made at the midfornix at approximately 5 mm below the inferior tarsal border. A 4-0 silk suture is used to retract the lower eyelid (Fig. 35–3*A*). Again, a proper tempo for depth of incision is needed so that the conjunctiva and lower lid retractor or capsulopalpebral fascia are incised in one

pass. The same 0.2–0.4 mm spot at 7–8 watts, either in continuous-wave or superpulsed mode, is used.

At this point, a toothed forceps is used to further separate the tissue, and again a sandblasted Desmarres retractor is used to retract the lower eyelid inferiorly. A 4-0 silk suture is passed to the eyelid retractor flap and is retracted superiorly. This exposes the orbital septum, which is incised with the laser hand piece, and the temporal fat pad is exposed first with intermittent gentle retropulsion of the contact lens and globe (Fig. 35–3*B*). The fat pad is incised and removed. It is again amputated by the laser incision to the base of the fat pad with a focused beam. With removal of the fat pad and simultaneous coagulation of all vessels and maintenance of hemostasis, a defocused hand piece is used for any additional coagulation necessary and for vaporizing the

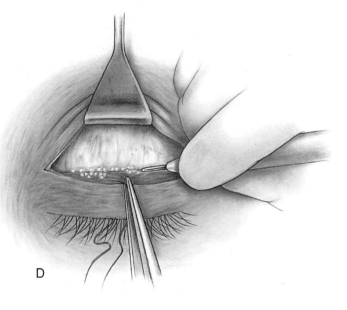

D, The CO_2 laser directly "fuses" the levator aponeurotic edge to the pretarsal orbicularis oculi muscle and skin.

D

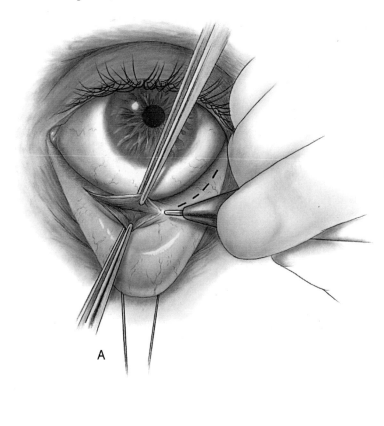

figure 35–3

Lower eyelid transconjunctival carbon dioxide (CO_2) laser blepharoplasty. *A,* A 4-0 silk suture is used to retract the lower eyelid. The CO_2 laser at 7 watts, continuous wave, at 0.4-mm beam makes midfornix conjunctival incision. (In vivo, a steel contact lens would be in place.)

A

B, The lower lid conjunctiva and margin are reflected under a Desmarres retractor in the transconjunctival approach. The postseptal herniated orbital fat is prolapsed and grasped with forceps and is excised and sealed directly with the CO_2 laser.

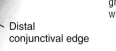

Distal
conjunctival edge

Proximal
conjunctival edge

Capsulopalpebral
fascia

B

Orbital septum

Herniated
orbital fat

remnants or contouring the shape of the fat pad to the orbital rim. The fat pad can actually be sculpted and shaped by the laser so that a natural and aesthetically acceptable contour from the cheek, orbital rim, and eyelid can be established.

The surgeon should use the *least movement* possible of the laser cutting beam in order to ensure safety and to avoid inadvertent laser delivery. Therefore, the fat pad is moved to and fro across a stationary laser cutting tip. The fat pad is amputated and incised by direct cutting with the laser beam and, in a defocused mode, is coagulated simultaneously (see Fig. 35–3*B*). Again, further contouring of the fat pad can be accomplished by direct application of the laser in the defocused mode to directly vaporize the fat pad until a smooth continuity from the orbital rim to the lid margin is achieved. The surgeon should look at the eyelid contour with the eyelid reopposed at various points during fat excision to ascertain the proper amount of fat pad removal and eyelid contouring and sculpting. Overaggressive fat removal should be discouraged because it leaves an unacceptable, cadaveric appearance.

To remove lower lid fat, the surgeon should take care to protect the inferior oblique musculature and to always identify the muscle. The surgeon uses moistened cotton swabs and/or a Desmarres retractor on the oblique muscle, and the nasal fat pad is incised with the same to-and-fro motion of the fat pad to a stable and stationary laser cutting tip. It should be noted that the nasal pads in both the upper and lower eyelids have specific large-caliber blood vessels. These vessels can be coagulated and contracted before cutting with a defocused laser hand piece to coagulate and contract the blood vessels before direct incision by the laser and amputation of the fat pad.

Lower Lid Transconjunctival Blepharoplasty Combined with Skin Resurfacing

Lower lid transconjunctival blepharoplasty can also be performed simultaneously with CO_2 laser skin resurfacing. Transconjunctival blepharoplasty is ideally combined with skin resurfacing for the treatment of skin laxity and rhytids (See Chapter 31). Whether to perform fat excision alone or fat excision with laser skin resurfacing needs to be decided individually. The quality, thickness, color, wrinkling, and amount of laxity of the skin are all factors.

COMPLICATIONS

Complications of laser incisional blepharoplasty are identical to those of conventional blepharoplasty (see Chapters 9, 10, and 20). They mainly relate to problems with overcorrection and overresection. Conservative techniques usually avoid ectropion, eyelid retraction, and eyelid level asymmetries.

The single additional complication I have found with laser technique is unexpected depth of incision. As the depth of incision is related to tempo—not tactile pressure—inadvertently deep or full-thickness wounds can be created.

RESULTS

Patient satisfaction with laser incisional blepharoplasty has greatly exceeded that with conventional techniques. I have performed more than 350 laser eyelid surgeries and consistently have seen marked reduction in postoperative morbidity. Cosmesis is restored in 4–6 days, and patients recuperate rapidly.

References

1. Waldorf HA, Kauvar AN, Geronemus RG: Skin resurfacing of fine to deep rhytides using a char-free carbon dioxide laser in 47 patients. Dermatol Surg 1995; 21:940–946.
2. Keller GS, Cray J: Laser-assisted surgery of the aging face. Facial Plast Surg Clin North Am 1995; 3:319–341.
3. Tu N: Dermabrasion, chemical peel and laser procedures. In Tu N (ed): Anesthesia and Facial Plastic Surgery. New York, Thieme, 1994.
4. Millman A: Comparison of histopathology of superpulse laser in carbon dioxide cosmetic skin resurfacing. Presented at the American Society of Plastic and Reconstructive Surgeons–American Academy of Ophthalmology Meeting, November 1996, Chicago.

Allen M. Putterman

Chapter **36**

Blepharoplasty with Neodymium:YAG Laser, Cautery, or Colorado Needle

The neodymium:YAG (Nd:YAG) laser can be used in cosmetic oculoplastic surgery to make skin incisions, sever the orbicularis oculi muscle, and remove orbital fat. It can also be used to make incisions for brow lifts and to excise tissue. It has the advantage over the scalpel or scissors of producing less bleeding and thereby saving intraoperative time by not requiring as much cauterization of bleeding vessels. It also enables removal of orbital fat without the need to clamp the fat, thereby producing less pain. However, the Nd:YAG laser is associated with the following disadvantages: (1) more preoperative time is required to set up the equipment, (2) less visualization is possible because of the need to wear goggles, and (3) the cost is higher. Therefore, I use this method only in patients who have known bleeding tendencies or who prefer laser treatment.

The carbon dioxide (CO_2) ultrapulse laser, I believe, is easier to use, requires glasses rather than goggles, and is less costly. However, it must be held away from tissues whereas the Nd:YAG laser is used like a scalpel, with direct touch of the tissues. Use of the CO_2 ultrapulse laser for blepharoplasty is described in Chapter 35.

An effect similar to that achieved by the Nd:YAG laser can be achieved with the Colorado needle. The Colorado needle is much easier to set up, is much less expensive than laser, and does not require wearing goggles. Although it can be used to incise skin and to remove orbital fat, I have used it only for penetrating the orbicularis muscle, orbital septum, and orbital fat capsule. It does produce more charring than either the Nd:YAG laser or CO_2 ultrapulse laser.

A disposable surgical cautery can be used not only to coagulate blood vessels but also to sever the orbicularis muscle, the orbital septum, and other soft tissues. It is readily available, does not require any additional set-up time, and is less expensive than the Nd:YAG laser, but it produces more charring than the Nd:YAG laser, CO_2 ultrapulse laser, or Colorado needle. I use this cautery at varying times along with the Colorado needle in cosmetic blepharoplasties, levator aponeurosis resection, and direct brow lifts.

ALLEN M. PUTTERMAN

NEODYMIUM:YAG LASER

The scalpel (*contact*) Nd:YAG laser has been shown to be useful in plastic surgical procedures.[1] The power of the Nd:YAG laser can be transmitted through a fiberoptic coil to a probe with a sapphire tip. The tip, when touched to tissue, creates an incision while simultaneously coagulating blood vessels. This differs from *noncontact* lasers, which rely on the transmission of laser energy through air to a direct spot.

Surgical Technique

Fiberoptic coils and sapphire tips are attached to a stationary Nd:YAG laser. A commercially available portable Nd:YAG laser unit is attached to the manufacturer's fiberoptic coils and sapphire tips. The sapphire tips are available in clear or frosted and vary in size. The clear tips are best for skin because they produce a finer incision and less charring of tissue than the frosted tips. The frosted tips are best for dissection of subcutaneous vascular tissue because they coagulate blood vessels better than the clear tips do. I most often use a 4-mm tip because the smaller tips produce a thinner incision.

The operating room staff should wear protective glasses with an optical density of at least 4.5 at 1064-nm wavelength. The patient's eyes are protected with large green scleral lenses that are used in routine oculoplastic surgical procedures.

The laser power source ranges from 0 to 60 watts. Usually, I use an 8-watt power setting for the skin incision and 10–12 watts of power for severing subcutaneous tissues.

A skin incision is made over the outlined area of upper eyelid skin with the sapphire tip of the Nd:YAG laser (Fig. 36–1). The laser power is transmitted when the surgeon steps on a foot pedal. Then an ellipse of skin and orbicularis muscle is resected with the laser tip (Fig. 36–2).

The surgeon removes orbital fat with the laser by lifting it up with forceps and lightly rubbing the laser tip over the base of the prolapsed fat as the power is turned on by pushing on the foot pedal (Fig. 36–3). This approach differs from the conventional technique of fat resection, which involves clamping the prolapsed fat with a hemostat, cutting it with a No. 15 Bard-Parker blade slid over the hemostat, placing cotton-tipped applicators under the hemostat, and applying a Bovie cautery to the hemostat.

Bleeding is controlled with the frosted sapphire tip or a disposable surgical cautery.

Results

Less bleeding occurs with the use of the scalpel Nd:YAG laser than during conventional surgery with a surgical blade and scissors, as shown in a comparative study I published in 1990.[1] Eighteen patients underwent oculoplastic surgical procedures (treatment of dermatochalasis and herniated orbital fat, levator aponeurosis resection, or brow lift) with the use of the sapphire-tipped Nd:YAG laser. Ten of the 18 patients received laser treatment on one side and conventional surgery on the other side. The operation performed on the laser-treated side was up to 20 minutes shorter because less time was spent controlling bleeding with the surgical cauteries.[1] Additionally, the patients reported that they experienced less pain on removal of orbital fat with the Nd:YAG laser than with conventional surgery.

Pathologic specimens were obtained during Nd:YAG laser treatment and surgical blade-scissors treatment in five patients. It was found that the Nd:YAG laser caused minimal charring of tissue compared with Bovie cauteries and other coagulative techniques. However, more

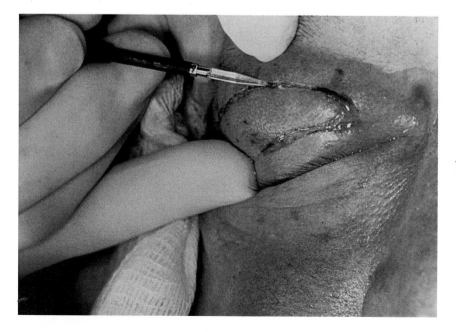

figure 36–1

Scalpel Nd:YAG laser used to incise skin during cosmetic blepharoplasty of the upper eyelids.

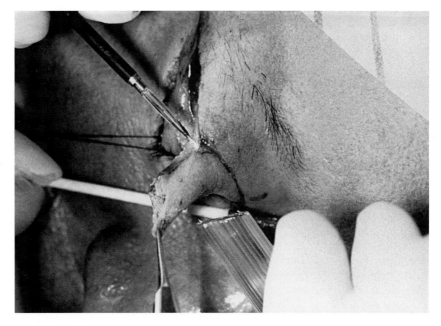

figure 36–2

Scalpel Nd:YAG laser severing the orbicularis muscle during resection of skin and orbicularis ellipse in upper blepharoplasty.

charring occurred compared with conventional surgery using a surgical blade.

Photographs of the patients were taken 1, 3, 6, and 12 weeks postoperatively. An unbiased physician observer compared these photographs and noted no significant difference in ecchymosis or edema between the Nd:YAG laser-treated side and the conventionally operated side.[1] The observer noted that the scars on the side that underwent the Nd:YAG laser procedures were more noticeable during the first few postoperative weeks. At 12 weeks, however, there was no noticeable difference between the two sides.

Nd:YAG LASER VERSUS COLORADO NEEDLE OR DISPOSABLE CAUTERY

My 1990 study showed that the Nd:YAG laser has the ability to incise and sever tissues with less bleeding and pain and shorter operating time compared with conventional surgery.[1] However, the equipment is expensive and takes additional time to set up, and it is difficult to visualize the operative field because the surgeon must wear goggles. Therefore, at present, I use the Nd:YAG laser in oculoplastic surgery only in selected patients who have a tendency to bleed excessively or who insist on this procedure.

Occasionally, I have used the CO_2 ultrapulse laser for blepharoplasty excision and dissection. The technique is described in detail in Chapter 35.

In most of my cosmetic oculoplastic surgery procedures, I use the Colorado needle (Colorado Biomedical, Inc., Evergreen, Colo.) or the Solan Accu-Temp disposable surgical cautery (Xomed Surgical Products, Jacksonville, Fla.). The advantages of both these instruments over the Nd:YAG laser are less expense, no need for a lengthy set-up time, and no need for the

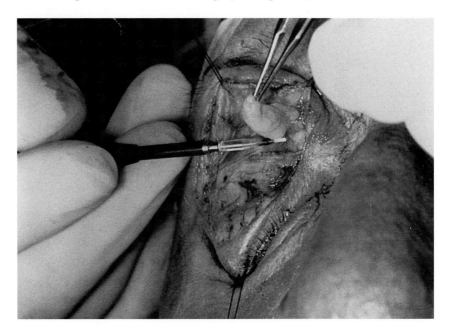

figure 36–3

Scalpel Nd:YAG laser severing herniated orbital fat in upper blepharoplasty.

surgeon to wear goggles. The disadvantage is more tissue scarring.

Colorado Needle

The Colorado needle comes in various sizes. It is inserted onto the Bovie cautery cord and plugged into the same equipment used for Bovie cauteries. I do not use this needle to penetrate skin, although with a cutting mode it can incise tissues very well. I switch between cutting and coagulating powers when using the Colorado needle. The coagulating mode produces better coagulation of blood vessels but causes more charring than the cutting mode does. The Colorado needle works on the principle of sending current through a very fine tip, which can produce an effect similar to that of the laser. In my experience, however, hemostasis is not quite as effective as with the laser.

I have not used the Colorado needle to sever fat, but I do use it to shrink minimal remaining fat after fat resection. I find it very useful in incising the orbicularis muscle and in excising the skin-muscle ellipse in upper blepharoplasties. I also use it to sever the suborbicularis fascia and orbital septum as well as the orbital fat capsule. Additionally, I use this instrument to excise brow fat in an internal brow lift (see Chapter 12).

Disposable Cautery

The disposable surgical cautery can be used in the same way as the Colorado needle to sever the orbicularis muscle, excise a skin-muscle flap, and penetrate the orbital septum and orbital fat capsule in upper blepharoplasties. It produces more charring, however, compared with the Colorado needle or the Nd:YAG laser.

Reference

1. Putterman AM: Scalpel neodymium:YAG laser in oculoplastic surgery. Am J Ophthalmol 1990; 109:581–584.

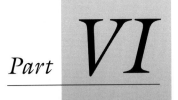

Part VI

POSTOPERATIVE
CONSIDERATIONS

Henry I. Baylis
Robert A. Goldberg
Martha C. Wilson

Chapter *37*

Complications of Upper Blepharoplasty

Complications of cosmetic oculoplastic surgery are rare but certainly can occur. It is therefore important for the surgeon to inform candidates for blepharoplasty of the possibility of complications so that they are completely prepared to handle them.

In this chapter, Henry Baylis, Robert Goldberg, and Martha Wilson discuss the possibility of retrobulbar hemorrhage and secondary blindness. They emphasize this potential complication to make sure that patients do not take anticoagulants, especially aspirin, for several weeks before surgery. I also believe that it is extremely important to avoid the use of patching therapy after surgery and to monitor visual function by the patient's ability to count fingers and to check for the presence of proptosis and pain for at least 10 hours after surgery. If a retrobulbar hemorrhage with loss of vision occurs, immediate medical attention is required.

Because reconstruction of the upper eyelid crease is becoming more popular, there are more postoperative occurrences of asymmetric creases and folds. I would like to emphasize the need for early observation of these complications. Many times the creases and folds will improve with time; also, if external sutures are used to unite skin to the levator aponeurosis, they can be removed from the higher crease as soon as asymmetry is seen. Finally, I have patients sit up on the operating table after reconstruction of upper eyelid creases, and if I note asymmetry at that time, I adjust it intraoperatively.

Dr. Baylis and colleagues describe a fat graft to lower a high upper eyelid crease. If the patient also has an upper eyelid ptosis (drooping eyelid), an internal or external levator aponeurosis ptosis procedure can create a lower crease while it simultaneously elevates the eyelid.

The authors also encourage us to err toward undercorrection rather than overcorrection because undercorrection is easier to revise with minimal touch-up surgery. New to this chapter is a discussion of the treatment of overcorrections and undercorrections that occur after surgery for upper eyelid retraction (see Chapters 15 and 16). In addition to the techniques recommended by the authors, I would like to emphasize downward massage of the residually retracted eyelid while the eyebrow area is being elevated and fixated.

411

Also, complications such as suture cysts, hypertrophic scars, superior sulcus syndrome, allergic reactions, wound dehiscence, lagophthalmos (inability to close the eye completely), lacrimal gland injury, and diplopia (double vision) are discussed. Lastly, ptosis can occur from direct laceration of the levator aponeurosis or even from swelling in the patients with a thin, friable levator aponeurosis.

ALLEN M. PUTTERMAN

Serious complications are unusual after blepharoplasty. However, minor complications or "nuisances" are encountered every day by the blepharoplasty surgeon.

AVOIDANCE OF COMPLICATIONS

The most common "complication" of cosmetic blepharoplasty is patient dissatisfaction with the results. The preoperative interview between the prospective patient and the surgeon is the best time to set the conditions that facilitate patient satisfaction. This interview helps patients define exactly what they wish to accomplish and what their expectations are and allows the surgeon to educate patients about what can be accomplished with blepharoplasty and how it can improve appearance. A thorough understanding of what surgery can achieve is a requisite for the blepharoplasty surgeon.

Patients should be made aware that a primary concern in cosmetic blepharoplasty is to enhance the appearance of the eyelids without producing a "surgical look." Because every effort is made not to produce an overdone appearance, surgery sometimes results in undercorrections. These are easily handled with a revision procedure, and the blepharoplasty surgeon is always willing to undertake small revisions because they represent the most powerful tool to fully please the patient. Patients also appreciate being able to make changes if the results are not completely satisfactory after a sufficient healing period (2–3 months).

COSMETIC COMPLICATIONS
Undercorrection

By far, the most common cosmetic complication of upper blepharoplasty is undercorrection. The most frequent presentation is that of a residual skin fold (Fig. 37–1). The surgeon can easily correct this complication by directly excising the skin fold after local infiltration of an anesthetic agent. There is no need to open the septum or excise fat unless a distinct bulge can be identified.

The surgeon initiates an additional excision of skin by outlining a segment of skin above and adjacent to the previous incision along the full length of the wound (Fig. 37–2A). The skin and underlying orbicularis oculi muscle are then excised, and the wound is closed with a running suture (Fig. 37–2B). A supratarsal fixation wound closure, which helps enhance the new crease, consists of a running suture in which a bite of levator aponeurosis is taken with every bite of skin. A fairly large impact can be produced with a moderate excision of skin and muscle (Fig. 37–2C and 2D).

An additional excision of fat is performed when a residual bulge can be clearly identified. Bulging occurs commonly at the site of the medial fat pad. A skin incision is made over the residual bulge unless there is also excessive skin, in which case an ellipse of skin and orbicularis muscle is excised. Under direct visualization, the orbital septum is incised while gentle posterior pressure is applied on the globe to cause the fat to prolapse

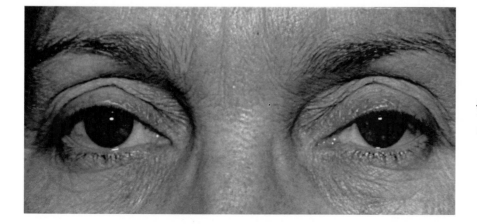

figure 37–1

The most common presentation of an undercorrection is a residual skin fold.

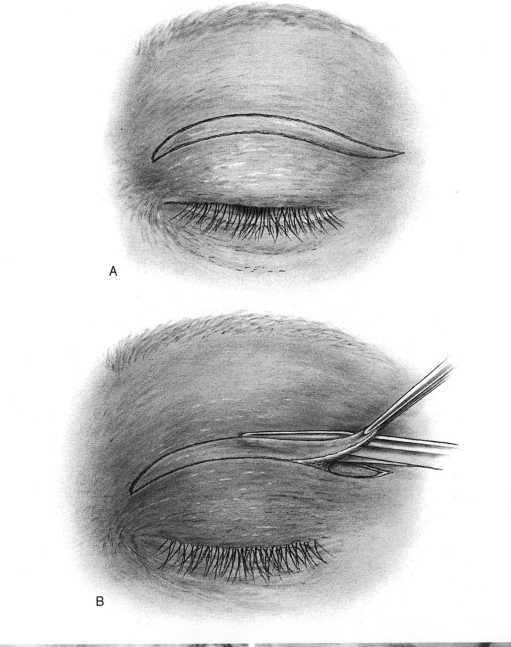

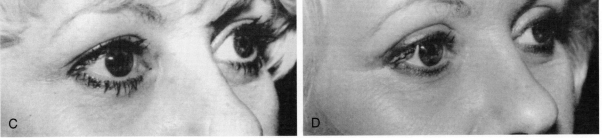

figure 37–2

Revision blepharoplasty with additional excision of skin. *A,* A 2-mm segment of skin is outlined. *B,* The skin and orbicularis oculi muscle are excised. *C* and *D,* Preoperative *(C)* and postoperative *(D)* appearances of a patient who underwent revision blepharoplasty with additional excision of skin and muscle.

(Fig. 37–3). The surgeon then excises the fat with scissors, cauterizing any bleeding vessels. The skin wound is closed as described previously.

High Eyelid Creases

A high eyelid crease is a common occurrence for the novice blepharoplasty surgeon and is difficult to correct

(Fig. 37–4). It is particularly important to avoid this complication in men because a high crease contributes to a feminine appearance. To prevent this complication, the surgeon should remember that most patients do not want drastic changes in their appearance. Only in rare instances should the new crease occur above the natural crease. It is relatively easy to raise a low crease surgically, but it is difficult to lower a high one. Therefore, it is better to err on the side of too low a crease. Minimally

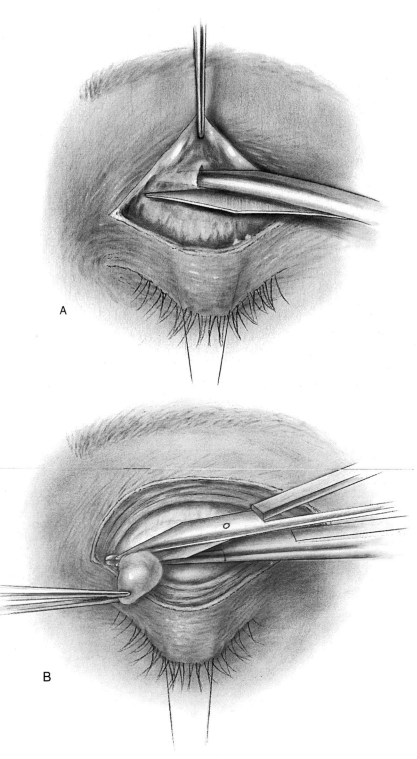

figure 37–3

Revision blepharoplasty with additional excision of fat. *A,* The skin and orbicularis muscle are lifted to uncover the fat still covered by the orbital septum. The orbital septum overlying the bulging fat is buttonholed under direct visualization, and the buttonhole in the septum is extended with scissors. *B,* The fat prolapses into the wound. Prolapsing fat is excised with scissors under direct visualization.

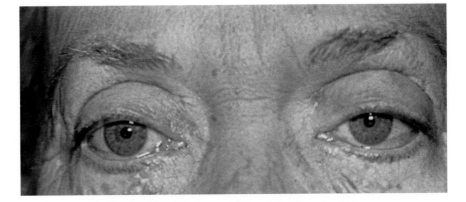

figure 37-4

High eyelid crease after upper blepharoplasty.

successful attempts at lowering an eyelid crease have required a fat graft between the septum and the levator aponeurosis to keep the structures from adhering to each other and a reformation of the crease at a lower level with an intentional overhang of the skin at the upper lip of the incision. This technique implies closure of the blepharoplasty wound with interrupted sutures. Each suture goes through the lower lip of the incision and takes a bite of the levator aponeurosis and then a bite of the upper lip, which has been allowed to roll in slightly. The result is tense skin inferiorly, and looser, slightly overhanging skin superiorly.

Asymmetric Eyelid Creases

Asymmetric eyelid creases are relatively common after surgery. Most often, one crease is higher than the other. The easiest way to approach this problem is to raise the crease that is too low. An ellipse of skin is marked at a level above the low crease. The lower line in the ellipse should be symmetric with the crease of the other eyelid. The skin and orbicularis muscle within the ellipse are then excised. A skin-muscle flap is dissected across the pretarsal eyelid, and any attachments of the levator aponeurosis inferior to the new crease line are disinserted. The surgeon then closes the skin using a lid crease enhancement technique (Fig. 37–5). With each pass of the needle, a bite of skin and underlying orbicularis muscle on the lower wound edge is taken, then a bite of levator about 1–2 mm above that, and finally, a bite of orbicularis muscle and skin at the upper wound edge.

Medial Tension Lines

Tension lines can be created when the nasal aspect of the wound is closed with a suture (Fig. 37–6). To prevent medial tension lines, the surgeon must place the first pass of the running suture. It is safest to start the running suture not at the medial-most corner of the wound but 3–4 mm lateral to it, with no suture placed medial to that. The needle passes through skin and orbicularis on the lower wound edge, then takes a bite of a few fibers of levator aponeurosis about 1–2 mm above the lower edge. The surgeon finally brings the

needle straight upward, rather than in a meridional fashion, to grasp orbicularis muscle and skin at the upper edge of the wound. This maneuver exerts a mild nasal pull on the upper aspect of the wound, thereby reducing the tension at the medialmost portion of the wound. If, despite these steps, stress lines are created by the first pass of the suture, the surgeon should remove and reposition the suture lateral to that point, without closing the nasal aspect of the wound.

Suture Milia

Suture milia occur relatively frequently and can be very distressing to patients (Fig. 37–7). Association with the suture is manifested by the occurrence of a cystic elevation at every site where the needle entered the skin, but the suture material employed is not consistently related to the occurrence of milia. Suture milia have been reported to occur more commonly when 6-0 silk suture material is used. However, we generally use 6-0 mild chromic gut and have experienced the occurrence of milia equally frequently. Changing to 6-0 polypropylene (Prolene) sutures seems to decrease but not eliminate the occurrence of milia.

Milia first appear approximately 1 week after surgery, and they disappear spontaneously; however, total resolution may take months. Some patients prefer to undergo surgical excision rather than to wait for spontaneous resolution. In those cases, a small needle or a scissors may be used to excise the cap of the cystic elevation, which allows for reepithelialization on the marsupialized surface. Some surgeons prefer to hyfrecate (electrolyze) the cysts or treat them with the carbon dioxide laser. Milia may be associated with hypertrophic scars, which also resolve spontaneously over several months (Fig. 37–8). The surgeon can minimize suture milia by using subcuticular sutures and by removing sutures early.

Superior Sulcus Syndrome

The superior sulcus syndrome occurs as a result of excessive excision of fat from the upper orbit. The area above the eyelid crease looks sunken, creating a significant cosmetic blemish that is difficult to correct (Fig. 37–9).

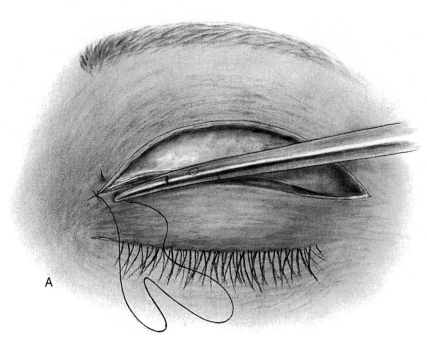

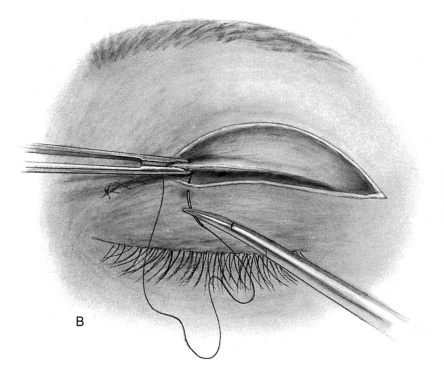

figure 37–5

Crease-enhancing suture. *A,* A running suture is begun medially through the lower skin and orbicularis muscle, catching a bite of the levator aponeurosis just 1 mm above the incision. The needle then goes through the skin in the upper incision.

Autogenous fat grafting by injection has been used to try to augment the superior orbital fat.[1] The technique involves removing fat from the donor site by liposuction, soaking the fat in regular insulin, and then injecting the fat in the desired site. A histologic specimen from a 2-month-old fat graft injected with this technique has been reported to show intact adipocytes surrounded by fibrovascular tissue.[1] The results of this technique, however, may be unpredictable because of postoperative shrinkage of fat grafts.

The surgeon can prevent this complication by excising only the fat that freely prolapses into the wound once the septum is open. The fat is never pulled; instead, it is allowed only to prolapse without pressure on the globe; it is then trimmed back to the level of the upper orbital rim. In men, it is particularly important for the surgeon to avoid excessive removal of fat because too much debulking gives a feminine appearance.

Complications of Blepharoplasty in Men

Although the objective of blepharoplasty in women is to highlight the contour of the eyelid margin and eye-

B, The suture is then run along the width of the eyelid from medial to lateral, until the lateral aspect of the levator aponeurosis is encountered. At the lateral edge of the wound, only skin and orbicularis muscle are closed.

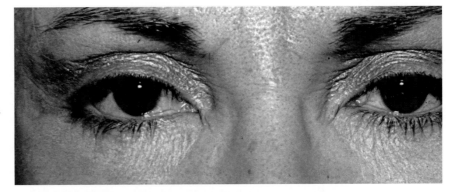

figure 37–6
Medial tension lines after upper blepharoplasty.

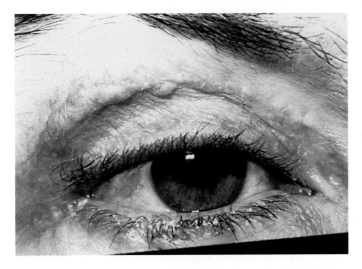

figure 37–7
Suture milia 3 weeks after operation.

figure 37–8
Suture milia may be associated with hypertrophic scars.

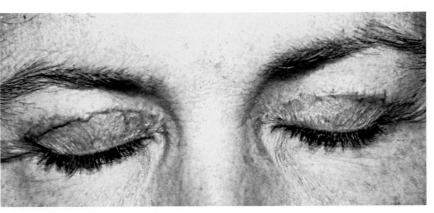

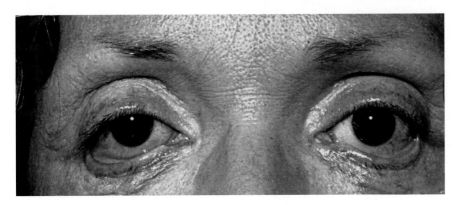

figure 37–9
Patient with superior sulcus syndrome resulting from excessive fat removal in the upper eyelids during upper blepharoplasty. She also has lower lid cicatricial ectropion from excessive removal of skin.

lashes, this result is not considered attractive in men. An overdone blepharoplasty in a man represents a serious cosmetic blemish because it contributes to a feminine appearance. Therefore, blepharoplasty in men is smaller in scope, and its objective is primarily to remove skin to the extent that it does not rest on the eyelashes. Blepharoplasty in men is planned according to how deep-set the eyes are. In about 50 per cent of male patients, the eyes are deep-set and there is an extreme amount of fullness; in those cases, the operation can be similar to that in women, except that the vertical dimension of the skin excision is about half of what it would be in a woman and the orbicularis muscle and fat are trimmed only conservatively. In the remaining 50 per cent of male patients, the eyes are prominent. In those cases, a conservative excision of skin and orbicularis muscle only, with cauterization of the underlying orbital septum and closure of the wound, may be all that is necessary. For male patients, the surgeon uses supratarsal fixation sutures to create a relatively deep eyelid crease without having to excise much skin.

Eyelid Retraction Overcorrections and Undercorrections in Patients with Graves' Disease

In a sophisticated patient population, ptosis, blepharoplasty, and thyroid eyelid surgery are all about revisions. The general unpredictability of eyelid recession, combined with the inflammatory nature of the underlying disease and the tendency for a drift in eyelid position, leads to frequent revisions. If patients do not understand this principle, they will be unhappy. If they understand, accept, and anticipate the possible need for enhancement surgeries, however, they become the partner of the physician and can tolerate the multiple operations that are sometimes necessary to achieve an optimal aesthetic result.

Timing of Revision

Undercorrections do not improve spontaneously, and as soon as the swelling has decreased, it is reasonable for the surgeon to perform additional recession, often within a month.

Overcorrections may improve over time, and even flattened contour abnormalities may improve somewhat as the central and temporal portions of the eyelid come back up preferentially. Waiting 2–3 months is prudent before overcorrections are treated, and if the overcorrection is small (<1.5 mm), it is reasonable to wait up to 6 months for possible improvement.

Technique of Revision

Small undercorrections (<2 mm) are treated with additional recession of the levator aponeurosis, either posterior or anterior. Larger undercorrections are treated by levator muscle Z-myotomy or, in the most intransigent cases, with the use of spacer grafts, such as hard-palate mucosa. Just as in the primary recession, contour is more important than position and segmental recession (or segmental grafts) are typically employed to address any abnormality in contour.

Overcorrections are best treated with full-thickness ptosis surgery. Full-thickness surgery has two advantages: it can control (1) eyelid contour (2) eyelid crease level, the two most important features for symmetry and aesthetics in thyroid eyelid surgery. The surgery is planned on the basis of contour and crease. The shape of the excised full-thickness eyelid is based on contour (e.g., a dumbbell shape for a peaked eyelid, a football shape for a flattened eyelid, or a pear shape wider medially for a medial droop).

The positioning relative to the crease is planned according to the position of the crease. For a high crease, the excision is below the existing crease; for a low crease, the excision is above the existing crease.

Full-thickness ptosis surgery is a powerful technique with the finesse to achieve good aesthetic results in any type of ptosis reoperation. In patients with thyroid disease, it is very important to use a *conservative* approach because it is easy to achieve an overcorrection and be right back to the starting point, with a retracted eyelid. For example, to address 2 mm of secondary ptosis, the surgeon might resect only 1.25 or 1.5 mm of full-thickness eyelid.

FUNCTIONAL COMPLICATIONS

Ptosis after Blepharoplasty

Ptosis is one of the most common functional complications of blepharoplasty (Fig. 37–10). It results from injury to the levator aponeurosis, which may occur by one of the following[2]:

- Direct laceration
- Stretching
- Restriction (tethering)

Direct laceration usually occurs at the lower half of the skin-muscle excision. At this location, the levator aponeurosis is merging with the septum and orbicularis muscle and is therefore more susceptible to injury (Fig. 37–11).[3] Avoidance of this complication has prompted several modifications in the surgical technique. During skin-muscle excision, the scissors blades are kept on a plane parallel to the levator complex. This reduces the risk of lacerating the levator aponeurosis. In addition, during septal excision, downward traction on the upper eyelid is exerted to tense the levator aponeurosis, thereby reducing the risk of direct injury to it. For the same reason, septal excision is performed at the superior lip of the wound because the preaponeurotic fat pad is thickest there and helps protect against direct levator injury (Fig. 37–12).[4]

Stretching of the levator aponeurosis can be caused by deep and persistent hematomas. The fibrosis that often accompanies this process may further restrict the normal excursion of the muscle. Both mechanisms can result in temporary or permanent ptosis.

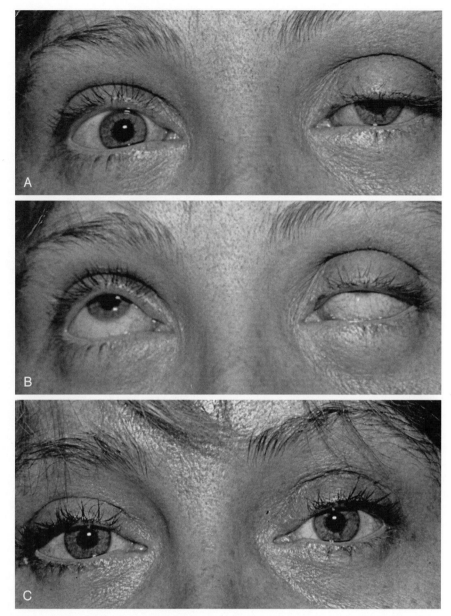

figure 37–10

Ptosis after blepharoplasty. *A,* The high eyelid crease suggests injury to the levator complex. *B,* Poor levator function confirms functional impairment of the levator complex. *C,* Postoperative appearance after repair of levator aponeurosis disinsertion.

Tethering, or restriction, of levator function can result in postoperative ptosis. This can occur if the orbital septum is inadvertently united to the levator aponeurosis during closure of a blepharoplasty wound. Ptosis ensues if the union is made on the levator superior to the original level of the septum or if the septum is foreshortened. To prevent this complication, the surgeon makes the running suture in such a way that the needle first grasps skin and orbicularis muscle below the wound, then a small amount of levator aponeurosis approximately 1 mm above the lower lip of the wound, and then the skin above the wound. The septum is left open and is not included in this closure. Grasping the levator more than 2 mm above the lower lip of the incision may also result in ptosis secondary to tethering of the levator muscle.

It is a common occurrence to observe a small rent in the levator aponeurosis during surgery, such that the Müller's muscle can be identified, because of its curlicue

vessels and beefy, muscular broad tissue, just where the glistening levator aponeurosis should be. If the rent is less than 5 mm above the upper margin of the tarsus, it does not need to be closed; instead, the upper edge of the rent can be included in the supratarsal fixation sutures during skin closure. If the rent is more than 5 mm above the upper edge of the tarsus, it may be closed but a conservative approach is warranted. The levator has many attachments and particularly in young people, a small rent has no effect on eyelid position. Aggressive intraoperative attempts to reattach the levator may produce eyelid retraction.

Treatment

Management of postoperative ptosis of less than 2 mm can involve just monitoring the patient, because most cases resolve spontaneously after days to weeks. Most of those cases are caused by edema. Swelling may cause

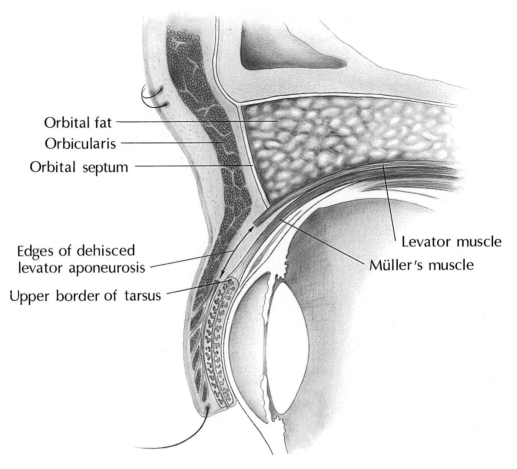

Orbital fat

Orbicularis

Orbital septum

Edges of dehisced
levator aponeurosis

Upper border of tarsus

Levator muscle

Müller's muscle

figure 37–11

An upper eyelid with dehiscence of the levator aponeurosis. (Adapted from Dryden RM, Leibsohn J: The levator aponeurosis in blepharoplasty. Ophthalmology 1978; 85:723. With permission.)

temporary ptosis by mechanical restriction. If the ptosis persists after 3 months, surgical correction is recommended. We prefer the Fasanella-Servat operation[5] or Müller's muscle-conjunctival resection for these cases (see Chapter 14).

The surgeon may best treat ptosis of more than 2 mm or ptosis with poor or absent levator function by prompt surgical exploration in order to avoid the difficult surgery associated with late fibrotic changes. A laceration of the levator aponeurosis is frequently found in these cases. Repair involves attachment of the levator aponeurosis to the anterior tarsal surface (Fig. 37–13). If this procedure does not fully correct the ptosis or if there is a contour abnormality, the full-thickness eyelid resection is used.[6]

Ptosis Before Surgery

Ptosis may be a preexisting condition in the blepharoplasty patient, and its recognition before surgery avoids patient disappointment and permits surgical planning to correct the ptosis during the same operation. A Fasanella-Servat operation, a Müller's muscle–conjunctival resection, or a levator aponeurosis procedure may be combined with blepharoplasty[3] (see Chapters 13 and 14). We prefer to scratch the incision line to mark it,

then perform ptosis surgery first through a posterior approach. The posterior approach (Müller's muscle–conjunctival resection or Fasanella-Servat) is more consistent and predictable than levator surgery and is less likely to cause a contour abnormality. We then proceed with a standard blepharoplasty. A single polypropylene suture can be used to close the posterior and anterior incisions.

Allergy to Topical Medications

In the patient with a known allergy to topical medications, it is easy to avoid an allergic reaction. However, sensitization in previously nonallergic patients cannot be predicted and results in added discomfort. The patient in whom an allergy to topical medications develops typically has had an uncomplicated blepharoplasty with the usual mild and easily tolerated postoperative discomfort. After 2–10 days, a delayed-type hypersensitivity reaction occurs, with progressively worsening edema, redness, and pruritus. Most patients are very distressed by the sudden worsening of what previously appeared to be a rapidly improving postoperative course.

Discontinuation of the topical medication halts the process, but the inflammatory reaction must run its

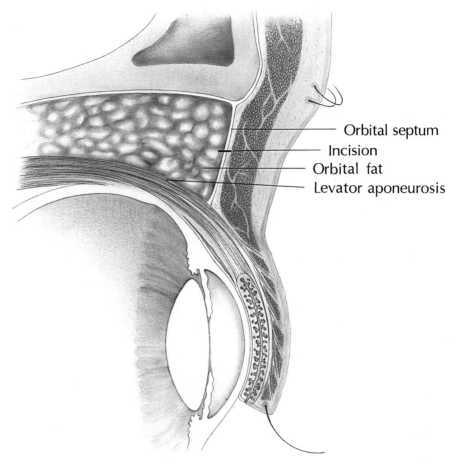

Orbital septum
Incision
Orbital fat
Levator aponeurosis

figure 37–12

High penetration of the orbital septum allows a margin of safety from injury to the levator aponeurosis because the preaponeurotic fat is between the septum and the levator aponeurosis. The lower the entry is on the septum, the greater the chance of penetrating the aponeurosis. (Modified from Wesley RE, Pollard ZF, McCord CD Jr: Superior oblique paresis after blepharoplasty. Plast Reconstr Surg 1980; 66:283–286. With permission.)

course and results in delayed healing, hypertrophic scars, and suture milia. Corticosteroid therapy may speed recovery. Neomycin and bacitracin zinc-polymyxin B (Polysporin) are frequently associated with allergic reactions (see Chapter 39).

Wound Dehiscence

Wound dehiscence is a fairly common occurrence after upper blepharoplasty, particularly when absorbable sutures are used (Fig. 37–14). It usually resolves spontaneously over a few days but may be associated with prolonged wound healing and a more noticeable scar. Exudation from the wound is common, but frank wound infection is rare (Fig. 37–15). Reapproximation of the recently dehisced wound may be helpful to speed healing, but long-standing dehiscence can be allowed to heal by secondary intention, with good results. If necessary, late prolonged dehiscence may be corrected by excision of the edges of the wound and reapproximation of the freshened edges with a suture.

Lagophthalmos

Although excision of large amounts of skin in blepharoplasty used to be common practice, surgeons now believe that the most important element of upper eyelid

blepharoplasty is the debulking of greater amounts of orbicularis muscle, septum, and fat and lesser amounts of excised skin. In addition, supratarsal fixation (anchor blepharoplasty) allows deepening of the eyelid crease without excessive removal of skin. This technique achieves a substantial debulking of the upper eyelid with minimal excision of skin, thus resulting in a dramatic change in appearance without the risk of excising too much skin.

When an excessive amount of skin has been removed, the postoperative manifestation is lagophthalmos (Fig. 37–16). Patients with good eye protection mechanisms (i.e., tear film and Bell's phenomenon) may have minimal symptoms, even though there is some lagophthalmos; however, if these mechanisms are compromised, symptoms of exposure keratopathy ensue. Management includes patching the eyes at night and instilling lubricants (either ointments or artificial tears) during the day until appropriate treatment can be instituted.

Milder cases may be managed conservatively with massage, time, and proper lubricants. At the stage during which tightness is maximum, the lagophthalmos may relax somewhat and may be tolerable without the need for further surgery. If the eye is compromised, however, a skin graft is necessary. The posterior auricular area is usually the best match for color and skin thickness (Fig. 37–17). Results are usually disappointing, and ptosis is a frequent complication.

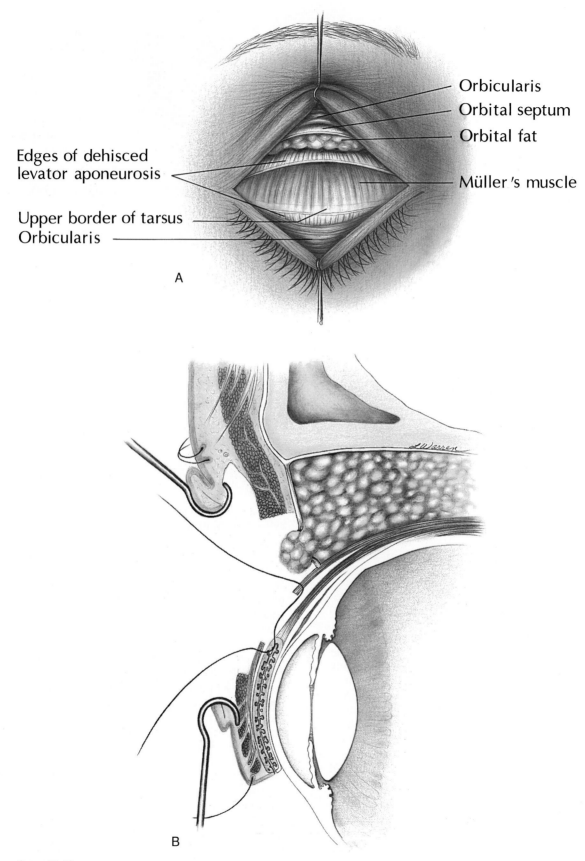

Orbicularis

Orbital septum

Orbital fat

Edges of dehisced
levator aponeurosis

Müller 's muscle

Upper border of tarsus
Orbicularis

A

B

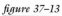

A, The levator aponeurosis is totally disinserted from the upper border of the tarsus. B, The aponeurosis is sutured to the upper tarsal border.

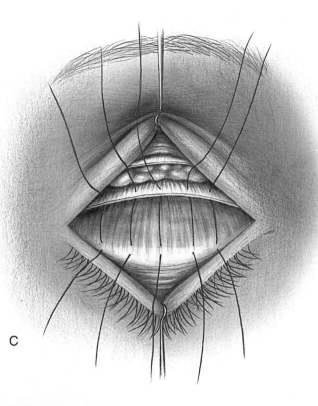

C, Multiple interrupted sutures from the edge of the levator dehiscence to the upper tarsal border.

C

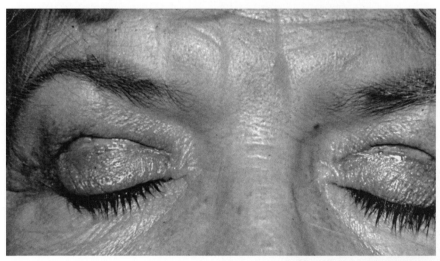

figure 37–14

Wound dehiscence after upper blepharoplasty.

figure 37–15

Wound dehiscence associated with wound infection approximately 2 weeks after blepharoplasty.

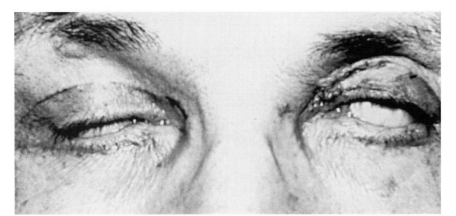

figure 37–16

Postblepharoplasty lagophthalmos from excessive skin removal.

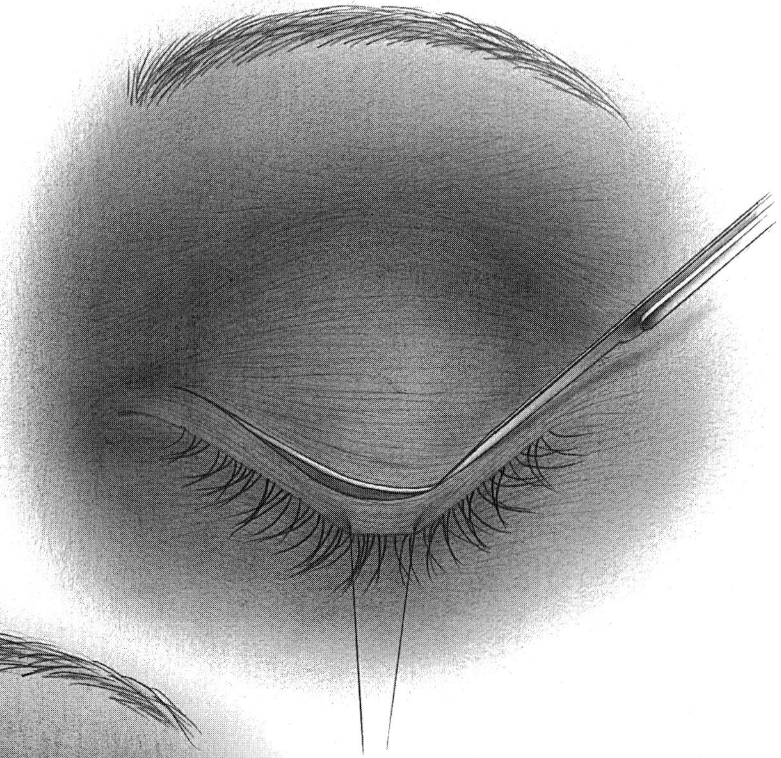

figure 37–17

A full-thickness skin graft is applied to the upper eyelid in severe cases of lagophthalmos following blepharoplasty. *A,* An incision is made just above the lash line along the entire width of eyelid. *B,* The skin is undermined above the incision to allow the upper skin edge to migrate toward the supratarsal crease area or higher.

A

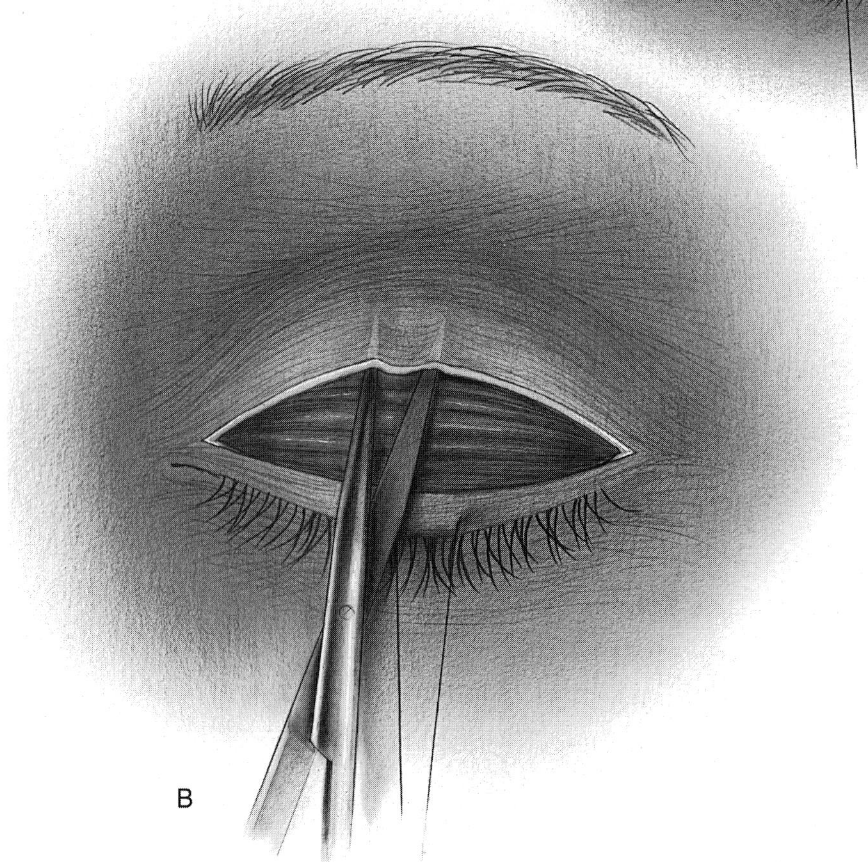

B

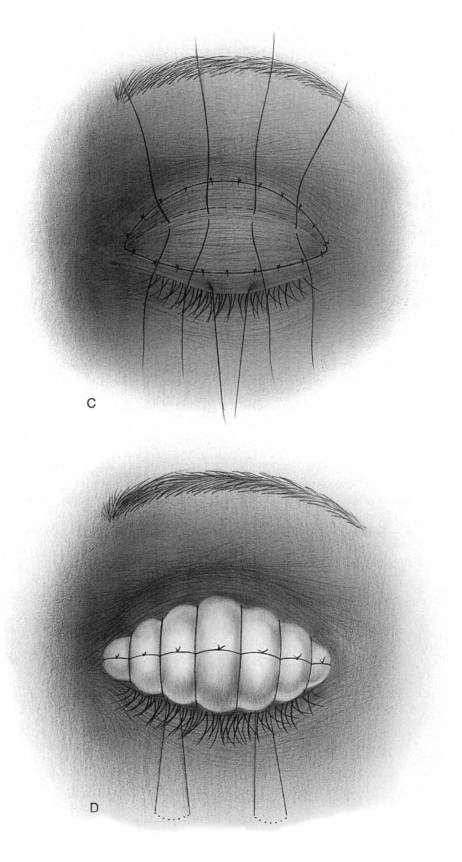

C, If the donor graft is somewhat larger than the tarsal plate, the graft is quilted along the area of desired supratarsal crease formation. Mattress sutures of 6-0 silk can be introduced through the graft at the desired crease formation, into either the superior tarsal border or the levator aponeurosis just above. *D,* The graft is fixated for 1 week with inter-marginal and traction sutures of 4-0 silk through the upper lid. Sutures are tied over the releasing gauze, cotton fluff, and/or dental wax dressing. Proper dressing and splinting of the graft are mandatory for success.

C

D

Lagophthalmos of the upper eyelid may also be caused by contracture of the orbital septum, either from fibrosis or from attempts to resuture the septum following removal of orbital fat. It is never advisable to resuture the orbital septum. The correction of lagophthalmos with septal scarring and contracture is difficult, and the repair necessitates a skin graft after extensive removal of subcutaneous scar tissue.

Lacrimal Gland Injury

In many cases of upper lid blepharoplasty, the lacrimal gland is encountered temporal to the preaponeurotic fat. The lacrimal gland can be identified as a firmer and grayish brown mass located in the temporal portion of the eyelid on the surface of the levator aponeurosis. In some cases, however, the gland has prolapsed to the level of the preaponeurotic fat pad, and it may be mistaken for fat and excised if it is not recognized. This results in a loss of some of the reflex secretors of the eye and the possible postoperative development of dry eyes, which requires treatment with artificial tears, ointments, and probably punctal occlusion.[7] A prolapsed lacrimal gland can be refixed with a suture, as detailed in Chapter 17.

VISION-THREATENING COMPLICATIONS

Bleeding

Although excessive bleeding during a blepharoplasty does not lead to significant depletion in blood volume, intraoperative bleeding might indicate that the patient will continue to bleed postoperatively, resulting in severe bruising and formation of hematomas. Orbital hematomas may cause compression of the optic nerve and ophthalmic or central retinal artery, with possible loss of vision. The preoperative history should have determined whether the patient has a history of bleeding or is taking medications that will cause excessive bleeding, such as aspirin, nonsteroidal anti-inflammatory drugs, and anticoagulants. By far, the most common cause of intraoperative and postoperative bleeding is the use of aspirin-containing products. Discontinuation of aspirin 2 weeks before surgery allows the platelet aggregation to return to normal.

Intraoperative Bleeding

Most of the bleeding during blepharoplasty comes from the orbicularis muscle, which is the most vascular structure of the eyelids.[8] Blood from the orbicularis can track posteriorly through an open septum to accumulate in the orbit and raise the intraorbital pressure to dangerous

levels. Securing hemostasis of the abundant orbicularis muscle vessels before wound closure helps avoid a postoperative orbital hemorrhage.

Some bleeding may also be encountered during fat excision, although the small nutrient vessels of the fat are unlikely to be responsible for appreciable bleeding.[8] During excision of the medial fat pads of both upper and lower eyelids, the superior and inferior medial palpebral vessels can be identified and gently teased away from the fat. The fat can then be excised and the vessels avoided. Excision can be done with scissors without the need of a clamp because the orbital fat does not retract into the orbit. If any bleeding is encountered, gentle retropulsion on the globe causes the orbital fat to prolapse and the bleeding vessels can then be cauterized under direct visualization.

Postoperative Bleeding

Postoperative bleeding may take the form of a (1) retrobulbar hemorrhage or (2) hematoma.

RETROBULBAR HEMORRHAGE

A retrobulbar hemorrhage is a true emergency, as it may lead to permanent visual loss.[9] The usual presentation is that of a patient in significant pain. The periorbital ecchymosis and subconjunctival hemorrhage are obvious. The orbit is tight, and proptosis may or may not be significant. There usually is some degree of visual loss, the intraocular pressure is increased, and there may be an afferent pupillary defect.

Management should be started immediately. The wound should be opened to release blood trapped in the orbit. If this is insufficient, a lateral canthotomy and cantholysis of the superior and inferior lateral canthal tendons should be performed.

The intervention of an ophthalmologist should be procured at once.

Hyperosmotic agents (mannitol, 1.0–2.0 g/kg intravenously) and carbonic anhydrase inhibitors (acetazolamide, initially 250–500 mg intramuscularly, followed by 250 mg orally every 6 hours) help reduce the intraocular pressure and reestablish flow in the ocular vessels. If the ocular circulation continues to be compromised, an emergency orbital decompression involving partial removal of the bony orbital walls is indicated. In an emergent situation, the thin floor or medial wall can be outfractured at the bedside with a sturdy instrument inserted through the conjunctiva.[10] Excellent reviews on the subject have been published.[11, 12]

HEMATOMA

A more common encountered form of postoperative bleeding is the formation of a hematoma with severe eyelid swelling (Fig. 37–18). As for other forms of bleeding during and after blepharoplasty, preoperative discontinuation of drugs associated with bleeding and intraoperative hemostasis help prevent this occurrence. Ice compresses during the first 48 hours are also helpful.

The patients most at risk for postoperative hematoma are heavy smokers, who are more likely to have coughing spells after surgery. Hematomas that are not associated with visual loss or an increase in the intraocular pressure can be treated conservatively.

If a hematoma is localized to the eyelid, it can often be expressed through the blepharoplasty incision or through a small stab incision with a No. 11 Bard-Parker blade. If signs of visual deterioration or progression of the hematoma are present to such a degree that they may compromise the final results, it is advisable to return the patient to the operating room, remove the sutures, evacuate the clots, and try to identify a source of bleeding that can be cauterized.[13]

Blindness after Blepharoplasty

Almost all cases of blindness after surgery are associated with tense orbital hemorrhage and resultant ischemic damage to the structures of vision. Funduscopic documentation of central retinal artery occlusion has been reported.[14, 15] However, most reports have associated the occurrence of visual loss with damage to the optic nerve, which is thought to be related to ischemia of the fine nutrient vessels at the interface of the nerve to the globe.[16–18]

Management includes documentation of the visual function in both eyes. A computed tomographic scan or orbital ultrasound examination may be considered if it can be obtained without delay, but these tests should never preempt emergent management of the tense orbit. Once the orbit is softened by draining the hematoma or performing cantholysis or bony decompression, medical therapy may be appropriately directed at reducing intraocular pressure with acetazolamide and mannitol and treating inflammation and modulating secondary injury with high-dose steroids.

Prevention of blindness after blepharoplasty is two-pronged: *hemostasis* and *monitoring*. Intraoperative hemostasis should always be careful and complete, with the surgeon bearing in mind that the orbicularis muscle is the most vascular structure encountered in blepharoplasty surgery. However, all surgeons recognize that a case that ends with perfect hemostasis can still lead to postoperative hemorrhage. The hemorrhage is most often in the first 24 hours although delays of days and even rarely weeks can occur. Routine postoperative vision checks allow early detection of any visual problems.[12] The nursing staff should be instructed to teach patients to check their vision after discharge and to report any changes immediately.

The nursing staff in the recovery room should also check for severe postoperative pain. The usual postoperative course of blepharoplasty is relatively painless, and severe pain should alert the surgeon to the possible presence of an orbital hematoma.

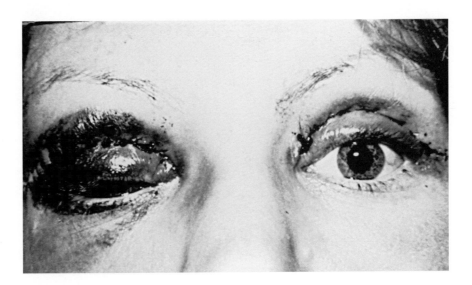

figure 37–18

Postoperative bleeding with formation of hematoma and severe eyelid swelling.

Diplopia: Superior Oblique Palsy

Wesley and associates[4] and others[19] reported cases of damage to the trochlea during upper blepharoplasty that produced permanent double vision (diplopia). In both cases, dissection of the superior nasal fat pad involved marked bleeding, and blind cauterization was applied to the upper nasal quadrant, damaging the trochlea. The trochlea is just under the superior orbital nasal fat pad, and the superior medial palpebral artery courses nasally, inferior to the medial fat pad of the upper eyelid, before dividing into marginal and peripheral eyelid arcades.[8] This vessel should be identified under direct visualization and gently teased away from the adipose tissue by blunt dissection.

Once the vessel is identified and spared, the fat can be excised. If bleeding does occur in this area, pressure is applied directly with a cotton-tipped applicator for 1–2 minutes; posterior pressure is then applied to the globe to produce protrusion of the fat. The bleeding vessel can then be visualized and cauterized under controlled conditions.

References

1. Silkiss RZ, Baylis HI: Autogenous fat grafting by injection. Ophthalmic Plast Reconstr Surg 1987; 3:71–75.
2. Baylis HI, Sutcliffe T, Fett DR: Levator injury during blepharoplasty. Arch Ophthalmol 1984; 102:570–571.
3. Dryden RM, Leibsohn J: The levator aponeurosis in blepharoplasty. Trans Am Acad Ophthalmol Otolaryngol 1978; 85:718–725.
4. Wesley RE, Pollard ZF, McCord CD Jr: Superior oblique paresis after blepharoplasty. Plast Reconstr Surg 1980; 66:283–286.
5. Fasanella RM, Servat J: Levator resection for minimal ptosis: Another simplified operation. Arch Ophthalmol 1961; 65:493–496.
6. Baylis HI, Axelrod RN, Rosen N: Full-thickness eyelid resection for the treatment of undercorrected blepharoptosis and eyelid contour defects. Adv Ophthalmic Plast Reconstr Surg 1982; 1:205–211.
7. Lamberts DW: Dry eyes. In Smolin G, Thoft RA (eds): The Cornea: Scientific Foundations and Clinical Practice, p 387. Boston, Little, Brown & Co, 1987.
8. Sutcliffe T, Baylis H, Fett D: Bleeding in cosmetic blepharoplasty: An anatomical approach. Ophthalmic Plast Reconstr Surg 1985; 1:107–113.
9. Smith B, Nesi FA: The complications of cosmetic blepharoplasty. Ophthalmology 1978; 85:726.
10. Liu D: A simplified technique of orbital decompression for severe retrobulbar hemorrhage [see comments]. Am J Ophthalmol 1993; 116:34–37.
11. DeMere M, Wood T, Austin W: Eye complications with blepharoplasty or other eyelid surgery: A national survey. Plast Reconstr Surg 1974; 53:634–637.
12. Mahaffey PJ, Wallace AF: Blindness following cosmetic blepharoplasty: A review. Br J Plast Surg 1986; 39:213–221.
13. Putterman AM: Temporary blindness after cosmetic blepharoplasty. Am J Ophthalmol 1975; 80:1081–1083.
14. Jafek BW, Kreiger AE, Morledge D: Blindness following blepharoplasty. Arch Otolaryngol 1973; 98:366–369.
15. Kelly PW, May DR: Central retinal artery occlusion following cosmetic blepharoplasty. Br J Ophthalmol 1980; 64:918–922.
16. Goldberg RA, Marmor MF, Shorr N: Blindness following blepharoplasty: Two case reports, and a discussion of management. Ophthalmic Surg 1990; 21:85–89.
17. Hepler RS, Sugimura GI, Straatsma BR: On the occurrence of blindness in association with blepharoplasty. Plast Reconstr Surg 1976; 57:233–235.
18. Goldberg RA, Markowitz B: Blindness after blepharoplasty (letter to the editor). Plast Reconstr Surg 1992; 90:929–930.
19. Levine MR, Boynton J, Tenzel RR, et al: Complications of blepharoplasty. Ophthalmic Surg 1975; 6:53–57.

Henry I. Baylis
Robert A. Goldberg
Michael J. Groth

Chapter **38**

Complications of Lower Blepharoplasty

Retraction (downward displacement) and ectropion (eversion) of the lower eyelid are the most common problems after lower blepharoplasty. They lead not only to an unsightly appearance but also to an uncomfortable eye.

In this chapter, Henry Baylis, Robert Goldberg, and Michael Groth thoroughly evaluate the possible complications of lower eyelid cosmetic surgery. They teach us how to avoid these problems, if possible, and how to handle them should they occur. The treatment of lower eyelid retraction is stressed because of the importance of this problem and the need for resolution. In fact, the steps for treating this complication are illustrated in more detail than any other technique in this textbook.

In the previous editions of *Cosmetic Oculoplastic Surgery*, ear cartilage graft was described as the method of relieving severe lower eyelid retraction; in this revised chapter, the hard-palate graft is emphasized as the graft of choice. Also, the advantage of early surgery to treat postoperative retraction is noted, and this differs from the treatment of most other complications, in which observation is necessary during the initial postoperative period.

Other complications described in this chapter are worsening of lower eyelid wrinkles, visual loss secondary to an orbital hemorrhage, inferior oblique injury, and underexcision and overexcision of orbital fat and skin. The tear trough deformity is another complication that can occur after aggressive orbital fat removal.

ALLEN M. PUTTERMAN

Complications of lower blepharoplasty are extremely distressing for both the patient and the surgeon. The objective of a lower blepharoplasty is usually an aesthetic improvement. Thus, the occurrence of postoperative *scleral show* due to lower eyelid retraction and rounding of the canthus is clearly undesirable. It is also distressing for the surgeon to confront a previously asymptomatic patient who now has *lagophthalmos* (inability to close the eyelids), and exposure keratopathy. Thus, prevention of complications should be the highest priority a lower blepharoplasty is performed.

Lower blepharoplasty has significantly changed over the past few years because of a better understanding of the complications and limitations of surgery. This procedure is most effective at reducing fullness of the lower eyelid, a condition that frequently is due to prolapse of orbital fat. This condition can manifest at a young age as a family characteristic that becomes more noticeable with age. During lower blepharoplasty, prolapsing fat can be excised by either a *transcutaneous* or *transconjunctival* approach (see Chapters 18–20).

Lower blepharoplasty is not very effective at correct-

429

ing skin folds or wrinkles. Skin folds are often secondary to redundant skin and underlying orbicularis oculi muscle. These folds can sometimes be reduced with modest results via a transcutaneous blepharoplasty or an alternative method, the *skin pinch technique* (described later). Skin wrinkles, however, are usually secondary to changes in the dermal collagen matrix from prolonged sun exposure (see Chapter 6). Attempts at placing the lower eyelid skin on tension by excising a large amount of skin often results in the persistence of the wrinkles in the remaining skin and risks lower eyelid retraction or ectropion. Skin wrinkles may be more amenable to resurfacing techniques, such as chemical peel or carbon dioxide laser resurfacing rather than surgery (see Chapters 30 and 31).

LOWER EYELID RETRACTION VERSUS CICATRICIAL ECTROPION

The technique of lower blepharoplasty performed via the *transcutaneous* route is associated with a significant incidence of lower eyelid retraction, probably because it necessitates an incision on the orbital septum to reach the orbital fat. The *transconjunctival* route, in contrast, avoids the septum and minimizes the risks of lower eyelid retraction. Therefore, avoiding the transcutaneous route is the best way to prevent the most common complication of lower blepharoplasty—lower eyelid retraction.

Certain patient characteristics increase the chance of complications and should be carefully noted. Lower eyelid retraction occurs more frequently in patients with shallow orbits and relatively prominent eyes. The larger area of the exposed inferior globe needs to be covered by the lower eyelid. The blepharoplasty surgeon must anticipate this by decreasing the amount of skin resected. Patients with *horizontal lower lid laxity* may be candidates for lateral canthal tightening in conjunction with

blepharoplasty (see Chapter 21). Horizontal laxity leads to lower eyelid instability and subsequent ectropion after a minimal amount of skin resection. The *distraction test*, whereby the lower eyelid is held away from the globe and then released, can identify excessive horizontal laxity (the eyelid does not immediately return to its normal position in apposition to the globe) (see Chapter 2).

EYELID MALPOSITION

The most common anatomic complications of lower blepharoplasty are lower eyelid retraction and cicatricial ectropion. Failure to distinguish ectropion from lower eyelid retraction reflects grave oversimplification because the predisposing anatomic factors, diagnostic tests, and methods of surgical correction for these two complications are different.

The surgeon must know the surgical anatomy of the lower eyelid in order to understand the pathophysiology of eyelid malposition after blepharoplasty. The normal eyelid is formed by an anterior lamella (layer) of skin and orbicularis muscle, a posterior lamella of tarsus, lower lid retractors and conjunctiva, and a middle lamella of orbital septum (see Chapter 7).

Lower eyelid retraction results from an incision in the middle lamella (orbital septum) that is followed by scar formation and contraction of the septum and adjacent tissues (Fig. 38–1). It may be accompanied by ectropion when excessive skin has been removed, but vertical shortage of skin is not necessary for lower eyelid retraction to occur.

Cicatricial ectropion (Fig. 38–2) results from an outward rotational force secondary to excessive removal of skin. The exposure of the conjunctiva induces a metaplastic change of the epithelium to a keratinized squamous epithelium, causing persistent irritation.

A mixed mechanism of scarring of the midlamella and

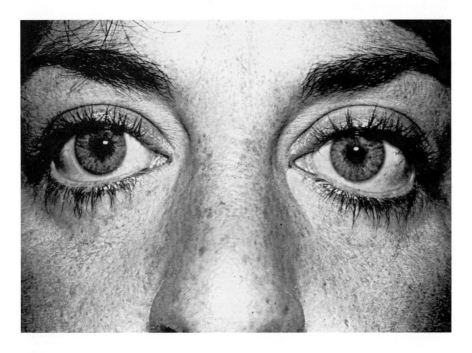

figure 38–1

Postblepharoplasty lower eyelid retraction.

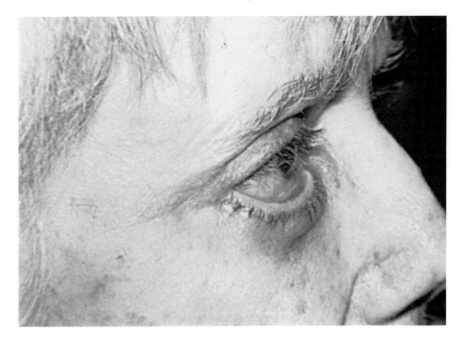

figure 38–2

Postblepharoplasty lower eyelid ectropion.

vertical shortening of the skin may be encountered in severe or long-standing cases (Fig. 38–3).

A careful preoperative evaluation can help in determining the relative contributions of midlamellar scarring versus skin insufficiency. The lower lid *traction test* serves to identify scarring of the midlamella. The surgeon applies upward traction to the eyelid and looks for tethering of the midlamella before the skin is pulled taut (Fig. 38–4). Tethering of the eyelid without evidence of skin shortage identifies scarring as the limiting factor in the eyelid position. The distinction is clinically pertinent because the treatment is different. Whereas tethering associated with skin shortage may indicate the need for a skin graft, eyelid retraction is treated with resuspension of the orbicularis muscle (see later).

LOWER EYELID RETRACTION

The patient with lower lid retraction typically presents with scleral show and rounding of the canthus that occurred after lower blepharoplasty (see Fig. 38–1). Whereas sophisticated patients clearly identify this specific eyelid deformity, many patients only express a dislike of the "surgical look" without being able to identify just what it is they do not like. Unless the retraction is severe and clearly disfiguring, they tend to seek repair several months or years after blepharoplasty. In contrast, patients with lower eyelid ectropion usually present with an uncomfortable eye as a result of constant irritation of the exposed conjunctiva, and they tend to seek medical

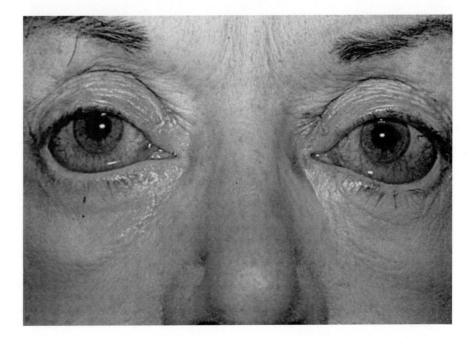

figure 38–3

Postblepharoplasty lower eyelid retraction and cicatricial ectropion.

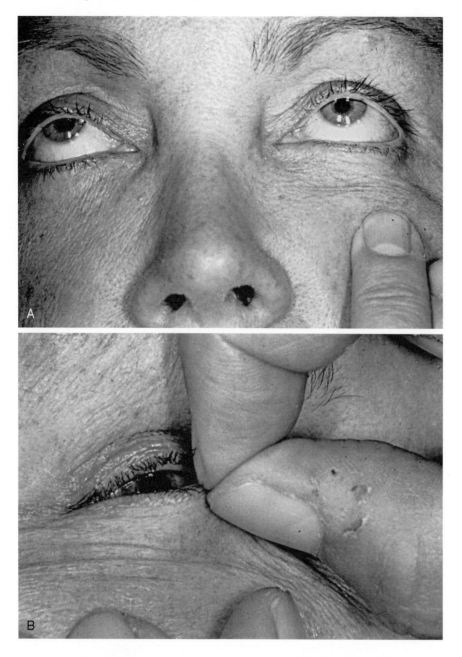

figure 38–4

Eyelid traction test. The examiner applies upward traction to the lower eyelid *(A)* while looking for tethering of the midlamella before the skin is pulled taut *(B)*.

attention shortly after blepharoplasty (see Figs. 38–2 and 38–3).

Lower eyelid retraction with scleral show, with or without ectropion, is by far the most common complication of lower blepharoplasty with the transcutaneous approach. Patients who undergo repeated transcutaneous blepharoplasties may be particularly prone to this complication; the complication has not been reported after transconjunctival blepharoplasty.[1, 2]

Lower eyelid retraction is due to the formation of scar tissue at the level of the septum (Fig. 38–5). Scar tissue formation at this level appears to be related to the violation of the septum and its delicate relationship to the orbicularis muscle and skin. Thus, minimizing injury to the septum appears to decrease the occurrence of lower eyelid retraction significantly.[3]

Management

The earlier lower eyelid retraction is recognized and treatment initiated, the better the prognosis for successful correction. When lower eyelid retraction is noted immediately after surgery, some cases may resolve after application of firm upward traction on the lower eyelid with traction sutures for 7–10 days (Fig. 38–6). (For placement of these sutures, see Suspension of the Lower Eyelid from the Brow.) Postoperative lower eyelid retraction of longer duration requires surgical correction that can be very involved.

Preoperative Evaluation

The preoperative evaluation includes an assessment of the anatomic and pathologic features that will determine

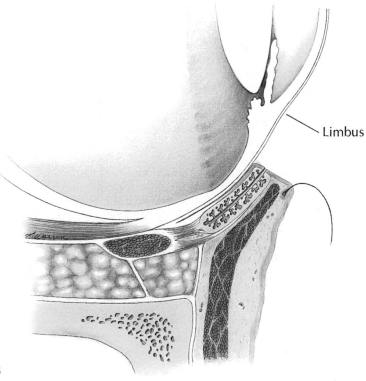

figure 38–5

Lower eyelid retraction. *A,* Normal inferior orbital septum. *B,* Shortened inferior orbital septum with lower eyelid retraction.

A

Limbus

B

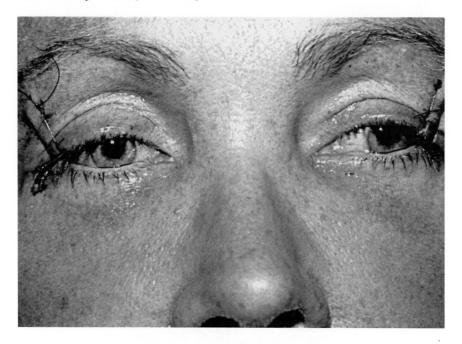

figure 38–6
Patient with lower eyelid retraction soon after blepharoplasty. In some cases, lower eyelid retraction detected within the first few postoperative days may resolve with firm upward traction in the lower eyelid.

the surgical approach and the prognosis for cosmetic and functional results. The lower eyelid traction test is performed to assess the relative contributions of vertical skin shortening or scarring in the plane of the septum (see Fig. 38–4). The time elapsed since blepharoplasty is taken into consideration because retraction that is managed early is more likely to respond to simple lysis of scar tissue and retractors and to a temporary traction suture to the brow.

Patients with prominent eyes present additional challenges in the correction of eyelid retraction. The relationship of the globe to the medial and lateral canthi is such that simple tightening of the inferior limb of the lateral canthal tendon may result in a lowering of the already retracted eyelid margin.

Surgical Technique for Early or Mild Cases*

Patients who present with lower eyelid retraction within 6 months of blepharoplasty are treated with division of scar tissue and lower eyelid retractors, followed by canthopexy. The orbicularis muscle of the lower eyelid is then suspended from the periosteum of the lateral orbital rim.

Adequate local anesthesia is obtained with 2 per cent lidocaine with epinephrine and hyaluronidase. Fifteen minutes are allowed for the vasoconstrictive effects of epinephrine to take place. This is particularly important when extensive lysis of scar tissue, with its attendant copious bleeding, is anticipated.

---

*Editor's Note: The description and illustrations used in the technique for lateral canthopexy are a combination of those of the authors and of Dr. Putterman (see Chapter 21). The authors usually use 5-0 polyglycolic acid (Dexon) or 6-0 polypropylene (Prolene) sutures for the tarsal strip, 6-0 polypropylene for the orbicularis muscle suspension, and 6-0 mild chromic for skin closure rather than the five sutures described in this section.

Lysis of Scar Tissue at the Level of the Septum

The surgeon repeats the lower eyelid traction test immediately before the beginning of the procedure to assess more accurately the degree of scarring at the level of the septum and how it limits the upward traction of the lower eyelid (see Fig. 38–4). A lateral canthotomy is performed to expose the lateral orbital rim and lateral canthal tendon (Fig. 38–7*A* and *B*). The lower limb of the lateral canthal tendon is cut with scissors at the orbital rim (Fig. 38–7*C*). A forceps is used to exert upward traction on the lower eyelid while the scissors is introduced within the midlamellar space, maintaining the integrity of the skin anteriorly and the conjunctiva posteriorly. The scissors is then used to palpate and divide the retracting scar tissue (Fig. 38–7*D*).

The surgeon maintains upward traction with the forceps throughout this step in order to continuously assess the degree of release of retraction obtained as the scar is divided (see Fig. 38–7*D*). When the lower eyelid can be freely drawn upward, the retraction is adequately relieved (Fig. 38–7*E*).

Lateral Canthopexy

The lower eyelid is drawn up into the desired position, and the location of the new lateral canthal angle is identified along the lower eyelid. A scratch is made with a No. 11 Bard-Parker blade at the aspect of the lower eyelid margin that is now adjacent to the temporal cut edge of the upper eyelid margin (Fig. 38–7*F*). A measurement is made with a ruler from the temporal cut end of the lower eyelid to the scratch incision, which determines the length of the tarsal strip.

The surgeon then divides the eyelid into two lamellae by cutting with scissors along the gray line from the temporal end of the eyelid to the scratch incision site (see Fig. 38–7*F*). A thin strip of the posterior eyelid

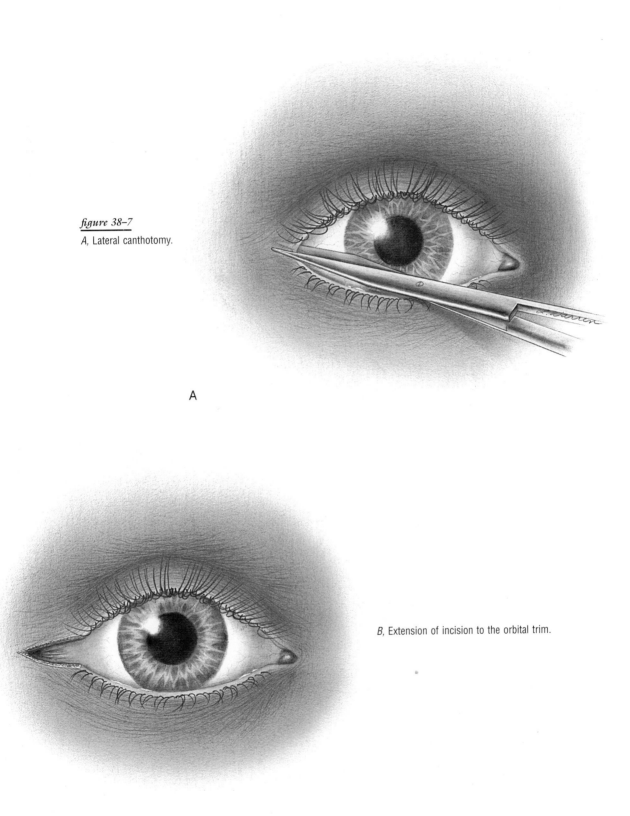

figure 38–7
A, Lateral canthotomy.

A

B, Extension of incision to the orbital trim.

B

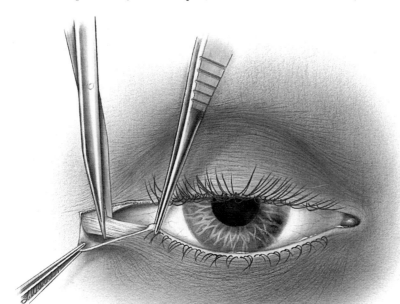

C, Lower limb of the lateral canthal tendon cut at the orbital rim.

C

D, Vertically shortened orbital septum within the lower eyelid is strummed and lysed close to the inferior orbital rim.

D

E, The lower eyelid, no longer tethered to the inferior orbital rim, is completely mobilized.

E

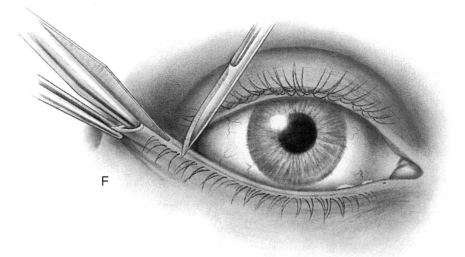

F, The eyelid is split at the gray line into anterior and posterior lamellae.

F

margin is excised with scissors (Fig. 38–7*G*). The conjunctiva is then cut from the inferior tarsal edge. Bleeding is controlled with monopolar or disposable cautery. Next, the surgeon scrapes off the conjunctival epithelium on the posterior surface of the tarsus with a No. 15 Bard-Parker blade to prevent epithelial inclusion cysts (Fig. 38–7*H*).

Each arm of a 4-0 polypropylene (Prolene) double-armed suture is then passed internally to externally through the tarsal strip at the junction of the strip and eyelid (Fig. 38–7*I*). The strip is then pulled temporally until the area of the polypropylene sutures is adjacent to the lateral orbital wall. The strip is drawn superiorly and internally until it seems to be at an acceptable position. The temporal lower eyelid should also be in contact with the eye and not displaced anterior to the eye. If the patient's eye is proptotic, as in thyroid disease, the

tarsal strip should be placed much more anteriorly than for a recessed or enophthalmic eye. Once the desired lateral position is determined, each arm of the 4-0 polypropylene suture is passed through the lateral orbital periosteum or the upper limb of the lateral canthal tendon at its position internally to externally (Fig. 38–7*J*).

The suture is then tied with the first tie of the surgeon's knot over a 4-0 black silk knot-releasing suture. The patient is then helped to sit up on the operating table, and the position of the lateral canthus is judged. If the lateral canthus is too high or low or too anterior or posterior, the knot-releasing suture is grasped with a forceps at each end of the suture and is pulled outward to release the knot. The suture arms are removed from the lateral wall periosteum or upper lateral canthal tendon and placed in a new position; this procedure is

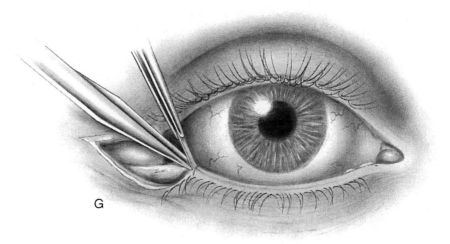

G, A thin strip of the posterior eyelid margin is cut with scissors.

G

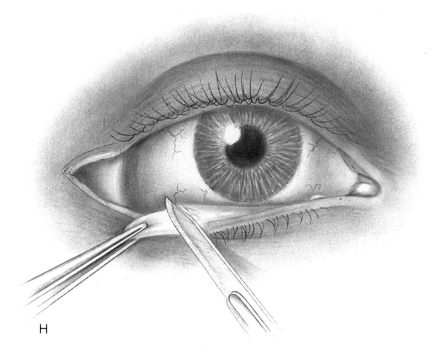

H, The conjunctiva is scraped off the tarsal strip to avoid burying epithelium.

repeated until the desired position of the lateral canthus and lower eyelid is achieved. The suture knot is again released.

Suspension of the Orbicularis Muscle of the Lower Lid from the Periosteum of the Orbital Rim

The lateral third of the lower eyelid orbicularis muscle is dissected from the overlying skin (Fig. 38–7*K*) and pulled superolaterally. The surgeon exposes the periosteum over the frontal process of the zygomatic bone and determines the site where the lower lid orbicularis muscle will be inserted by drawing the lateral aspect of the muscle upward into the desired position and by excising a triangle of muscle from the overlapping lateral segment (Fig. 38–7*L*). A 6-0 polypropylene suture is then used in a whip stitch fashion to attach the undersurface of the orbicularis flap to the periosteum at the previously selected site; the tension in the suture is adjusted as necessary to achieve the desired amount of traction on the orbicularis muscle (Fig. 38–7*M*).

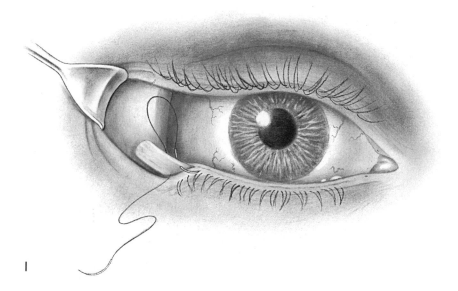

I, Each arm of a 4-0 polypropylene (Prolene) double-armed suture is passed through the tarsal strip at the location of the new lateral canthal angle.

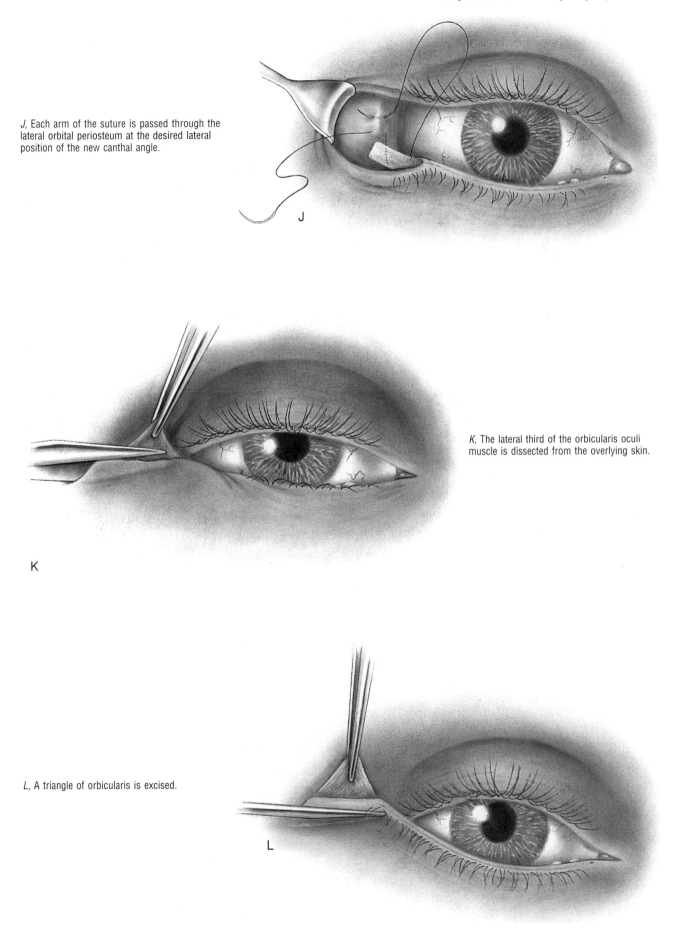

J, Each arm of the suture is passed through the lateral orbital periosteum at the desired lateral position of the new canthal angle.

K, The lateral third of the orbicularis oculi muscle is dissected from the overlying skin.

L, A triangle of orbicularis is excised.

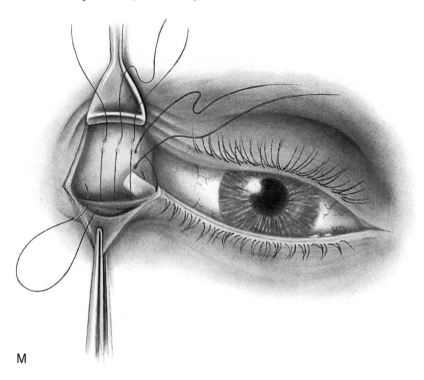

M, A 6-0 polypropylene suture is used in a whip stitch fashion to attach the undersurface of the orbicularis muscle to the lateral orbital periosteum. Tension in the suture is adjusted to achieve the desired muscle traction.

Securing the Tarsal Strip

The tarsal strip is secured to the lateral orbital wall by tying the 4-0 polypropylene sutures. A 4-0 polyglactin (Vicryl) suture is passed through the periosteum adjacent and temporal to the polypropylene knot (Fig. 38–7N). It is passed through the tarsal strip internally to externally and then externally to internally (Fig. 38–7O). When drawn up and tied, this suture further secures the tarsal strip to the periosteum and buries the polypropylene suture. The tarsal strip temporal to the polyglactin suture is then severed (Fig. 38–7P). The orbicularis suspension suture is then tied.

Securing the Lateral Canthus

A 6-0 black silk suture is placed through the temporal corner of the upper eyelid, and another sure is passed through the temporal corner of the lower eyelid (Fig. 38–7Q). The 6-0 black silk sutures are drawn up and tied, forming the lateral canthal angle. The suture ends are left long and are eventually tied over the 6-0 silk sutures in the lateral canthal skin so that the knot can be easily found and the ends do not drag over the eye. (An alternative is to reform the lateral canthal angle with a 5-0 chromic catgut suture entering the temporal upper and lower eyelid gray line and exiting the severed tem-

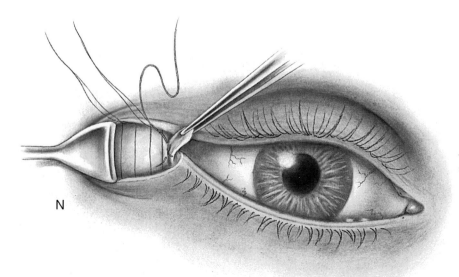

N, A 4-0 polyglactin (Vicryl) suture is passed through periosteum and then through the tarsal strip.

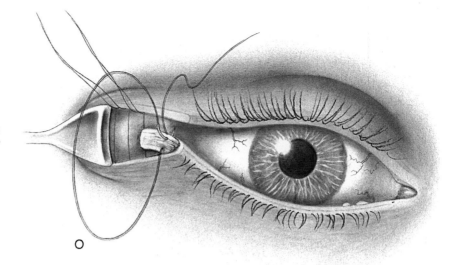

O, The suture is passed through the tarsal strip internally to externally and then externally to internally.

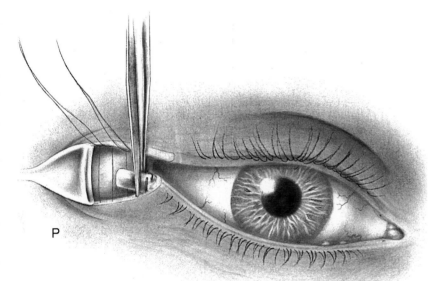

P, The tarsal strip temporal to the polyglactin suture is severed.

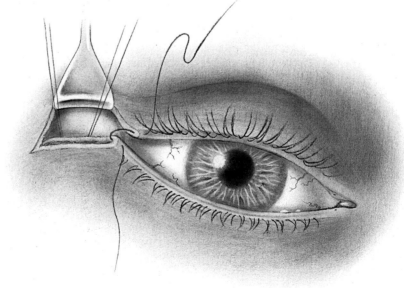

Q, A 6-0 black silk suture is placed through the temporal corners of the upper and lower eyelids, and the 6-0 polypropylene sutures connecting the orbicularis muscle to periosteum are tied.

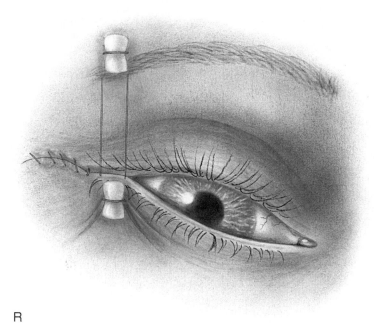

R, The lower eyelid is suspended from the brow for at least 7 days.

R

poral edges of upper and lower eyelid. This buries the suture and avoids the difficult, sometimes painful postoperative removal of the angle suture.)

The surgeon ties the 6-0 polypropylene sutures connecting the orbicularis muscle to the periosteum to provide uniform support to the lower eyelid across the lateral canthal incision while minimizing distortion of the lateral canthus (see Fig. 38–7*Q*). (An alternative to the tarsal strip is to remove a full-thickness section of the temporal lower eyelid, as described in Chapter 24.)

Suspension of the Lower Eyelid from the Brow

A 4-0 double-armed polypropylene suture is used to suspend the lateral lower eyelid from the lateral brow for at least 7 days. The needle enters through the skin and the orbicularis muscle and exits through the gray line of the lower eyelid margin; the suture is then passed through the skin and the orbicularis muscle near the brow and tied (Fig. 38–7*R*).

Postoperative Care

Antibiotic steroid ointment is applied to the cul-de-sac and the skin incision three times daily. Ice compresses are applied for 48 hours, followed by warm compresses for 5 days. The 4-0 polypropylene traction sutures are removed after 7–14 days (Fig. 38–8).

Technique for Severe or Long-Standing Cases

Most cases of lower eyelid retraction can be repaired by the technique just described. In those uncommon cases

in which the posterior lamella is so short that a posterior lamellar spacer is necessary, an ear cartilage graft or a hard-palate graft may be used to augment the posterior lamella. A spacer is more likely to be required if:

1. Blepharoplasty was performed 6 or more months before retraction repair.
2. The patient has prominent eyes.
3. The patient has severe retraction.
4. Retraction does not improve with lateral canthal surgery alone.

An ear cartilage graft is easy to obtain, intraoperative bleeding is minimal, and the postoperative discomfort is moderate. A hard-palate graft may be associated with significant intraoperative and postoperative bleeding, and it is usually uncomfortable for several days postoperatively.

The disadvantages of the ear cartilage graft are that it lacks a mucosal surface, it may buckle or warp, and cartilage may continue to grow, resulting in a "lumpy" surface. In contrast, the hard-palate graft has a mucosal surface, remains smooth, and is flexible.

The advantages and disadvantages of each technique must be considered in relation to the specific characteristics of each patient. Hard-palate mucosal grafts are cosmetically superior and generally preferable.

Obtaining Ear Cartilage

So that ear cartilage is obtained for grafting, a local anesthetic agent is infiltrated in the subcutaneous tissues of the helix. A skin incision is made on the posterior surface of the helix (Fig. 38–9*A* and *B*). After the skin is undermined and freed from its attachment to the underlying cartilage, an incision is made through the

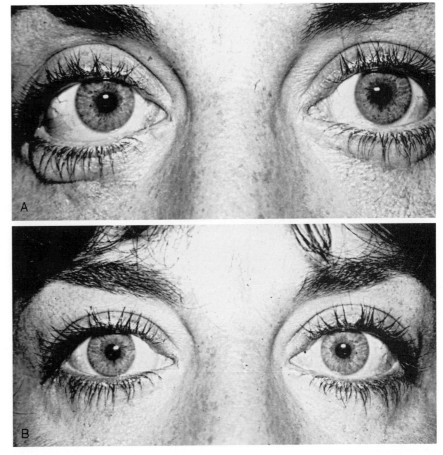

figure 38–8

Patient with postblepharoplasty lower eyelid retraction before *(A)* and after *(B)* correction by scar lysis and resuspension of the lateral orbicularis.

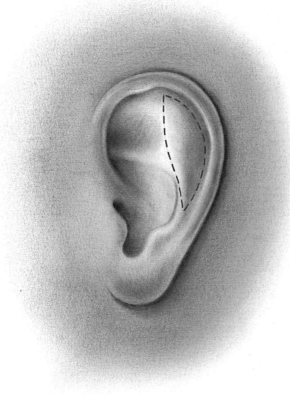

A

figure 38–9

A, Outline of an ear cartilage graft, anterior view.

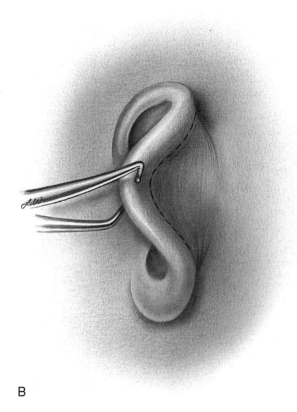

B, Skin incision on the posterior aspect of the ear.

B

cartilage, leaving at least 2 mm of lateral cartilage to support the helix (Fig. 38–9C). Next, the cartilage is elevated and dissected from the skin of the anterior surface of the ear (Fig. 38–9D).

Once the desired amount of cartilage is mobilized, it can be removed from the donor bed with scissors or knife (Fig. 38–9E). The skin incision is then closed with 6-0 polypropylene suture, and a dressing is applied over the external ear.

Obtaining Hard Palate

Before hard palate is obtained for grafting, 1–2 ml of 2 per cent lidocaine with epinephrine and hyaluronidase is injected at the greater palatine foramen of the operative side. The foramen can be palpated medial to the second molar tooth, at the junction of the vertical and horizontal plates of the palate. Alternatively, bilateral infiltration can be used and may provide better anesthesia because some crossing over of innervation may occur. The four corners of the donor site are marked with cautery. The site is chosen as peripheral and as anterior as possible, avoiding the 2–3 mm closest to the teeth laterally, the rugae anteriorly, and the greater palatine vessels and nerves posteriorly.

Obtaining the graft as far from the midline as possible decreases the amount of bleeding. The graft is first outlined with a superficial incision with a No. 15 Bard-Parker or similar blade. The graft is then dissected with the same blade to a thickness of approximately 1 mm (Fig. 38–10). Deeper dissection is associated with more bleeding.

Once the graft is separated, the donor site is covered with an absorbable gelatin sponge (Gelfoam) or packed with oxidized regenerated cellulose (Surgicel), and the patient is asked to push his or her tongue against a soaked gauze pad placed against the palate. If bleeding continues after a few minutes, hemostasis can be obtained with a monopolar cautery.

Creation of Recipient Bed

A lateral canthotomy and cantholysis and a tarsal strip procedure are performed as described for mild cases. The recipient bed is then fashioned in the lower eyelid by a transverse incision of conjunctiva and eyelid retractors (Fig. 38–11A). A horizontal incision on the conjunctiva and lower eyelid retractors all along the lower border of the tarsus releases the vertical tethering of the eyelid, since the lower eyelid retractors join the orbital septum at the lower tarsal margin. As the eyelid is mobilized, superiorly, the orbicularis muscle is visualized. This flat, well-vascularized tissue plane is ideal for supporting a graft made from either ear cartilage or hard palate.

Preoperative determination of the amount of vertical shortening of the eyelid dictates the width of the graft. Typically, the maximum vertical height is needed along the lateral eyelid. The graft is the same size as the defect in the posterior lamella.

Graft Placement

The graft is placed on the recipient site and is trimmed to fit the shape of the defect between the lower eyelid

C, Dissection of ear cartilage from the posterior ear surface.

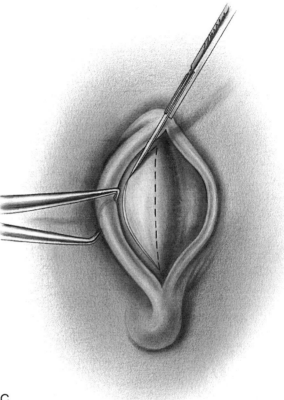

C

D, Dissection of the cartilage from the anterior skin of the ear, leaving the skin intact.

D

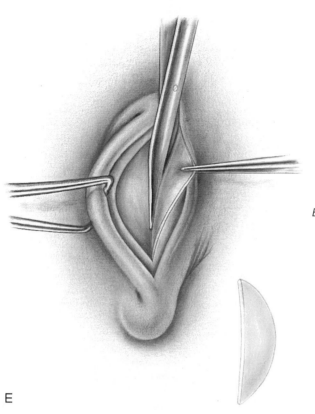

E, Removal of the cartilage from the donor site.

E

retractors inferiorly and the tarsus superiorly. The graft is sutured to the retractors below and the tarsus above with interrupted sutures of 6-0 mild chromic gut (Fig. 38–11*B*). The lateral canthal tightening operation then proceeds as described for mild cases.

With the use of a spacer, it is advisable to plan for the operation to be done in two stages. In the first stage, the graft is placed and the eyelid is suspended at a moderate height. In the second stage, 2 or 3 months after the graft has adequately taken, the eyelid is sus-

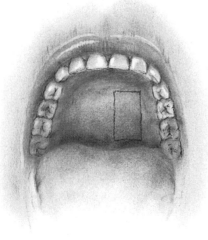

figure 38–10

Obtaining a hard-palate mucosal graft: The graft is determined on a millimeter-per-millimeter basis. A strip of hard palate is obtained to match the bed graft.

pended again. The presence of a fibrotic scar provides a firm tissue that can be pulled under more tension during the second stage of the operation (Fig. 38–12). A slight modification of the hard-palate graft is demonstrated in Chapter 25.

Patients who have prominent eyes frequently require the use of spacers for the correction of lower eyelid retraction. Simple horizontal shortening and resuspension of the lower eyelid result in a further lowering of the retracted eyelid. Patients with marked proptosis of the eyeball (e.g., Hertel measurements > 22 mm) are less likely to achieve satisfactory results from soft-tissue repositioning alone. In these cases, non-Graves' orbital decompression or orbital rim onlay advancement should be considered.

LOWER LID ECTROPION

Lower lid ectropion is a less commonly encountered complication than lower eyelid retraction, but it is often more symptomatic. Lower eyelid ectropion results from excessive excision of skin and orbicularis muscle during transcutaneous lower blepharoplasty with skin removal.[4, 5] The ectropion is caused by outward rotation secondary to excessive vertical shortening of the anterior lamella (Fig. 38–13). Replacement of the missing skin is accomplished through skin grafting. In some cases, however, cicatricial ectropion after blepharoplasty coexists with lower eyelid retraction and the contracting tissue must be divided at the midlamellar level as described previously, followed by skin grafting.

figure 38–11

A, Creation of a recipient bed along the inferior tarsal border.

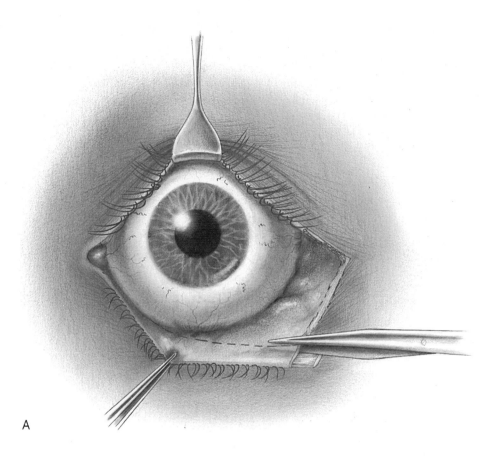

A

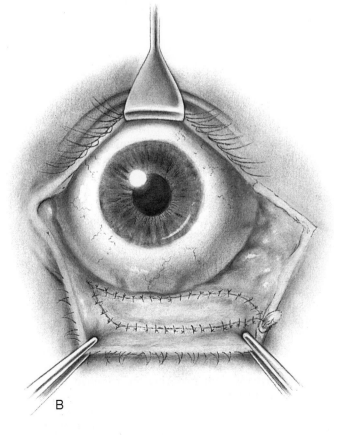

B

B, The graft is sutured to the retractors below the tarsus above with interrupted 6-0 polyglycolic acid (Dexon) suture.

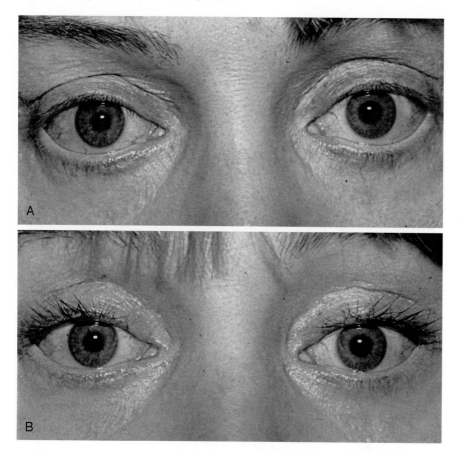

figure 38–12

Patient with postblepharoplasty lower eyelid retraction before *(A)* and after *(B)* a two-stage ear cartilage graft procedure.

Skin Grafting

Before the graft is obtained, the surgeon determines its size by preparing the recipient bed.

Preparing the Bed for the Graft

Local anesthesia is obtained by subcutaneous infiltration of 2 per cent lidocaine with epinephrine and hyaluronidase. Three traction sutures of 4-0 polypropylene are used to keep the lower eyelid on stretch during and after skin grafting. The sutures are passed horizontally through the lower eyelid margin at the gray line and through the skin above the eyebrow and then tied with temporary knots.

A skin incision is made 1–2 mm below and along the entire length of the eyelash line (Fig. 38–14*A*). The skin is undermined from the orbicularis muscle to the inferior orbital rim (Fig. 38–14*B*). This allows the vertically shortened skin to recede inferiorly, thereby relaxing the force that is causing the ectropion. The traction sutures to the brow can then be tied permanently, exerting upward traction on the lower eyelid and exposing the area to be covered by the skin graft.

During the dissection of the skin flap toward the orbital rim, an above-average amount of bleeding may be encountered because of previous surgical changes in the area. The surgeon must obtain meticulous hemostasis in order to prevent subsequent hematoma formation under the free skin graft, which would preclude vascu-

larization of the graft. The skin defect remaining superiorly with a flat bed of well-vascularized orbicularis muscle provides an ideal recipient site for grafting (Fig. 24–14*C*).

Horizontal Lid Shortening

In most cases, horizontal eyelid laxity is associated with cicatricial ectropion. A horizontal shortening is then indicated and can be accomplished by the lateral tarsal strip technique (see earlier and Chapter 21) or by a full-thickness temporal eyelid resection (see Chapter 24).

Obtaining the Skin Graft

Once the lower eyelid is in a proper position in relationship to the globe, the size of the skin graft can be determined. It should be measured with calipers or a ruler in the vertical and horizontal dimensions. Additional skin should be harvested to allow easy surgical closure. Full-thickness skin is used instead of split-thickness skin because of less secondary contraction after revascularization. Unfortunately, full-thickness skin does have greater primary contracture immediately after it is removed from the donor site. Therefore, the surgeon should harvest at least 30–40 per cent more skin than needed. Excess graft may then be trimmed when it is sutured to its bed.

The upper eyelid, if it has redundant skin, is the ideal donor site. To harvest the graft, the surgeon applies the

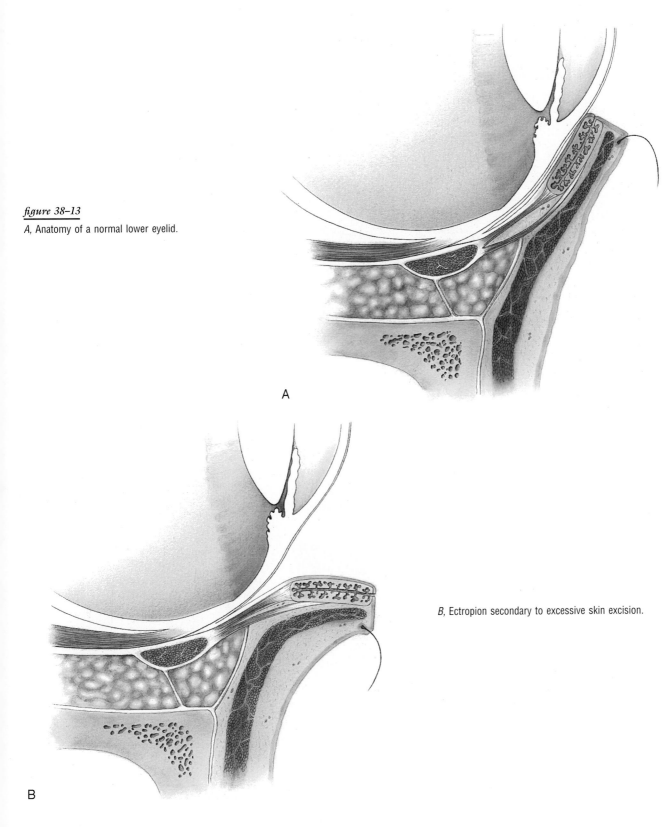

figure 38–13

A, Anatomy of a normal lower eyelid.

A

B, Ectropion secondary to excessive skin excision.

B

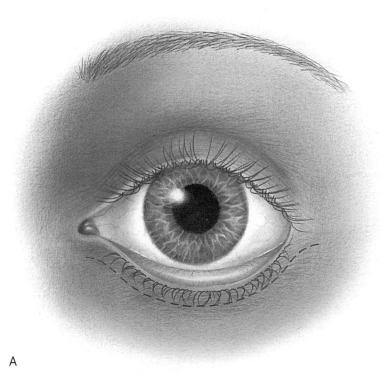

A

figure 38–14
Lower eyelid skin graft. *A*, Proposed skin incision.

B, Relaxing the skin incision with a skin flap.

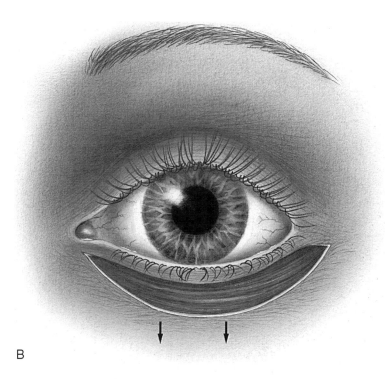

B

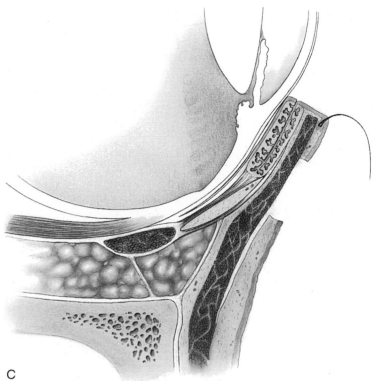

C, Sagittal section of the recipient bed of the orbicularis muscle.

C

D, Skin incision for harvesting a skin graft from the retroauricular areas.

D

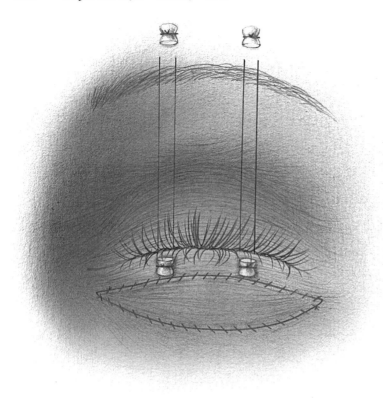

E, Suturing of the skin graft into the recipient bed in the lower eyelid.

same technique as used for a skin-only blepharoplasty (see Chapter 9). The surgeon then thins the skin graft by removing any adherent orbicularis muscle in order to facilitate revascularization. Unfortunately, patients frequently have had previous upper blepharoplasty, which eliminates the upper eyelid as a donor site for skin grafting.

Complications

All patients have some cosmetic blemish because of the skin grafts (Fig. 38–15). The second most common complication is inadequate vascularization of the skin graft with subsequent necrosis. In such cases, the recipient bed heals by secondary intention with scarring and recurrence of cicatricial ectropion. The area may be grafted again after healing is complete, in approximately 2 months.

WORSENING OF LOWER LID WRINKLES AFTER TRANSCONJUNCTIVAL FAT EXCISION

After transconjunctival lower blepharoplasty, the skin retracts spontaneously to a certain degree. In most patients, the main cosmetic improvement achieved by blepharoplasty is the reduction of lower eyelid bulges by fat excision. Usually, the skin wrinkles are no more prominent after lower blepharoplasty and patients understand the concept that skin quality cannot be changed with surgery. Chemical peeling or carbon dioxide laser resurfacing may be better able to achieve the

desired improvement (see Chapters 30 and 31). However, some patients request surgical reduction of lower eyelid wrinkles. In individuals in whom a skin fold is easily identifiable, an excision of the fold by the "pinch" technique can be performed safely and sometimes results in cosmetic improvement without noticeable scars.

The *skin pinch technique* requires, first, the identification of a distinct skin fold within the area of thin skin in the lower eyelid. Local anesthesia is obtained with infiltration of 2 per cent lidocaine with epinephrine and hyaluronidase (Wydase). A Brown-Adson forceps is used to crush the skin fold along its horizontal length (Fig. 38–16A). The use of hyaluronidase allows the skin to tent up where it has been crushed with the forceps. The surgeon uses scissors to excise the tented-up skin (Fig. 38–16B). The incision is closed with 6-0 polypropylene on a running, everting suture (Fig. 38–16C).

ORBITAL COMPLICATIONS OF LOWER BLEPHAROPLASTY

Orbital complications of lower blepharoplasty relate to specific orbital structures adjacent to the lower eyelid and to orbital tissues in general. Many orbital complications of lower blepharoplasty are the same as those of upper blepharoplasty (Chapter 37).

The etiology of *visual loss* after blepharoplasty is not fully understood. There appears to be an association between postoperative orbital hemorrhage and loss of vision following blepharoplasty.[6–8] The mechanism of the visual loss may be optic nerve damage, from (1) compression of the optic nerve by the hemorrhage or (2) occlusion of its vascular supply.[9]

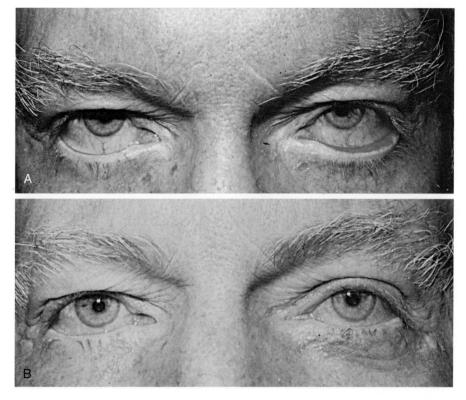

figure 38–15

A, Preoperative photograph showing cicatricial left lower eyelid ectropion secondary to blepharoplasty. *B*, Postoperative results of skin graft to lower eyelid.

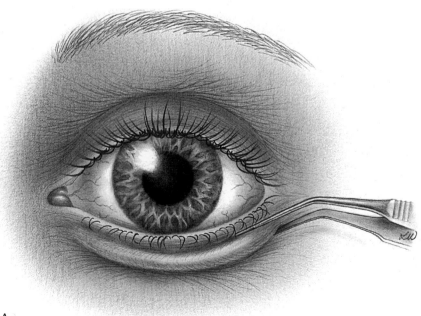

A

figure 38–16

Pinch technique. *A*, A skin fold is identified and crushed with forceps.

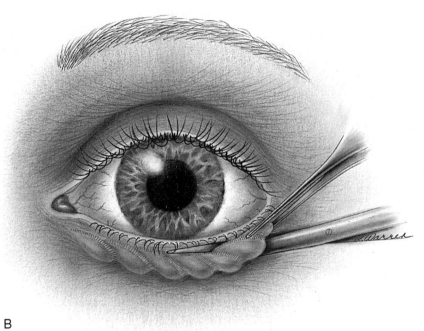

B, The tented-up fold of skin is excised.

C, The wound is closed with an everting suture.

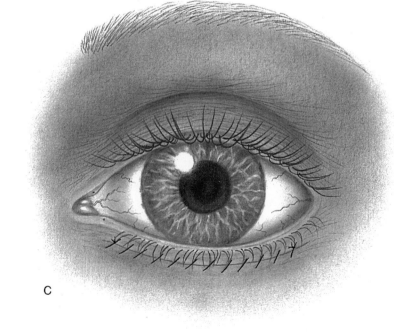

C

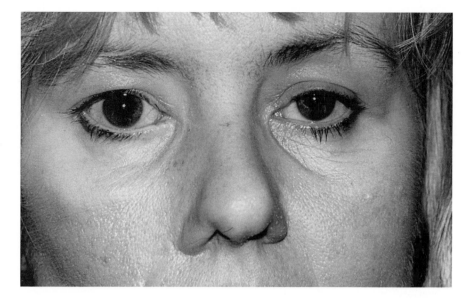

figure 38–17

Prominent tear trough deformity (palpebrojugal fold and inferior orbital rim) in patient with aggressive fat removal (transconjunctival blepharoplasty and canthoplasty).

Management is initiated by opening the wound for drainage and performing a canthotomy and cantholysis for release of tension. Ocular hypotensives are used as an adjunct. If this is not enough, exploration and evacuation of the hematoma and orbital decompression may be necessary and are best done without delay.

Prevention of postoperative hemorrhage is achieved by meticulous hemostasis before closure of the wound. Most of the bleeding during blepharoplasty comes from the orbicularis muscle. The bleeding points can be easily visualized and directly cauterized. In the case of bleeding from the orbital fat, gentle retropulsion of the globe causes the fat to prolapse, allowing for direct visualization and cauterization of the bleeding vessels.

INFERIOR OBLIQUE MUSCLE INJURY

Specific to lower eyelid surgery is the anterior orbital location of the inferior oblique muscle and its nerve. During removal of the medial fat pad, the inferior oblique muscle is frequently identified. So that damage to the muscle or its nerve is avoided, dissection and fat removal in this area must be performed under direct visualization with meticulous hemostasis. If the inferior oblique muscle or its nerve has been damaged, the patient will complain of vertical diplopia (double vision) that will increase in gaze to the contralateral side. Corrective extraocular muscle surgery should be delayed, because this complication may spontaneously resolve.

UNDEREXCISION OR OVEREXCISION OF FAT

Whereas underexcision of upper eyelid fat is encountered relatively often, excessive removal of fat from the lower eyelid is very rare. Because the orbital contents tend to move inferiorly when the patient is in the up-

right position, a concavity of the lower eyelid, analogous to a deep superior sulcus in the upper eyelid after upper blepharoplasty, is not observed except when the patient is supine. Rather, overexcision of fat creates an increased definition of the bony orbital rim and palpebrojugal fold, called a tear trough deformity (Fig. 38–17). Free fat grafts can be placed into this defect transconjunctivally, although variable absorption may occur. Elevating cheek fat into the deformity can also rejuvenate the lower eyelid and orbital rim (see Chapter 24).

Much more frequently, undercorrection of fat removal occurs in the lower eyelid, requiring revision surgery for correction. Treating an overcorrection may require placement of subperiosteal material to augment orbital volume.

RESULTS

The repair of lower eyelid retraction after blepharoplasty is a challenge for the oculoplastic surgeon, and multiple operations are frequently necessary. We recently reviewed 30 consecutive cases managed as described here; all patients had undergone blepharoplasty with the transcutaneous approach. For nine patients, one procedure satisfactorily corrected the problem; for 21 patients, however, repeated operations were required, with seven patients needing as many as four procedures for optimal correction.[10] The reoperation rate was lower for retraction of less than 6 months' duration.

Avoiding this difficult problem is preferable to treating it. In our experience, transcutaneous blepharoplasty of the lower eyelid may result in eyelid retraction even if minimal or no skin was removed. The percentage of transcutaneous blepharoplasties that result in retraction is difficult to estimate, because only patients with severe retraction seek medical attention, but the transconjunctival approach has not been associated with retraction.[1]

References

1. Baylis HI, Long JA, Groth MJ: Transconjunctival lower eyelid blepharoplasty: Technique and complications. Ophthalmology 1989; 96:1027–1032.
2. Goldberg RA, Lesner AM, Shorr N, Baylis HI: The transconjunctival approach to the orbital floor and orbital fat: A prospective study. Ophthalmic Plast Reconstr Surg 1990; 6:241–246.
3. Smith B: Postsurgical complications of cosmetic blepharoplasty. Trans Am Acad Ophthalmol Otolaryngol 1969; 73:1162–1164.
4. Hamako C, Baylis HI: Lower eyelid retraction after blepharoplasty. Am J Ophthalmol 1980; 89:517–521.
5. Edgerton MT Jr: Causes and prevention of lower lid ectropion following blepharoplasty. Plast Reconstr Surg 1972; 49:367–373.
6. DeMere M, Wood T, Austin W: Eye complications with blepharoplasty or other eyelid surgery: A national survey. Plast Reconstr Surg 1974; 53:634–637.
7. Mahaffey PJ, Wallace AF: Blindness following cosmetic blepharoplasty: A review. Br J Plast Surg 1986; 39:213–221.
8. Putterman AM: Temporary blindness after cosmetic blepharoplasty. Am J Ophthalmol 1975; 80:1081–1083.
9. Goldberg RA, Marmor MF, Shorr N: Blindness following blepharoplasty: Two case reports and a discussion of management. Ophthalmic Surg 1990; 21:85–89.
10. Nelson E, Baylis HI, Goldberg RA: Lower eyelid retraction following blepharoplasty. Ophthalmic Plast Reconstr Surg 1992; 8:170–175.

Marianne Nelson O'Donoghue

Chapter *39*

Ocular and Facial Cosmetics

The immediate postoperative period is difficult for most patients undergoing eyelid, brow, and facial surgery. They have gone through the trauma of an operation to improve their appearance and now must contend with the unpleasant look of eyelid and facial edema, cysts, blemishes, subcutaneous lumps, asymmetry, upper eyelid ptosis (drooping eyelid), and scars. Hair loss is another possible consequence. Makeup at this point is an important adjunct to cosmetic oculoplastic and facial surgery.

Marianne O'Donoghue is a dermatologist with expertise in facial cosmetics. She begins with tips on preparing the eyelids for cosmetic surgery, with emphasis on preventing mechanical trauma to the eyelids, ruling out contact dermatitis, and treating seborrheic blepharitis. She then describes how our patients can use eye shadow, eyeliner, mascara, and eyebrow pencil to camouflage postoperative bruising, swelling, and asymmetries. Last, she describes how eye cosmetics can deemphasize eyelid and brow deformities in patients who are unable to have surgery; she discusses how to diminish the appearance of proptosis (eyeball protrusion), wide-set eyes, narrow eyes, dark circles, bags, and infrabrow fullness.

I have found cosmetics to be invaluable for patients after blepharoplasty. They give the patient a chance for a speedier improvement in appearance and are extremely useful in dealing with asymmetries. I find that the main asymmetries following cosmetic oculoplastic surgery are of the upper eyelid creases and folds, eyelid levels, and brows. Dr. O'Donoghue tells us how we can teach our patients to deal with asymmetric creases and folds by blotting out the abnormal crease and penciling in one at a more normal level. Also, applying heavier eyeliner on the side with a greater distance between eyelid margin and fold also helps reduce the asymmetry.

For this edition, Dr. O'Donoghue has added a new section on the use of cosmetics after facial and brow surgery and after laser resurfacing. This provides us with useful suggestions on handling the postoperative disfigurement that occurs in other parts of the face as we begin to expand to more extensive facial surgery.

This chapter is important for the cosmetic surgeon. Reading it has led me to recommend the use of makeup to more of my patients.

ALLEN M. PUTTERMAN

457

This chapter discusses how to prepare for and complement eye surgery with care of the skin around the eyes. It describes the use of ocular cosmetics before, after, and in place of oculoplastic surgery. The use of cosmetics to camouflage bruising and swelling after laser resurfacing, facelifts, and brow lifts is also addressed.

The skin on the eye is much thinner than skin elsewhere and reacts much more quickly to allergy or irritation than skin on the hands, legs, or arms. Several periorbital conditions cause problems in this area.

PREPARING THE EYELIDS FOR COSMETIC SURGERY

Avoid Mechanical Trauma

The first condition relates to mechanical trauma. If someone has itchy eyes from hay fever or a cold, rubbing the eyes may result in edema and erythema. It is important to instruct patients to apply cold compresses to pruritic eyes instead of rubbing them.

Rule Out Contact Dermatitis

Contact dermatitis may represent an allergic reaction to ingredients in eye makeup or drops, or to external allergens present on the hands or scalp. The most common manifestation of allergy to nail polish or hand cream is erythema and scaling around the eye. This occurs because most people touch their upper eyelids several times a day with their hands. The skin on the eyelid reacts to a fragrance or chemical ingredient in hand cream more quickly than the skin on the hands.

The resin in nail polish and methyl methacrylate in artificial nails may cause a problem. Because the periungual skin is quite thick, it usually is the last to react to an offending ingredient in nail cosmetics.

Allergy to perfumes or certain preservatives in shampoos usually manifests as eyelid edema and erythema or similar reactions in the ears. Hair dyes also may cause eyelid reactions.

Because most health care workers wear gloves today, patients have a fair amount of exposure to latex. Additionally, many cases of contact dermatitis have occurred from rubber-tipped cosmetic applicators. It is advisable for these patients to use a cotton swab (e.g., a Q-tip) to apply cosmetics.

All of the eye cosmetics that contain water, such as most eye shadows, water-washable mascara, and many eyelid creams, contain preservatives. Most eye makeup is formulated without fragrance, but the preservatives can cause contact dermatitis. If a patient is allergic to one preservative, she can usually use another. For example, if she is unable to tolerate imidazolidinyl urea or Quaternium-15, she may be able to tolerate thimerosal or parabens. (These preservatives are also found in contact lens preparations.) Table 39–1 lists the sensitizers, preservatives, and antibiotics likely to be found in cosmetics or eye drops.[1, 2]

Because of the incidence of contact dermatitis, all eye preparations that are to be used after surgery should be used or tested before surgery. Fresh products with new applicators should be used to avoid irritation from dried-up products or excessive contamination by bacteria.

Treat Seborrheic Blepharitis

In my practice, the most common cause of erythema and scaling in the upper eyelid is seborrheic blepharitis. This condition, called "dandruff" of the eyelids, is most prevalent when the ambient humidity drops and perspiration evaporates into the dry air, leaving thick, gummy sebum on the eyelids, central forehead, and nares. This substance irritates these areas and causes a flaky, red dermatitis.

One easy way of thinning out the sebum and clearing the dermatitis and blepharitis is to use an antiseborrheic shampoo. Hair products containing zinc pyrithione, selenium sulfide, salicylic acid, or tar appear to alleviate

table 39–1
Common Sensitizers, Preservatives, and Antibiotics

Preservatives	**Resins**
Dimercaprol	Colophony
Ethylenediaminetetraacetic acid (EDTA)	Dihydroabietyl alcohol
Merthiolate	
Benzalkonium chloride	**Pearlescent Additives**
Parabens	Bismuth oxychloride
Phenyl mercuric acetate	
Imidazolidinyl urea	**Emollients**
Quaternium-15	Lanolin
Potassium sorbate	Propylene glycol
Antioxidants	**Antibiotics**
Butylated hydroxyanisole	Sulfisoxazole
Butylated hydroxytoluene	Neomycin
Propyl gallate	Sulfacetamide
Di-*tert*-butyl-hydroquinone	

this condition. Ideally, the shampoo should be used twice a week to obtain therapeutic success. Occasionally, a 1 per cent hydrocortisone cream, in addition to the shampoo, may be used. Some ophthalmologists use a product called I-scrub for this problem.

Seborrheic blepharitis also occurs in elderly patients when they decrease the frequency of shampooing to less than once weekly. This condition may also develop in patients with Parkinson's disease or other neurologic disorders.

In preparation for any eye surgery, it is important that the patient have healthy eyelid skin. It may be wise to have the patient use an antiseborrheic shampoo prophylactically during the immediate preoperative and postoperative periods.

EYE COSMETICS AFTER SURGERY

Eye cosmetics, including eye shadow, eyeliner, mascara, and eyebrow pencil, can be used to camouflage postoperative bruising and swelling.

Eye Shadow

Eye shadow functions to give depth to the eye and to enhance the color of the eye. It is available in powder, cream, emulsion, pencil, and stick. The choice of base depends on the presence or absence of extra eye folds and on the patient's skin type, age, and adeptness in applying makeup. The best way to apply eye shadow is with a soft eye sponge. Clean cotton swabs may also be used.

Darker eye shadows can camouflage postoperative edema and erythema. Products are available to cover most discoloration, for example, Flori Robert's Dermablend and Lydia O'Leary's Covermark. The former seems a little easier to apply. It is wise to attempt only about 80 per cent coverage so that the makeup does not look artificial.[3] If lighter coverage is desired, regular foundation may be used over cream in the color opposite to that of the bruising; for example, a thin green cream can cover red bruises or yellow can camouflage purple bruises. The color wheel should be consulted in the selection of the camouflage (Fig. 39–1). An exception to the color wheel is that orange should be avoided in the case of bluish bruises. Orange always accentuates skin problems, looks harsh, and is difficult to blend with the rest of the makeup.[3]

Because the eyelid skin is tender after surgery, it may be necessary to first apply a moisturizing eyelid cream to allow for easy application of the makeup. Any makeup intended for use after surgery should be fresh and should have been tested on the patient before surgery.

Frosted eye shadow should not be used in older patients because it accentuates lax skin. In addition, this product should not be used immediately postoperatively because it contains rough particles, such as pearlized mica, that may irritate and cause small cuts in healing skin.

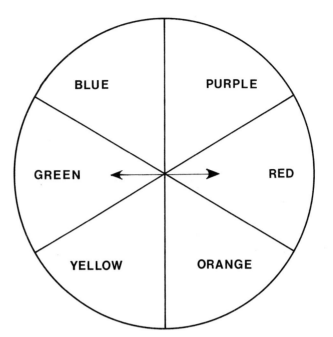

figure 39–1

A color wheel is used to determine what color makeup should be used to camouflage bruises and skin discolorations

Eyeliner

Eyeliner is designed to enhance the eyelashes on both the upper and lower eyelids. The products come in three formulations: (1) cake, (2) liquid, and (3) pencil. Fashion dictates the way eyeliners are used.

Cake liners seem to be out of vogue because the addition of water and a separate brush to use it are required.

Liquid liners are very convenient because a brush is included inside the cylindrical container. The liquids contain a water-soluble latex or a polymer, such as ammonium acrylate. Because water-soluble latex needs a preservative, liquid eyeliner may cause contact dermatitis.

Pencil liners are the most popular today. They contain natural and synthetic waxes combined with oils and pigments. The waxes are then formed into rods and encased in wood. Because there is no preservative or fragrance in these eyeliners, there is almost no incidence of contact dermatitis. The eyeliner is applied with several soft strokes, which give the eye softness.

If the eyelashes have been disturbed during surgery, the liner can be an asset to camouflage their absence. Some older women are able to use only liquid liner, which goes on easily over tender edematous eyelids. The disadvantage is that liquid liner sometimes gives the eyes a harsh appearance.

If *ectropion* (eyelid eversion) occurs postoperatively, the application of an eyeliner just above the eyelashes camouflages the problem. White eyeliner makes the eye look brighter. Black or dark brown liner makes the lashes appear thicker at the base. Blue or violet liner might complement the eye color.

In the event of a slight unilateral *ptosis*, the same eye shadow would be applied to both eyelids, but white eyeliner would be applied directly to the lid margin above the iris on the ptotic eyelid. No other eyeliner on the upper eyelid should be used, because it would call attention to the asymmetry.

If the *creases are asymmetric*, the crease that is less attractive can be blotted out with Dermablend or a touch base made of clay (e.g., Clinique's Touch Base for Eyes). A crease that matches the level of the good crease on the other eye is then drawn. Eyeliner or a dark thin line of eye shadow can be used for this purpose. The eye with the good crease is then covered with approximately the same color eye shadow, and its natural crease is accentuated with a thin line of dark shadow or eyeliner.

Another way of managing asymmetry is to place thicker eyeliner on the eyelid with the higher crease. This creates the illusion that the distance from eyeliner to eyelid fold is more symmetric because on the more normal eyelid there is a finer line. A cosmetician should assist the patient in learning these techniques.

Mascara and Eyelash Dye

Mascara enhances the lashes, making them longer and thicker. There are two types of mascara: (1) water-based and (2) waterproof.

Water-based mascara consists of waxes and pigments suspended in water with the aid of an emulsifier. It must contain preservatives in relatively large concentrations and thus may cause some allergic reactions. Because this mascara does wash off very easily with soap and water, however, it is the preferred choice for healthy eyelashes. Most women are not allergic to all preservatives, and if one ingredient causes a problem, another mascara can be selected. As with other cosmetics, it is important to ascertain any allergy before surgery.

Patients with tearing eyes or an ectropion may need to use *waterproof* mascara. This also may be a choice for swimmers or people who reside in hot, humid climates. Waterproof products are less likely to clump than water-based products. They are composed of waxes and pigments in a petrolatum distillate requiring cold cream or a solvent for removal. Although waterproof mascara does not encourage the growth of bacteria as much as water-washable mascara does, *Pseudomonas* organisms can still contaminate the product; as a result, waterproof mascara contains some preservatives. The gentle eye makeup remover products available from many cosmetic houses rarely cause allergy but may cause irritation.

Any type of mascara can have lash-building additives. These can be particles of keratin or talc or fibers of rayon or nylon. In patients who have just had surgery and in contact lens wearers, these additives may present a problem because particles or fibers may drop into the eye. These additives may even induce a conjunctivitis. It is best to avoid these additives in the first few months after surgery.

If a patient has very pale eyelashes, the lashes may be accidentally cut during surgery. To avoid this possibility, such a patient may wish to have the eyelashes dyed brown before the surgical procedure. However, this dye procedure may be against the law in some states.

An eyelash curler may also be necessary after surgery to train eyelashes that have taken on a new angle.

Eyebrow Pencil

Before I discuss the final type of eye cosmetic, the eyebrow pencil, a review of the classically proportioned face is needed (Fig. 39–2).

According to Cristian,[3] "Eyes are considered to be in proportion if the space between the two eyes is equal to the width of one eye and the distance from the upper eyelid crease to the eyebrow is approximately equal to the diameter of the cornea (i.e., 12 mm)." The cosmetician should strive for this proportion with highlighting and contour just as the surgeon should with the scalpel.

The ideal eyebrow should begin at a point defined by a line drawn from the corner of the nose superiorly. It should arch maximally at a point drawn from the corner of the nose through the pupil. The eyebrow should end at a point defined by a line drawn from the corner of the nose to the lateral canthus.[1] The standard bird's wing eyebrow gives the most open look to the eyes.

Eyebrows should match hair color or should be only one shade lighter or darker. Too much tweezing, coloring, or drawing on the brow looks artificial and is distracting. It is important to leave as much of the natural eyebrow as possible before surgery in case the shape needs to be changed after surgery.

Eyebrow pencils are fairly easy to use. They should be applied with small, short strokes for a natural appearance. The pencils contain pigment in petrolatum, lanolin, and waxes and are encased in wood or plastic. Ideally, they can be used to fill out sparse eyebrows or to help change eyebrow shape.

After surgery, if the eyebrows droop, the lower part can be plucked and pencil can be added to the upper part. This may be especially necessary if a brow lift was not performed at the same time as the blepharoplasty.

If asymmetry occurs, it can be corrected with pencil and shaping. A cosmetician should work with the patient to achieve the most natural appearance.

If eyebrow hairs are going in a different direction after surgery, the patient can train them by brushing the hairs with a toothbrush or cosmetic brush and holding them in place with the aid of hair spray. The hair spray should be sprayed on the thumb and index finger and then applied to the wayward hairs.

If the patient has chosen to lighten her hair color after surgery, facial bleach can be used on the eyebrows to lighten them slightly. Dark brown eyebrows with light hair present a harsh appearance.

All of the cosmetics and medicines used postoperatively should have been tried and found to be nonallergenic for that patient. This includes the patient's hand cream, nail polish, hair products, and any eye drops that may be used.

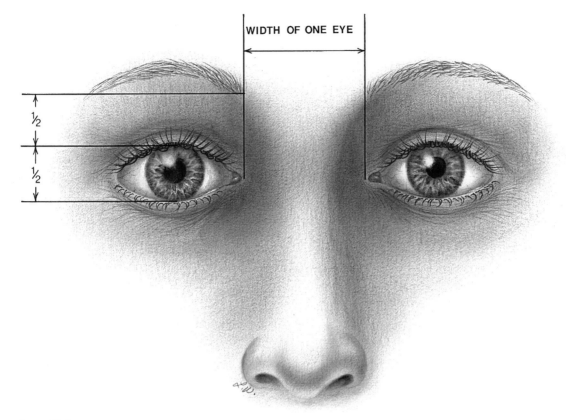

figure 39–2

The classically proportioned face. The space between the eyes is equal to the width of one eye. The distance from the upper eyelid crease to the eyebrow is equal to the diameter of the cornea (~12 mm).

USE OF EYE COSMETICS INSTEAD OF SURGERY

A few cosmetic maneuvers can be useful for patients with eyelid or brow deformities who are unable to have surgery.

Eyeliner and Abnormal-Appearing Eyes

Eyeliner can be used to make the eyes symmetric, imparting the illusion that eyes are set farther apart or closer together. Eyeliner used just on the lower eyelid makes the eyes seem more open and alert.

For example, the technique for making narrow eyes appear to be set farther apart involves lining the upper eyelid and the lower eyelid only from the outer corner to the middle of the eye—not lining the inner section of either eyelid.[4] For eyes set too far apart, lining the inner sections of the eyelid or only the center of the eyelids, and not the outer corners, makes them appear more closely set together.[4]

Eye Shadow

In a patient who has "crepey" (wrinkled) eyelids or in patients who desire longer-lasting eye color, a touch base made of clay should be applied first. This makes it easier for powder eye shadow to stay in place. Another way to achieve long-lasting eye shadow without accentuating lax skin is to moisten the powder eye shadow with a wet sponge to create a paste that is thicker and stays in place.

After the first layer is applied to the eyelid, an appropriate light powder eye shadow may be applied. Powder rather than cream eye shadow is selected because the cream-based shadow would likely collect in the creases of lax eyelids. In the patient with dermatochalasis (excessive skin), a thin line of color just above the lash line would be less likely to exaggerate the drooping eyelid.

Eye shadow can minimize the following deformities.

Proptosis. Proptosis (exophthalmos) can be camouflaged if the subtle or darker eye shadow is carried all the way to the brow line to give the illusion of depth.

Enophthalmos. For deeply sunken eyes, light eye shadow is extended almost to the brow line to bring the eyelids out.

Infrabrow Puffiness. Puffy skin under the brows can be made to appear smaller if a darker shade of eye shadow is applied just under the brow and a lighter shade is applied on the eyelid.

Circles and Bags. Patients can alleviate dark circles or bags under the eyes by applying a light highlighter, such as an eraser stick, under the eye. The eraser stick should be applied to the crease above and below the bags, with regular foundation then applied over the entire area.

Narrow-Set Eyes. Narrow-set eyes can be made to appear farther apart if lighter eye shadow is applied above the medial canthus and eyeliner is applied only on the outer edges of the eye.[4]

Small Eyes. Small eyes may appear larger if the patient avoids using dark liner around the eyes. Eye shadow that is similar in color to the color of the eyes may also make small eyes appear larger.

Sometimes eyes appear small because of a wedge resection for basal cell carcinoma. To enlarge the appearance of these eyes, the patient can apply a dark eye shadow. The eye shadow should be placed along the lateral orbital ridge and eyebrow, with a small amount placed beneath the lateral lower lash line. To give the eye a more open appearance, the patient should then place light eye shadow medially beneath the eyebrow.[5]

Eyelash Curler

If a patient has dermatochalasis and is unable to undergo blepharoplasty, besides using a thin line of color instead of regular eye shadow, an eyelash curler may be of assistance. For a more alert appearance, the eyelashes can be curled up and over the sagging skin before mascara is applied.

There are a few precautions concerning the use of eyelash curlers:

1. The rubber liner should be soft and should contain no old pieces of hardened mascara.
2. The curler should not be used by persons sensitive to rubber or nickel (the major components of the metal frame).
3. If the rubber liner gets old, the entire curler should be thrown away. Replacement rubber strips might be put on incorrectly and therefore cut some of the lashes.
4. The curler should always be used *before* mascara is applied.

CAMOUFLAGE COSMETICS AFTER FACELIFT AND BROW LIFT

Before applying any cosmetic, the postoperative patient must receive permission from the surgeon. The application of cosmetics to any break in the skin, such as suture lines, should be avoided. The same color wheel that is appropriate for eyelid surgery applies to face lifts (see Fig. 39–1).

Several products available at the department or drugstore can conceal discolorations. Physician's Formula cosmetics contain yellow, green, and mauve concealers; these are easily found at most drugstores and are reason-ably priced. These products should be new and uncontaminated. Application with a cotton swab is less likely to infect the newly operated on skin.

There are two steps to application:

1. Concealing the bruise or hemorrhage with green, yellow, or mauve depending on the defect.
2. Covering the entire face with heavy, concealing makeup.

Chanel and Estée Lauder make some skin tone–colored concealing makeup products, which may be sufficient for minor discolorations. Because most of these products contain titanium dioxide, they act to protect the new skin from sun damage. For major concealment, Dermablend or Covermark may be needed.

For minor discoloring, all of the major cosmetic houses (e.g., Yves Saint Laurent, Estée Lauder, Chanel, Revlon, or Clinique) make a concealer cover stick. These can be used to touch up minor flaws before a regular foundation is applied. A cover stick would be used later in the recuperation process.

Removal of concealer makeup should be performed with the oil cleanser that is sold with the major concealers (e.g., Dermablend or Covermark). If the concealer is a cosmetic product, it should be removed with a lipid-free cleanser, such as Cetaphil (Galderma) or Aquanil (Person & Covey).

CAMOUFLAGE COSMETICS AFTER LASER RESURFACING

The major change in skin after laser surgery is its extremely violaceous color. After telangiectasis treatment, the hemorrhage into the skin is too great to try to cover for the first week or so. Afterward, some of the green products may be appropriate.

After laser resurfacing, the immediate postoperative care requires lubrication. Something as simple as Crisco shortening (Procter & Gamble, Cincinnati), Aquafor (Beiersdorf, Norwalk, Conn.), Eutra, polymyxin B sulfate; bacitracin zinc-polymyxin B (Polysporin, Glaxo Wellcome, Research Triangle Park, N.C.), or bacitracin ointment may be used for the first 10–20 days. Some laser surgeons use biologic-type dressings, whereas others choose to use only water and simple emollients. The interval between the surgery and the application of camouflage cosmetics depends on the type and depth of the laser procedure.

Initial cream or stick preparations with no water content can be applied to neutralize the violaceous color. Over the green neutralizer, a heavier concealer type of makeup is then used (see previous topic).

As the weeks pass by, a thinner green cover, such as Physician's Formula Self Defense lotion with green tint or Ultima II aqua tint, can be used. Often these are enough for male patients to use to tone down the violaceous color. Women may want to use their normal foundation over the thinner green base.

COSMETIC CONSULTATION

We as physicians cannot begin to take the place of a good cosmetician in caring for patients and advising them about the use of cosmetics before and after surgery. However, we should inform our patients of the value of a good cosmetician and we should know some of the possible solutions so that we can suggest them to our patients. The use of cosmetics and surgery is an excellent combination of tools for achieving aesthetically pleasing eyes.

References

1. Draelos ZK: Eye cosmetics. Dermatol Clin 1991; 9:1–7.
2. Engasser PG, Maibach HI: Dermatitis due to cosmetics. In Fisher AA (ed): Contact Dermatitis, 3rd ed, pp 368–393. Philadelphia, Lea & Febiger, 1986.
3. Cristian S: Corrective eyelid makeup technique for cosmetic surgery. In Putterman AM (ed): Cosmetic Oculoplastic Surgery, pp 307–319. New York, Grune & Stratton, 1982.
4. Balfour LA: The Professional Model's Handbook, pp 77–85. Bronx, NY, Milady Publishing Co, 1990.
5. Draelos ZD: Cosmetics in Dermatology, 2nd ed, p 36. New York, Churchill Livingstone, 1995.

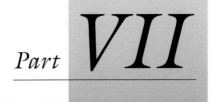

Part **VII**

MARKETING IN COSMETIC OCULOPLASTIC SURGERY

David R. Fett

Chapter 40

Cosmetic Oculoplastic Surgery Marketing

Because of my medical training, I earlier questioned whether advertising and marketing was in good taste or even ethical. For these reasons, I did not include a chapter on marketing in the first two editions of *Cosmetic Oculoplastic Surgery.* Later, when David Fett was my oculoplastic fellow, I became interested in marketing, took courses on the subject, developed a logo for my practice, and created a marketing brochure. Additionally, I advertised in local magazines on several occasions, with effective results.

Today, it is obvious that marketing plays an important part in our medical practices. Many of us lecture and write scientific articles, include a listing of our practices in the telephone book's Yellow Pages, and have brochures. This is one end of the spectrum of marketing, and Dr. Fett discusses all the other methods and extensions of this tool.

With managed care decreasing physicians' incomes, more and more doctors are likely to gravitate toward performing cosmetic surgery as a way of increasing their revenues. As the marketplace becomes more competitive, marketing will definitely play a deciding role in which practices survive and which do not. Therefore, I believe that this chapter will benefit us all, and I commend Dr. Fett on writing a thorough discussion of marketing.

ALLEN M. PUTTERMAN

Most medical schools turn physicians out into the world who are filled with medical knowledge but little business knowledge. Yet many doctors eventually go into private practice, which is by any definition very much a business.

It is the goal of this chapter to familiarize you with the basics of marketing, one of the more useful business skills in today's competitive world. Marketing means taking your product or service to the marketplace in a way that encourages customers to buy it.

Until recently, medicine and marketing were considered to be in conflict. Medicine is a profession born out of a desire to heal; marketing is a skill born out of a desire to succeed in conducting commerce. Thus, the subject of marketing a physician's services begs the question, "Why should a doctor be involved in marketing?"

There are three realistic answers to that question:

1. To make a living.
2. To make a good living.
3. To make a very good living.

Making a living after you complete your medical education is often a challenge filled with unexpected obstacles. There are 630,000 physicians in the United States, most of whom are concentrated in urban areas; therefore, there is a great deal of competition. In addition to ophthalmologists and ophthalmic plastic surgeons, thousands of physicians with varying degrees of qualifications also perform cosmetic and reconstructive eyelid surgery. By and large, the patient population does not really understand the differences in medical training. In addition, health maintenance organizations (HMOs) and preferred provider organizations (PPOs) make sure that patients see doctors within their own physician network. As you seek referrals from doctors in private practice, you may well run into an *old-boy network* (see later), which tends to exclude you or ignore your abilities.

A good, solid knowledge of marketing is your best chance for navigating through these obstacles, being in charge of your own destiny, and reaching your business goals.

Once you have some marketing experience under your belt, you will see that there really is no conflict between a desire to help and heal and making a good living, as long as the latter does not take precedence. In fact, one might argue that the better living one makes, the more patients one has helped.

Marketing involves common sense. What makes for good marketing, however, is organizing that common sense and directing it toward the accomplishment of a marketing goal.

To market your practice successfully, you must stay objective. To stay objective, try to think of yourself and the service you offer as a product. A product is anything, including services, that can be offered to a market to satisfy a need.[1] Also, think of your patients as customers. In fact, smart marketers know that their success in marketing is directly proportional to their ability to remain customers themselves. Indeed, thinking like your customers allows you to view a problem from the patient's point of view and makes you a more competitive marketer.

A step-by-step template follows for creating a marketing plan that will work for you.

DEFINING YOUR MARKET

In marketing terms, your customers are referred to as the "target group." The more you can define the target group, the more you will understand it. The more you understand your target group, the better focused and more successful your entire marketing effort will be.

Most marketers recognize that they have more than one target group. Therefore, thinking about separate targets, each one with their own characteristics, is the smarter course.

As a physician with a specialty, you have basically three different target groups or markets that are important to you:

1. Your colleagues in medical practices, hospitals, and medical schools.
2. Your existing patient base.
3. New patients brought in through your own commercial marketing efforts.

Maximizing the potential from any of these target groups can form the basis of a thriving medical practice. However, maximizing all three can result in an extremely successful practice.

We now take a closer look at each of the three target groups.

Your Colleagues as a Target Group

It is common sense that the more doctors who know you and your work, the more patients will be referred to you. Developing a doctor-to-doctor referral network takes the most personal time of all your marketing efforts, often years. Once established, however, this network will be the most durable and dependable of all your new-patient resources.

You may often hear doctors and other businesspeople refer to an old-boy network. This term is most often used by people who are not in it. To those not part of a network, exclusion can represent a frustrating and seemingly unjust experience. However, to be fair to the doctors in such a network, that network is often the natural result of years of cultivating professional relationships and friendships. From a business standpoint, it is part of a real (and salable) asset called *goodwill*, and "membership" is not to be merely given away to the next doctor who shows up in town.

Of course, you should make attempts to break into the network in your area. You would be better off, in a marketing sense, however, by establishing your own new old-boy network. Keep in touch with your medical school classmates, former fellow interns, and fellow residents. Start the ball rolling by referring patients whenever you can to other new physicians in different disciplines or subdisciplines. Reciprocity will follow.

Market yourself to your colleagues. Whether you open your own practice or join an already existing practice, send announcements about this event to as many physicians as possible.

As an ophthalmic plastic surgeon, your practice is not geographically limited. Draw a circle encompassing an hour to an hour and a half's drive from your location. Call your local county medical association, and buy mailing lists of every family physician, internist, and ophthalmologist within that circle. Use your Yellow Pages, and add every optometrist within that area to your list. Send the announcement of your new practice to your entire mailing list. In addition, develop a "hit list." Pick 100 specific doctors based on reputation, specialty, hospital affiliation, and location, and write a personal letter to each describing your practice. Write to five of these doctors each week.

While your practice is still not overflowing with patients, telephone or try to meet with those doctors who may be of particular help to you. Remember, one colleague in your corner can result in hundreds of referrals over the years.

Join and stay active in as many medical associations as you can handle. Become an instructor to other physicians at the postgraduate level. Publish and lecture at every opportunity.

The points listed above are easy to put off doing. This is exactly why they often end up in the file folder marked "good intentions." Write them down, formalize your efforts to do them, and check up on yourself weekly.

Your Patients as a Target Group

Patients talk about their doctors a great deal. When they really like a doctor or the results of a treatment, they tell everyone they can. The reverse is also true. Therefore, there is no more powerful (or inexpensive) marketing tool than patients' word of mouth. This is especially true in surgery that involves the eyes and face. The face is where everybody looks. It is the billboard of your work. When a friend or relative of a patient says to that patient, "You look terrific," or "You look younger," you want your patient to reply, "Yes, and my doctor was terrific! You should go to Dr. (your name here) yourself!"

Here is one of the most valuable pieces of marketing advice I can give you for getting that kind of response from your patients: *Never forget that you are not only in medicine but also in the service business.*

The service business is a challenging one. You can do 19 things right and one thing wrong, and the one thing wrong can negate the positive effects of everything else. This is not fair, but it is true. A telephone call that is not returned, a rude receptionist, or a flippant, arrogant answer can cost you thousands of dollars in referrals that you will not get from your patient.

The organization you arrange, the people you hire, and the tone you set are not just there for your convenience; they are there to work for you in marketing your practice to your biggest potential fans, your patients. I cover this in detail later (see Sales).

The Community as a Target Group

Where your colleague referral target group is somewhat finite, and your patient referral target group is proportional to your years in business, the outside community is your volume target group. This group is immense, always changing, and—the expense of advertising notwithstanding—quite easy to reach. Imagine you live in a community of 1 million residents. Statistically, between one third and one half of that population will be between 35 and 75 years of age and will have bags, lines, wrinkles, and skin problems that an ophthalmic plastic surgeon can treat. Most of those would-be patients will not be referred to you by your colleagues. Nor will they be referred to you by friends and relatives of your patients. You must reach out to them and refer yourself. In this instance, I am talking about physician advertising. You cannot personally talk to hundreds of thousands of would-be baby-boomer patients, so you reach them by sending out an advertisement.

At its best, advertising can build a physician's practice into a recognized brand name. Brand familiarity is a bulwark of successful marketing. People tend to buy products and services that are familiar to them. You can use newspapers, magazines, radio, television, direct mail, the Internet, or any combination of these media to tell patients about you and your practice.

In summary, it is important to recognize colleagues in hospitals and medical schools, your patient base, and your entire community as distinct marketing target groups. Formalize your plans to reach each of them through a targeted, ongoing effort.

THE FUNDAMENTALS OF MARKETING

Once you appreciate the role that marketing can play in building a practice and recognize your target groups, you can write and implement a solid marketing plan. To do so, you must have a grasp of marketing fundamentals.

Bringing any product (this also includes a service) to the marketplace often involves efforts and expertise in the following areas:

- Product—formulating a product (or service) that your would-be customers want and need
- Positioning—positioning that product so that it has a unique and desired place in the market
- Packaging—dressing up that product so that at the time and point of purchase, it (rather than someone else's) is bought
- Pricing—pricing the product so that the selected target group regards it as the best value for the money
- Sales—reaching out to your target group to initiate and to close sales
- Promotion—making sure that everyone in your target group knows that your product exists and is available
- Distribution—making sure your product is readily available to would-be buyers

Many businesses have separate staff or hire marketing consultants to handle each of these areas.

At first glance, some of these marketing fundamentals might not seem readily applicable to ophthalmology and plastic surgery. As you develop your marketing plan, you can decide the importance and the scale that each of these will have in your business.

Next, we look at each aspect of marketing in detail.

Product

Before you do anything, you have to understand exactly what it is that you are bringing to the market.

- Is it you and your skill and expertise?
- Are you the product?
- Is it a medical or technical procedure?

For example, the laser is a great technologic breakthrough. In the consumer's mind, it is the closest thing plastic surgery has to a magic bullet. Is your laser procedure the product? Or is your product a solution to a consumers' needs or problems?

The answer, of course, is that all of these elements are your product. However, the degree to which each element is emphasized depends on which target group you are addressing at the time.

To your colleagues in a publishing or lecturing venue, your credentials and expertise are a greater part of your product.

To referring physicians who will receive feedback and some credit or blame from their patients, the results you get and the quality of service you give are a more important aspect of your product.

To a consumer considering laser eyelid surgery and reading an ad, the main product may be the prospect of ending up looking younger by undergoing an easier, less painful procedure.

Positioning

Positioning is actually an offshoot of product. Car models, for example, are positioned to blue-collar workers, professionals, women, men, outdoor enthusiasts, young people, seniors, and so on. You are no different. You can position yourself as an "all things to all people" doctor. You can be a "doctor's doctor." You can be the reconstructive doctor, you can be "the doctor to the stars," you can be the doctor to a specific ethnic or cultural community, and you can be all of the above or none of the above. Your choice depends on your inclinations, the size of the community you serve, and the competition that already exists for each positioning.

If one of these positionings appeals to you, recognize it and include it as part of your marketing plan. Your positioning will skew the tone of what you do and say, influence where you locate your office, determine who you associate with, and even dictate what your advertising looks like.

Packaging

For marketing purposes, packaging means your office and staff. When you approach a shelf in a store and see 10 different brands that you can buy, you are most often attracted to the packaging with which you identify. If you were to buy a bottle of wine, you would perceive that the bottle with the more sophisticated label is a better wine than the bottle with a colorful label and you likely would be willing to pay more for it. Marketers call this place and time the "point of purchase." It is important because it is literally the last time they can influence your buying decision. That is why good marketers spend as much time on their packaging as on anything else.

One of the last things that patients do in the process of making their buying decision is to visit your office. Your office, in a very real sense, becomes your point of purchase. It is your packaging.

Because patients frequently shop around for doctors, they often visit more than one office. This is especially true for patients seeking an expensive, out-of-pocket, elective procedure such as cosmetic surgery. One can assume that patients who can afford cosmetic surgery are demographically skewed upscale and have fairly good furniture and carpeting in their homes. Your office should reflect this economic reality. This will not turn off middle-class or lower-middle-class patients. In addition, patients spend a lot of time in your waiting room. They should not become fatigued by sitting on poorly made furniture. Office furniture is all part of your packaging.

My office has a "sophisticated" but understated look, with contemporary, warm colors, high-quality carpeting, and good furniture that one can comfortably sit in for a long time. One of my competitors, also an aggressive marketer, has an office that is somewhat shabby and tattered and without much attention paid to comfort. When a patient visits both offices, the purchase decision is almost always made in my favor.

Because your office is your point of purchase, design it with thought and invest in it. It will pay you back.

Pricing

Pricing is often the single biggest factor in making any purchase decision. This is especially true if a patient is paying for part or all of the procedure. To do everything else right and then lose a patient over too high a price is unacceptable. On the other hand, do not undersell your services. There is a segment of the market who thinks that if a price is below others, the product cannot be as good.

Pricing should reflect your target and your positioning. Gather information about what your competitors are charging. You have to know what the market is bearing in order to successfully compete.

Sales

Sales are integral to marketing. In fact, by definition, marketing has to end in a sale. When a patient calls your office for an appointment, the person he or she first talks to automatically becomes your opening salesperson. This staff member sets the tone for everything that will follow. Good salesmanship dictates that your would-be patient feels welcome from the first "hello."

Therefore, it is a good idea to designate one or two of your staff members to handle incoming inquiries. An even better idea is to hire specifically for this function. Either way, write a script for them to follow when someone calls. Rehearse them. Surprise them with questions they might not expect. Work out the answers to these questions. The more answers you can make standard policy, the better off you will be.

Have you ever been annoyed by a rude office employee on the telephone? An overaggressive salesperson who will not take no for an answer? An arrogant, aloof doctor? If so, you understand the importance of good telephone etiquette.

Everybody in your office, including you, is part of your sales team. So hire for energy and positiveness, qualities that transmit easily to your patients. Do not hide in your medical "inner sanctum." Wander out to the reception desk and talk with your patients who are coming and going. Address them by name. If they are there to see someone else, greet them and even take a quick look at their progress. The patients in the waiting room see and hear this. Patients want a good relationship with their doctor, so it is smart marketing to demonstrate your interpersonal skills.

It is easy to forget that you and your staff are still making a sales impression after surgery. Sales in a service business is a process with a beginning, a middle, and no end. Your patients can be your best fans and your least expensive and most effective advertising. Call them every so often just to see how they are doing after surgery. Imagine how patients feel when a surgeon calls 3 or 6 months postoperatively to check on their progress. You would have to spend thousands of dollars in advertising and pubic relations to buy the kind of goodwill that a genuine interest in your patients can generate.

When a patient's friends mention how good they look, you don't just want them to say, "Oh, yes, I had eyelid surgery!" You want them to say, "Yes, I went to Dr. So and So." Everything you and your staff do in front of a patient before, during, and after the procedure can be part of good salesmanship and, hence, effective marketing.

Promotion

Advertising

Advertising is your most visible foray into the marketplace. The trick is to think of an ad as a sales opportunity. Because you cannot sell in person to numerous potential customers, you instead publish, broadcast, or mail your sales proposition. The principles of selling, however, remain much the same. If you have ever sold anything, you know that the first rule in selling is not to talk about yourself or your product. Instead, you should first talk about your potential customer's needs and desires. Once the needs are established, you show the customer how your product or service meets these needs. The sale follows. An ad should be no different.

In an ad, the emphasis must be on the solution to a consumer need or problem rather than your expertise or the procedure. Even though your product is a mixture of all three, nothing attracts a consumer to an ad more than a headline that promises a benefit he or she desires. Your expertise and the procedure are reasons why the person should go to you to receive the benefit. They are the tie-breakers.

The quality of your ad tells the consumer all about you, your office, and the quality of your work. If your ad looks unattractive, it subconsciously communicates your taste. If your taste in advertising is poor, how can the quality of your work be any better?

On the other hand, if your ad appears classy, contemporary, graceful, and sophisticated, it will transfer those attributes to the quality of your work. It is an easy choice to hire a professional graphic designer if you are unable to communicate this image yourself.

Do not make your ad a large version of a business card, with a "laundry list" of your services. Your patients want information. Do not be afraid to use long copy. Some people believe that consumers will not read long ad copy and that you must be brief. That's true if you are selling a $49 tire. However, people who have entered the cosmetic surgery purchase cycle are hungry for information and will read everything you can say in an ad. The more you can communicate, the better. This is your chance to be more interesting and persuasive than your competitors.

Bear in mind that comprehensive does not mean wordy or complex. Copy should be well-written, succinct, and clear.

Run your ads over and over again. People often say, "I ran an ad, and nobody called. Advertising doesn't work!" Think about it. Unless you have a product that everybody wants and nobody else is offering and you offer it at a price that is incredibly affordable, why should people call the first time they see your ad? Advertising does not work like that; it works by repetition over months (*frequency*).

People who are interested in laser eyelid surgery, for example, go through a purchase decision process that lasts up to a year. They often "follow" the ads, reading them over and over again, trying to convince themselves to actually go ahead and do it. For your ad to be followed, it must become familiar to those involved in a purchase cycle. The day a potential patient finally decides to have the surgery, you want them to see your ad, not another surgeon's. If you run ads infrequently, chances are that will not happen.

Choice of Media

Should you use newspaper, magazines, radio, television, or direct mail advertising? I like newspaper advertising because I can react quickly to market trends or experiment with a new idea almost as soon as I get it and because the consumer can save the ad and not have to remember the telephone number. I think newspaper is the best medium to target the prospective patient who is shopping around for a surgeon.

Drive-time radio can also be very effective because the prospective patient is often alone in a car and thus there is nothing to compete with your commercial. This is a good time to plant the idea of having cosmetic surgery.

Television is good for building brand-name recognition. If you are appearing on television, many will consider you to be famous. In fact, few major brands have not used television as the centerpiece for building name recognition. Television is a targeted medium. You can appear on programming that is specifically skewed to your target group demographics. The "down side" is that air time on shows watched by audiences that can afford cosmetic surgery can be expensive.

Direct mail is even more targeted. Good mailing lists can reach specific consumers with amazingly narrow criteria. Mailing lists are relatively inexpensive to buy, but postage is expensive. Besides great targeting, direct mail can allow you to communicate much more information than any other advertising media. Direct mail works at its best when combined with an offer. If your direct mail ad works, it can give you an excellent return on your investment. If it does not work or is targeted incorrectly, it can be a waste of money.

A brochure, a direct mail piece, can serve a dual function. It can be an important part of your response package to prospective patients calling for more information. It can also serve as reinforcement to those who visited your office for a consultation and are trying to remember everything they found out. Therefore, your brochure should be both a *selling* piece, which includes your qualifications and the benefits of the procedures, and an *information* piece, which features the important questions and answers that no doubt took place during the patient's visit.

Yellow Pages advertising is essential because the telephone book is often the first and last place a patient will look. You can assume that everyone looking up ophthalmic or plastic surgery in the telephone book is interested in having a procedure done. Therefore, your listing or ad will be displayed in a highly competitive environment. Do not run a display ad that is merely a business card in print. This is a good time and place to outdo your competition by stressing your unique qualifications and formal ophthalmic training. If you do no other promotion, make sure you have a noticeable and persuasive presence in the Yellow Pages.

Distribution

Distribution involves making your product available to be purchased. The closest analogy a doctor would have to this aspect of marketing is the location of his or her office and hospital. Ideally, both the office and hospital should be in areas that are easy to reach, that are safe, and that reflect the economic status of the targeted patient base.

Budget

I look at money as a tool with which to make money. Many doctors, when setting up an advertising budget, try to spend as little as possible. They consider this task a rather suspect venture. The truth is, many professionals invest in significantly higher risk ventures than marketing their own practices. Physicians must change their attitude. To paraphrase the above expression, it takes money to make money.

Spend the most you can afford on advertising initially. If need be, hire one less person or take home less money and use the savings for advertising. When your practice is established, target 6–7 per cent of your revenue on advertising. Done with thought and intelligence, advertising can give you a significant return on your investment.

DEVELOPING A MARKETING PLAN

Tucking away marketing knowledge in your head will do you no good. Your ideas must be formalized into a plan of action. Make your marketing effort concrete by writing a plan, budgeting for marketing, following your plan, and checking your progress periodically to keep yourself on track.

A simple, but good marketing plan consists of the following:

- Background—everything you know about your market

- Objectives—what you are trying to accomplish
- Strategy—specifically how you are going to accomplish those objectives
- Critical path—when you are going to accomplish those objectives
- Budget—how much you expect to spend, when you will spend it, and from where the money will come

Background

Write down everything you can think of regarding your market, as if you were an outside consultant. Be realistic. State the background, credentials, talents, and desires of the doctor (you). Describe the nature of the procedure the doctor is offering to the public. Describe the competition.

Describe the mind-set of the consumer regarding the procedure or procedures. Write it so that a lay person, seeing it for the first time, will understand the nature of the ophthalmic surgery marketplace.

Objectives

Next, state your marketing objectives clearly and in order of priority. Be sure to include all three target groups—colleagues, your patients, and the community—to some degree in your objectives. Remember, no one need see your plan except yourself.

Table 40–1 gives an example of an oculoplastic surgeon's marketing objectives.

Strategy

Strategy defines how you will accomplish your stated objectives. This is the action-oriented section of your plan and is very specific. You should develop strategies for each of your objectives and target groups. Remember that positioning, packaging, pricing, promotion, and sales are also critical parts of the strategy you design to meet your objectives. Write a specific plan of action for each under this section.

Table 40–2 presents an example of strategies.

---

table 40–1

Sample Marketing Objectives for the Oculoplastic Surgeon

---

1. To become the leading ophthalmic plastic surgeon catering to corporate executives in the greater St. Louis area.
2. To get referrals from all the physicians affiliated with St. Louis General Hospital.
3. To develop a reputation for my practice as the place to go for cosmetic laser surgery.
4. To receive five inquiries from doctor-referred patients each week.
5. To receive five inquiries from patient-referred patients each week.
6. To receive 10 inquiries from newspaper advertisements each week.

---

table 40–2

Sample Marketing Strategies for the Oculoplastic Surgeon

For the objective "To become the leading ophthalmic plastic surgeon catering to corporate executives in the greater St. Louis area":

1. I will reach St. Louis corporate executives by developing a series of seminars on laser surgery for the middle-aged man. The series will be advertised via direct mail to the chief executive officers of the leading 500 companies in the area.
2. The direct-mail piece will stress the importance of youthful appearance in closing sales for the corporations. A special discount will be made available only to employees of these companies.
3. A salesperson will be hired to follow up by telephone on each of the mailings.

Positioning:

1. I will position myself as a leading expert in laser eyelid surgery.
2. I will position myself as having the best training available for this procedure.

Packaging:

1. The office will be set up to give an aura of professionalism.
2. Staff will be trained to be friendly and approachable.
3. Staff meetings will be held weekly to review and discuss matters relating to patients.

Pricing:

1. I will gather information on the pricing used by physicians performing the same procedures in my geographic and economic area.
2. I will try to maintain a pricing structure 10 percent less than that of my competition.

Sales:

1. I will hire a full-time, in-office salesperson with experience in telephone sales.
2. I will target a 50 per cent call-to-consultation success ratio.

Promotion:

1. Advertising will emphasize experience.
   a. Copy points will be experience and technology.
   b. The advertising tone will be serious yet friendly.
2. Media used will be radio; advertising will run weekly, twice a month, and so forth.

Critical Path

Since the strategy section will be lengthy and detailed, include a calendar or critical path in your marketing plan. Mark each step of each strategic action, from inception through implementation and follow-up, with specific dates. Think of each critical path as an unstoppable arrow heading straight toward a target. If obstacles arise that seem to force changes in your goals, change them but do not delete them from your plan.

Budget

Estimate all costs and earmark funds. Include costs of creating ads and mailings, printing, telephone calls, postage, time allotted for yourself and staff toward marketing, lunches with colleagues, membership and association dues, subscriptions, mailing lists, and mass media advertising.

Do not overextend yourself financially, but do not underestimate the wisdom of investing in yourself either.

EVALUATING YOUR MARKETING PLAN

Do not shortchange your marketing plan by losing faith in it. Stick with your plan, but do analyze your goals versus actual performance and make changes where necessary. You will find that some aspects of your plan are working better than others. An important decision you will face is whether to try to fix those aspects that are not working or whether to put more effort and money into those that are working. One of the best things a business owner can do is to figure out what he or she is doing right and do it even more.

CONCLUSION

Marketing is important enough to today's private practice physician to require a formalized course of action rather than "making it up as you go." Remember your target groups, and maximize your presence to all. Familiarize yourself with the various fundamentals of marketing: product, positioning, packaging, pricing, promotion, sales, and distribution.

Write a formal marketing plan and use it from day 1. Remember, it's hard to get where you're going if you don't know where it is.

Reference

1. Kotler P: Marketing for Nonprofit Organizations, 2nd ed., p 261. Englewood Cliffs, NJ, Prentice-Hall, 1982.

Allen M. Putterman

Chapter 41

Patient Satisfaction in Cosmetic Oculoplastic Surgery*

Achieving patient satisfaction in a cosmetic oculoplastic surgery practice is an extremely important marketing consideration. Whereas a satisfied patient commonly will refer a few patients, a dissatisfied patient often will discourage many more patients from visiting the surgeon.

Patient satisfaction must be measured in ways other than an increase in the number of patients and patient retention. Patient satisfaction surveys, frequently used in health care, can help practitioners measure the satisfaction of their patients and learn which changes are needed to increase satisfaction.

In 1990 I conducted a survey of patient satisfaction in my own practice and in several other cosmetic oculoplastic surgery practices throughout the United States. Results of this survey show other cosmetic oculoplastic surgeons how to improve patient satisfaction in their practices.

Most patients surveyed were happy with their surgical results. They rated the results achieved as being more important to satisfaction than other factors, including the cost of treatment. In addition, the patients emphasized the need for oculoplastic surgeons to be more compassionate about the pain and discomfort associated with the surgery. Patients also wanted shorter waiting times in the surgeon's office as well as more postoperative communication with their surgeon.

ALLEN M. PUTTERMAN

In judging the outcome of cosmetic surgery, various patients perceive the same operative result differently because of differences in personality and expectations. In an effort to measure patient satisfaction in oculoplastic surgery, I embarked on a survey. With the help of a marketing firm, I devised three questionnaires to be sent to patients, referring physicians, and oculoplastic surgeons. I engaged the help of seven colleagues in data collection, four of whom gave me information about patients and referring doctors.

One of my motivating factors in performing this study was my perception that the government, health maintenance organizations (HMOs), and insurance companies are emphasizing decreased costs at the expense of quality of medical care. It was my belief that patients value quality and are willing to pay for it. The study proved that this was true far beyond what I had imagined.[1] Also, the study clearly showed that patients are more concerned with pain and discomfort and with waiting time in the surgeon's office than are the oculoplastic surgeons who perform these procedures, a not unexpected finding. Patients found that communication with their surgeons decreased postoperatively and were unhappy about that. The results of this study therefore

*This chapter was modified, with permission of Slack, Inc., from Putterman AM: Patient satisfaction in oculoplastic surgery. Ophthalmic Surg 1990; 21:15–21.

suggest that to improve patient satisfaction, surgeons should address the issues of pain, discomfort, and waiting time and improve their postoperative communication with patients.

MATERIALS AND METHODS

The study evaluated satisfaction after one of two oculoplastic surgical procedures: correction of acquired blepharoptosis and cosmetic blepharoplasty. I chose these two procedures because they had cosmetic considerations in their outcome. Acquired blepharoptosis was defined as ptosis (drooping eyelid) that developed after birth, usually as a result of a levator aponeurosis disinsertion. Congenital and neurogenic ptoses, such as external ophthalmoplegia, myasthenia gravis, and third nerve paralysis, were excluded from the study. The procedures performed to treat acquired ptosis were not delineated, but it was assumed in most cases that the procedures consisted of a levator aponeurosis advancement, tuck, or resection procedure, a Müller's muscle–conjunctival resection procedure, or a Fasanella-Servat operation.[2–4] The procedures were performed to improve vision and appearance.

Cosmetic blepharoplasty consisted of the excision of skin and fat of the upper eyelids, lower eyelids, or all four eyelids. Usually, the operation was performed to improve appearance but, at times, to improve vision as well. Sometimes, these procedures were combined with reconstruction of the upper eyelid creases. In some cases, only skin was removed; in other cases, orbicularis oculi muscle and fat were removed as well.

Initially, the plan was to send a questionnaire only to patients who had undergone acquired blepharoptosis and cosmetic blepharoplasty procedures in an attempt to evaluate their satisfaction with the surgery. Because I soon realized that the satisfaction of the referring physician also could be used to measure patient satisfaction, another questionnaire was designed and sent to these physicians. Finally, to gain an even greater perspective, a third questionnaire was sent to a group of randomly selected oculoplastic surgeons to learn what they deemed important in patient satisfaction. I hoped that this variety of viewpoints would provide the most objective conclusion possible as to how the needs of patients in oculoplastic surgery can best be satisfied.

I sent questionnaires to my patients who had undergone surgery for acquired blepharoptosis or cosmetic blepharoplasty. Questionnaires also were sent to seven other oculoplastic surgeons with a request that they send them to their patients.

After the questionnaires were returned, a statistician analyzed the accumulated data.

RESULTS

Questionnaires from 145 patients, 85 referring physicians, and 69 oculoplastic surgeons were returned. Two of the original eight targeted surgeons did not send any questionnaires back before the deadline, and a third surgeon claimed he had not received the questionnaires. Thus, the patient and referring physician surveys came from five surgeons: one practicing in Los Angeles, one in Minneapolis, one in Cleveland, one in Atlanta, and one in Chicago (me).

Of the patients who completed the questionnaires, 42 per cent had undergone cosmetic blepharoplasty and 55 per cent had undergone surgery for blepharoptosis. Three per cent of patients underwent both procedures.

Of the five satisfaction factors measured, patients judged the results achieved to be the most important (Table 41–1). Communication was rated second most important; pain and discomfort, third; patient treatment cost, fourth; and waiting time in the surgeon's office, last. There was a remarkable disparity between the patients' perception of the importance of the results achieved (55 per cent) and their perception of the importance of the treatment cost (8 per cent) (see Table 41–1). This difference was further emphasized by the mean rating scores for results achieved, 9.8, compared

table 41–1

Patient Satisfaction Survey Ratings of Most Important Factors in Oculoplastic Surgery

Measure of Satisfaction	% of Responses in Each Procedure Category		
	Total	*Blepharoplasty*	*Ptosis Procedures*
Results achieved	55	60	50
Communication	20	17	20
Pain–discomfort	11	12	13
Patient treatment cost	8	6	9
Waiting Time	6	5	8
Total	100	100	100
Total No. of patients*	145	79	79
Base (No. of responses)†	231	113	135

*There is a total of only 145 patients but 158 cases (79 blepharoplasty and 79 ptosis procedures) because 13 patients had both procedures.

†The base, or number of responses, is greater than the total number of patients because many patients listed several measures of satisfaction as most important.

table 41–2

Mean Importance Ratings of Patient Satisfaction with Oculoplastic Surgery*

| Measure of Satisfaction | Mean Importance Rating by Respondent Group | | |
	Patients	Referring Physician	Oculoplastic Surgeon
Results achieved	9.8	9.8	8.8
Communication	8.4	8.5	9.1
Pain–discomfort	6.8	6.2	4.2
Treatment cost	6.6	4.7	5.8
Waiting time	4.4	3.1	2.6

*The scale to determine the mean importance ratings was derived by ranking the most important factor as 10, the next most important factor as 8, and the least important as 2.

with the scores for treatment costs, 6.6 (Table 41–2). There was no significant difference in these responses as they pertained to either cosmetic blepharoplasty or ptosis procedures (see Table 41–1).

The referring physicians, in evaluating the relative importance of these same five factors, ranked them nearly the same as their patients did. They considered results achieved the most important factor, followed by pain and discomfort, patient treatment costs, and waiting time. These factors were ranked slightly differently by the oculoplastic surgeons, who rated communication as the most important and results achieved as the second most important factor (see Table 41–2). These surgeons judged pain and discomfort and waiting time as less important than did their patients (see Table 41–2).

Seventy-nine per cent of patients were either extremely or very satisfied with their overall treatment. Generally, satisfaction levels of the referring physicians were rated much higher than were those of their patients. This was particularly true for the categories of overall satisfaction, functional improvement, appearance, and length of time required for treatment. These physicians judged that the surgical results obtained were the most satisfying aspect of the treatment, and few of them made any comments about what was least satisfying. Virtually all (99 per cent) of these referring physicians and 80 per cent of their patients indicated that they were extremely or very likely to recommend other patients to the oculoplastic surgeon to perform similar surgery.

Patients rated the level of communication with the surgeon before and at the time of surgery as "very high" (85–87 per cent and 88–89 per cent, respectively), but they were less satisfied with communication after surgery (76 per cent) (Table 41–3). Patients also indicated decreasing satisfaction with the amount of pain and discomfort at the time of their surgery (74 per cent) and postoperatively (63 per cent) (see Table 41–3).

The oculoplastic surgeons indicated that they communicated with their patients mostly in person, and they rated this the most effective method of doing so (Table 41–4). They also said they communicated through their staff and by instruction sheets, rating staff communication as much more effective than the latter. Finally, although they indicated that they did not use the telephone extensively to communicate with their patients, they believed telephone communication was very valuable and effective (see Table 41–4).

No demographic evaluation of the data was completed. The statistician judged that the group of five physicians whose patients and referring doctors were surveyed was too small to allow any significant conclusion to be drawn about demographic data.

CONCLUSIONS

This study statistically demonstrated that oculoplastic surgical patients perceived the results achieved as the

table 41–3

Patient Treatment Satisfaction Ratings

| Measure of Satisfaction | % of Patients Who Were Extremely or Very Satisfied | | |
	Before Surgery	At Surgery	After Surgery
Overall communication			
By surgeon	87	90	76
By staff	85	88	76
Pain–discomfort	—*	74	63

*Not applicable.

table 41–4

Communication Ratings of Oculoplastic Surgeons

Type of Communication	Always/Almost Always Used	Rated Very Effective	Index of Mean Use/Effectiveness*
In person			
By surgeon	99%	80%	105
By staff	49%	38%	97
Instruction sheets	44%	19%	97
Telephone			
By surgeon	22%	44%	76
By staff	35%	13%	100

*The index of mean use/effectiveness relates the type of communication used to its perceived effectiveness.

most important factor determining their satisfaction with the treatments they received for acquired blepharoptosis and cosmetic blepharoplasty. "Results achieved" had a 55 per cent rating and a 9.8 mean rating score (see Tables 41–1 and 41–2). These figures were sharply higher than those for other factors of importance, such as communication (20 per cent), pain and discomfort (11 per cent), patient treatment cost (8 per cent), and waiting time in the surgeon's office (6 per cent), which had mean rating scores from 8.4 to 4.4. Confidence in these results was strengthened by the referring physicians' nearly equal ranking of the importance of these factors (see Table 41–2).

The responding patients were much more concerned with the results achieved than with treatment expenses. Although the government, third-party payers, and the media continue to stress the need for cost containment at the possible sacrifice of quality of care, this study demonstrated, at least in the treatment of ptosis and blepharoplasty, that patients regarded quality of care as paramount and that they are willing to pay for it. If these data are supported by studies of patient satisfaction for other medical procedures, it is probably just a matter of time before patients begin to demand a return to higher-quality medical care, even if they have to pay more for it.

In addition, patients and referring doctors were satisfied with the blepharoptosis procedures and cosmetic blepharoplasty they received. Eighty per cent of the patients indicated that they would recommend the same type of surgery to a close friend or relative, and 99 per cent of the referring physicians indicated that they would refer other patients for the same treatment. This high level of patient satisfaction implies that satisfaction of patients and referring doctors is an excellent marketing tool to increase an oculoplastic surgical practice.

In general, patients tended to be more concerned than the oculoplastic surgeons about the pain and discomfort they experienced, both at surgery and postoperatively, as well as about the amount of time they had to wait in the surgeon's office (see Table 41–2). On the basis of this study, then, in order to increase patient satisfaction, oculoplastic surgeons should strive to decrease the pain and discomfort of their patients as well as the amount of time they have to wait for services.

Patients were dissatisfied with the falloff in communication with the surgeon after surgery (see Table 41–3). Obviously, they wanted more communication at that time. The surgeons seemed to recognize that the telephone is an effective means of communication that they should use more often (see Table 41–4). Therefore, on the basis of the study, another way for surgeons to increase patient satisfaction would be to communicate more often with their patients postoperatively and to use the telephone to do so.

The inclusion of five oculoplastic surgeons in a primary sampling frame constitutes a nonprobability sample of convenience. As such, the results of the questionnaires returned by their patients and by the physicians who referred them are not necessarily representative of the responses that would have been received had all patients who underwent these treatments and all the physicians who referred such patients for surgery participated in the survey. The sample was too small. By contrast, the 69 oculoplastic surgeons participating in the surgeon-patient satisfaction survey were chosen at random, and the results of that survey were representative of the results that would have been achieved if all oculoplastic surgeons had been surveyed.

Even though the respondents' names were not included on these questionnaires, the fact that the questionnaires were returned to the oculoplastic surgeon who sent them out may have decreased the freedom of the responses and thus biased the results. In retrospect, it would have been better to have the questionnaires returned to me or to a person not participating in the study.

References

1. Putterman AM: Patient satisfaction in oculoplastic surgery. Ophthalmic Surg 1990; 21:15–21.
2. Jones LT, Quickert MH, Wobig JL: The cure of ptosis by aponeurotic repair. Arch Ophthalmol 1975; 93:629–634.
3. Putterman AM, Urist J: Müller muscle-conjunctival resection: Technique for treatment of blepharoptosis. Arch Ophthalmol 1975; 94:619–623.
4. Fasanella RN, Servat J: Levator resection of minimal ptosis: Another simplified operation. Arch Ophthalmol 1961; 65:493–496.

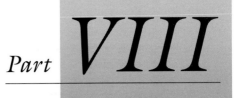
NEW DEVELOPMENTS

Robert A. Goldberg

Chapter 42

Fat Repositioning

Fat repositioning is a new cosmetic technique that only recently has begun to be used for correction of palpebrojugal fold depressions. These depressions occasionally occur over the nasal inferior orbital rims. Also, the cheek descends downward and inward with age, producing a depression at and under the inferior orbital rims. Alloplastic implants and soft-tissue augmentation as well as cheek lifts (described in Chapter 24), have been used in the past to improve these deformities. Fat repositioning, a useful adjunctive technique for correction of palpebrojugal fold depressions, involves repositioning the patient's own inferior nasal and central herniated orbital fat into the areas of the depression.

In this chapter, Robert Goldberg explains how to perform fat repositioning for correction of palpebrojugal fold depressions. I have used this technique in a few patients and am excited about the potential results. Until now, I have not been able to satisfactorily address patients' complaints of these facial depressions. Now I have a treatment to offer these patients that appears to be effective.

ALLEN M. PUTTERMAN

The technique of lower blepharoplasty has evolved substantially. Thirty years ago, we viewed lower blepharoplasty as an operation to remove skin and fat from the lower eyelid. This produced rounding of the lateral canthal angle and lower eyelid retraction with scleral show, and did not improve skin quality in the lower eyelid. Twenty years ago, we switched to transconjunctival fat removal, and 10 years ago we began simultaneously treating skin quality, first with chemical peeling and more recently with carbon dioxide (CO_2) laser resurfacing. The newest stage of evolution of lower blepharoplasty is an understanding of the concept of fat preservation.[1]

Loss of fat in the face is an age-related change. Some young patients do have a true excess or atypically prolapsed orbital fat compartment with a substantial bulge in the lower eyelid that is treated with fat removal. Many older patients, however, who come in for rejuvenation of the lower eyelid and midface have contours that are characterized by descent of the midfacial structures and loss of fat over the orbital rim. This contour is related to the bony support of the underlying maxilla and is accentuated when the maxilla is relatively hypoplastic.[2]

A tear trough deformity develops along the inferior orbital rim between the demarcation of the septal attachment above and the cheek fat pad and levator muscles of the lip below.[3] Removal of orbital fat alone in this circumstance only accentuates the tear trough deformity. For these patients, who present with a double-convexity contour of the lower eyelid and cheek, the orbital fat can be advantageously repositioned over the rim rather than being excised.

PREOPERATIVE EVALUATION

The depth of the tear trough deformity, or palpebrojugal fold, is assessed and graded preoperatively with regard to the medial lateral extent and depth. If there is significant descent of the cheek fat, orbital fat repositioning will not improve the midfacial contours. In this circumstance, a midface lift can be performed simultaneously with orbital fat repositioning to restore the single-convexity youthful contour of the lower eyelid and cheek (see Chapter 24). I have heard some surgeons suggest that the tear trough deformity can be filled by cheek fat via

481

an aggressive lift of suborbicularis oculi fat (SOOF). This has not been my experience, however. The tear trough deformity, or palpebrojugal fold, lies along the orbital rim, and I have not found it possible to lift or redistribute the cheek fat sufficiently to fill in this very high medial deformity.

Preoperative assessment must also take into account the distribution and contour of the medial, central, and lateral fat pockets. Typically, these fat pads are conservatively debulked at the time of orbital fat repositioning of the medial pad into the tear trough deformity. In some cases, the palpebrojugal fold extends laterally into the central eyelid, and in these cases the surgeon may elect to carry the release of the arcus marginalis into the central eyelid and redistribute part of the central fat pad over the rim. I have not had the occasion to distribute the lateral fat pad over the rim. In fact, descent of the zygomatic subcutaneous fat into the lateral inferior rim area often leads to fullness outside the rim in this area, and redistribution of fat outside the orbit in this region might only exacerbate this aesthetically negative contour.

SURGICAL TECHNIQUE

The tear trough (palpebrojugal fold) is marked with a surgical marking pen on the skin surface to guide the intraoperative placement of the fat pedicle. The initial portion of the surgery is identical to any other transconjunctival blepharoplasty, with an incision in the conjunctival fornix and wide-open sky exposure of the individual fat pockets (see Chapter 20). The lateral fat pocket is debulked to the extent determined by the preoperative plan, and the central fat pocket is also typically debulked.

The medial orbital rim is palpated with the tips of a Stevens scissors. A cut is made with the scissors through the orbital septum just at the junction of the arcus marginalis, at the orbital rim. This exposes the periosteum of the maxilla near the origin of the levator labii superioris alaeque nasi muscle. Dissection is then carried out over the orbital rim for a distance of approximately 1–1.5 cm. The entire area that is intended for placement of the fat pedicle is undermined.

There are two potential planes. The first plane that the surgeon may establish is the *subperiosteal plane*. This plane has the advantages of being both relatively free of blood and straightforward. The periosteum in this area is fairly loose, and I have found that the fat is easily repositioned into the subperiosteal pocket.

Alternatively, the dissection may be carried out in the *suborbicularis plane*. The disadvantage of this plane is that significant bleeding can be encountered within the highly vascular orbicularis muscle and labial elevators. The angular vasculature sometimes runs across this area in the muscular plane and can be an additional source of bleeding.

Once the plane is completely dissected, the fat pedicle is created from the medial fat pocket. Although there are some large vessels in the medial fat pad and care must be taken to avoid cutting across them, the fat pedicle is essentially a random flap. The stalk of the pedicle should be large enough to provide reasonable blood supply (usually 5 mm in diameter) but small enough to avoid pulling on the orbital connective tissue system as the pedicle is transposed over the rim. Usually,

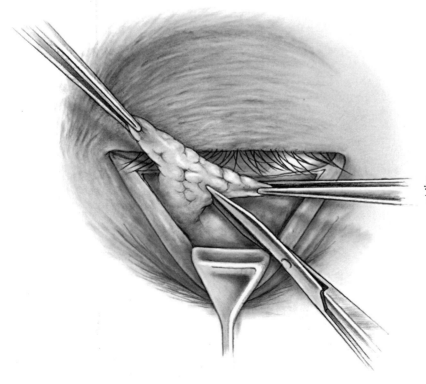

figure 42–1

The fat pedicle is dissected into a T-shaped wedge.

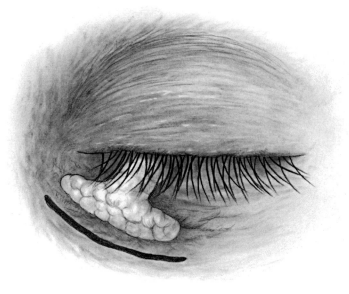

figure 42–2

The pedicles are ready to be placed into the subperiosteal pocket.

I construct a T-shaped pedicle by dissecting the leading edge of the pedicle into the desired shape (Fig. 42–1).

The pedicle is transposed over the orbital rim (Fig. 42–2). It is then placed into the predissected pocket and distributed evenly within it.

Next, I check forced ductions of the globe to be sure that the fat pedicle is not attached to the motility system of the orbit. There should be no movement or tugging on the pedicle as the globe is rotated.

I fixate the pedicle into the flap using an externalized 6-0 polypropylene (Prolene) suture on a PC-1 needle. Three lazy loops are passed from the lower eyelid, across the pedicle touching the bony orbital rim, and exiting on the upper cheek. These suture passes form a "cage" that keeps the pedicle in position during the early healing phase (Fig. 42–3).

POSTOPERATIVE CARE

The sutures are removed 3–5 days after surgery.

COMPLICATIONS

The complications from fat repositioning are the same as for any other variation of transconjunctival blepharoplasty. To date, in 38 cases, I have noted no complications specific to this technique and no reabsorption of fat.

RESULTS

The technique of fat repositioning provides a subtle but long-lasting change in the contour of the lower eyelid

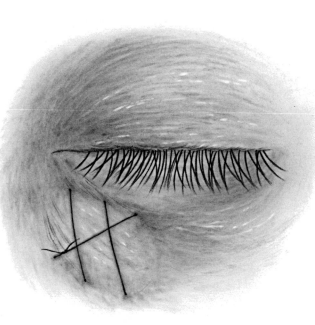

figure 42–3

Construction of the 6-0 polypropylene (Prolene) "cage."

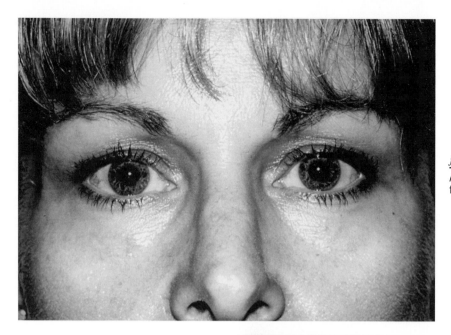

figure 42–4

A young patient with a prominent tear trough deformity before surgery.

figure 42–5

Four days postoperatively, the polypropylene cage is ready to be removed from the patient shown in Figure 42–4.

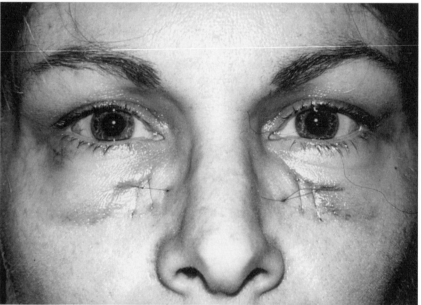

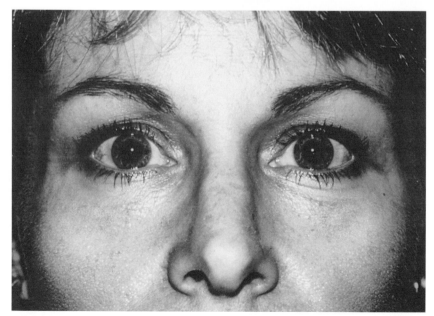

figure 42–6

Postoperative photograph demonstrating improvement in lower eyelid contour.

(Figs. 42–4 to 42–6). It is not as powerful as an alloplastic implant, which other authors have suggested,[4, 5] but it has the advantage of vascularized autogenous tissue.

References

1. Hamra ST: The role of orbital fat preservation in facial aesthetic surgery: A new concept. Clin Plast Surg 1996; 23:17–28.
2. Goldberg RA, Relan A, Hoenig JH: Relationship of the eye to the bony orbit. Presented at the American Society of Ophthalmic Plastic and Reconstructive Surgery Scientific Symposium, Chicago, October 26, 1996.
3. Kikkawa DO, Lemke BN, Dortzbach RK: Relations of the superficial musculoaponeurotic system to the orbit and characterization of the orbitomalar ligament. Ophthalmic Plast Reconstruct Surg 1996; 12:77–88.
4. Steinsapir KD, Shorr N: Suborbital augmentation. In Bosniak S (ed): Ophthalmic Plastic and Reconstructive Surgery, vol 1, pp 484–503. Philadelphia, WB Saunders, 1996.
5. Flowers RS: Tear trough implants for correction of tear trough deformity. Clin Plast Surg 1993; 20:403–415.

Allen M. Putterman

Chapter 43

Excision of Corrugator Muscles: Upper Blepharoplasty Approach

As I was completing this text, new techniques were being developed, including excision of the corrugator muscles through an upper blepharoplasty approach.

Overaction of the corrugator muscles leads to frown lines above the bridge of the nose, a common cosmetic disturbance to patients. These lines have been successfully treated in the past through brow-lifting techniques as well as with botulinum toxin (Botox) injections. Another simple way of managing this problem is to excise the corrugator muscles through an upper blepharoplasty approach. This is a relatively simple technique that can be combined with the excision of orbicularis oculi muscle and fat and lid reconstruction of the upper eyelids, without the need to resort to the invasiveness of endoscopic or coronal brow lifts.

So far, I have found patient satisfaction with this technique to be quite high.

ALLEN M. PUTTERMAN

Overaction of the corrugator muscles leads to frown lines above the nose, which many patients find objectionable. Weakening or excision of these muscles is commonly done as part of the coronal or small-incision endoscopic brow lift (see Chapters 27 and 28). These muscles can also be weakened by botulinum toxin injections (see Chapter 33). Another relatively simple way of weakening these muscles consists of excising them through an upper blepharoplasty approach.

I have performed an upper blepharoplasty for approximately 15 years as part of the Anderson[1] orbicularis muscle extirpation procedure in the treatment of essential blepharospasm. For the past few years, I have performed this procedure with small-incision scalp endoscopic brow lifting (see Chapter 28). When I perform endoscopic brow lifts, I routinely release the periosteum from the superior orbital rim and excise the corrugator muscles through an upper eyelid approach; then I dissect the periosteum upward until I meet the periosteum that was released through the scalp incision approach. It is only recently that I have begun excising the corrugator

muscles in the upper eyelid as part of an upper blepharoplasty without orbicularis muscle extirpation and without endoscopic brow lifting. This technique was brought to my attention by Guyuron, who with his associates popularized it as an entity in itself.[2] Knize[3] has also documented this technique.

SURGICAL TECHNIQUE

Skin Marking

The upper eyelid crease and amount of skin–orbicularis muscle resection is marked (see Chapter 10 and Fig. 10–1*A* to *C*). A methylene blue mark and line are also drawn at the site of the supraorbital canal to mark the site of the supraorbital nerve.

Anesthesia

Two per cent lidocaine (Xylocaine) with 1:100,000 epinephrine is injected subcutaneously over the entire up-

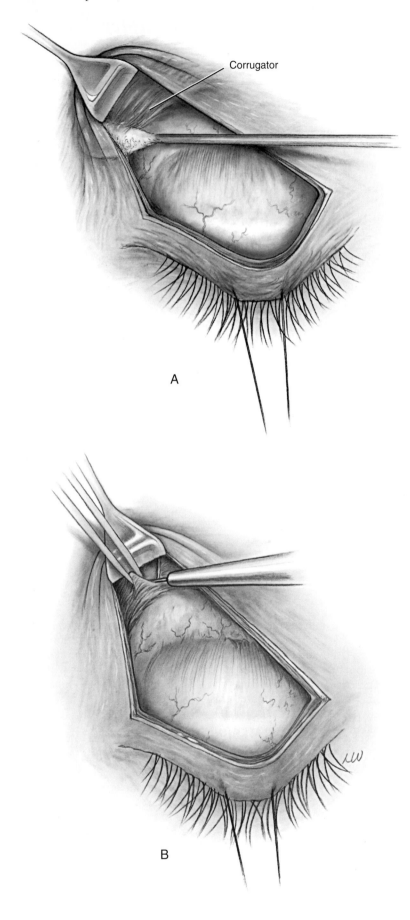

figure 43–1

A, After excision of an ellipse of skin and orbicularis oculi muscle reflecting the orbicularis from orbital septum to the superior orbital rim, a small Desmarres retractor is used to reflect the skin-muscle flap over the nasal superior orbital rim while the traction suture is pulled downward. Cotton-tipped applicators are used to reflect the orbicularis muscle above and over the superior orbital rim to isolate the corrugator muscle. *B,* A forceps is used to grasp the isolated corrugator muscle as a Colorado needle is used to excise a section of the muscle.

per eyelid and beneath the brow. Injections are also given over the corrugator muscles.

Incision and Excision

A 4-0 black silk traction suture is placed through the center of the upper eyelid through skin, orbicularis muscle, and superficial tarsus slightly above the eyelashes. A No. 15 Bard-Parker blade is used to incise skin at the site of the marked elliptical resection site. The 4-0 black silk traction suture is pulled downward while the eyebrow is pulled upward, and an ellipse of skin and orbicularis muscle is excised with a Westcott scissors, Colorado needle, or carbon dioxide (CO_2) pulse laser. During this resection, there is an attempt to leave the orbital septum intact so that the levator aponeurosis and orbital fat are not exposed at this time. The Westcott scissors, Colorado needle, or a neodymium (Nd):YAG laser is then used to dissect between the orbicularis muscle and the orbital septum to the level of the superior orbital rim (see Chapter 12 and Fig. 12–4A and B). However, it is unnecessary to dissect above the superior orbital rim, as is done with the internal brow lift.

A Desmarres retractor is then used to reflect the skin-muscle flap upward to expose the superior orbital rim (Fig. 43–1A).

The previous steps also are used in the small-incision endoscopic brow lift. In that procedure, however, the periosteum at this point would be released from the superior orbital rim, along with corrugator muscle excision. In this chapter, I emphasize only the corrugator muscle excision.

Corrugator Muscle Isolation and Excision

With the 4-0 black silk traction suture pulling the upper lid downward by attaching it to the inferior drape, the assistant uses a small Desmarres retractor to gently ele-

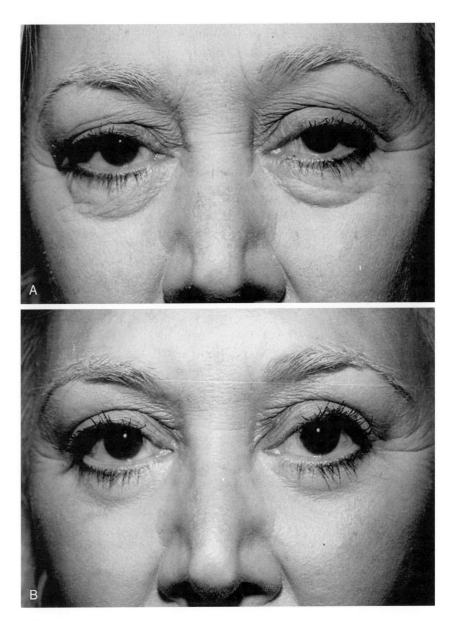

figure 43–2

A, Preoperative photograph of a patient with prominent frown lines and wrinkles above the nose. The patient also has bilateral upper eyelid ptosis (drooping) as well as dermatochalasis (excess skin) and herniated orbital fat of all four eyelids. *B,* Postoperative photograph of the same patient after excision of corrugator muscles through an upper blepharoplasty approach, with improvement of the frown lines and wrinkles above the nose. She also underwent a bilateral upper eyelid Müller's muscle–conjunctival resection–ptosis procedure and excision of the excess skin and fat from all four eyelids.

vate the skin-muscle flap upward to expose the nasal superior orbital rim. Cotton-tipped applicators are then used to gently dissect under the orbicularis muscle over and above the superior orbital rim, just nasal to the supraorbital canal. As this dissection proceeds, the corrugator muscle becomes visible. The dissection is carried out until the mass of the muscle is isolated. A toothed forceps is used to grasp the corrugator muscle over its midbelly.

A piece of the corrugator muscle is excised, with either a Colorado needle or a disposable cautery (Fig. 43–1*B*). Usually, I remove at least a 4–5-mm section of the midcorrugator muscle. One may also weaken the muscle by stretching it with two toothed forceps pulled in opposite directions or with a partial severing of the muscle with the Colorado needle or disposable cautery. As this release of corrugator muscle occurs, the branches of supratrochlear nerve become visible. Any remaining fibers can also be excised. At this point, it should be evident that there is an opening in the entire horizontal dimension of the muscle.

Opening of Orbital Septum and Isolation of Levator Aponeurosis and Orbital Fat

While the assistant pulls the 4-0 traction suture in the upper eyelid downward, the orbital septum–suborbicularis fascia is grasped with forceps and pulled upward and outward. A Westcott scissors is then used to sever the septal suborbicularis fascia at its inferior position, just above the superior tarsal border. Once the opening is made in this tissue, the septum–suborbicularis fascia is severed at its most inferior extent (see Chapter 12 on Putterman's modification of the internal brow lift and Fig. 12–9*A* to *C*). After the orbital fat is excised, the surgeon reconstructs the eyelid crease by uniting the levator aponeurosis to the orbicularis muscle (see Chapter 10).

Skin Closure

Three 6-0 polyglactin (Vicryl) sutures unite the skin edges to the levator aponeurosis and the inferior edge of the septal suborbicularis fascia (see Chapter 12, Fig. 12–9*D*). The surgeon enters the septum–suborbicularis fascia after excising the corrugator and suturing it back in place in order to avoid a high upper eyelid crease by the orbicularis muscle attaching to the levator aponeurosis. Having the septum–suborbicularis fascia between the orbicularis muscle and the levator aponeurosis, presumably, prevents this. The skin is then closed with a continuous 6-0 silk suture, as described in Chapter 10.

COMPLICATIONS

Many patients have localized numbness above the nose because of a disturbance to the supratrochlear nerve.

RESULTS

I have performed this procedure in at least 15 cases with an upper eyelid blepharoplasty and in an additional 50 or more patients also receiving endoscopy-assisted brow lifts. In my experience, the corrugator excision through an upper blepharoplasty approach has improved the appearance of frown lines (Fig. 43–2).

Patient acceptance of this procedure is quite high, since the patient does not have to go through an extremely invasive procedure and does not need repeated botulinum toxin injections.

References

1. Anderson R: Myectomy for blepharospasm and hemifacial spasm. Adv Ophthalmic Plast Reconstr Surg 1985; 4:331–347.
2. Guyuron B, Michelow B, Thomas T: Corrugator supercilii muscle resection through blepharoplasty incision. Plast Reconstr Surg 1995; 95:691–696.
3. Knize DM: Transpalpebral approach to the corrugator supercilii and procerus muscles. Plast Reconstr Surg 1995; 95:52.

Index